KEY NOTES

&

RED LINE SYMPTOMS

OF

THE MATERIA MEDICA

Dr. ADOLPH VON LIPPE

Professor of Materia Medica at the Homœopathic College of Pennsylvania.

B. JAIN PUBLISHERS (P) LTD.

An ISO 9001 : 2000 Certified Company
USA — EUROPE — INDIA

Reprint Edition: 2006, 2008

© Copyright with the Publisher

Published by
KULDEEP JAIN

for

B. Jain Publishers (P) Ltd.

1921, Chuna Mandi, St. 10th, Paharganj,
New Delhi-110 055
Phones: 2358 0800, 2358 1100, 2358 1300, 2358 3100,
Fax: 011-2358 0471   *Email:* bjain@vsnl.com
Website: **www.bjainbooks.com**

Printed in India by
J.J. Offset Printers
522, FIE, Patpar Ganj, Delhi-110 092

ISBN : 978-81-319-0526-5

FOREWARD

The name and fame of the world-renowned Homœopath, Dr. Adolph von Lippe needs no introduction to the Homœopathic Fraternity. With our claim on their appreciation, we now present before them the author's masterpiece, " Key Notes of the Materia Medica," adding thereto the characteristic symptoms of the most important remedies under the style, " Red Line Symptoms," gleaned from the author's writings, appearing in several old foreign journals, together with the other important ones, collected from the writings of the great Homœopaths of the by-gone days.

The book with these additions is in no sense a treatise now, and must not be considered as such. Each sterling symptom in the context other than that of Dr. Lippe has the name of its author indicated against it in abbreviatory form. The book is now as accurate and reliable a compilation and the fullest collection of the most common remedies as it is possible to obtain within its compass.

It may be claimed that the book supplements every other work on the subject, and if used as a ready reminder of the common important facts of our vast Materia Medica, it will fulfil its purpose and prove the greatest aid to the profession and students alike.

LIST OF THE NAMES OF AUTHORITIES
AND THEIR ABBREVIATIONS.

Dr. H. C. Allen (A.).
Dr. A. P. Angel (An.).
Dr. Bæhr (Bhr.).
Dr. Bayes (Ba.).
Dr. J. B. Bell (Be.).
Dr. Bers (Brs.).
Dr. W. H. Biglers (Bg.).
Dr. A. L. Blackwood (Bl.).
Dr. Bœnninghausen (Bn.).
Dr. W. Boericke (Br.).
Dr. C. M. Boger (B.).
Dr. Bowen (Bw.).
Dr. C. W. Boyce (Bo.).
Dr. Boyd (By.).
Dr. W. H. Burt (Bt.).
Dr. Chapusat (Ch.).
Dr. Clarke (Cla.).
Dr. S. H. Collum (Cl.).
Dr. J. W. Cook (Co.).
Dr. R. T. Cooper (Cp.).
Dr. A. C. Cowperthwaite (C.).
Dr. W. A. Dewey (D.).
Dr. J. S. Douglas (*Dg.*).
Dr. C. Dunham (Dn.).
Dr. Dunn (Du.).
Dr. Farrington (F.).
Dr. Franklin (Frn.).
Dr. Freleigh (Frl.).
Dr. Frost (Fr.).
Dr. L. Gross (Gr.).
Dr. H. N. Guernsey (G.).
Dr. Hahnemann (Hn.)
Dr. Hale (Ha.).

Dr. Hall (Hl.).
Dr. Helmuth (Hlm.).
Dr. Hempel (Hm.).
Dr. C. Hering (Hr.).
Dr. Hill (Hi.).
Dr. Holcombe (Ho.).
Dr. R. Hughes (Hg.).
Dr. Hunt (Ht.).
Dr. Jahr (J.).
Dr. Kenderick (Kn.).
Dr. J. T. Kent (K.).
Dr. Kenyon (Ken.).
Dr. King (Kg.).
Dr. C. B. Kuler (Kl.).
Dr. S. Lilienthal (L.).
Dr. Marcy (Ma.).
Dr. H. N. Martin (Mr.).
Dr. J. C. Mullier (Ml.).
Dr. E. B. Nash (N.).
Dr. Neidhard (Nd.).
Dr. W. E. Payne (Py.).
Dr. Pearson (P.).
Dr. Preston (Pr.).
Dr. Rane (Ra.).
Dr. Renwick (Rn.).
Dr. Rogers (Rg.).
Dr. G. Royal (R.).
Dr. Shaw (S.).
Dr. A. E. Small (Sm.).
Dr. C. C. Smith (Smi.).
Dr. Teste (T.).
Dr. R. C. Vance (Vn.).
Dr. P. P. Wells (W.).
Dr. J. H. Woodbury (Wd.).
Dr. J. A. Young (Y.).

CONTENTS.

PART I.

A

				Page
Abrotanum	..	..	..	17
Acetic Acid	..	..	..	19
Aconitum Napellus	..	..	..	21
Actea Racemosa	..	..	..	24
Aesculus Hippocastanum		..	..	27
Aethusa Cynapium	..	..	..	30
Agaricus Muscarius	..	..	..	32
Agnus Castus	..	..	..	36
Allium Cepa	..	..	..	39
Aloe Socotrina	..	..	..	42
Alumina	..	..	..	46
Ambra Grisea	..	..	..	50
Ammonium Carbonicum	..	..	..	53
Ammonium Muriaticum	..	..	..	57
Amyl Nitrite	..	..	..	60
Anacardium Orientale	..	..	..	63
Angustura Vera	..	..	..	67
Anthracinum	..	..	..	70
Antimonium Crudum	..	..	..	72
Antimonium Tartaricum		..	..	76
Apis Mellifica	..	..	..	82
Apocynum Cannabinum	..	..	..	86
Argentum Metallicum	..	..	..	88
Argentum Nitricum	..	..	..	91
Arnica Montana	..	..	..	97
Arsenicum Album	..	..	..	102
Arsenicum Metallicum	..	..	..	108
Arum Triphyllum	..	..	..	109
Asafoetida	..	..	..	112
Asarum Europoeum	..	..	..	115
Asterias Rubens	..	..	..	117
Aurum Metallicum	..	..	..	119

B

				PAGE
BAPTISIA TINCTORIA	..	..	..	123
BARYTA CARBONICA	.;	..	..	127
BELLADONNA ..	..	..	..	131
BENZOIC ACID ..	..	..	..	137
BERBERIS VULGARIS	..	..	..	140
BISMUTH ..	..	..	..	144
BLATTA ORIENTALIS	..	..	..	147
BORAX ..	..	..	..	148
BOVISTA ..	..	..	..	152
BROMIUM ..	..	..	..	156
BRYONIA ALBA	..	..	..	160

C

CACTUS GRANDIFLORUS	..	..	..	166
CALADIUM SEGUINUM	..	..	..	169
CALCAREA ARSENICA	..	..	..	172
CALCAREA CARBONICA	..	..	..	174
CALCAREA PHOSPHORICA	..	..	..	181
CALCAREA SULPHURICA	..	..	..	185
CALENDULA OFFICINALIS	..	..	..	187
CAMPHORA ..	..	..	..	189
CANNABIS INDICA	..	..	..	194
CANNABIS SATIVA	..	..	..	198
CANTHARIS ..	..	..	..	203
CAPSICUM ..	..	..	..	209
CARBO ANIMALIS	..	..	..	215
CARBO VEGETABILIS	..	..	..	220
CARBOLIC ACID	..	..	..	229
CARDUUS MARIANUS	..	..	..	232
CASCARILLA ..	..	..	..	234
CASTOR EQUI ..	..	..	..	236
CASTOREUM ..	..	..	..	236
CAULOPHYLLUM	..	..	..	238
CAUSTICUM ..	..	..	..	241
CEANOTHUS AMERICANUS	..	..	..	249
CHAMOMILLA ..	..	..	..	250
CHELIDONIUM ..	..	..	..	255
CHINA ..	..	..	..	260

PAGE

CHININUM ARSENICUM 266
CICUTA VIROSA 269
CINA 273
CINNABARIS 278, 339
CINNAMONUM 339
CLEMATIS ERECTA 280
COCA 284
COCCULUS INDICUS 287
COFFEA CRUDA 292
COLCHICUM 297
COLLINSONIA 301
COLOCYNTH 304
CONIUM MACULATUM 308
CORALLIUM RUBRUM 313
CRATAEGUS OXYACANTHA 316
CROCUS SATIVUS 318
CROTALUS HORRIDUS 320
CROTON TIGLIUM 324
CUPRUM ARSENICOSUM 329
CUPRUM METALLICUM 330
CYCLAMEN 335

D

DIGITALIS PURPUREA 341
DIOSCOREA VILLOSA 344
DIPHTHERINUM 347
DROSERA 348
DULCAMARA 351

E

ECHINACEA ANGUSTIFOLIA 354
EQUISETUM HYMALE 355
ERIGERON CANADENSE 356
EUPATORIUM PERFOLIATUM 357
EUPHORBIUM 360
EUPHRASIA 361

F

	PAGE
FERRUM METALLICUM	363
FLUORIC ACID	366

G

GELSEMIUM	368
GLONOINE	372
GNAPHALIUM	375
GOSSYPIUM	376
GRAPHITES	377
GUAIACUM	382

H

HAMAMELIS	384
HELLEBORUS NIGER	387
HELONIAS DIOICA	390
HEPAR SULPHUR	392
HYDRASTIS CANADENSIS	396
HYOSCYAMUS NIGER	398
HYPERICUM	401

I

IGNATIA	402
IODIUM	407
IPECACUANHA	411

K

KALI BICHROMICUM	415
KALI BROMATUM	420
KALI CARBONICA	422
KALMIA LATIFOLIA	428
KREOSOTUM	429

L

LAC CANINUM	433
LAC DEFLORATUM	436
LACHESIS	438
LATRODECTUS MACTANS	446

		PAGE
LAUROCERASUS	.. .. ..	447
LEDUM PALUSTRE	.. .. ..	449
LILIUM TIGRINUM	.. .. ..	451
LOBELIA INFLATA	.. .. ..	454
LYCOPODIUM CLAVATUM	.. .. ..	456
LYSSIN	.. .. ..	463

M

MAGNESIA CARBONICA	.. .. ..	466
MAGNESIA MURIATICA	.. .. ..	469
MAGNESIA PHOSPHORICA	.. .. ..	472
MANGANUM	.. .. ..	474
MEDORRHINUM	.. .. ..	476
MELILOTUS ALBA	.. .. ..	480
MENYANTHES	.. .. ..	481
MERCURIUS BINIODIDE	.. .. ..	483
MERCURIUS CORROSIVUS	.. .. ..	484
MERCURIUS CYANATUS	.. .. ..	488
MERCURIUS DULCIS	.. .. ..	489
MERCURIUS PROTOIODIDE	.. .. ..	490
MERCURIUS SOLUBILIS	.. .. ..	492
MERCURIUS SULPHURICUS	.. ..	497
MEZERIUM	.. .. ..	498
MILLEFOLIUM	.. .. ..	500
MOSCHUS	.. .. ..	502
MUREX PURPUREA	.. .. ..	505
MURIATIC ACID	.. .. ..	507

PART II.

N

NAJA TRIPUDIANS	.. .. ..	1
NAPHTHALINUM	.. .. ..	3
NATRUM CARBONICUM	.. .. ..	4
NATRUM MURIATICUM	.. .. ..	7
NATRUM SULPHURICUM	.. .. ..	13

	PAGE
NITRIC ACID	17
NITRUM	23
NUX MOSCHATA	24
NUX VOMICA	28

O

OLEANDER	36
OPIUM	38

P

PARIS QUADRIFOLIA	42
PASSIFLORA INCARNATA	45
PETROLEUM	46
PETROSELINUM	51
PHOSPHORIC ACID	53
PHOSPHORUS	59
PHYSOSTIGMA	67
PHYTOLACCA	69
PICRIC ACID	73
PLANTAGO MAJOR	75
PLATINUM METALLICUM	76
PLUMBUM METALLICUM	80
PODOPHYLLUM PELTATUM	84
PULSATILLA	89
PYROGEN	95

R

RADIUM BROMIDE	98
RANUNCULUS BULBOSUS	100
RANUNCULUS SCLERATUS	102
RATANHIA	103
RHEUM	105
RHODODENDRON	107
RHUS TOXICODENDRON	110
RUMEX CRISPUS	117
RUTA GRAVEOLEUS	119

S

	PAGE
SABADILLA	121
SABINA	123
SAMBUCUS NIGRA	126
SANGUINARIA CANADENSIS	128
SANIGULA	132
SARRACENIA PURPUREA	135
SARSAPARILLA	136
SECALE CORNUTUM	139
SELENIUM	143
SENEGA	147
SEPIA	150
SILICEA	158
SPIGELIA ANTHELMINTICA	165
SPONGIA TOSTA	168
STANNUM METALLICUM	171
STAPHISAGRIA	176
STRAMONIUM	180
STRONTIANA CARBONICA	186
STRYCHNINUM	188
SULPHUR	190
SULPHURIC ACID	199
SYMPHYTUM	203
SYPHILINUM	204

T

	PAGE
TABACUM	208
TARANTULA HISPANIA	212
TARANTULA CUBENSIS	214
TARAXACUM	215
TARTARUS EMETICUS	217
TEREBINTHINA	223
TEUCRIUM MARUM VERUM	227
THERIDION CURASSAVICUM	228
THLASPI BURSA PASTONIS	231
THUJA OCCIDENTALIS	232
THYROIDINUM	238
TRILLIUM PENDULUM	239
TUBERCULINUM	241

U

		PAGE
URTICA URENS	.. .. ..	245
UVA URSI ..	.. .. ..	247

V

VACCININUM ..	.. .. ..	248
VALERIANA ..	.. .. ..	249
VARIOLINUM ..	.. .. ..	252
VERATRUM ALBUM	.. .. ..	254
VERATRUM VIRIDE	.. .. ..	260
VERBASCUM THAPSUS	.. .. ..	263
VIOLA ODORATA	.. .. ..	265

X

| X-RAY .. | .. .. .. | 267 |

Y

| YOHIMBINUM .. | .. .. .. | 268 |

Z

| ZINCUM METALLICUM | .. .. .. | 269 |

LIPPE'S KEY NOTES
&
RED LINE SYMPTOMS

PART I.

ABROTANUM to MURIATIC ACID

Abrotanum.

COMMON NAME : SOUTHERN WOOD.

Marasmus of children, with marked emaciation, especially of legs (*Iod., Sanic., Tub.* emaciation of neck—*Nat-M., Sanic.*). The skin is flabby and hangs loose in folds (A.).

The child is cross and depressed (G.).

RAVENOUS HUNGER ; LOSING FLESH WHILE EATING WELL (*Iod., Nat-M., Sanic., Tub.*) (A.).

Alternate diarrhœa and rheumatism (metastatic rheumatism) (N.).

Alternate constipation and diarrhœa ; lienteria (*Aloe, Nux-V., Podo., Sulph.*) (A.).

Epistaxis, hydrocele or emaciation of little boys (G.).

Numb, weak, tremulous and paretic (B.).

MARASMUS OF LOWER EXTREMITIES ONLY (*Amm-M., Arg-N.*) (A.).

Rheumatism of heart (K.).

Nightly backache (B.).

Child is ill-natured, irritable, cross and despondent ; violent, inhuman, would like to do something cruel (A.).

BLOATED ABDOMEN (B.).

Face old, pale, wrinkled (*Arg-N., Lyc., Op.*) (A.).

Darting or twitching in either or both ovaries (G.).

In marasmus, head weak, cannot hold it up (Æth.).

Cutting pains in stomach, gnawing, burning (G.).

2

Painful contractions of the limbs from cramps or following colic (A.).

Vomits much offensive fluid (B.).

Rheumatism : *for the excessive pain before the swelling commences* ; *from suddenly checked diarrhœa or other secretions* ; *alternates with hæmorrhoids, with dysentery* (A.).

Great weakness and prostration after influenza (G.).

Gout : joints stiff, swollen, with pricking sensation : wrists and ankle-joints painful and inflamed (A.).

Very lame and sore all over (*Arn., Bapt., Pyrog., Rhus-T.*) (A.).

Blood and moisture oozing from the navel of new-born children (G.).

Itching chilblains (*Agar.*) (A.).

Distended veins on forehead (B.).

Great weakness and prostration and a kind of hectic fever with children ; unable to stand (A.).

AGGRAVATION : In cold air or from getting wet ; from checked secretions ; in fogs ; during night.

AMELIORATION : From loose stool ; from motion.

RELATIONSHIP : After *Hepar* in furuncle ; after *Acon.* and *Bry.* is pleurisy, when a pressing sensation remains in affected side impeding respiration.

Acetic Acid.

COMMON NAME : GLACIAL ACETIC ACID.

Adapted to pale, lean persons with lax, flabby muscles (A.).

Passes large quantities of pale urine (N.).

Marasmus and other wasting diseases of children (*Abrot., Iod., Sanic., Sars., Tub.*) (A.).

Emaciation, especially of the face, hands and thighs (Selen.) (N.).

Vomits after every kind of food (*Ars., Phos., Sep.*) (G.).

Anguish and anxiety (Ars.) (K.).

FACE PALE, WAXY (*Fer.*) (A.).

Dyspnœa : while lying, especially on the back ; and on ascending (K.).

Diphtheria : false membranes in the throat (G.).

Foul eructation, or hot eructation (Ars., Caust., Cop., Hep., Naja, Phos., Puls.) (K.).

Hæmorrhage : from every mucous outlet, nose, throat, lungs, stomach, bowels, uterus (Fer., Mill., Phos.) ; metrorrhagia ; vicarious ; traumatic epistaxis (Arn.) (A.).

Chronic diarrhœa of children, with great emaciation (G.).

Aversion to food, especially salted food (K.).

Great prostration : after injuries (*Sulph-Ac.*) ; after surgical shock ; after anæsthetics (A.).

Colliquative sweat (K.).

THIRST : INTENSE, BURNING, INSATIABLE EVEN FOR LARGE QUANTITIES IN DROPSY, DIA-BETES, AND CHRONIC DIARRHŒA ; BUT NO THIRST IN FEVER (A.).

Vertigo during headache (*Apis, Bell., Calc., Con., Nux-V., Sil.*) (*K.*).

Sour belching and vomiting of pregnancy. Burning water-brash and profuse salivation, day and night (Lact-Ac. ; salivation worse at night—*Merc.*) (A.).

Phthisis pulmonalis (*Agar., Calc., Calc-P., Fer-P., Hep., Iod., Kali-C., Kali-S., Lyc., Phos., Puls., Sil.*) (*K.*).

Diarrhœa ; copious, exhausting ; with great thirst ; in dropsy, typhus, phthisis ; with night sweats (A.).

Cannot sleep lying on the back (sleeps better on the back—*Ars.*) ; sensation of sinking in the abdomen causing dyspnœa ; rests better lying on belly (*Am-C.*) (A.).

Hectic fever : skin dry and hot ; red spot on left cheek and drenching night sweats (A.).

AGGRAVATION : From lying on the back, during night and after eating.

AMELIORATION : From lying on the belly, during rest and in the day time.

RELATIONSHIP : It aggravates the symptoms of *Arn., Bell., Lach.* and *Merc.*); especially the headache from *Belladonna*. It antidotes anæsthetic vapours (*Amyl*) ; fumes of charcoal and gas ; *Opium* and *Stramonium*.

Cider Vinegar antidotes *Carbolic Acid*.

It follows well : after *Cinchona* in hæmorrhage ; after *Digitalis*, in dropsy.

Aconitum Napellus.

COMMON NAME : MONK'S HOOD.

Is generally indicated in acute or recent cases occurring in young persons, especially girls of a full, plethoric habit, who lead a sedentary life ; persons easily affected by atmospheric changes ; dark hair and eyes, rigid muscular fibres (A.).

THE PAIN IS INSUPPORTABLE, DRIVING TO DESPAIR (*Coff.*).

THE PATIENT IS FULL OF FEARS, AND TOSSES ABOUT, AS IF IN AGONY (*Ars.*).

RESTLESSNESS AND INCONSOLABLE ANXIETY.

IS AFRAID TO GO OUT, TO GO INTO A CROWD, WHERE THERE IS ANY EXCITEMENT OR MANY PEOPLE ; TO CROSS THE STREET (A.).

SUDDEN AND GREAT SINKING OF STRENGTH (*Ars., Camph., Hydro-Ac.*).

Sensation of soreness of the body, and of heaviness in inner parts.

Tearing in outer parts (*Rhus.*).

Tingling in the fingers, œsophagus and back (*Sec.*).

Painfulness of the whole body to contact (he does not wish to be touched) (*Arn.*).

Pulsating pain in the head and teeth (*Bell.*).

Inflammation of inner parts (*mucous membranes*).

Stitches in internal organs. (*Apis.*, *Bry.*, *Kali-C.*, *Sulph.*).

Tightness of the muscles (acute rheumatism).

THE MOST VALUABLE FEBRIFUGE IN THE ENTIRE RANGE OF THERAPEUTIC AGENTS.

PULSE FULL AND HARD, OR IMPERCEPTIBLE.

DRY, BURNING SKIN.

HEAT, WITH INCLINATION TO UNCOVER ONESELF (*Sulph.*).

MILIARIA LIKE THE ERUPTION OF MEASLES (*Bry.*, *Puls.*).

WHEN RISING PALENESS OF THE FACE.

PRODUCES AND CURES DRENCHING SWEATS (*Chin.*).

Bad effects from catching cold, from anger, or from fright, especially with females during menstruation.

Most symptoms disappear while sitting quietly, but at night and in bed they are insupportable.

Cough, croup ; dry, hoarse, suffocating ; loud, rough, croaking ; hard, ringing, whistling ; on expiration (*Caust.* ; on inhalation—*Spong.*) ; from dry, cold winds, or drafts of air (A.).

RETENTION OF URINE IN NEW BORN INFANTS (*Apis, Ars., Camph., Caust.. Lyc., Puls.*) (*K.*).

DYSENTERY : WHEN THE DAYS ARE WARM AND THE NIGHTS ARE COOL ; SCANTY, LOOSE,

FREQUENT STOOLS WITH TORMINA AND TENES-MUS; SMALL, BROWN, PAINFUL, AT LAST BLOODY, OR PURE BLOOD PASSES WITHOUT FÆCES (L.).

Desire for bitter drinks (Dig., Nat-M., Tereb.) (K.).

Pneumonia : first stage in robust persons ; chill of more or less severity, followed by intense fever, hot, dry skin ; laboured and incomplete respiration ; and dry, hard cough (L.).

Everything tastes bitter except water *(Stann.)* (K.).

Convulsions : of teething children ; heat, jerks and twitches of single muscles ; child gnaws its fist, frets and screams ; skin hot and dry ; high fever (Bell., Stram.) (A.).

PALPITATION : FROM ANXIETY ; DURING FEVER (*Ars., Calc., Nit-Ac., Puls.*) ; AFTER FRIGHT ; FROM MOTION ; AND ON WAKING (*Lach., Naja, Phos.*) (K.).

Uncomplicated cardiac disease, especially with numbness of left arm ; tingling in fingers ; faintings (N.).

Great aversion to light *(Bell., Con., Merc., Sulph.).* Sufferings from foreign bodies, as speck of dust or iron in the eyes (G.).

Beside himself, frantic from intensity of pain (B.).

Music is intolerable, makes her sad *(Sab.* ; during menses—*Nat-C.)* (A.).

AGGRAVATION : In the evening and night ; in a warm room ; when rising from bed ; and lying on the left or affected side **(***Bell., Hep., Nux-M.***).**

AMELIORATION : In the open air (*Alum., Mag-C., Puls., Sab.*).

RELATIONSHIP : Complementary to *Coffea* in fever, sleeplessness and intolerance of pain ; to *Arnica* in traumatism ; to *Sulphur* in all cases.

Aconite is the acute of *Sulphur*, and both precedes and follows it in acute inflammatory conditions.

Actæa Racemosa.

COMMON NAMES : SQUAW ROOT ; BLACK COHOSH ; CIMICIFUGA.

GLOOMY, SAD, SLEEPLESS ; THINKS SHE WILL GO INSANE (N.).

Puerperal mania ; tries to injure herself.

Weeping mood ; melancholia.

Mania following disappearance of neuralgia (A.).

In all her mental symptoms there is a want of natural coherence (G.).

SENSATION AS IF A HEAVY, BLACK CLOUD HAD SETTLED ALL OVER HER AND ENVELOPED HER HEAD, SO THAT ALL IS DARKNESS AND CONFUSION (A.).

Visions of rats, mice, etc. (D.).

MUSCULAR RHEUMATISM ; STIFF NECK, DRAWING HEAD BACK ; CAN'T TURN THE HEAD ; RHEUMATISM OF THE BELLY OF MUSCLES BY PREFERENCE (N.).

Nervous symptoms, twitchings, spasms, convulsions, neuralgias ; chills without shaking, worse at menstrual period (N.).

Angina pectoris : pains radiate all over the chest, and are associated with cerebral congestion and unconsciousness ; the face is livid, and the arm feels as if bound tightly to the body (F.).

Palpitation from the least motion (R.).

Choreic movements, accompanied by rheumatism (Br.).

Headache of drunkards and students (L.).

HEADACHE PRESSING OUTWARD ; OR UP-WARD, AS IF TOP OF HEAD WOULD FLY OFF, OR INTO EYES (CILIARY NEURALGIA), OR DOWN NAPE INTO SPINE (N.).

Prolapsus uterus during menses (Lach., Lil-T., Nat-C., Puls., Sep.) (K.).

Menses irregular in time and amount (B.).

Ovarian neuralgia, with other reflex left-sided pains (D.).

Rheumatic dysmenorrhœa (Bell.) (A.).

Menorrhagia ; pains run through hips into thighs, passing down (N.).

Pregnancy : nausea, sleeplessness ; false labour-like

pains ; sharp pains across abdomen ; abortion at third month (*Sab.*) (A).

Climacteric ; infra-mammary pains left side, persistent (N.).

After-pains, worse in the groins (A.).

DURING LABOUR : SHIVERS IN THE FIRST STAGE ; CONVULSIONS, FROM NERVOUS EXCITEMENT ; RIGID OS ; PAINS SEVERE, SPASMODIC, TEDIOUS, AGGRAVATED BY LEAST NOISE (A.).

Lochia suppressed (*Acon., Bry., Sec.*) (C.).

The patient cannot sleep because of pain ; he tosses about ; is extremely restless ; and should he fall asleep, it is full of unpleasant dreams ; never is the sleep restful or refreshing (R.).

Dry, short cough, worse from speaking and at night (Br.).

Tickling in the throat, with violent cough (*Bell., Hyos., Phos., Rumx.*) (C.).

Cough excited by every attempt to speak, so that one is obliged to desist (N.).

Excessive muscular soreness, after dancing, skating, or other violent muscular exertion (A.).

ACHING PAINS IN THE EYEBALLS, OR IN TEMPLES, EXTENDING TO EYES (N.).

Periodical colicky pains, better bending double and after stool (*Coloc.*) (C.).

Brain feels too large for the cranium (*Arg-N Glon.*) (C.).

Heart troubles from reflex symptoms of uterus or ovaries. Heart's action ceases suddenly ; impending suffocation (A.).

Sinking in epigastrium (Sep., Sulph.). Gnawing pain. Nausea and vomiting caused by pressure on spine and cervical region (Br.).

Hysterical or epileptical spasms at the time of menses (C.).

PLEURODYNIA (*Bell., Bry., Ran-B.*) (B.).

AGGRAVATION : During menstrual period and climacteric ; the more profuse the flow, the greater the suffering ; from cold, damp air ; sitting and alcohol.

AMELIORATION : In open air ; gentle, continued motion ; pressure ; and warm covering.

RELATIONSHIP : Similar to *Caul.* and *Puls.* in uterine and rheumatic affections ; to *Agar., Lil-T.* and *Sep.*

Æsculus Hippocastanum.

COMMON NAME : HORSE CHESTNUT.

For persons with hæmorrhoidal tendencies, and who suffer with gastric, bilious or catarrhal troubles (A.).

SENSATION OF FULLNESS IN VARIOUS PARTS, AS HEART, LUNGS, STOMACH, ANUS, BRAIN, PELVIS, ETC.

Prolapsus ani with constipation (Bt.).

Follicular pharyngitis : violent burning, raw sensation in throat ; dryness and roughness of throat (A.).

PILES ; PURPLE, PAINFUL, EXTERNAL, WITH BACKACHE (*Nux-V.*) (B.).

Sensation as if a foreign body was in the rectum, or as if it was full of small sticks, with fruitless efforts at evacuation and pains through hips and sacrum (N.).

STOOL FOLLOWED BY FULLNESS OF RECTUM AND INTENSE PAIN IN ANUS FOR HOURS (*Aloe, Ign., Mur-Ac., Nit-Ac., Sulph.*) (A.).

Large hæmorrhoids, which quite block up the rectum, without much hæmorrhage (Hg.).

Constipation : large stool voided with difficulty and followed hours with severe pain in back, lumbar or sacral region (N.).

Pain from occiput to frontal region, with bruised sensation of the scalp.

SEVERE DULL BACKACHE IN LUMBO-SACRAL ARTICULATION ; MORE OR LESS CONSTANT ; AFFECTING SACRUM AND HIPS (A.).

Nose sensitive to inspired air (B.).

Severe fluent coryza, with burning and raw feeling in the nostrils.

FREQUENT INCLINATION TO SWALLOW WITH BURNING, PRICKING, STINGING AND DRY CONSTRICTED FAUCES (*Apis, Bell., Lach.*) (N.).

Depressed and irritable state of the mind (G.).

Dull aching pains in the right hypochondriac region and region of the gall-bladder.

Jaundice (*Chel.*, *Iod.*, *Merc.*, *Sep.*). Congestion of the liver and portal system (*Aloe.*, *Podo.*, *Sulph.*).

THROBS, DEEP IN ABDOMEN (B.).

Weak feeling at the sacro-iliac symphysis, as though the legs were about to give out (F.).

Discharge of prostratic fluid at stool (Br.).

With uterine troubles constant backache across the hips and sacrum, aggravated by walking or stooping (N.).

Pulsation in the hypogastrium of the female (Calc-P.) (K.).

Old cases of leucorrhœa, of a dark yellow colour, thick and sticky, worse after menstrual period, increased by walking, corrodes the labia, with aching in the sacrum and knees (G.).

Vertigo, when sitting and walking (Br.).

Violent vomiting (*Ant-T.*, *Ipec.*, *Verat.*) ; great burning distress in the stomach (*Ars.*, *Canth.*, *Iris.*, *Phos.*, *Sulph.*). Pressure as from a stone in the pit of the stomach (*Acon.*, *Ars.*, *Bry.*, *Nux-V.*, *Puls.*) (C.).

AGGRAVATION : From inhaling cold air ; by motion ; by walking ; from stooping ; after washing in water ; in winter.

AMELIORATION : In summer ; chill better from heat.

RELATIONSHIP : Similar to *Aloe, Coll., Ign., Mur-Ac., Nit-Ac., Nux-V.* and *Sulph.* in hæmorrhoids.

After *Coll.* has improved piles, *Æsc. often cures.*

Useful after *Nux-V.* and *Sulph.* have improved, but failed to cure piles.

Æthusa Cynapium.

COMMON NAMES : FOOL'S PARSLEY ; GARDEN HEMLOCK.

Useful in gastro-intestinal troubles, especially in gastro-intestinal catarrh and convulsions of children during dentition (C).

Dozing of child after vomiting spells (Ant-T.), or *after the stool (Nux-M.)* (C.).

Head feels bound up, or in a vise (Arg-N.) (Br.).

Regurgitation of food an hour or so after eating ; copious greenish vomiting (A.).

VIOLENT VOMITING OF CURDLED MILK (*Calc., Mag-C., Iris*) AND CHEESY MATTER (C.).

Complete absence of thirst (*Apis, Puls.* ; reverse of *Ars.*) (A.).

CANNOT BEAR MILK IN ANY FORM (A.).

INTOLERANCE OF MILK ; IT IS FORCIBLY EJECTED ALMOST AS SOON AS SWALLOWED :

THEN WEAKNESS CAUSES DROWSINESS ; IN NUR-
SING CHILDREN (C.).

*Cholera infantum : after much purging and vomiting
the child becomes cold, clammy, stupid, loses consciousness,
and often lies with staring eyes and dilated pupils* (G.).

HUNGRY AFTER VOMITING ; EATS AND VOM-
ITS AGAIN (N.).

The buccal cavity is usually very dry (G.).

Stool : undigested or partly so *(Ant-C.)* ; green, thin,
bilious, with violent tenesmus before and after stool ;
bright yellow, or greenish. watery, slimy stools, with
crying and drawing up of the feet in infants (G.).

*An expression of great anxiety and pain, with a
drawn condition and well-marked linea nasalia* (A.)

Herpetic eruption on the tip of nose (Br.).
Deathly aspect ; blue white pallor about lips (B).
Sweat with aversion to uncovering (B.).

Vertigo, during and after rising from a seat (L.).

Idiocy in children *(Bar-C.)* ; incapacity to think ;
confused (A.).

Awkwardness *(Apis, Bov., Ign., *Lach., Nat-M.,
Nux-V.)* (F.).

Headache : violent pain, as if the brain were dashed
to pieces, with a desire to have a band fastened tightly
around head (L.).

*Great weakness ; children cannot stand ; unable to
hold up the head (Abrot.) ; prostration with sleepiness.*

Epileptic spasms, with clenched thumbs, red face, eyes turned downwards, pupils fixed and dilated ; foam at the mouth. jaws locked ; pulse small, hard and quick (A.).

BRAIN-FAG (*Anac., Kali-P.*) (Br.).

STUDENTS CANNOT CONCENTRATE THEIR MIND ON THEIR WORK AND PREPARE FOR AN EXAMINATION (*Kali-P., Nux-V.*) (*Bl.*).

INABILITY TO THINK OR TO FIX ATTENTION (Br.).

Profound exhaustion and lack of reaction (B.).

AGGRAVATION : After eating or drinking, after vomiting ; after stool ; after spasm ; during dentition ; from milk ; and during hot weather.

AMELIORATION : From covering ; from tightly bandaging the head ; and during rest.

RELATIONSHIP : Similar to : *Ant-C., Ars., Calc. Cic., Sanic., Sep. and Sulph.*

Complementary : *Calc-C.*

Agaricus Muscarius.

COMMON NAMES : BUG AGARIC ; FLY AGARIC ; TOAD STOOL.

It acts as an intoxicant to the brain, producing more vertigo and delirium than alcohol, followed by profound sopor with lowered reflexes.

GREAT DEBILITY AND HEAVINESS IN THE LIMBS.

Nervous prostration, after sexual debauchery (A.).

Boring or dull pains.

Every motion, every turn of body, causes pain in the spine. Single vertebra sensitive to touch (A.).

Great sensitiveness of the body to pressure and cold air.

SPINAL IRRITATION, DUE TO SEXUAL EXCES-SES (*Kali-P.*).

Seminal emissions, without dreams (*Anac., Camph. Con., Dios., Phos.*) (K.).

Sensation as if ice touched or ice-cold needles were piercing the skin ; as from hot needles (A.).

Reeling and staggering to and fro, when walking in open air (G.).

ITCHING, WITH BURNING AND REDNESS, AS IF FROST-BITTEN, OF THE NOSE, EARS, FINGERS AND TOES.

Chilblains, that itch and burn intolerably (A.).

Sensation of soreness in the nose and mouth.

Epistaxis of old people (*Carb-V., Ham., Sec., Sulph-Ac.*) (K.).

Fluent coryza (C.).

Nosebleed, when blowing the nose, early in the morn-ing (Ambr., Bry.) (C.).

Tearing pains in the limbs, which : are continuous while at rest, but disappearing on moving about.

Uncertainty in walking ; stumbles over everything in the way ; feels pain as if beaten, when standing (A.).

Motion of type, with flickering, when reading (R.).

TWITCHING OF THE EYELIDS.
BLEPHAROSPASMUS (F.).

Dim-sightedness ; everything seems obscured (G.).

Asthenopia, caused by prolonged strain (R.).

Palsy of upper and lower limbs, from incipient softening of spinal cord (L.).

CLONIC SPASMS (*Cup.*, *Nux-V.*).

Epilepsy, from suppressed eruptions (*Caust.*, *Psor.*, *Sulph.*) (A.).

Delirium, with constant raving ; tries to get out of bed (Bell., Hyos., Stram.) ; in typhoid or typhus (A.).

RAGE, WITH GREAT EFFORTS OF STRENGTH (*Bell.* ; *Canth.* ; *Stram.*).

Sings, talks, but does not answer (Br.).
Disinclination to work (G.).

THE PATIENT IS EXCESSIVELY FANCIFUL AND FULL OF ECSTACY (*Coff.*).

Self-willed, stubborn (G.).

Profuse sweat when walking, or from the least exertion (C.).

In old people with indolent circulation, or drunkards, especially for their headaches (N.).

THE SYMPTOMS FREQUENTLY APPEAR DIAGONALLY, AS IN THE RIGHT ARM AND LEFT LEG.

A sudden and violent stitch comes in the sacrum, whilst walking in the open air (G.).

Sense of languor, as if the body were bruised and the joints dislocated (L.).

INVOLUNTARY MOVEMENTS WHILE AWAKE, CEASE DURING SLEEP ; CHOREA, FROM SIMPLE MOTIONS AND JERKS OF SINGLE MUSCLES TO DANCING OF WHOLE BODY ; TREMBLING OF WHOLE BODY (A.).

Senile tremor (L.).

Tingling and formication in the back (D.).

Convulsive shocks in various muscles (C.).

Spasmodic, convulsive, nervous cough (R.).

Menses : too profuse ; with titillation in the genital organs and desire for embrace (Bt.).

FAINTNESS, AFTER COITION (*Asaf.*, *Dig.*, *Nat-P.*, *Sep.*) (K.).

Leucorrhœa, with much itching (Br.).

Post-climacteric prolapsus (A.).

Bearing down pains of a violent character (at once benefited by the action of this medicine).

Complaints, following parturition and coitus (Br.).

AGGRAVATION : After motion ; after eating ; after coitus ; from mental application ; before a thunder-storm ; and in cold air.

AMELIORATION : When moving about slowly.

RELATIONSHIP : Similar to *Act.*, *Calc.*, *Cann-I.*, *Hyos.*, *Kali-P.*, *Lach.*, *Nux-V.*, *Op.* and *Stram.*, in delirium of alcoholism (delirium tremens) ; and to *Mygl.*, *Tar.* and *Zinc.*, in chorea.

Agnus Castus.

COMMON NAME : CHASTE TREE.

Especially useful in premature old age, which arises in young persons from abuse of the sexual powers (C.).

Mental distraction ; self-contempt (A.).

Melancholic and hypochondriacal mood.

Sad and despairing (B.).

Desires death (*Aur., Lac-C., Nux-V.*) Lack of courage (Br.).

ABSENT-MINDEDNESS (*Alum., Apis, Bar-C., Cann-I., Caust., Cham., Graph., Hell., Kali-P., Lach., Mez., Nat-M., Nux-M., Plat., Puls., Sep., Verat.*).

FORGETFUL (*Con., Kali-P., Nux-V.*) (Br.).

Cannot recollect ; has to read a sentence twice before he can comprehend (*Lyc., Phos-Ac., Sep.*) (A.).

Illusion of smell—herring or musk (Br.).

Retention of urine, from paralysis of the bladder (*Caust., Op., Sulph.*) (Bt.).

Rumbling of flatulence, during sleep.

Thirstlessness, and aversion to all drink.

Nausea, first in the pit of the stomach, later in the stomach, with the sensation as if all the intestines were pressing downward.

Swelling and induration of the spleen, often with soreness, after intermittent fever (*Cean.*) (G.).

COMPLAINTS OF JADED RAKES (B.).

Corrosive itching of the perineum and difficulty of passing soft motions.

Gleety discharge (*Kali-B.*, *Nat-M.*, *Sep.*) (Br.).

Sexual desire lessened, almost lost ; penis so relaxed that voluptuous fancies excite no erection (*Calad.*) (N.).

Impotence, after frequent attacks of gonorrhœa(*Cob.*, *Cub.*, *Hydr.*, *Med.*, *Sulph.*, *Thuj.* ; impotence from syphilis—*Merc.*) (A.).

THE SEXUAL DESIRE IS SUPPRESSED.

DIMINUTION OF SEXUAL POWERS ; THE PENIS IS SMALL AND FLACCID (*Bar-C.*, *Berb.*, *Caps.*. *Lyc.*, *Sulph.*) AND THE TESTICLES ARE COLD (*Aloe*, *Berb.*, *Brom.*, *Camph.*, *Caps.*, *Cer-S.*, *Gels.*, *Merc.*, *Zinc.*).

COMPLETE IMPOTENCE (*Calad.*, *Calc.*, *Chin.*, *Con.*, *Lyc.*, *Med.*, *Nux-V.*, *Phos.*, *Sel.*, *Sep.*, *Sulph.*) (A.).

Spermatorrhœa in old sinners (*F.*).

When pressing at stool there is a discharge of prostatic fluid (*Agar.*, *Anac.*, *Calc.*, *Caust.*, *Con.*, *Hep.*, *Kali-B.*, *Nat-C.*, *Nat-M.*, *Nux-V.*, *Petr.*, *Phos-Ac.*, *Phos.*, *Sel.*, *Sep.* *Sil.*, *Sulph.*, *Zinc.*).

DRAWING ALONG THE SPERMATIC CORDS (*All-C.*, *Berb.*, *Chel.*, *Clem.*, *Con.*, *Ham.*, *Ind.*, *Mang.*, *Merc.*, *Nux-V.*, *Ox-A.*).

ITCHING ON THE GENITAL ORGANS, WITH YELLOW DISCHARGES FROM THE URETHRA (A.).

In old men, who, having spent their youth and early manhood in the practice of excessive venery, are just as excitable in their sexual passion at sixty as at eighteen or twenty, and yet they are physically impotent, *Agnus Castus* is a good remedy (F.).

HISTORY OF REPEATED GONORRHŒAS (*Thuj.*) (*Br.*).

Sterility (*Aur.*, *Bor.*, *Graph.*, *Nat-C.*, *Nat-M.*, *Sep.*) (*Br.*).

In the female, there is suppressing of the menses, with drawing pain in the abdomen and lack of sexual desire (*Sep.*).

THERE IS DEFICIENT SECRETION OF MILK IN LYING-IN-WOMEN (*Bry.*, *Calc.*, *Carb-V.*, *Caust.*, *Cham.*, *Hyos.*, *Iod.*, *Lac-D.*, *Lach.*, *Merc.*, *Puls.*, *Rhus-T.*, *Sec.*, *Sil.*, *Sulph.*, *Urt-U.*, *Verat.*).

Milk entirely suppressed (N.).

LEUCORRHŒA : STAINING YELLOW ; TRANSPARENT (Br.).

Leucorrhœa, passing imperceptibly from the very relaxed parts (A.).

Difficulty of passing soft stools (*Alum.*) (G.).

Sometimes stools seem inclined to re-enter the rectum (Sil.).

AGGRAVATION : From seminal losses.

AMELIORATION : By scratching (itching) ; by pressure (aching in the dorsum of the nose).

RELATIONSHIP : *Calad.* and *Selen.* follow well after *Agnus* in weakness of sexual organs or impotence.

ANTIDOTE : *Camph.*

Allium Cepa.

COMMON NAME : RED ONION.

HEADACHE, BETTER IN THE OPEN AIR (*Apis, Ars., Bell., Coff., Ferr., Lyc., Puls.*) ; GETS WORSE ON RETURNING TO A WARM ROOM (*Apis, Carb-V., Kali-S., Phos., Plat., Puls., Seneg., Sep., Sulph.*) (G.).

HEADACHE, WITH CORYZA (*Calc-S., Dulc.,Euphr., Gels., Graph., Hep.*) (C.).

Headache ceases during menses ; returns when flow disappears (*Lach., Zinc.*) (Br.).

Coryza, from odour of peaches, or flowers (K.).

Acrid, watery discharge dropping from tip of the nose (*Ars., Ars-I.*) (A.).

FLUENT CORYZA (*Amm-C., Ars., Kali-A.*) (C.).

COPIOUS WATERY DISCHARGE FROM THE NOSE, WITH LACHRYMATION (G.).

EXCESSIVE, NON-EXCORIATING LACHRYMATION (excoriating lachrymation—*Euphr.*) (C.).

FREQUENT AND VIOLENT SNEEZING, PARTICULARLY ON ENTERING A WARM ROOM (*Puls.*) (G.).

EXCORIATING NASAL DISCHARGE, WITH BLAND DISCHARGE FROM THE EYES (K.).

NASAL DISCHARGE BURNS AND CORRODES NOSE AND UPPER LIP (A.).

EXCORIATING DISCHARGE FROM THE LEFT NOSTRIL (K.).

Sensation of weakness in the bladder and urethra.

Pressure and other pains in the region of the bladder.

Increased secretion of urine, with coryza.

Dysuria (*Acon.*, *Bell.*, *Cop.*, *Dig.*, *Lil-T.*) (K.).

Urine red, with much pressure and burning in the urethra.

Eyes sensitive to light (Br.).

Redness of the eyes, with itching, burning and stinging.

Cough, when inhaling cold air. Incessant, hacking, tickling cough (*Nux-V.*, *Squil.*) (B.).

Breathing oppressed, from pressure in the middle of the chest, worse in the evening (*Bry.*, *Phos.*).

Senile bronchitis (*Ars.*, *Bar-C.*, *Calc.*, *Carb-V.*, *Lyc.*, *Seneg.*, *Sil.*, *Sulph.*) (Br.).

Cold extends to the bronchi, with profuse secretion of mucus ; coughing and much rattling (*Chel.*, *Phos.*) (N.).

Sensation as of a lump in the throat (*Asaf.*, *Ign.*, *Lach.*, *Nat-M.*, *Psor.*, *Sep.*).

Sore, tired feeling of the limbs, especially arms (C.).

Soreness of the lower extremities.

Sore and raw spots on feet, especially heel, from friction (A.).

Constrictive pain in fore part of the throat, in the region of os hyoides, then low down posteriorly on the right side (C.).

Rough and raw feeling in the throat (F.).

CATARRHAL HOARSENESS (*Arum-T.*, *Carb-V. Caust.*, *Phos.*) (C.).

CATARRHAL LARYNGITIS : COUGH COMPELS THE PATIENT TO GRASP THE LARYNX (*Bell.* ; to grasp the head—*Bry.* ; to hold the abdomen—*Nux-V.*) ; SEEMS AS IF IT WOULD TEAR IT (A.).

Aching throughout the body (*Arn., Bapt., Bell., Bry., Eup-P., Rhus-T.*) (C.).

NEURALGIC PAINS, FOLLOWING AMPUTATIONS OR INJURIES TO NERVES (*Hyper.*) (Br.).

NASAL POLYPUS (*Calc., Con., Graph., Kali-B., Lem-M., Lyc., Merc., Phos., Psor., Sang., Sep., Sil., Sulph., Teucr., Thuj.*) (A.).

Panaritium ; *with red streaks up the arm* ; *pains drive to despair* (A.).

Diarrhœa, after midnight and in the morning.

Colic : from cold, by getting feet wet ; overeating ; from cucumbers ; salads ; hæmorrhoidal ; of children ; worse from sitting, better from moving about (A.).

Itching at the anus (worms).

Heat, with rumbling in the abdomen, coryza and thirst.

Sensation of glowing heat, on different parts of the body (Br.).

Hay-fever (*Psor., Sabad., Sil.*) (Br.).

Pulse full and accelerated.

Gaping in deep sleep (Br.).

AGGRAVATION : In the evening ; in a warm room.

AMELIORATION : In the open air ; in a cold room.

RELATIONSHIP : Similar to *Euphr.*, but coryza and lachrymation are opposite.

COMPLEMENTARY : *Phos., Puls.,* and *Thuj.*

Aloe Socotrina.

COMMON NAME : SOCOTRINE ALOES.

Aloe is frequently called for in correcting the bad effects from sedentary life and habits (Nux-V.), and is especially suitable to persons of a lymphatic and hypochondriacal constitution.

DISEASES OF MUCOUS MEMBRANES ; CAUSES THE PRODUCTION OF MUCUS IN JELLY-LIKE LUMPS FROM THROAT OR RECTUM ; AFFECTS MUCOUS MEMBRANES OF RECTUM (A.).

Mental dissatisfaction and bad humour about himself, more especially during the state of costiveness, or when he suffers from pain.

Disinclined to perform either physical or mental labour (G.).

Acts most prominently in the region of the liver. Has many symptoms of portal congestion (D.).

The taste is bitter and sour and tasteless eructations are present, with portal congestion and a sense of abdominal fullness, heaviness and heat.

It should be remembered in chronic types of jaundice that attend bilious states, when the tongue is coated, the breath foul, and there is a sensation of fullness and heaviness in the hepatic region (Bl.).

Sensation of a plug between the symphysis pubis and os coccygis, with urging to stool (R.).

Bloated abdomen, more on the left side, or along the colon, and worse after eating.

Profuse menstruation (Chin., Ferr., Sab.) (Bt.).

Pressing down in the rectum, during catamenia (G.).

Pain around the navel, worse from pressure (Mang. ; better from pressure—Plb.).

Is of great value in atonic condition of the uterus, uterine hæmorrhages, etc. (C.).

Great weakness and weak pulse, after vomiting.

Abdominal plethora, with feeling of fullness and pressing down, or weight in anus and bladder (N.).

Lumbago, alternating with headache (C.).

Backache (Bell., Cimic., Nux-V., Puls., Sep.) (C.).

A DISCHARGE OF MUCH FLATULENCY, BURN-ING AND SMELLING OFFENSIVELY, WHICH RELIEVES THE PAIN IN THE ABDOMEN.

Itching and burning in anus, preventing sleep (*Ind., Merc., Sulph.*) (A.).

Giddiness on moving (Agar., Amm-C., Bry., Calc-P., Con., Glon., Phos., Sil.).

Longing for juicy things (Br.).

HUNGRY, DURING DIARRHŒA (hungry, during dysentery—*Nux-V.*) (A.).

Desire for apples (*Ant-T., Guai., Sulph., Tell.*).

Itch appears each year, as winter approaches (Psor.) (A.).

Golden coloured skin (C.).

Feeling of weakness in abdomen, as if diarrhœa would come on ; heaviness in hypogastrium and rectum (N.).

Headache across the forehead, aggravated by every foot-step (Bell., Bry.) ; with heaviness of eyes and nausea (A.).

Headache : pain is situated over the eyes and is attended by a sensation as though a weight were pressing down the eyelids. Relief comes from partially closing the eyelids (F.).

HEADACHE : WORSE FROM HEAT, BETTER FROM COLD APPLICATIONS (*Ars.*, *Bell.*, *Bry.*, *Calc.*, *Ferr.*, *Ferr-P.*, *Glon.*, *Lach.*) ; ALTERNATING WITH LUMBAGO ; AFTER INSUFFICIENT STOOL (A.).

Menses too early and copious ; cramp, in uterus ; determination of blood to uterus (R.).

Colic, before and during stool (*Coloc.*) (Br.).

AFTER STOOL, FEELS EXTREMELY WEAK AND PROSTRATED (*Ars.*, *Ars-M.*, *Bism.*, *Con.*, *Merc.*, *Nat-S.*, *Nit-Ac.*, *Phos.*, *Pic-Ac.*, *Podo.*, *Sec.*, *Verat.*) (G.).

HÆMORRHOIDS PROTRUDE LIKE GRAPES ; VERY SORE AND TENDER ; BETTER FROM COLD WATER APPLICATION (Br.).

The hæmorrhoids bleed often and profusely (Bt.).

Stool contains a jelly-like mucus, and there is a colic, which is relieved by bending double (F.).

Stools are often very hot (*Calc-P.*, *Cham.*, *Dios.*, *Merc.*, *Merc-C.*, *Nux-V.*, *Phos.*, *Sulph.*) (G.).

Solid stool and masses of mucus pass involuntarily (A.).

Constant urging to stool, during the day (C.).

EVERY MORNING, ON RISING, HAS A HASTY DESIRE FOR STOOL, WITH RUMBLING IN THE ABDOMEN, AND FINALLY SPUTTERING STOOL (EUG., NAT-S.) (G.).

Fear lest stool should escape with flatus (*Carb-V.,* *Nat-P.*, *Nat-S.*, *Olnd.*, *Phos-Ac.*, *Podo.*, *Sulph.*, *Verat.*) (R.).

FEELING OF WEAKNESS AND LOSS OF POWER OF SPHINCTER ANI. SENSE OF INSECURITY IN RECTUM, WHEN PASSING FLATUS (Br.).

FÆCES AND URINE WILL PASS AT THE SAME TIME ; CANNOT PASS ONE WITHOUT THE OTHER (*Alum.*, *Canth.*, *Merc.*, *Mur-Ac.*, *Nux-V.*, *Puls.*, *Staph.,* *Thuj.*) (G.).

Liquid, yellow, copious, involuntary stool, with passing of flatus or urine, falling out without exertion (R.).

ONE MUST GO TO STOOL SOON AFTER A MEAL (*Ars.*, *Chin.*, *Coloc.*, *Crot-T.*, *Lyc.*, *Podo.*).

Dysentery : Stools are covered with blood and accompanied by griping in the epigastric region (D.).

Prolapsus recti (*Podo.*, *Sulph.*) (B.).

Fistula in ano (*Calc-P.*, *Sil.*) (By.).

AGGRAVATION : In early morning ; during hot, dry, weather after eating or drinking ; on standing or walking.

AMELIORATION : From cold water ; during cold weather , from discharge of flatus and stool.

RELATIONSHIP : Like *Sulphur* in many diseases, with abdominal plethora and congestion of portal vein ; develops suppressed eruptions.

Similar to Amm-M., Gamb., Nux-V., and *Podo.*

Alumina.

COMMON NAME : PURE CLAY.

Spare, dry, thin subjects (A.).

Dryness of membranes ; the conjunctiva, the nose and the intestinal tract are all very dry (D.).

Constant, dry, hacking cough ; interrupts breathing (B.).

Throat feels full of sticks or constricted (B.).

Eyes : Agglutination in the morning on waking, with burning when opened, and dread of light ; dim vision, obliging her to wipe her eyes constantly (R.).

Useful for granular lids (*Graph., Sep., Sulph.*), *or chronic blepharitis* (*Bor., Calc., Graph., Sep., Sil., Sulph., Thuj.*) (R.).

Dry, tettery, itching eruption, worse in winter (*Psor.*) (A.).

Chapped skin and eczematous eruptions.

Intolerable itching of the whole body, when getting warm in bed (*Sulph.*) ; *scratches until bleeds, then becomes painful* (*A.*).

ECZEMA (*Ars., Graph., Merc., Mezer., Sulph.*) *(B.).*

ABNORMAL APPETITE ; WANTS STARCH, CHALK, CHARCOAL, COFFEE OR TEA GROUNDS, ACIDS, INDIGESTIBLE THINGS ; POTATOES DISAGREE (N.).

Bruised feeling in the back. Pain in the lower vertebræ, as if a hot iron were thrust through. Shooting pains in back (R.).

No desire for stool (*Bry., Op., Sulph.*) (Br.).

Constipation of children ; the rectum is dry, hard, inflamed and bleeding (D.).

THE STOOLS MAY BE DRY, HARD AND KNOTTY, LIKE SHEEP DUNG, OR SOFT (D.).

Constipation, from great dryness of the mucous follicles of the rectum, with long-lasting pain in the rectum:(Bt.).

Very efficient in the cure of intractable costiveness in women of an extremely sedentary habit.

INACTIVITY OF THE RECTUM ; EVEN A SMALL STOOL REQUIRES GREAT STRAINING (*Anac., Graph., Op., Plb., Sep., Sil., Sulph.*) (N.).

Weakness of memory and inability to think coherently.

The patient is tired and faints easily (*Sep.*), and must lie down (Bl.).

Confused as to personal identity (*Anac.*) (Br.).

Sad thoughts constantly crowd upon the mind ; everything is viewed in a sad light (G.).

TIME PASSES TOO SLOWLY ; AN HOUR SEEMS HALF A DAY (*Cann-I.*) (A.).

He feels as if some parts of the body were enlarged.

AS SOON AS SHE SEES BLOOD OR A KNIFE, WANTS TO KILL HERSELF (Dg.).

Vertigo on opening the eyes ; everything turns with him in a circle ; with white stars (G.).

There is a sensation as if there was a cobweb on the face (D.).

INTESTINAL HÆMORRHAGE ; PROFUSE DIS-
CHARGE OF COAGULATED BLOOD IN A MASS,
RESEMBLING LIVER AND SERUM, WITHOUT
PAIN, BUT GREAT WEAKNESS (TYPHOID) (N.).

Chlorosis, with pale and scanty menses and craving
for indigestible substances (D.).

Unpleasant want of animal heat (Sil.).

Pain in the back, as if a hot iron were thrust through
the lower vertebræ.

Great debility from exercise, as in walking.

Bearing down pains, as though everything would
fall through the vagina (Dg.).

PROFUSE, TRANSPARENT, ACRID LEUCOR-
RHŒA, RUNNING DOWN TO THE HEELS IN
LARGE QUANTITIES (G.).

After the menses, she is so weak in body and mind,
that a little exercise prostrates her (G.).

Leucorrhœa : acrid, worse after the menses, with
burning in the genitals and rectum, which parts seemed
inflamed and corroded, so that walking was difficult ;
better from washing with cold water (R.).

Chronic eructations for years ; worse in the
evening (A.).

Great dryness of the throat (Bt.).

Clergyman's sorethroat (Br.).

*There is present tearing pain in the limbs and a
sensation of constriction of the internal organs (œsophagus).*

SENSE OF CONSTRICTION, FROM PHARYNX DOWN TO STOMACH ; SEEMS AS IF FOOD COULD NOT PASS (*Æsc.*, *Alumn.*, *Arg-M.*, *Ars.*, *Bell.*, *Cact.*, *Cupr.*, *Hyos.*, *Ign.*, *Kali-C.*, *Lyss.*, *Merc-C.*, *Nat-M.*, *Phos.*, *Plb.*, *Sabad.*, *Zinc.*).

Involuntary motions (jerking of the head and other parts are associated in this condition).

INABILITY TO WALK, EXCEPT WITH THE EYES OPEN, AND IN THE DAY TIME ; TOTTERING AND FALLING WHEN CLOSING EYES (*Arg-N.*, *Gels.*, *Kali-P.*, *Phos.*, *Sil.*) (A.).

When sitting the nates go to sleep (G.).

HE FEELS AS IF HE WAS WALKING ON CUSHIONS (D.).

THERE IS CREEPING, AS IF ANTS WERE CRAWLING ON HIS LEGS AND BACK (D.).

Has proven useful in cases simulating locomotor ataxia. The lower limbs appear heavy ; can scarcely drag them along ; staggers when walking (Bl.).

Muscles of bladder paretic ; difficult starting (Br.).

Involuntary urination with the stool, or urine can be passed only during stool (N.).

Retention of urine. Can only void urine while straining at stool (N.).

AGGRAVATION : In cold air ; during winter ; while sitting ; from eating potatoes ; after eating soups ; in the afternoon ; periodically ; on alternate days ; at new and full moon ; and during the act of micturition.

4

AMELIORATION : Mild summer weather ; from warm drinks ; while eating ; in wet weather ; during moderate exercise ; in the open air ; in the evening ; and on alternate days.

RELATIONSHIP : *Alumina* is the chronic of *Bryonia*.

Similar to Bar-C., Con., Pareira and *Sep.* in ailments of old people.

Complementary to Bryonia.

Follows well after Bry., Lach. and *Sulph.*

Alumina is one of the chief antidotes for lead poisoning ; painter's colic ; and ailments from lead.

Ambra Grisea.

COMMON NAME : AMBERGRIS.

Nervous affections of old people ; nerves worn out (A.).

Especially called for young girls, who are excitable, nervous and weak (A.).

Forgetful ; cannot remember the simplest fact (*Anac., Kali-P., Lyc., Sil.*) (F.).

Intensely shy, blushes easily (Br.).

Time passes slowly (D.).

Does everything in a hurry (*Arg-N.*) (D.).

Great sadness, sits for days weeping (*Ign., Nat-M., Stann.*) (A.).

Dwells on unpleasant things (**Br.**).

Is especially suitable for lean or aged persons.

Asthma of children, or old people (*Ant-T.*, *Carb-V.*, *Lyc.*, *Phos.*, *Sulph.*).

Asthma, worse during coition (*Æth.*; worse after coition—*Asaf.*, *Cedr.*, *Kali-B.*) (**K.**).

Many complaints appear while sleeping and disappear after rising (*Lach.*).

Itching and burning in the skin.

Suppressed cutaneous eruptions (*Amm-C.*, *Ars.*, *Bry.*, *Cup.*, *Phos.*, *Psor.*, *Sil.*, *Sulph.*, *Zinc.*).

Weakness in the morning and at night, when awakening.

Cough is followed by eructation (*Ang.*, *Sulph-Ac.*, *Verat.*). (**F.**).

Whooping cough (*Arn.*, *Bell.*, *Dros.*, *Ipec.*, *Kali-C.*) (**A.**).

Violent cough, worse from talking or reading aloud (**A.**).

COUGH, WORSE WHEN STRANGERS ARE PRE-SENT (*Ars.*, *Bar-C.*, *Phos.*) (**D.**).

Spasmodic cough (*Ars.*, *Bell.*, *Cup.*, *Dros.*, *Hep.*, *Kali-M.*, *Lyc.*, *Merc.*, *Nat-S.*, *Phos.*, *Sil.*) (**N.**).

EXTERNAL NUMBNESS OF THE WHOLE BODY, IN THE MORNING.

The presence of others, even the nurse, is unbearable during stool (**A.**).

Nose-bleed during menses (*Bry.*, *Nat-S.*, *Puls.*, *Sep.*, *Sulph.*) (**B.**).

Hysteria, with fainting fits (*Ign.*, *Nat-M.*, *Phos-Ac.*, *Sep.*) (Bt.).

Itching, from the small of the back through the right leg, and burning, especially where the skin turns into the mucous membranes.

Ebullitions and pulsations in the whole body, after walking in the open air.

Sleeplessness, arising from worriment of mind, as from business troubles (F.).

Fetid odour from the mouth (*Arn.*, *Bry.*, *Kali-P.*, *Nux-V.*, *Puls.*, *Sulph.*) (C.).

Spasms and twitches in the muscular parts.

Frequent ineffectual desire for stool (*Anac.*, *Nux-V.*, *Puls.*, *Sulph.*) (C.).

The urine deposits a brown sediment (C.).

Menses too early and too profuse (C.).

Falling off of the hair (*Graph.*, *Hep.*, *Lyc.*, *Nat-M*, *Phos.*, *Sep.*) (C.).

One-sided complaints (perspiration, tearing, numbness and sensation of coldness in the abdomen).

Tearing in the muscles of the joints, often one-sided.

Defective reaction, from nervous weakness (*Amm-C.*, *Ars.*, *Brom.*, *Calc.*, *Caps.*, *Con.*, *Gels.*, *Hell.*, *Hydr-Ac.*, *Laur.*, *Med.*, *Olnd.*, *Op.*, *Phos-Ac.*, *Psor.*, *Sulph.*) (D.).

DISCHARGE OF BLOOD BETWEEN PERIODS, AT EVERY LITTLE ACCIDENT (Br.).

Bluish-white discharge from the vagina (Bl.).

Itching of the pudendum, with soreness and swelling (Br.).

Nymphomania (*Apis, Bell., Hyos., Lach., Orig., Plat., Stram.*) (Bl.).

Copious nose-bleeding, early every morning (G.).
Ranula (*Calc.. Fluor-Ac., Merc., Thuj.*) (G.).

Is of service in the male, when there is voluptuous itching on the scrotum and burning in the region of the spermatic vesicles, priapism, and painful rawness between the thighs (Bl.).

AGGRAVATION : In the evening ; while lying in a warm place ; from being in a warm room ; from warm drinks ; from music ; on lying down ; on awakening ; when reading or talking aloud ; after walking ; and from the presence of many people.

AMELIORATION : After eating ; in cold air ; from cold food and drinks ; on rising from bed ; while lying on the painful part ; and from slow motion in open air.

RELATIONSHIP : Similar to *Act-R., Asaf., Coca, Ign., Mosch., Phos., Valer., Zinc.*).

Ammonium Carbonicum.

COMMON NAME : SMELLING SALTS.
Long-lasting coryza (A.).

NOSE-BLEED : WHEN WASHING THE FACE AND HANDS IN THE MORNING ; FROM LEFT NOSTRIL ; AFTER EATING (A.).

Ozæna : blowing bloody mucus from the nose frequently (A.).

Blood rushes to the tip of nose, when stooping (A.).

Great sensitiveness to the cold (*Hep.*, *Psor.*, *Sil.*).

Children dislike washing (*Ant-C.*, *Sulph.*) (A.).

STOPPING OF THE NOSE, MOSTLY AT NIGHT. MUST BREATHE THROUGH THE MOUTH (*Lyc.*, *Nux-V.*, *Stict.*) (A.).

SNUFFLES OF INFANTS (*Hep.*, *Nux-V.*, *Samb.*, *Stict.*) (A.).

Profuse, watery coryza (*All-C.*, *Nat-M.*) (B.).

Tearing in the joints, relieved by the heat of the bed.

Lies in profound stupor ; the breathing is stertorous, and the vitality is greatly weakened (Bl.).

Tendency to gangrenous ulceration (*Ars.*, *Bapt.*, *Carb-Ac.*, *Lach.*, *Nit-Ac.*, *Phos.*) (Bt.).

Stinging and tearing pains (*Apis*, *Bry.*, *Kali-C.*, *Nit-Ac.*, *Phos.*).

The teeth loosen and gums ulcerate (F.).

Toothache ; *after taking sweets* (*Nat-C.*, *Phos.*, *Sep.*) ; from touch of tongue ; before, during and after menses ; better from external warmth (K.).

TENDER, BLEEDING GUMS (*Kreos.*, *Merc.*, *Nat-M.*) (B.).

Drawing and tension, as from the shortening of the muscles

MALIGNANT SCARLATINA : DARK RED, SORE-THROAT, PAROTID AND CERVICAL GLANDS MUCH SWOLLEN ; SKIN RED, WITH MILIARY RASH OR FAINTLY DEVELOPED ERUPTIONS (N.).

CHOLERA-LIKE SYMPTOMS AT THE BEGINNING OF MENSTRUATION (N.).

Inclination to stretch the limbs (*Ars.*, *Bell.*, *Calc.*, *Caust.*, *Cham.*, *Nux-V.*, *Puls.*, *Rhus-T.*).

Pain, as of dislocation in the joints.

Pain, as from sub-cutaneous ulceration.

Menses composed of clots; premature and abundant (*Calc.*, *Ferr.*, *Sab.*) (Bt.).

DIARRHŒA AND VOMITING, DURING MENSTRUATION.

Debility, which only permits to lie down.

At every menstrual period, there is a discharge of blood from the bowels (N.).

Disinclination to walk in the open air, and from it aggravation of many complaints.

Weak, anæmic. flabby women, addicted to the smelling bottle (N.).

Restlessness of the body in the evening.

The right side of the body is mostly affected (*Lyc.*, *Merc.*).

Dry cough, as from dust in the throat (*Ars.*, *Dros.*, *Lyc.*, *Puls.*, *Sulph.*).

Cough only at night, or only in day time.

Dyspnœa, from retrocession of an eruption (*Ant-T.*, *Ars.*, *Bry.*, *Phos.*, *Sulph.*) (Bt.).

Incessant cough, excited by a sensation as of feathers down in the larynx, from 3 to 4 A. M. (Bt.).

Exanthemata of a scarlet colour (*Bell.*, *Rhus-T.*, *Sulph.*).

Erysipelas of old, debilitated persons. Cerebral symptoms, simulating a drunken stupor, are present (N.).

Itching eruptions ; desquamations of the skin.

Panaritium ; fingers inflamed ; deep-seated periosteal pain (*Fluor-Ac., Sil.*) (N.).

Talking and hearing others talk affect him greatly.

Mistakes in writing and speaking (*Lyc., Nat-M., Phos.*) (G.).

Ill humour during wet, stormy weather (A.).

Disposed to weep, particularly in the evening (*Puls., Sep.*) (G.).

Pain at pit of stomach, with heart-burn, nausea, water-brash, and chilliness (Br.).

There is a feeling as of a lump in the throat (*Ign., Lach., Nux-M.*) (F.).

Swollen veins and bluish colour of the extremities (*Carb-V., Lach.*) (R.).

GREAT OPPRESSION OF BREATHING, ESPECIALLY IN GOING UP EVEN A FEW STEPS (*Ars., Calc., Phos.*) (C.).

Hoarseness (*Arg-N., Carb-V., Phos., Rhus-T.*) (C.).

Bleeding hæmorrhoids ; varices protrude during stool, which are very painful a long time after, hindering walking (*Ign., Nit-Ac., Thuj.*) (G.).

Violent palpitation of the heart, followed by syncope (*Lach., Nux-M., Verat.*) (G.).

Dilatation of the heart (*Dig., Lach., Phos.*) (F.).

Chronic bronchitis. with atony of the bronchial tubes (F.).

Much disturbed by night-mare nearly every night (G.).

Emphysema (Ant-A., Ant-T., Ars., Brom., Carb-V., Hep., Lach., Lob., Phos., Sulph.) (Br.).

Asthenic pneumonia (Carb-V., Lyc., Phos.) (Br.).

The pulse is very weak (F.).

Much oppression in breathing ; worse after any effort, and entering a warm room, or ascending even a few steps (Br.).

AGGRAVATION : From washing ; in the evening ; during cold, wet weather ; from wet poultices ; and during menses.

AMELIORATION : From lying on the abdomen ; from lying on painful side ; and in dry weather.

RELATIONSHIP : It antidotes poisoning with *Rhus Tox.* and stings of insects.

Is also useful in p isoning by charcoal fumes *(Arn., Bov.).*

Affects the right side most.

Inimical to *Lachesis.*

Ammonium Muriaticum.

COMMON NAME : SAL AMMONIAC.

Especially adapted to those, who are fat and sluggish ; or whose bodies are large and fat, but legs too thin (A.).

Nasal catarrh : the discharge is watery and acrid,

making the inside of the nostrils and the upper lip sore
(*All-C.*, *Ars.*, *Merc-C.*, *Nat-M.*) (C.).

Sensation of soreness in different parts of the body
(*Apis*, *Arn.*, *Bell.*, *Eup-P.*, *Rhus-T.*, *Pyrog.*).

SENSATION OF COLDNESS IN THE BACK,
BETWEEN THE SCAPULÆ (*Lach.*) (A.).

CONSTIPATION : STOOL HARD AND CRUMB-
LING (*Nat-M.*). REQUIRING GREAT EFFORT TO
EXPEL (*Alum.*, *Plb.*, *Sep.*) (C.).

Constipation, alternating with diarrhœa ; hard stool,
followed by a loose stool (*Ant-C.*) (G.).

Chronic congestion of the liver (*Chin.*, *Iod.*, *Merc.*,
Podo., *Sep.*, *Sulph.*) (Br.).

Hæmorrhoids : sore and smarting ; with burning
and stinging in the rectum, for hours after stool (A.).

Burning, stinging and throbbing, as from a boil
(*Apis*, *Ars-I.*, *Hep.*).

LEUCORRHŒA : LIKE WHITE OF AN EGG, PRE-
CEDED BY GRIPING PAIN ABOUT THE NAVEL ;
BROWN, SLIMY, PAINLESS, AFTER EVERY
URINATION (A.).

Prolapsus uteri (*Nat-M.*, *Sep.*) (B.).

*Tension in the joints, as from shortening of the
muscles.*

Contraction of the hamstring tendons (Br.).

Neuralgic pains in the stumps of amputated limbs
(*Hyper.*) (Bl.).

Offensive sweat on the feet (*Alum.*, *Graph.*, *Psor.*,
Sanic., *Sil.*) (A.).

SCIATICA : WORSE SITTING, BETTER LYING (Br.).

Ebullition, with anxiety and weakness. Irregular circulation (B.).

Chilly, as often as he wakes (B.).

Night sweat over the whole body, most copious after midnight and early in the morning (*Ars., Chel., Ferr., Phos., Psor., Sil., Tub.*) (G.).

Regurgitation of food (*Nux-V., Puls., Sep.*) (G.).

Hiccough (*Ars., Bell., Carb-V., Cic., Cup., Mag-P., Nux-V., Phos., Puls., Sulph., Verat.*).

Blisters on the tongue (*Ars., Nat-M., Rhus-T.*).

Sorethroat, with viscid phlegm, so tough that it cannot be hawked up (*Alum., Bor., Kali-B.*).

Cough, with salivation (*Ambr., Ars., Carb-V., Cycl., Lach., Merc.*) or liver symptoms (B.).

Many group of symptoms are accompanied by cough.

Noisy, rattling, tenacious mucus in the chest (*Carb-V., Hydr., Nat-S.*) (B.).

In the morning hours she feels stiff, but is relieved by walking in the open air.

Menses too early, with pain in the abdomen and small of back (C.).

During menses : diarrhœa and vomiting ; bloody discharge from the bowels (*Phos.*) ; *neuralgic pains in the feet* ; *flow more profuse at night* (*Bov. :* on lying down— *Kreos.*) (A.).

Moving the arms with force, or even stooping, excites asthma (G.).

Complains of heaviness in the chest (*Bry.*, *Phos.*) (F.).

Backache, as if in a vise, when sitting (Br.).

Hoarseness, with burning in region of the larynx (*Caust.*, *Phos.*) (G.).

Throbbing in the tonsils (*Bell.*) (F.).

Hæmorrhoids, after suppressed leucorrhœa (Br.).

Hard stool, covered with mucus (*Graph.*) (C.).

Profuse and frequent discharge of urine at night (*Ambr.*, *Phos-Ac.*) (C.).

AGGRAVATION : Of the head and chest symptoms, in the morning ; of the abdominal symptoms, in the afternoon ; and of the skin and fever symptoms, in the evening.

AMELIORATION : In the open air.

RELATIONSHIP : Similar to *Alum.*, *Amm-C.*, *Arg-N.*, *Ars.*, *Kali-C.*, *Mur-Ac.*, *Nat-M.*, *Phos.*, *Sil.* and *Sulph.*

Antidotes : *Camph.*, *Coff.*, *Hep.*, and *Nux-V.*

Antidotes to large doses : *Vinegar* or *Vegetable Acids.*

To be followed by *Ant-C.*, *Phos.*, *Puls.*, and *Sanic.*

Amyl Nitrite.

COMMON NAME : NITRITE OF AMYL.

For nervous, sensitive, plethoric women, during or after the menopause (A.).

Anxiety, as if something might happen ; must have fresh air (C.).

Sea-sickness (*Cocc., Petr., Phos., Tab.*) (Br.).

FLUSHINGS : START FROM FACE, STOMACH, VARIOUS PARTS OF BODY, FOLLOWED BY SWEATINGS, OFTEN HOT, PROFUSE (*Glon., Graph., Lach., Sang., Sep., Sulph.*) ; ABRUPTLY LIMITED, PARTS BELOW ARE ICY COLD ; FOLLOWED BY GREAT PROSTRATION (A.).

FLUSHES OF HEAT, AT CHANGE OF LIFE (*Graph., Sep., Sulph.*) (F.).

Constant stretching for hours ; impossible to satisfy the desire ; would seize the bed and call for help to stretch (A.).

Spasmodic, suffocative cough (*Bell., Cup., Dros., Hyos., Kali-C., Phos., Sulph.*) (Br.).

Much throbbing in the ears (C.).

Craves fresh air, opens clothing, removes bed covering and opens windows in the coldest weather (*Arg-N., Lach., Phos., Sulph.*) (A.).

Puerperal convulsions, immediately after delivery (*Bell., Cup., Sec.*) (A.).

Exophthalmic goitre (*Spong.*) (C.).

FACE FLUSHES AT THE SLIGHTEST EMOTION (*Bell., Coca, Ferr.*) (A.).

Visible, pulsating throbbing in the temples (*Glon.*) (C.).

Sudden and intense rush of blood to the head and face, flushing the face deeply (N.).

Migrane (Glon., Sang., Spig.). (B.).

Bursting sensation in the head (*Arg-N., Bry., Glon., Meli., Nat-M.*) (C.).

INTENSE SURGING OF BLOOD TO FACE AND HEAD (*Acon., Bell., Ferr-P., Sang.*) (A.).

Heat and throbbing in the head, with feeling of intense fullness in the head (C.).

Eyes protruded, staring ; conjunctival vessels injected as well as the fundus (N.).

Collar seems too tight ; *must loosen it* (*Lach.*) (A.).

ANGINA PECTORIS : TUMULTUOUS HEART ACTION ; INTENSE THROBBING OF HEART AND CAROTIDS (*Glon.*) (A.).

Aching pain and constriction around the heart (C.).

Pulse variable, irregular and jerking (C.).

Fluttering, at the slightest excitement (Br.).

It has quite a reputation for **arresting paroxysms of** epilepsy and resuscitating patients sinking under anæsthetics. (It is given here by olfaction.) (N.).

Laryngismus stridulus (*Brom., Lach., Phos., Samb., Spong.*) (Bl.).

Profound and repeated yawning (*Kali-C., Nux-V.*) (A.).

Flushing heats ; *then drenching* (*unilateral*) *sweats* (B.).

AGGRAVATION : From mental or physical exertion ; in a closed room ; and during climacteric.

AMELIORATION : In the open air ; from taking rest.

RELATIONSHIP : Similar to *Acon.*, *Bell.*, *Cact.*, *Coca*, *Ferr.*, *Ferr-P.*, *Glon.*, *Graph.*, *Lach.*, *Meli.*, *Sang.*, *Sep.*, *Sulph.* and *Verat-V.*

Anacardium Orientale.

COMMON NAME : MARKING NUT.

Excessive anger at slight offence, breaking out in personal violence (*Nux-V.*, *Sulph.*). (R.).

Fixed ideas ; that he is double ; that there is no reality in anything, all appears like a dream ; and that the mind and body are separated (G.).

MALICIOUSNESS (*Ars.*, *Bell.*, *Canth.*. *Cupr.*, *Hep.*, *Hyos.*, *Lach.*, *Nux-V.*, *Stram.*).

Imagines that he hears voices afar off (*Hyos.*) (D.).

CURSING AND SWEARING (*Ars.*, *Bell.*, *Cann-I.*, *Canth.*, *Hyos.*, *Lyc.*, *Nit-Ac.*, *Nux-V.*, *Stram.*).

VACILLATING (*Ign.*, *Lyc.*, *Puls.*) (B.).

LOSS OF MEMORY (*Ambr.*, *Arg-N.*. *Ars.*, *Bar-C.*, *Bufo*, *Caust.*, *Cocc.*, *Con.*. *Glon.*, *Hell.*. *Hyos.*, *Kali-P.*, *Lach.*, *Lyc.*, *Med.*, *Merc.*, *Nit-Ac.*, *Nux-M.*. *Phos-Ac.*, *Phos.*, *Plat.*, *Plb.*, *Sep.*, *Verat.*).

He fears demons, is suspicious, endeavours to escape, refuses to eat and fears being poisoned (Bl.).

WHEN WALKING, FEELS AS IF SOME ONE WERE PURSUING ; SUSPECTS EVERYONE AROUND, AND IS CONSTANTLY APPREHENDING TROUBLE FROM EVERYTHING, WHICH GIVES HIM NO PEACE (G.).

Lack of confidence in himself and others.

FEELS AS THOUGH HE HAD TWO WILLS, ONE COMMANDING HIM TO DO WHAT THE OTHER FORBIDS (A.).

Crampish pains in the muscles (*Cup., Mag-P., Sec.*).

Ugly, irritable (*Cham., Nux-V., Stram.*) (N.).

Paralytic weakness (*Cocc., Plb., Sep.*) (Br.).

Contraction of the joints.

BRAIN-FAG (*Kali-P., Phos-Ac., Sil.*) (Br.).

SENSATION OF A BAND OR HOOP AROUND THE PARTS.

Bad effects of over-use of the mind (*Kali-P., Nux-V., Phos.*) (F.).

PAIN IN DIFFERENT PARTS, AS IF A PLUG HAD ENTERED.

Has unpleasant dreams of fire (*Ars., Hep.*), being near dead bodies (*Calc., Mag-M., Thuj.*) and tombs (Bl.).

Mental exertion brings on a tearing headache, the pains being situated mostly in the forehead and back part of the head (F.).

Trembling debility and paralytic weakness (*Gels., Kali-P., Lach., Phos., Sep., Sil., Sulph., Zinc.*).

The knees feel paralyzed (F.).

Has a feeling, as though the knees were bandaged tightly (F.).

Incomplete paralysis of the voluntary muscles (Bl.).

DIMINUTION OF THE SENSES (SMELL, SIGHT AND HEARING).

Loss of comprehension, with confusion and empty feeling in the head (R.).

Liability to catch cold, and sensitiveness to the draft of air (*Bell., Hep., Rumx., Psor., Sil*).

Palpitation of the heart, associated with pericarditis, especially of a rheumatic character ; there are stitching, sticking pains referred to the parts (Bl.).

Periodicity of symptoms (*Ars., Kali-B., Nat-M., Sulph.*).

The eruption of Anacardium is analogous to that of variola (T.).

Warty excrescences, with thickened epidermis (D.).

Wheals, exuding a viscid, yellowish fluid (*Rhus-T.*) (D.).

Intense itching and pustular eruptions; parts swollen, with burning pains (D.).

DERMATITIS *(Canth., Ran-B., Rhus-T., Sulph.)* (B.).

Warts on palms of hands (*Nat-M.*) (A.).

Itching of the skin, worse from scratching (*Rhus-T.*).

White, herpetic spots (C.).

Tasteless or sour eructations (D.).

GREAT DESIRE FOR STOOL, BUT WITH THE EFFORT THE DESIRE PASSES AWAY WITHOUT

5

EVACUATION ; RECTUM SEEMS POWERLESS, PARALYZED, WITH SENSATION AS IF PLUGGED UP (A.).

Can't evacuate, even a soft stool (*Alum.*, *Plat.*, *Sep.*) (B.).

Hæmorrhage during stool. Painful hæmorrhoids (Br.).

GASTRIC PAIN, RELIEVED BY EATING (*Brom.*, *Graph.*, *Kali-B.*, *Med.*, *Phos.*, *Sep.*, *Stann.*), BUT AGAIN WORSE IN 3 HOURS (B.).

Pain around the navel, as if a blunt plug were squeezed into the intestines (N.).

Faint feeling in the stomach, one or two hours after eating, extending to the spine (D.).

Violent gastralgia, and urging to stool, which passes off on going to stool (D.).

Symptoms are prone to go from right to left (*Lyc.* ; *left to right—Lach.*, *Rhus-T.*) (A.).

Swallows food and drink hastily (A.).

ALL SYMPTOMS ARE RELIEVED BY EATING, BUT THEY RETURN AND CONTINUE UNTIL THE PATIENT EATS AGAIN (D.).

Many symptoms appear after eating, while more of them appear during dinner.

Vertigo, as if turning in a circle, aggravated from stooping (*Bell.*, *Calc.*, *Caust.*, *Graph.*, *Lach.*, *Nux-V.*, *Puls.*, *Sulph.*) (R.).

Vomiting of ingesta, during pregnancy, ameliorated by eating (R.).

Very faint, on going upstairs (C.).

Male sexual organs : *Voluptuous itching* ; *increased desire* ; *seminal emissions, without dreams* ; *prostatic discharge during stool* (Br.).

AGGRAVATION : When lying on the side ; from rubbing ; from taking hold of anything ; from remaining without food : and from mental occupation.

AMELIORATION : From eating.

RELATIONSHIP : Similar to : *Canth.*, *Ran-B.*, *Rhus-R.*, *Rhus-T.*, *Rhus-V.*, and *Sulph.*

Follows well after : *Lyc.*, *Plat.*, and *Puls.*
It antidotes *Rhus-T.*

Angustura Vera.

COMMON NAME : GALIPŒA CUSPARIA.

Very painful ulcers, which affect the bone and extend into the marrow of it (*Asaf.*, *Fluor-Ac.*, *Hep.*, *Nit-Ac.*, *Sil.*).

Weakness of the whole body, as if the marrow of the bones was stiff.

CARIES OF LONG BONES, AS THE HUMERUS, TIBIA, FEMUR, ETC. (*Fluor-Ac.*) (N.).

Paralytic diseases and tetanus (Bt.).

LOCK-JAW, THE LIPS ARE DRAWN BACK, SHOWING THE TEETH (*Bell.*, *Caust.*, *Hyos.*, *Ign.*, *Œna.*, *Plb.*, *Sec.*, *Stram.*, *Strych.*, *Verat.*).

Cracking in the joints (*Ant-C.*, *Calc.*, *Caps.*, *Led.*, *Nit-Ac.*, *Petr.*, *Rhus-T.*).

SPASMODIC BREATHING, PALPITATION OF THE HEART, WITH ANGUISH *(Ars., Cact., Dig., Kali-P., Spig.).*

Spasmodic twitching (Bell., Hyos., Ign., Mag-P., Stram.).

Stiffness and stretching of the limbs *(Nux-V., Rhus-T.).*

Bends himself backward (Bell., Cupr., Nux-V., Strych.).

Twitching and jerking along the back, like electric shocks.

CARIES *(Calc-F., Fluor-Ac., Sil.).*

INTERMITTENTS : CHILL EVERY DAY AT 3 P. M. *(Ant-T., Apis, Ars., Chin-S., Staph., Thuj.)* *(Bt.).*

Thirst and vomiting of bile, with hot stage *(Eup-P., Ipec., Nat-S.)* (G.).

TETANIC SPASMS, CAUSED BY CONTACT, NOISE AND THE DRINKING OF LUKE-WARM WATER.

In impending tetanus it may be used as a preventive, if the wound is suppurating, or has suddenly ceased to discharge pus *(Bell., Cic., Sil.)* (F.).

CHEEKS AND LIPS BECOME BLUE *(Dig., Lach., Verat.).*

Burning in anus *(Aloe, Ars., Merc., Nat-M., Sulph.).* (Br.).

Chronic diarrhœa, with debility and loss of flesh (Br.).

Tenesmus recti, with soft stool *(Aloe., Nux-V., Sulph.)* (F.).

THE BREATHING IS HEAVY AND DURING THE SPASMS THERE IS GROANING AND CLOSING OF THE EYES.

Atonic dyspepsia (*Chin.*, *Hep.*, *Puls.*) (Br.).

ABNORMAL CRAVING FOR COFFEE (*Alum.*, *Ars.*, *Aur.*, *Bry.*, *Caps.*, *Chin.*, *Con.*, *Lach.*, *Nux-V.*, *Sel.*) (N.).

Necrosis of the lower jaw (*Hep.*, *Merc.*, *Phos.*, *Sil.*) (F.).

Urging to urinate, with copious flow (*Apis*, *Merc.*, *Phos-Ac.*, *Sulph.*) (F.).

Drawing, tension and stiffness of muscles and joints, with contused, sore feeling, as after a blow (*Arn.*, *Phyt.*, *Rhus-T.*) (F.).

Sharp cutting pains, from just beneath the right scapula to the breast, near the nipple (*Chel.*) (F.).

BELCHING, WITH COUGH (*Ambr.*, *Sulph-Ac.*, *Verat.*) (Br.).

Pain in articulation of jaw, in masseter muscles, as if fatigued by chewing too much (Br.).

Very much fatigued, most in the thighs (G.).

AGGRAVATION : From touching the affected part ; from noise ; and drinking lukewarm water.

AMELIORATION : From rest.

RELATIONSHIP. Similar to : *Ign.*, *Nux-V.*, and *Strych.*

To be followed by : *Bell.*, *Ign.*, *Lyc.*, and *Sep.*

ANTIDOTE : *Coffea.*

Anthracinum.

COMMON NAME : ANTHRAX POISON.

It is one of the most efficacious remedies for boils, abscesses, felons, or swellings of any kind, when there are intense burning pains (*Ars., Tarant-C., Sulph.*) (N.).

Hæmorrhages : black, thick, tar-like, rapidly decomposing, from any orifice (*Lach., Lept.*) (C.).

Malignancy : Terrible burning pains, with great prostration (Apis, Ars., Lach., Phos., Sulph., Tarant-C.) (B.).

THE AFFECTED PARTS BURN, AS THOUGH ON FIRE (Bl.).

WE HAVE SWELLINGS ON ALL PARTS OF THE BODY, AND ONE OF THE MOST CHARACTERISTIC CONDITIONS IS THE COLOUR OF THEM. THEY ARE BLUISH, VERGING INTO BLACK (*Lach., Tarant-C.*) (N.).

Black and blue blisters (C.).

Bad effects from inhaling foul odours (C.).

Succession of boils (*Merc., Sil., Sulph.*) (B.).

Discharge of ichorous, offensive pus (*Ars., Carb-Ac., Merc-C., Nit-Ac.*) (A.).

Glands swollen, cellular tissues œdematous and indurated (*Apis, Brom., Carb-An., Merc-I., Rhus-T., Sil., Tarant-C.*) (C.).

"Erysipelas" of a malignant type (A.).

"In all cases, simulating septic fever or poisoning, *Arsenicum*, **Anthracinum** and *Pyrogen* should be remembered. The horrible BURNING PAINS of the first two are prominent" (N.).

Gangrenous parotitis (*Apis*, *Ars.*, *Lach.*, *Tarant-C.*) (C.).

SEPTIC FEVER : RAPID LOSS OF STRENGTH, SINKING PULSE, DELIRIUM AND FAINTING (*Pyrog.*) (A.).

Suspicious insect stings. If the swelling changes colour and red streaks from the wound map out the course of lymphatics (*Lach.*, *Pyrog.*) (A.).

Gangrenous ulcers (*Ars.*, *Carb-Ac.*, *Carbo-V.*, *Kali-P.*, *Lach.*, *Lyc.*, *Merc-C.*, *Nit-Ac.*, *Phos.*, *Sec.*, *Sulph.*) (A.).

Dissecting wounds : especially if tendency is to become gangrenous (*Ars.*, *Pyrog.*) (A.).

Felon ; the worst cases, with sloughing and terrible burning pains (Ars., Carb-Ac., Lach.) (A.).

Arsenicum sometimes fails in "carbuncles". Then we have to resort to *Anthracinum*, chiefly in the thirtieth potency. It has precisely the same symptoms as *Arsenicum*, but to a more intense degree (F.).

AGGRAVATION : From cold application (better from cold application—*Apis*, *Flour-Ac.*, *Led.*, *Phos.*, *Puls.*, *Sec.*).

AMELIORATION : From hot application. (Worse from cold application : *Ars.*, *Lach.*, *Sil.*, *Syph.*).

RELATIONSHIP. Similar to : *Ars.*, *Carb-Ac.*, *Crot-H.*, *Echin.*, *Lach.*, *Pyrog.*, *Rhus-T.*, *Sec.*, and *Tarant-C.*

Silicea follows it well.

Antimonium Crudum.

COMMON NAME : SULPHIDE OF ANTIMONY.

For children and young people, inclined to grow fat (*Calc., Graph.*), for the extremes of life (*Ant-T., Lyc., Op., Sil.*) (A.).

SENTIMENTAL MOOD IN THE MOON-LIGHT, PARTICULARLY ECSTATIC LOVE (N.).

Gastric derangement, with tongue coated thickly white, accompanying different complaints, such as eruptive fevers, rheumatism, gout, hydrocephalus, etc. (N.).

AVERSION TO BE LOOKED AT (*Ant-T., Ars., Cham., Chin., Cina, Iod., Mag-C., Nat-M., Nux-V., Rhus-T., Stram., Sulph.*) AND TO BE TOUCHED (*Acon., Ant-T., Ars., Bell., Bry., Cham., Chin., Cina, Coff., Kali-C., Kali-I., Lach., Med., Nux-V., Sil., Stram., Tarant-C., Thuj., Verat.*).

He is much concerned about his fate.

The greatest sadness and woeful mood, with intermittent fever (N.).

CHILD IS FRETFUL, PEEVISH, SULKY ; DOES NOT WISH TO SPEAK OR TO BE SPOKEN TO (*Ant-T., Iod., Sil.*) ; ANGRY AT EVERY LITTLE ATTENTION (A.).

Loathing life (*Ars., Aur., Hep., Naja, Nit-Ac., Nux-V.*) (A.).

Abject despair ; wants to commit suicide by drowning (A.).

Bad effects of disappointed affection (*Calc-P.*, *Gels.*, *Ign.*, *Nat-M.*, *Phos-Ac.*) (A.).

Cross and contradictive ; whatever is done fails to give satisfaction (*Sulph.*) (Br.).

Menses suppressed, from cold bathing, with feeling of pressure in the pelvis (Br.).

Toothache, before the menses (*Amm-C.*, *Ars.*, *Bar-C.*, *Nat-M.*, *Phos.*, *Puls.*, *Sulph.*, *Thuj.*) (G.).

Nausea, vomiting and diarrhœa, during pregnancy (G.).

Disposition to grow fat (*Amm-M.*, *Calc.*, *Caps.*, *Ferr.*, *Graph.*, *Kali-B.*, *Kali-C.*, *Lyc.*, *Puls.*, *Sil.*, *Sulph.*).

SORE, CRACKED AND CRUSTY NOSTRILS, AND CORNERS OF THE MOUTH (*Graph.*, *Nat-M.*, *Nit-Ac.*, *Petr.*) (N.).

Inflammation of the muscles (*Bell.*, *Bry.*, *Merc.*, *Sulph.*).

Suppurating and long-lasting eruption on cheeks (*Caust.*, *Cic.*, *Dulc.*, *Euph.*, *Kreos.*, *Merc.*, *Nat-M.*, *Rhus-T.*, *Sil.*, *Staph.*, *Viol-T.*) (N.).

Crushed finger-nails grow in splits ; and like warts, and with horny spots (N.).

HORN-LIKE EXCRESCENCES AND DISPOSITION TO ABNORMAL ORGANIZATIONS OF THE SKIN.

Corns and callosities in the soles of the feet ; *very sensitive* ; *can't walk* (N.).

TONGUE COATED, LIKE WHITEWASH (B.).

TONGUE COATED THICK, MILKY WHITE (*Kali-M.*) (N.).

Longing for acids and pickles (*Hep., Lach., Sulph., Sulph-I., Verat.*) (A.).

Gastric symptoms, worse in the afternoon and at night (*Calc., Carb-V., Lyc., Puls., Sep., Sulph.*).

Gastric and intestinal affections : from bread and pastry ; acids, especially vinegar ; sour or bad wine ; after cold bathing ; over-heating ; and in hot weather (A.).

ERUCTATIONS, TASTING OF THE INGESTA (*Carb-An., Caust., Chin., Graph., Lyc., Nat-M., Puls., Sulph.*) (Br.).

After nursing, the child vomits its milk in curds, and refuses to nurse afterwards, and is very cross (Br.).

Constant belching (*Arg-N., Carb-V., Lyc., Puls., Sulph.*) (Br.).

DIGESTIVE TROUBLES, FROM OVERLOADING THE STOMACH (*Puls.*) (D.).

Complaints after bathing, especially in cold water (N.).

Feels as if something had lodged in the throat, which causes a frequent desire to swallow (*Ign., Lach., Phyt.*) (G.).

Decayed teeth ache, generally worse at night (*Kreos., Merc., Puls., Sep.*) ; cannot bear to be touched by the tongue (*Amm-C., Bry., Carb-V., Ign., Merc., Mezer., Nat-C., Phos., Sep., Thuj.*).

Headache : after river bathing ; from taking cold ; alcoholic drinks ; deranged digestion, acids, fat, fruit ; suppressed eruption (A.).

Great sleepiness during the day; can hardly rise in the morning—so sleepy (G.).

When the symptoms reappear they change their locality, or go from one side of the body to the other.

ALTERNATE DIARRHŒA AND CONSTIPATION (*Aloe, Nux-V., Podo., Sulph., Tub.*) (N.).

Diarrhœa at night, with great thirst for cold water (diarrhœa worse during night, with little or no thirst—*Puls.*) (Bt.).

STOOLS OFTEN LIQUID, CONTAINING PORTIONS OF SOLID MATTER (SOMETIMES INVOLUNTARY, IN OLD PEOPLE) (N.).

Hard and loose stools, with nausea (N.).

Much mucus secretion from the anus, staining the linen, with burning, tingling and itching (*Pœon.*).

Redness and inflammation of the lids; itching in canthi; chronic blepharitis, of cross children (*Alum., Arg-N., Graph., Sulph.*) (N.).

Much rumbling in the abdomen (*Carb-V., Crot-T., Lyc., Podo., Sulph.*) (C.).

Mucus piles (*Aloe, Kali-B., Merc., Nit-Ac., Sulph.*) (C.).

Itching of the anus (*Calc, Cina, Nux-V., Sep., Sulph.*) (C.).

Burning in the urethra, during urination (*Acon., Canth., Nat-M., Sulph.*) (C.).

Loss of voice, from becoming over-heated (A.).

LOOKING INTO THE FIRE INCREASES THE COUGH (N.).

The irritation to cough is felt in the abdomen (N.).

Cough after rising in the morning, in paroxysms ; as if arising from the abdomen ; the first paroxysm always most severe ; the subsequent ones weaker and weaker, until the last only resembles a hacking (C.).

Tenderness over the ovarian region, with nausea, vomiting and white tongue (N.).

Measles-like eruptions, with marked, gastric disturbance (*Kali-M., Puls.*) (G.).

Urticaria white, with red areolæ, which itch fearfully (*Apis, Nat-M., Rhus-T., Urt-U.*) (G.).

Solid lumps in a watery leucorrhœa, which sometimes causes a smarting down the thighs (G.).

AGGRAVATION : From drinking sour wine ; in the heat of the sun ; after eating (pork) ; at night ; after bathing ; from extremes of cold or heat ; and from acids.

AMELIORATION : During rest ; in the open air ; and after a warm bath.

RELATIONSHIP. Similar to : *Bry., Ipec., Kali-M., Lyc., Puls.*, and *Sep.* in gastric complaints. Follows well after *Ant-C.* : *Merc., Puls.*, and *Sulph.*

Complementary : *Squil.*

Antimonium Tartaricum.

COMMON NAME : TARTAR EMETIC.

Through the pneumo-gastric nerve it depresses the respiration and circulation (A.).

Diseases originating from exposure in damp basements or cellars (*Aran.*, **Ars.**, *Dulc.*, *Nat-S.*, *Tereb.*) (A.).

GREAT DEBILITY AND WEAKNESS (*Apis*, *Ars.*, *Bism.*, *Chin.*, *Dig.*, *Ferr.*, *Gels.*, *Kali-P.*, *Lach.*, *Mosch.*, *Nat-C.*, *Op.*, *Phos.*, *Phos-Ac.*, *Sel.*, *Sep.*, *Sulph.*, *Verat.*).

Attacks of fainting and syncope (*Ars.*, *Camph.*, *Kali-P.*, *Nux-V.*, *Phos.*, *Verat.*).

Internal trembling (*Calc.*, *Graph.*, *Iod.*, *Rhus-T.*, *Stann.*, *Staph.*, *Sulph-Ac.*).

FAN-LIKE MOTION OF THE ALÆ NASI (*Amm-C.*, *Brom.*, *Chel.*, *Iod.*, *Kreos.*, *Lyc.*, **Phos.**, *Sulph.*).

Is indicated in affections of old people, and particularly in orthopnœa, or threatening paralysis of the lungs in the aged. You hear loud rattling in the chest, and yet the patient cannot get up the phlegm (F.).

THE CHILD WANTS TO BE CARRIED (*Ars.*, *Brom.*, *Carb-V.*, **Cham.**, *Cina*, *Ign.*, *Kali-C.*, *Lyc.*, *Puls.*, *Rhus-T.*, *Sanic.*, *Staph.*, *Sulph.*, *Verat.*), AND DOES NOT WISH TO BE TOUCHED (*Acon.*, *Ant-C.*, *Ars.*, *Bell.*, *Cham.*, *Cina*).

Great despondency (*Ars.*, *Aur.*, *Calc.*, *Coff.*, *Hell.*, *Ign.*, *Psor.*) (Br.).

Fear of being alone (*Arg-N.*, *Ars.*, *Crot-C.*, *Hyos.*, *Kali-C.*, *Lyc.*, *Phos.*) (Br.).

THE CHILD CLINGS TO THOSE AROUND ; CRIES AND WHINES IF ANY ONE TOUCHES IT ; WILL NOT LET YOU FEEL THE PULSE (*Ant-C.*, *Cham.*, *Cina*, *Nat-M.*).

GREAT SLEEPINESS OR IRRESISTIBLE IN-CLINATION TO SLEEP, WITH NEARLY ALL COM-PLAINTS (*Æth.*, *Apis*, *Gels.*, *Nux-M.*, *Op.*) (A.).

It produces pustules very nearly identical with those of small-pox ; hence, it may be a very useful remedy in that disease (F.).

CONVULSIONS, WHEN SMALL-POX FAILS TO BREAK OUT (K.).

Muttering delirium and stupor (*Arn.,* *Hyos., Rhus-T.*) (Br.).

One-sided complaints (rheumatic pains in the left chest, pulsation in one side of the forehead and one-sided headache).

Soreness all over the chest (*Arn., Bell., Bry., Eup-P., Nat-S., Nux-V., Phos., Ran-B., Rhus-T.*).

CONSTANT AND DISTRESSING COUGH, DISPOSED TO BE LOOSE WITH MUCH EXPECTORATION (*Lyc., Nat-S., Puls., Sil.*).

Excessive vomiting in intermittent (K.).

Diarrhœa in eruptive diseases (*Puls.*) (Br.).

Appetite variable : sometimes great for apples, with thirst for cool water ; again lost, with no thirst ; anxious nausea after eating ; vomiting difficult, with trembling of hands, frequent stools and weakness (R.).

Croup, with whistling and rattling, extending into trachea (D.).

A remedy of great utility in cases of pneumonia

When of service, there is rattling of mucus in the chest, catarrhal ophthalmia, and marked gastro-enteric disturbance.

Face cold, blue, pale, covered with cold sweat (*Camph., Tab., Verat.*) (A.).

WHEN THE PATIENT COUGHS, THERE AP-
PEARS TO BE A LARGE COLLECTION OF MUCUS
IN THE BRONCHI; IT SEEMS AS IF MUCH
WOULD BE EXPECTORATED, BUT NOTHING
COMES UP (A.).

Icterus, with pneumonia (Chel., Dig., Iod., Merc.,
Nat-S.), especially of the right lung (A.).

It may be used in the pneumonia of drunkards (F.).

Antim Tart. produces a perfect picture of pleuro-
pneumonia (Bry., Kali-C., Phos., Sulph.).

Certain portions of the lungs are paralyzed. Fine
rales are heard, even over the hepatized portions.
There is great oppression of breathing, particularly towards morning. The patient must sit up, in order to
breathe. The pit of the stomach is very sensitive to
touch or pressure. There are meteorism, nausea and
vomiting (F.).

(In LYCOPODIUM there is greater and more distressing dyspnœa, many mucous rales present, stitching
and stabbing pleuritic pain and a tendency to abdominal
distension).

Coughs and yawns alternately. Thick expectoration.
Capillary bronchitis.

COUGH, WORSE WHEN THE CHILD IS ANGRY,
OR WHEN EATING; IT CULMINATES IN VOMI-
TING OF MUCUS AND FOOD (D.).

Pleuro-pneumonia. Paralytic depression of heart and
lungs (Bar-C.) (B.).

FORCIBLE VOMITING, THEN EXHAUSTION
AND SLEEP (Æth.). VIOLENT RETCHING, SINK-
ING AT STOMACH (B.).

(In *Lycopodium* !there is! present marked weakness, but there is great struggling on the part of the patient to get his breath, with a flaying of the alæ nasi'.

Asphyxia neonatorum (F.).

Child at birth pale, breathless, gasping. Relieves the death-rattle (Laur.) (A.).

Torpid, cool, sweaty skin. Delayed or receding, blue or pustular eruptions (*Cup., Hyos., Lach., Zinc.*) (B.).

Tongue coated, pasty, thick, white, with reddened papillæ and red edges ; red in streaks ; very red, dry in the middle (A.).

Long lasting dyspeptic symptoms, with loss of appetite (Bry., Chin., Hep., Kali-C., Lyc., Puls., Sep.).

Extraordinary craving for apples (*Aloe, Guai., Sulph., Tell* ; for acids and pickles—*Ant-C., Hep., Lach., Sulph., Sulph-I., Verat.*) (A).

NAUSEA, WITH FREQUENT VOMITING OF BITTER, SOUR SUBSTANCES—A MARKED CHARACTERISTIC.

Vomiting ; in any position except lying on the right side ; until he faints ; followed by drowsiness and prostration (A.).

Painful urging to urinate ; scanty discharge, dark red, or the least bloody, with stitches in the bladder, and burning in the urethra (Bt.).

Cannot keep her eyes open ; irresistible drowsiness, and deep, stupefied sleep ; when awake, hopelessness and despair, or chill and fever, or vomiting of food (N.).

Cold, clammy sweat over the whole body (Ars., Camph., Carb-V., Sec., Verat.) (C.).

Palpitation of the heart (*Acon., Ars.; Cact., Calc., Dig., Kali-P., Spig.*) (C.).

Pulse : rapid, weak, trembling ; full and slow ; or contracted and hardly perceptible (C.).

Colic, as if the bowels would be cut to pieces ; labour-like tearing from above downward, with rumbling and looseness (N.).

Leucorrhœa of watery blood, liable to occur in paroxysms, worse while sitting (N.).

Violent pains in sacro-lumbar region (*Æsc., Kali-C., Rhus-T.*) ; *the slightest effort to move causes retching and cold sweat* (N.).

Eyes are!sunken, surrounded by dark circles (*Cina, Staph.*) (G.).

Rheumatic ophthalmia (*Calc., Hep., Kali-B., Rhus-T., Sep., Sulph.*) (G.).

Inflamed lids, with catarrhal conjunctivitis (*All-C., Euphr., Rhus-T.*).

AGGRAVATION : In damp, cold weather ; lying down at night ; warmth of room ; change of weather ; and in spring.

AMELIORATION : In cold open air ; sitting upright ; expectorating ; and lying on the right side.

RELATIONSHIP. Similar to *Lycopodium ;* but spasmodic motion of alæ is replaced by dilated nostrils ; to *Veratrum* ; both have diarrhœa, colic, vomiting, coldness and craving for acids ; to *Ipecac*, but more drowsiness from defective respiration ; nausea, but better after vomiting.

6

When lungs seem to fail, patient becomes sleepy, cough declines or ceases, it supplants *Ipecac*.

For bad effects of vaccination, when *Thuja* fails and *Silicea* is not indicated.

Children not easily impressed, when *Antim Tart.* seems indicated in coughs, require *Hepar*.

Antidotes : *Puls.* and *Sep.*

Apis Mellifica.

COMMON NAME : THE HONEY BEE.

Cancer of the tongue (Br.).

BURNING AND STINGING PAINS.

Scarlatina, dry nose and throat, with hydrocephalic symptoms (Hr.).

A most important remedy in hydrothorax and also in basilar meningitis of children, after effusion (Fr.).

SENSATION OF SORENESS, AS IF BRUISED (*Arn., Bell., Lach.*).

VERY BUSY ; RESTLESS ; CHANGING THE KIND OF WORK, WITH AWKWARDNESS ; BREAKING THINGS (Bt.).

Great sensitiveness to the touch and to external pressure, especially on the abdomen (*Lach.*).

Uvula swollen, sac-like. Throat swollen inside and outside.

Tonsils swollen, puffy, fiery red (Br.).

Great debility, as if he had worked hard ; he must lie down on the ground (Bapt., Kali-P., Sep.).

Much yawning and uneasiness (Ra.).

Incontinence of urine, with great irritability of the parts ; worse at night and when coughing (Ra.).

Dark coloured and scanty urine (Bt.).

Tension over the eyes, behind the ears, in the neck, and a tension involving the head of the left side.

ASCITES : URINE SCANTY AND DARK COLOURED ; GREAT SORENESS OF THE ABDOMINAL WALLS, WITH STINGING, BURNING PAINS (Bt.).

PERITONITIS (*Bell., Bry., Lach.*) (Bt.).
Very tired feeling of the brain (Bt.).

Declares she is well, during delirium (Arn., Ars.) (K.).

Heaviness and pressure in the head, especially when rising from a recumbent position, or from a seat, worse in a warm room and relieved by pressing the head with the hands.

Child lies in a torpor ; delirium ; sudden shrill cries ; squinting ; grinding teeth ; boring head in pillows ; one half of the body twitching, the other lame ; head wet from sweating ; urine scanty (Hr.).

Pale red, erysipelatous inflammations.
Urticaria, worse during night (K.).

ERUPTIONS, LIKE HIVES (*Rhus-T., Urt-U.*).
Urticaria, especially during chill (*Cop., Ign., Rhus-T., Sulph.*) (K.).

Could bear nothing to touch his neck ; could hardly breathe, from suffocation (*Bor.*).

DROPSICAL SWELLINGS, WITHOUT THIRST.

Œdematous swelling of the eyelids with stinging and burning pains ; lids turned inside out, with granulations on their edges ; cornea especially involved ; falling out of the eyelashes (*Bor.*, *Graph.*, *Sep.*, *Sulph.*) (Bt.).

INFLAMMATION OF THE EYES, WITH INTENSE PHOTOPHOBIA AND INCREASED SECRETIONS (*Bell.*, *Canth.*, *Merc-C.*, *Rhus-T.*, *Sulph.*).

Styes, particularly on the left eyelid (G.).

KERATITIS, WITH INTENSE CHEMOSIS OF OCULAR CONJUNCTIVA (*Merc-C.*) (Br.).

GREAT OPPRESSION AND BURNING IN THE CHEST, AS THOUGH THE PATIENT WOULD SMOTHER.

SENSATION, AS THOUGH HE WOULD NOT BE ABLE TO BREATHE AGAIN (W.).

Rapid, painful, spasmodic respiration ; aggravated by lying down, and relieve1 by inhaling fresh air, in an upright position (Fr.).

SKIN USUALLY WHITE AND ALMOST TRANS-PARENT (OVARIAN DROPSY) (N.).

Alternate sweat with dryness of the skin (N.).

Frequent, involuntary, deep breathing (*Ign.*, *Phos-Ac.*) ; long and sighing respiration (N.).

Œdema of hands, legs and feet ; *pale and waxy* (N.).

With heart troubles great feeling of suffocation, as if he could never breathe again (N.).

PANARITIUM OR FELON, WITH BURNING,

STINGING AND THROBBING ; VERY SENSITIVE TO TOUCH (N.).

Diarrhœa : of drunkards ; in eruptive diseases, especially if eruption be suppressed ; involuntary, from every motion, as though anus was wide open (*Phos.*) (A.).

Gaping, after coughing (N.).

Affects right side ; enlargement or dropsy of right ovary ; right testicle (A.).

Is serviceable in acute nephritis, when the urine is scanty and of a dark colour (Bl.).

Metritis, with stinging, thrusting pains. Ulceration and engorgement of os uteri. Uterine dropsy. Menses too profuse or too scanty. Ovarian tumours, with stinging pains, like bee-stings (G.).

Chill anticipates. with dyspnœa (B.).

Heat of one part, with coldness of another (B.).

INTERMITTENT FEVER : CHILL AT 3 P. M. WITH THIRST, ALWAYS (*Ign.*). WORSE IN A WARM ROOM AND FROM EXTERNAL HEAT (A.).

Chill begins in front of chest, abdomen and knees. Sleep and urticaria as chill passes off. Heat without thirst, with inclination to uncover (L.).

AGGRAVATION : In a warm room ; after sleeping ; from getting wet ; from hot application ; in the evening ; and from pressure.

AMELIORATION : In an open air ; from cold water or cold bathing ; from uncovering ; and when sitting erect.

RELATIONSHIP. Complementary : *Nat-M.*

Disagrees, when used either before or after *Rhus-T.*

Ars. and *Puls.* follow *Apis* well.

Apocynum Cannabinum.

COMMON NAME : INDIAN HEMP.

Low spirited (*Aur., Ign., Puls., Sep.*) (Br.).

Excretions diminished, especially urine and sweat (*Apis, Sep., Sulph.*) (A.).

All kinds of dropsies, with a sinking feeling at the pit of the stomach (Hl.).

GENERAL ŒDEMA (*Apis, Ars., Dig., Merc., Phos., Sep., Sulph.*) (Bt.).

Ascites, with bruised feeling in the abdomen (Bt.).

Dropsy of serous membranes ; acute, inflammatory (*Apis, Ars-I., Bry., Phos., Merc-Sulph., Sulph.*) (A.).

DROPSY : WITH THIRST (*Acet-Ac., Ars., Iod., Nat-M., Phos., Sulph.*), ; dropsy without thirst—*Apis, Nux-V., Puls., Sep.*) ; WATER DISAGREES OR IS VOMITED (*Ars., Phos.*) ; AFTER TYPHUS, TYPHOID, SCARLA-TINA, OR CIRRHOSIS ; ALSO AFTER ABUSE OF QUININE (R.).

Hydrocephalus : sutures opened ; forehead projecting ; sight of one eye totally lost, the other slightly sensible ; stupour ; constant involuntary motion of one leg and arm (*Hell.*) ; urine suppressed ; vomiting, with stupour (Rn.).

Skin dry and husky (Hl.).

URINE EXCESSIVELY SCANTY, THICK, YEL-
LOW AND TURBID (Frl.).

WATERY DIARRHŒA, OR CONSTIPATION (Rg.).

*Obliged to sit up ; lying down produces violent dysp-
nœa (Ars., Lyc., Phos., Sulph.) (Bt.).*

Amenorrhœa in young girls (*Ferr., Puls., Sep.*), with
bloating or dropsical extension of abdomen and extremities (A.).

Metrorrhagia : continued or paroxysmal flow ; fluid or
clotted ; nausea ; vomiting ; palpitation ; pulse feeble
quick, when moved ; vital depression ; fainting, when
raising head from pillow (A.).

Sometimes cures nocturnal enuresis (G.).

*Hydro-thorax (Apis, Ars., Aur., Lach., Lyc., Merc-
Sulph., Nat-S., Sulph.)* (G.).

Penis and scrotum swollen, dropsical (*Dig., Merc.,
Rhus-T.*) (G.).

Should be remembered in dropsy, that is dependent
upon a feeble heart, when the blood pressure is lowered,
also in the later stages of heart disease, when a general
anasarca is present (Bl.).

Cough, short and dry, or deep and loose (*Hep.,
Nat-S., Spong.*), during pregnancy (*Caust., Con.,
Kali-Br., Nux-M., Phos., Puls., Sep.*) (A.).

Excessive vomiting. Food or water is immediately
ejected (*Ars., Bism., Phos.*) (Br.).

RENAL DROPSY (*Apis, Dig., Kali-C., Merc-C.,
Phos., Sep., Sulph.*) (Br.).

Oppression of the chest (*Ars.*, *Cact.*, *Dig.*, *Kali-Ars.*, *Lach.*, *Lyc.*, *Phos.*) (B.).

Great restlessness and little sleep (Br.).

COPIOUS, YELLOW OR BROWNISH DIARRHŒA, EXPELLED WITH GREAT FORCE (*Crot-T.*, *Gamb.*, *Nat-S.*, *Podo.*, *Sulph.*) (D.).

A weak, all-gone feeling in the abdomen (*Carb-An.*, *Kali-P.*, *Sep.*, *Sulph.*) (D.).

AGGRAVATION : In cold weather ; from cold drinks ; from uncovering ; and on lying down.

AMELIORATION : From sitting up.

RELATIONSHIP. Similar to : *Acet-Ac.*, *Apis*, *Ars.*, *Dig.*, *Hell.*, *Lyc.*, *Phos.*, *Sep.*, and *Sulph.* in dropsical affections.

Cymarin is the active principle of *Apocynum.* It lowers the pulse-rate and increases the blood-pressure.

Argentum Metallicum.

COMMON NAME : SILVER.

Has strong effects upon the secretions of the mucous membranes (*Hydr.*, *Kali-B.*, *Nat-M.*, *Puls.*, *Rhus-T.*). *Produces spasms, which simulate those of epilepsy. The* attacks are *followed by delirious rage* (*Stram.*). *The patient jumps about and tries to strike those near him* (*Bell.*, *Canth.*, *Stram.*) (F.).

Sensation of soreness and rawness in the internal organs (*Caust.*).

Spasmodic twitching of the heart muscle, particularly when lying on his back (F.).

BAD EFFECTS FROM ONANISM (*Bufo, Calad., Calc., Con., Kali-P., Nux-V., Staph.*).

IS EXTREMELY FORGETFUL (*Cann-I., Con., Kali-P., Lyc., Nat-M., Phos., Sil.*) (F.).

DISCHARGE OF URINE TOO FREQUENT AND TOO COPIOUS (*Nat-M., Phos-Ac.*).

DIABETES (*Apis, Merc., Phos-Ac., Sulph., Thuj., Uran-N.*) (C.).

Turbid urine (*Calc., Cina, Phos-Ac.*) (C.).

Has a particular affinity for the cartilages of joints (*Calc.*) (F.).

SENSATION OF SORENESS IN THE JOINTS (*Apis, Arn., Bry., Colch., Kali-C., Lach., Rhus-T.*).

Tearing in the joints of the hands and feet, through the fingers and toes.

Ailments, from abuse of *Mercury* (*Aur., Hep., Nit-Ac., Thuj.*) (A.).

Boring in the joints (*Bry., Nit-Ac.*).

Bruised pain in the left ovary, and a feeling as though it was growing large (F.).

Prolapsus uteri (*Helon., Nat-M., Sep.*) (F.).

Pricking, from within outwards.

GENERAL WEARINESS, FORCING THE PATIENT TO LIE DOWN (F.).

Viscid gray, jelly-like mucus in the pharynx, easily hawked up, early in the morning (N.).

Sensation of numbness, and as if asleep in the limbs (*Alum., Caust., Con.*).

Pressing, tearing pain, mostly in the head (*Bell., Ign., Kalm., Rhus-T., Sep.*).

HEADACHE: PAIN GRADUALLY INCREASES, AND, AFTER REACHING ITS ACME, SUDDENLY CEASES (F.).

CRUSHED PAIN IN THE TESTICLES (*Acon.*). CLOTHING INCREASES THE PAIN, ON WALKING (*Puls.*) (C.).

Chronic gleet (*Cop., Kali-B., Nat-M.*) (C.).

Heat of the whole body, except the head, without thirst.

Yellowish, greenish gonorrhœa (C.).

Seminal emissions, almost every night (*Nat-P., Phos., Sulph.*), *without erection, with atrophy of the penis* (*Lyc.*)*; after onanism* (*Nux-V., Phos-Ac., Staph.*) (C.).

PAINS INCREASE GRADUALLY, AND DISAPPEAR SUDDENLY (*Caust., Puls., Sulph-Ac.*; pains appear suddenly, and disappear gradually—*Asaf., Calc., Fluor-Ac., Puls., Ran-S.*) (N.).

Hurried feeling; *time passes too slowly* (Br.).

Easy expectoration, looking like boiled starch (*Nat-M.*) (Br.).

On reading aloud, must hem and hawk (Br.).

Alteration in timbre of voice (Br.).

The legs are trembling and weak (*Alum.*, *Con.*, *Nux-V.*, *Phos.*, *Pic-Ac.*) (Bl.).

Excessive fluent coryza, often with sneezing, tickling and crawling sensation in the nose (*All-C.*, *Ars.*) (G.).

Great weakness in the chest (*Phos.*, *Stann.*) (A.).

Raw spot over bifurcation of the trachea ; worse when laughing, talking or singing (A.).

HOARSENESS, ESPECIALLY OF PROFESSIONAL SINGERS, SPEAKERS, ETC. (*Arg-N.*, *Arum-T.*, *Carb-V.*, *Caust.*, *Phos.*) (C.).

Laughing produces mucus in the larynx, and excites cough (Phos.) (C.).

AGGRAVATION : Towards noon ; from riding in a carriage ; when touched or pressed upon ; and from laughing, talking, singing or reading aloud.

AMELIORATION : In the open air ; from taking rest ; and from keeping quiet.

RELATIONSHIP. Antidotes : *Merc.*, and *Puls.*

Similar to : *Phos.*, *Puls.*, and *Stann.*

Follows well : after *Alum.*

Argentum Nitricum.

COMMON NAME : SILVER NITRATE.

Think of this remedy on seeing a withered and dried-up person (G.).

Acute or chronic diseases, from unusual or long continued mental exertion (A).

Weakness of mind and inability to express himself suitably and coherently (R.).

IMPULSIVE, TIME SEEMS TOO SHORT, WANTS TO DO THINGS IN A HURRY, MUST WALK FAST—IS ALWAYS HURRIED (G.).

Does not undertake anything, lest he should not succeed (R.).

Time passes too slowly (*Cann-I.*) (A.).

MEMORY IMPAIRED (*Agn., Calc., Kali-P., Lyc., Nat-M, Nux-M., Phos.*) (R.).

STAGE FRIGHT (*Gels.*).

Apprehensive of some incurable disease (R.).

APPREHENSION, WHEN READY FOR CHURCH OR OPERA, DIARRHŒA SETS IN (A.).

The high notes cause cough (*Alum., Arg-M., Arum-T.*) (A.).

CHRONIC LARYNGITIS OF SINGERS AND SPEAKERS (D.).

Hoarseness, rawness and burning in the larynx, and a copious exudation into the larynx, looking like boiled starch ; it is easily expectorated (D.).

Coition painful, in both sexes ; followed by bleeding from the vagina (*Arn., Ars., Hydr., Kreos., Nit-Ac., Sep., Tarant-C.*) (A.).

Ulceration of vagina, os and cervix, with frequent

bleeding from points of ulceration ; *copious, yellow, corroding discharge* (*Calc., Kreos., Nit-Ac., Sep.*) (R.).

Metrorrhagia : in young widows ; in sterility ; with nervous erethism at change of life (*Lach.*) (A.).

PALPITATION : PRESSURE WITH THE HAND AMELIORATES (K.).

PALPITATION, WORSE, FROM LYING ON THE RIGHT SIDE (*Alumn., Bad., Kali-N., Lil-T., Plat., Spong.* ; better from lying on the right side—*Glon., Lach., Phos., Psor., Tab.*) (B.).

PALPITATION, AFTER EXCITEMENT OR FROM EXERTION (K.).

Burning in the urethra during micturition, with swollen feeling and difficulty in passing the last part of urine (*Nat-M., Sars., Thuj.*) (R.).

WANT OF SEXUAL DESIRE ; THE ORGANS SEEM MUCH SHRIVELLED (*Agn., Calad., Lyc., Phos-Ac.*) (G.).

IMPOTENCE : ERECTION FAILS, WHEN COITION IS ATTEMPTED (*Agn., Calad., Graph., Nux-V., Phos., Selen., Sulph.*) (A.).

Sugar in the urine (*Merc., Phos-Ac., Sulph.*) (Bt.).

Chilly when uncovered, yet feels smothered if wrapped up ; craves fresh air (*Puls.*) (A.).

Violent pains from kidneys to bladder (*Berb., Canth., Lyc., Nux-V., Ocimum-C.*) (B.).

Cutting in the urethra, with painful priapism (*Cann-S., Canth.*) (B.).

In ophthalmia neonatorum, gonorrhœal ophthalmia, granulated eyelids, and in purulent conjunctivitis, it is of the greatest service, and should be employed both locally and internally (Bl.).

VIOLENT, PURULENT OPHTHALMIA, WITH THICK, YELLOW, BLAND DISCHARGE ; THE CHARACTERISTIC IS THE PROFUSENESS OF THE DISCHARGE (D.).

Canthi, as red as blood ; swollen, standing out like a lump of red flesh (N.).

Eye-strain from sewing, worse in a warm room and better in an open air (*Nat-M.*, *Ruta*) (A.).

Blurred vision (*Chin.*, *Kali-P.*, *Phos.*) (Br.).

Chronic ulceration of margin of the lids (Br.).

Diseases of the eyes, due to defective accommodation (*Agar.*, *Aur-M.*, *Hydr.*, *Morph.*, *Nat-M.*) (A.).

It should be studied in cases of locomotor ataxia ; there is the ataxic gait, which is aggravated from closing the eyes ; he cannot walk in the dark without reeling ; the legs feel as if made of wood (Bl.).

Vertigo : as if turning in a circle, accompanied by headache (G.).

Vertigo, with buzzing in the ears, and weakness and trembling (N.).

EXCESSIVE CONGESTION TO THE HEAD, WITH THROBBING CAROTIDS, OBLIGING ONE TO LOOSEN THE CRAVAT (G.).

Hemicrania, a boring pain which is relieved by binding the head up tightly—even the wearing of a tight hat relieves ; it is worse over left frontal eminence ; the head sometimes feels enormously large, and there is a feeling as if the bones of the skull would separate (D.).

Palpitation of heart, with nausea and faintness (*Dig., Lob., Verat.*) (G.).

There is severe gastralgia, the pains radiate from the stomach in all directions (*Dios.*) ; they are relieved by hard pressure and by bending double (*Bell., Coloc., Mag-P.*) ; the pains often increase gradually and decrease gradually, as under *Stannum* ; vomiting of glairy mucus relieves (D.).

SENSATION AS OF A SPLINTER IN THE THROAT, WHEN SWALLOWING (*Bell., Hep., Nit-Ac., Sil.*) (G.).

There is flatulence, which presses up and causes dyspnœa (*Lyc.*) (D.).

Craves fresh air (*Apis, Phos., Sulph.*) (N.).

Gums tender and bleed easily (*Hep., Kreos., Merc., Nat-M., Sulph.*) (Br.).

Emaciation, progressing every year ; most marked in the lower extremities (*Amm-M. *) ; *marasmus* (A.).

Faintish, nauseated feeling in P. M., with palpitation of heart (R.).

Eructates ingesta (*Chin., Ferr., Ferr-P., Phos., Phos-Ac., Puls.*) (Br.).

CRAVES SUGAR ; CHILD IS FOND OF IT, BUT DIARRHŒA RESULTS FROM EATING (craves salt or smoked meat—*Calc-P.*) (A.).

Nausea, retching and vomiting of glairy mucus (Br.).

FLATULENT DYSPEPSIA : BELCHING AFTER EVERY MEAL ; STOMACH, AS IF IT WOULD BURST WITH WIND ; BELCHING DIFFICULT, FINALLY AIR RUSHES OUT WITH GREAT VIOLENCE (A.).

Gastritis of drunkards (Carb-V., Nux-V., Puls., Sep., Sulph-Ac.) (Br.).

Ulceration of stomach, with radiating pain (*Dios.*) (Br.).

Diarrhœa : green mucus, like chopped spinach in flakes ; turning green after remaining on diaper ; after drinking ; after eating candy or sugar ; masses of muco-lymph in shreddy, strips, or lumps ; with noisy flatus (Aloe, Calc-P., Nat-S., Podo.) (A.).

Vomiting and diarrhœa, with violent colicky pains (*Coloc., Nux-V., Verat.*).

Bloody stools (*Acon., Canth., Merc-C., Nux-V., Sulph.*).

Stools expelled forcibly, with much fuss (*Crot-T., Gamb., Nat-S.*) (G.).

Advanced dysentery, with suspected ulceration (C.).

Itching in the anus (*Æsc., Aloe, Calc.. Cina, Merc., Nat-P., Sulph.*) (C.).

Copious fluid stool (Podo , Verat.) (C.).

Chorea-like convulsive motion of all the limbs (C.).

Epilepsy and epileptiform convulsions (C.).

AGGRAVATION : After eating candy or sugar ; from drinking ; from taking ice-cream ; from cold food ; from unusual mental exertion ; and from emotion.

AMELIORATION : In the open air ; from cold application ; from cold bathing ; and from pressure or tight bandaging.

RELATIONSHIP. *Nat-M.*, for the bad effects of cauterizing with *Nitrate of Silver*.

Coffea increases the nervous headache.

Similar to : *Aur.*, *Cupr.*, *Dios.*, *Lach.*, *Lyc.*, *Nat-M.*, *Nit-Ac.*, *Sep.*, and *Sulph.*

Lyc. follows it well in flatulent dyspepsia.

Arnica Montana.

COMMON NAME : LEOPARD'S BANE.

Over-sensitiveness of the whole body (*Coff.*, *Kali-C.*, *Nux-V.*).

SORE, LAME, BRUISED FEELING ALL THROUGH THE BODY, AS IF BEATEN (*Bapt.*, *Eup-P.*, *Ham.*, *Pyrog.*) (A.).

Pricking from without inwards.

Loud blowing inspirations and expirations (C.).

Tearing and drawing in outer parts.

Tingling in outer parts (*Acon.*, *Arg-N.*, *Nux-V.*, *Puls.*, *Zinc.*).

Pain, as if beaten or bruised, in outer parts.

Pain, as if sprained in outer parts and the joints.

Brown streak through the middle of the tongue(C_i).

7

Pressing in inner parts.

Involuntary stool and urine ; brown or white diarrhœa, with distention of the abdomen before and rumbling in the abdomen during stool (C.).

Gout, with the greatest fear of being struck by persons coming towards him across the room (Hr.).

RETENTION OF URINE, DURING DYSENTERY (*Merc.*) (A.).

Twitching of the muscles (*Hyos., Lach., Mygale, Tarant-C.*).

TRAUMATIC AFFECTIONS OF MUSCLES (A.).

Myalgia of the intercostal muscles after great exertion, with a sensation as if all the ribs were bruised ; short breath ; pain in the chest, with anxiety (Ra.).

Ebullitions, with burning of the upper part of the body, but coldness of the lower part.

Tendency to small boils ; ecchymosis on various parts of the body (Hr.).

Dysentery : with ischuria ; fruitless urging ; long interval between the stools (A.).

BAD EFFECTS FROM MECHANICAL INJURIES (FALLS, BRUISES AND CONTUSIONS).

In all acute diseases, brought on by mechanical injuries, *Arnica* should be studied thoroughly (Bt.).

MECHANICAL INJURIES, ESPECIALLY WITH STUPOUR FROM CONCUSSION ; INVOLUNTARY FÆCES AND URINE (A.).

Bleeding of external and internal parts (*vomiting of blood*).

Useful after injuries with blunt instruments (*Symph.*) (A.).

Petechiæ (*Bapt., Ham., Sulph-Ac.*).

COMPOUND FRACTURES AND THEIR PROFUSE SUPPURATION (*Calend.*) (A.).

Traumatic ophthalmia (Bt.).

Traumatic injuries of the testicles (*Con.*) (Bt.).

Hæmoptysis, from mechanical injuries (*Mil., Ruta*) (Bt.).

Hoarseness, caused by over-exertion of the voice, in persons who constantly speak or sing (K.).

Conjunctival or retinal hæmorrhage, with extravasation, from injuries or cough (*Led., Nux-V.*) (A.).

Concussions of the brain and spine (D.).

Sudden wrenching of muscles from strains (D.).

EVERYTHING ON WHICH HE LIES SEEMS TOO HARD; COMPLAINS CONSTANTLY OF IT, AND KEEPS MOVING FROM PLACE TO PLACE IN SEARCH OF A SOFTER SPOT (A.).

UNCONSCIOUSNESS; WHEN SPOKEN TO ANSWERS CORRECTLY, BUT UNCONSCIOUSNESS AND DELIRIUM AT ONCE RETURN (A.).

Irritable and angry, wants to be let alone (C.).

Morose, repelling mood (B.).

Physically restless, but mentally prostrate or apathetic; says nothing ails him (*Op.*) (B.).

SAYS HE IS WELL, WHEN VERY SICK (*Apis, Ars., Cinnb., Hyos., Kreos., Merc., Puls.*) (K.).

FEARS, BEING STRUCK OR APPROACHED
(*Ambr., Bell., Ign., Kali-C., Lach., Stram., Thuj.*) (B.).

Answers slowly, with an effort (B.).

Sopor ; drops to sleep as he answers (B.).

Belchings, tasting like rotten eggs (Bt.).

Feeling of nauseous repletion, after eating (G.).

Vomiting of dark, clotted blood (Hm.).

Gout, with extreme soreness (*Colch.*) (D.).

Cannot walk erect on account of a bruised, sore feeling in the uterine region (Hr.).

Abortion, from mechanical injuries (Bt.).

Paralysis (left sided) ; pulse full, strong ; stertor, sighing, muttering (A.).

The patient feels as if he had been pounded (D.).

Rheumatism, resulting from exposure to dampness, cold and excessive muscular strain combined ; the parts are sore and bruised (D.).

Retention or incontinence of urine after labour (*Op.*). (A.).

THIRST DURING CHILL (*Apis, Caps., Cina, Eup-P., Ign., Nat-M., Nux-V., Pyrog., Sep., Sil., Tub., Verat.*) (B.).

Hot head, with cool body (*Bell.*) (B.).

Typhoid fever, with the greatest indifference ; putrid breath ; and red spots, like suggilations on the body (Hr.).

Ailments from spirituous liquors, or from charcoal vapours (A.).

May be used as a preventive of pyæmia (F.).

It tends to relieve the soreness following parturition and promotes proper contraction of the uterus and expulsion of coagula and of any portions of the membranes that may have been retained (F.).

Whooping cough; violent tickling cough, which seems to be excited whenever the child becomes angry (Ant-T., Bry., Cham., Nux-V., Staph., Verat.). The child loses its breath when it cries. Before a paroxysm it begins to cry. Why ? (Because) the lungs and trachea are sore. The little sufferer knows what is coming on and dreads it (F.).

Ribbon-like stools, from enlarged prostate or retroverted uterus (A.).

AGGRAVATION : In the evening and through the night ; from contact ; from motion ; from noise ; during rest ; when lying down ; and from wine.

AMELIORATION : From motion.

RELATIONSHIP. *Complementary to : Acon., Bry., Hyper., Nux-V., and Rhus-T.*

Similar to : Bapt., Bell., Bry., Chin., Eup-P., Ham., Kali-P., Phyt., Pyrog., Rhus-T., Ruta, Staph., and *Sulph-Ac.*

It follows well after : *Acon., Apis, Ham., Ipec.,* and *Verat.* ; and is to be followed by *Sulph-Ac.*

Arsenicum Album.

COMMON NAME : WHITE OXIDE OF ARSENIC. SYMPTOMS GENERALLY WORSE FROM 1 TO 2 P. M. OR 12 TO 2 A. M. (A.).

There is amelioration from heat of all complaints except headache, which is temporarily relieved by cold bathing (*Nux-V.*, *Spig.*) ; burning pain relieved by heat (A.).

ANXIETY AND RESTLESSNESS VERY HIGHLY MARKED.

DELIRIUM TREMENS (*Bell.*, *Hyos.*, *Stram.*) (Br.).

FEAR, FRIGHT AND WORRY MORE MARKED THAN IN ANY REMEDY KNOWN.

DREAD OF DEATH AND YET A DISPOSITION TO SUICIDE (*Aur.*, *Hep.*, *Nit-Ac.*, *Nux-V.*) (R.).

Despair ; driving him from place to place for relief ; weeps (R.).

Fear of being left alone (*Ka'i-C.*, *Phos.*) (N.).

Hears voices and sees animals after having taken alcohol (N.).

Very great anguish and restlessness ; cannot rest anywhere, moves from place to place ; wants to go from one bed to another (N.).

Avarice (*Bry.*, *Calc.*, *Calc-F.*, *Cina*, *Coloc.*, *Lyc.*, *Meli.*, *Nat-C.*, *Puls.*, *Sep.*).

Hallucination of smell and sight (Br.)

Thinks it is useless to take medicine, is incurable, is surely going to die (A.).

Burning pains of an excruciating character (*Apis, Anthr., Canth., Phos., Sec., Sulph.*).

The discharges are usually thin, acrid and offensive (*Kreos., Merc-C., Nit-Ac.*) (R.).

Hæmaturia (*Canth., Colch., Ham., Phos., Tereb.*) (C.).
Albuminuria (*Apis, Canth., Colch., Phos.*) (C.).

Tearing pains in the limbs, worse during the night and while at rest, after previous powerful exertion, and only relieved by walking about and by external heat.

Face deathly pale ; pale yellow, cachectic look ; swollen, covered with cold sweat ; hippocratic (N.).

EXCESSIVE EXHAUSTION, FROM LEAST EXERTION (A.).

FREQUENT SPELLS OF UNCONSCIOUSNESS (*Bapt., Hyos., Ign., Merc-Cy., Nat-M., Phos.*).

Periodical pains, with coldness, chills, debility and anxious despair.

Sudden sinking of strength highly prominent in the sphere of drug's curative usefulness.

WATERY CORYZA ; DISCHARGE CAUSES BURNING ; OR SMARTING OF NOSTRILS, AS IF SORE (*All-C., Arum-T., Merc-C., Nat-M.*) (N.).

Nose feels stopped up (*Lyc., Nux-V., Puls., Stict.*) (Br.).
Bloatedness or emaciation (*Nat-M., Phos., Sulph.*).

Conjunctivæ inflamed ; extreme redness and dryness of inner surface of lids ; they rub painfully against the ball (*Bor., Graph., Nat-M., Sep., Sulph.*) ; *burning pains* (N.).

Eyelid swollen and œdematous, firmly closed and looks as if distended with air (N.).

THE LACHRYMAL DISCHARGES BURN AND EXCORIATE THE CHEEKS (N.).

Twitching of single parts of the body, when going to sleep.

Grinding of teeth while asleep (*Bell., Bry., Calc., Cann-I., Cina, Hyos., Kali-P., Merc., Nat-P., Podo., Sant., Stram., Tub., Verat., Zinc.*) (C.).

WATER TASTES BITTER (*Calc-P., Chin-A.*) (K.).

Violent burning on the tongue (C.).

VOMITING OF WHAT HAS BEEN EATEN OR DRUNKEN, OR OF BLACK MATTER WITH IT.

Sensation as if food lodged in the œsophagus (*Bar-C., Calc., Caust., Chin., Dig., Gels., Kali-C., Puls.*) (K.).

GURGLING IN THE ŒSOPHAGUS WHEN DRINKING (*Çina, Cupr., Hell., Hydr-Ac., Laur.*) (K.).

WATERY AND OFFENSIVE DIARRHŒA (*Aloe, Bry., Chin., Kali-P., Podo., Sec., Sulph.*).

Hæmorrhoids, with intense burning, relieved by heat (relieved by cold water—Aloe) (R.).

Phagedenic ulceration, constantly extending its breadth (Bt.).

ULCERS, TURNING BLACK, BURNING, WITH HIGH EDGES (*Anthr.*).

GANGRENE (*Canth., Carb-Ac., Kali-P., Lach., Phos., Plb., Rhus-T., Sec., Sil.*).

Burns (*Canth., Sulph.*).

Nettlerash or urticaria, caused by eating shell-fish. Wheals attended with burning, itching and restlessness (L.).

Bad effects, like croup, from repercussion of nettlerash or hives (L.).

Leprosy : yellow or white spots ; tubercular swelling in the nose ; burning ulcers at the ends of the fingers, at the toes, soles of feet, navel and cheek ; raised up tubercles ; hyperæsthesia and anæsthesia alternating (*Alum., Anac., Hydrocot., Lach., Phos.*) (L.).

Bran-like, dry, scaly eruptions, with itching and burning ; the latter increased by scratching and followed by bleeding (Hr.).

Skin : dry and scaly ; cold, blue and wrinkled ; with cold, clammy perspiration ; like parchment ; white and pasty ; black vesicles and burning pain (A.).

Bad effects from decayed food or animal matter, whether by inoculation, olfaction or ingestion (A.).

General anasarca, with white, waxy paleness of the face and great debility (Bt.).

Diarrhœa is renewed after eating or drinking (*Aloe, Crot-T., Nat-M.*) (G.).

Diarrhœa of a cadaverous smell, scenting the whole atmosphere of the room (Ra.).

Great thirst for cold water (*Bry., Nat-M., Phos., Sec., Sulph.*) (A.).

Drinks often, but little at a time (A.).

ASTHMA, WITH CONSTRICTION OF THE CHEST AND ANGUISH, AGGRAVATED BY MOTION ; WORSE EVENINGS (*Phos.*) (Bt.).

CANNOT LIE DOWN, FOR FEAR OF SUFFOCA-
TION ; HIGHEST DEGREE OF DYSPNŒA (G.).

GREAT ENERVATION AFTER STOOL (*Aloe,
Phos., Verat.*) (Hm.).

*Intense burning sensation, like coals of fire, in the abdo-
men (Carb-V.)* (Bt.).

*Sensation as if a stone was in the stomach (Bry.,
Nux-V., Puls.)* (Bt.).

Violent vomiting of ingesta, serous liquids with flakes,
also brown or b'ack substances, with violent burning
pains in the stomach and watery diarrhœa, accompanied
with cramps of the abdominal muscles and extremities (Ra.)

Stomach disordered, after eating ice-cream or fruit
(*Ipec., Phos.*) (Hr.).

*The stomach does not seem to assimilate cold water ;
it is wanted, but cannot drink it* (Ra.).

Desire for pungent things, acids, acid fruits, milk, and
coffee (K.).

COMPLAINTS RETURN ANNUALLY (*Carb-V.,
Lach., Sulph., Thuj.*). (A.).

Retention of urine after confinement (*Arn., Caust.,
Hyos., Op., Sec.*) (K.).

*Cholera Asiatica ; intense vomiting and purging ; in-
tense thirst ; the surface of the body is as cold as ice, but
internally, the patient feels as if full of fire* (F.).

Arsenic should be thought of in ailments from
chewing tobacco, alcoholism, sea-bathing, sausage

poisoning, dissecting wounds, anthrax poison and stings of venomous insects.

AGGRAVATION : Periodically at night ; after midnight (from 1 to 2 A. M.) ; on entering a cold place ; from cold food or drinks ; from rapid walking ; from the use of milk ; from cold ; and when lying on the affected side, with the head low.

AMELIORATION : From external heat ; when moving about : from warmth ; from hot drinks ; and from hot food.

RELATIONSHIP. COMPLEMENTARY : *All-S., Anthr., Carb-V., Phos., Pyrog., Rhus-T., Sec.,* and *Thuj.*

ANTIDOTES : *Camph., Carb-V., Chin., Chin-S., Ferr., Hep., Iod., Ipec., Lach., Nux-V., Samb., Tab.,* and *Verat.* To large doses : *Sesquioxide of Iron, Hydrated Peroxide of Iron, or Precipitated Carbonate of Iron ; juice of sugar cane or honey water ; lime water in copious draughts ; emetics of Sulphate of Zinc. : Carbonate of Potash and Magnesia, shaken in oil ; infusion of astringent substances ; and large quantities of diluent drinks.*

ARSENICUM ANTIDOTES : *Carb-V., Chin., Ferr., Graph., Iod., Ipec., Lach., Merc., Nux-V.,* and *Verat.* Also lead poisoning and evil effects of alcohol.

Arsenicum Metallicum.

COMMON NAME : THE METAL ARSENIC.

Arouses latent syphilis (*Syph.*). (Br.).

Periodicity very marked (*Alum.*, *Arg-M.*, *Ars.*, *Cedr.*, *Chin.*, *Chin-A.*, *Chin-S.*, *Ipec.*, *Nat-M.*, *Nit-Ac.*, *Sep.*, *Sil.*, *Sulph.*) (Br.).

Symptoms recur every two or three weeks (Br.).

Low-spiritedness and weakness of memory (Kali-P.).

Desire to be let alone—the patient is annoyed by visions, which cause her to cry.

Sensation of fullness in the head, as if the head were too large.

Left-sided headache up to the eyes and into the ear.

Headache, aggravated when stooping and when lying down.

Œdematous swelling of forehead and face with itching, which can only be allayed by pinching.

The face is, red, itching, burning and bloated (Apis, Bell., Stram.).

Eyes swelled and watery (with coryza).

Eyes burn with coryza.

The eyes are weak—day and gas-light are very unpleasant.

Mouth sore and ulcerated (*Aur.*, *Kali-B.*, *Lach.*, *Lyc.*, *Merc.*, *Nit-Ac.*, *Sil.*) (Br.).

Tongue coated white and showing imprints of teeth (*Chel., Merc., Podo., Rhus-T., Sep., Stram.*) (*Br.*).

Diarrhœa : *burning, watery stools, with relief of pain* (*Gamb.*) (*Br.*).

AGGRAVATION : From stooping ; when lying down ; and from light.

AMELIORATION : In darkness ; by pinching ; and from sitting erect.

RELATIONSHIP. Similar to : *Anac., Ign., Gels., Phos.,* and *Sulph.*

Arum Triphyllum.

COMMON NAME : INDIAN TURNIP.

Coryza : *acrid, fluent* ; *nostrils raw* (*Ars., Nat-M., Nit-Ac., Rhus-T.*).

CORYZA, PARTICULARLY AFFECTING THE LEFT NOSTRIL (*All-C., Jug-C., Mang.*) (K.).

Coryza, especially in the afternoon (*Calc-P., Kali-C., Mag-S., Plb., Sulph.* ; especially during evening— *All-C.*) (K.).

CORYZA , DURING DIPHTHERIA (*Amm-C., Ars., Carb-Ac., Kali-B., Merc-C., Merc-Cy., Mur-Ac., Nit-Ac.*) (K.).

Nose feels stopped up, inspite of the watery discharge (*Amm-C., Ars., Samb., Sinap.*) (A.).

Sneezing, worse at night (A.).

EXCORIATING (NASAL) DISCHARGE; THE NOSE IS VERY SORE AND EXCORIATED (D.).

CONSTANTLY PICKING THE NOSE, UNTIL IT BLEEDS (*Cina, Con., Lach.*) (Bl.).

Boring with the finger into the side of the nose (*Aur., Bufo, Cina, Phos., Phos-Ac., Stict., Verat., Zinc.*) (A.).

Hoarseness and rawness in the larynx (*Caust., Phos.*); *the control over the voice is lost* (*Amm-Caust.*); *the voice suddenly changes*; *dry cough*; *the patient cringes under it, it hurts so* (D.).

An excellent remedy in clergyman's sorethroat.

Must breathe with the mouth open (*Ant-T., Hyos., Lach., Lyc., Op., Sulph.*). (Bl.).

Sorethroat of public speakers (*Arg-N.*) (Bl.).

PICKS LIPS UNTIL THEY BLEED (*Bry., Cina, Con., Hell., Nit-Ac., Nux-V., Phos-Ac., Rheum, Zinc.*) (A.).

CORNERS OF THE MOUTH SORE, CRACKED, AND BLEEDING (A.).

Diphtheria the mouth and fauces are covered with a deposit. Ulcers are to be seen at different points. The secretions are acrid and excoriating. The glands of the neck are swollen and painful (Bl.).

Excessive salivation; saliva acrid.

Throat sore; feels as if excoriated; cannot swallow.

Has relieved cases of stomatitis, when there are burning pains and excessive salivation. The mucous surfaces are raw and sore; the tongue is red, like a beet, and the papillæ are prominent (Bl.).

Swelling of the sub-maxillary glands. The corners of the mouth, buccal cavity, and even the throat become raw and sore, emitting blood ; so sore in fact, that the patient refuses all food and drink, in consequence of the suffering occasioned by mastication or swallowing (G.).

Putrid odour emanating from the mouth (*Ars.*, *Aur.*, *Bapt.*, *Carb-V.*, *Kali-P.*, *Lach.*, *Mur-Ac.*, *Nit-Ac.*) (G.).

DISCHARGE OF BURNING, ICHOROUS FLUID FROM THE NOSE, EXCORIATING THE NOSTRILS AND UPPER LIP.

Accumulation of mucus in the trachea (*Calc.*, *Ipec.*, *Kali-B.*, *Lyc.*, *Nat-S.*).

After a long paroxysm of cough, he raises mucus, traversed with yellow threads (Dg.).

EXANTHEMATA LIKE SCARLET-RASH ; THE SKIN PEELS OFF AFTERWARDS.

Bites nails until fingers bleed (A.).

Patients pick and bore into the raw bleeding surfaces, though very painful ; scream with pain, but keep up the boring (*in diphtheria, scarlatina, or typhoid*) (A.).

Excessively cross and stubborn (B.).

Mouth burns and is so sore that they refuse to drink, and cry when anything is offered (N.).

Chronic hoarseness, from speaking or singing (clergyman's sorethroat, acute cases—*Ferr-P.*, *Rhus-T.*) (*Arg-M.*) (N.).

Urine scanty or suppressed, in scarlatina (C.).

AGGRAVATION : From north-west wind ; from lying

down ; during night ; from talking, speaking or singing ; and in the afternoon.

AMELIORATION : From warmth.

RELATIONSHIP. Useful after *Hep.* and *Nit-Ac.* in dry, hoarse, croupy cough ; after *Caust.*, and *Hep.* in morning hoarseness and deafness, and in scarlatina.

Similar to : *Ailan.*, *All-C.*, *Amm-C.*, *Ars.*, *Bor.*, *Cina,* *Merc-C.*, *Nit-Ac.*, and *Sulph.*

ANTIDOTES : Butter milk ; also *Acet-Ac.* and *Puls.*

Asafœtida.

COMMON NAMES : GUM OF THE STINKASAND ; DEVIL'S DUNG.

Hysterical attacks (*Ign.*, *Nux-M.*, *Sep.*).

Hysteria, where the throat symptoms predominate, with all kinds of spasms and nervous irritability, such as fits of great joy and laughter, or anxious sadness ; constant change of position ; flushes in the face, etc. (Bt.).

Leucorrhœa ; profuse, greenish, thin and offensive (G.).

Menses scanty and too early (G.).

Hysterical spasms, with much trouble about the œsophagus (G.).

SENSATION OF PRESSURE, AS IF A BODY OR LUMP WERE ASCENDING IN THE ŒSOPHAGUS, OBLIGING FREQUENT DEGLUTITIONS (G.).

Caries of nasal bones (*Ars., Aur., Calc-F., Hep., Merc., Nit-Ac., Sil.*) (Br.).

INTOLERABLE SORENESS AROUND THE ULCER (*Hep.*) (F.).

Bluish ulcers, with high edges (*Lach.*) (B.).

SYPHILITIC OZŒNA (*Aur-M., Calc., Hep., Kali-B., Kali-I., Merc., Puls., Sep., Sil.*), WITH VERY OFFENSIVE, PURULENT DISCHARGE (Br.).

Is employed as a galactagogue, in sensitive, hysterical females (Bl.).

Fetid or purulent discharge from the ears (*Calc., Calc-S., Hep., Merc., Sil.*) (G.).

Sometimes indicated for iritis following mercurialization ; extreme soreness of the bones around the eyes (F.).

ERUCTATIONS OF GAS, SMELLING LIKE GARLIC OR FÆCES (Bt.).

Pulsation in the pit of the stomach (*Acon., Ant-T., Calc., Chin., Cic., Ferr., Glon., Kali-C., Nux-V., Phos., Puls., Sep., Sil.*) (Bt.).

Painful inflammation of the bones (*Aur., Hep., Nit-Ac.*). *Caries, with thin, offensive pus* (*tibia*).

Swelling of the glands (*Calc., Merc-I., Tub.*).

Sense of rigor.

Greasy taste in the mouth (*Puls.*) (D.).

Body heavy and bloated.

St. Vitus's dance (*Agar., Ign., Nux-V., Sep.*).

Dark red and hot swellings.

Pains on the inside of the joints of the limbs.

TWITCHING AND JERKING IN THE MUSCLES
(*Bell., Hyos., Ign., Lach., Nux-V., Stram.*).

*Pricking, stinging and darting pain, which is periodic
from within outwards ; by touch relieved or changed.*

SYPHILITIC IRITIS (*Merc-C., Nit-Ac., Sil.*) (Br.).
*Sensation as if peristaltic motion were taking place
from below upwards* (G.).

An empty gone feeling in the stomach at 11 A. M.
(*Sulph.*) (F.).

Particularly adapted to syphilitic patients, who have
taken much mercury, or to nervous, hysterical individuals (C.).

*Extreme sensitiveness around the diseased portion of
bone* (F.).

Painfulness of the periosteum, accompanied with great
sensitiveness ; enlargement of bones (G.).

Nervous palpitation (*Cocc.*), like a tremor when sitting,
with small, quick, irregular pulse (C.).

*Spasmodic tightness of the chest, as if the lungs could
not be fully expanded* (*Crot-T., Ign., Laur., Phos.*) (C.).

Hysteria arising from the sudden suppression of
discharges.

*A bursting feeling upwards, as though everything in the
abdomen was coming out at the mouth* (*Arg-N.*) (F.).

Burning in the stomach and œsophagus (*Carb-V., Iris-
V., Sulph.*) (D.).

AGGRAVATION : While sitting ; at night ; during

rest ; from warm application ; and from dressing the wound.

AMELIORATION : In the open air ; from motion and from pressure.

RELATIONSHIP. *Similar to* : *Aur.*, *Chin.*, *Merc.*, *Mosch.*, *Nit-Ac.* and *Sil.*

Antidotes : *Chin.*, *Merc.*

Asarum Europœum.

COMMON NAME : EUROPEAN SNAKE ROOT.

Hyperæsthesia of the senses (*Bell.*, *Coff.*, *Nux-V.*, *Op.*, *Phos.*) (Bl.).

OVERSENSITIVENESS OF THE NERVES ; THE SCRATCHING ON LINEN OR SILK IS INSUPPORT-ABLE (*Ferr.*, *Tarant-C.*).

Cold "shivers" from any emotion (A.).

Nervous irritability and exaltation. Asthmatic breathing, worse from odour or cold (B.).

Sensation of tightness in the limbs ; *when she walks she thinks she is gliding through the air.*

When reading, sensation in eyes as if they would be pressed asunder or outward ; relieved by bathing them in cold water (A.).

Great faintness and constant yawning (A.).

Vomiting, with violent retching and anxiety (*Ars.*, *Cupr.*, *Ipec.*, *Tab.*).

It is of service in gastric derangements, such as mucous colitis, when the patient craves alcoholic stimulants. There is loss of appetite with eructations and vomiting, while the stools consist of undigested food and strings of mucus (Bl.).

Eructations putrid or sour, setting the teeth on edge. "Horrible sensation" of pressing, digging in the stomach when walking in the morning (after a debauch) (A.).

Menses : too early, long lasting ; black ; with violent pains in small of back (Br.).

Tenacious, yellow leucorrhœa (*Hydr.*) (Br.).

Smoking tobacco tastes bitter (G.).

Unconquerable longing for alcohol ; a popular remedy in Russia for drunkards (A.).

Chilliness ; single parts get cold. Easily excited perspiration (Br.).

Prolapsus ani during stool (*Podo.*).

Gelatinous or shreddy mucous stool (B.).

Cold air or cold water very pleasant to the eyes ; sunshine, light and wind are intolerable (A.).

AGGRAVATION : In the evening ; in cold and dry weather ; and from penetrating sounds.

AMELIORATION : From washing the face in cold water ; from wetting the affected part ; and from damp, wet weather.

RELATIONSHIP. *Similar to* : *Caust. in modalities,* and *to Aloe, Arg-N., Graph., Kali-B., Merc., Podo., Puls.* and *Sulph-Ac*, in stringy, shreddy stools.

Asterias Rubens.

COMMON NAME : STAR FISH.

Easily excited by any emotion, especially by contradictions (*Anac.*, *Bell.*, *Con.*, *Nux-V.*, *Sulph.*) (A.).

Weeps from least emotion (*Ign.*, *Puls.*, *Nat-M.*, *Sep.*) (B.).

Irritable temperament (*Nux-V.*) (A.).

Gait unsteady ; muscles refuse to obey the will (*Alum.*, *Arg-N.*, *Gels.*).

Hysterical and neuralgic symptoms predominate (C.).

Sexual erethism (*Aur.*, *Hyos.*, *Phos.*, *Pic-Ac.*, *Sulph.*, *Zinc.*) (B.).

Sexual desire increased in women (*Canth.*, *Con.*, *Fluor-Ac.*, *Hyos.*, *Lach.*, *Murx.*, *Nux-V.*, *Orig.*, *Phos.*, *Plat.*, *Puls.*, *Verat.*) (A.).

SANGUINEOUS CONGESTION TO THE BRAIN (A.).

RUSH OF BLOOD TO THE HEAD ; IT FEELS SURROUNDED BY HOT AIR (B.).

APOPLEXY : FACE RED ; PULSE HARD, FULL, FREQUENT (*Acon.*, *Bell.*, *Gels.*, *Glon.*, *Nat-M.*, *Op.*, *Verat-V.*) (A.).

Stools of brown, gushing water (B.).

Diarrhœa ; stools gushing out in a violent jet (*Crot-T.*, *Grat.*, *Gum.*, *Jatr.*, *Podo.*, *Thuj.*) (A.).

Constipation : obstinate ; ineffectual desire ; stools of hard, round balls, like olive (A.).

Pulsations in head, womb, chest, etc. (B.).

Epilepsy : twitching over the whole body four or five days before the attack (A.).

Red face (*Amyl-N., Bell., Ferr., Meli., Sang., Stram., Verat-V.*).

CANCER OF THE MAMMÆ : ACUTE, LANCINAT-ING PAIN ; DRAWING PAIN IN BREAST ; SWOLLEN, DISTENDED, AS BEFORE THE MENSES ; BREAST FEELS DRAWN IN (A.).

A livid, red spot appeared, broke and discharged ; gradually invaded the entire breast ; very fetid odour ; edges pale, elevated, mammillary, hard, everted ; bottom covered with reddish granulations (A.).

Colic and other sufferings cease with the appearance of the menstrual flow (Br.).

A remedy for the sycotic diathesis (*Med., Nat-S., Sep., Thuj.*) (Br.).

Numbness of hand and fingers of the left side (Br.).

Axillary glands swollen, hard and knotted (Br.).

AGGRAVATION : From contradiction ; in cold, damp weather ; in left side ; from coffee ; and at night.

AMELIORATION : From the appearance of menses.

RELATIONSHIP. *Similar to* : *Murx., Sep.*

COMPARE : *Ars., Ars-I., Carb-An., Condur., Con.,* and *Sil.* in mammary cancer ; an *Bell., Calc.,* and *Sulph.* in epilepsy.

ANTIDOTES : *Plb.* and *Zinc.*

Aurum Metallicum.

COMMON NAME : GOLD.

GREAT HOPELESSNESS ; HARASSED, WITH A DESIRE TO COMMIT SUICIDE ; WEARY OF LIFE (N.).

Peevish and vehement ; wrath at least contradiction (*Bry.*, *Nux-V.*, *Sulph.*) (R.).

MELANCHOLY (*Ign.*, *Nat-M.*, *Puls.*, *Stann.*).

QUARRELSOME (*Anac.*, *Bell.*, *Bry.*, *Hyos.*, *Nit-Ac.*, *Sulph.*) (R.).

Imagines that he is not fit for this world, and longs for death, which he contemplates with delight (R.).

FEAR EVEN TO SUICIDE (*Ars.*, *Merc.*, *Nit-Ac.*).

Sad, gloomy, taciturn (A.).

Imagines he cannot succeed in anything (*Arg-M.*) (R.).

RELIGIOUS MELANCHOLIA : THEY THINK THEY ARE TO BE DAMNED FOR SOMETHING THEY HAVE DONE. THEY WEEP, CRY AND BEMOAN THEIR IMAGINARY FATE (R.).

Weeping, because he imagines he has lost the affections of his friends *(Puls.)* (R.).

Oversensitive to pain, to smell, taste, hearing and touch (*Anac.*, *Coff.*, *Nux-V.*) (A.).

Caries of the mastoid process ; obstinate fetid otorrhœa (*Calc-F.*, *Caps.*, *Hep.*, *Merc.*, *Nit-Ac.*) (N.).

Broken down constitutions from syphilis and mercury (N.).

GREAT EBULLITION AND PALPITATION OF THE HEART (*Acon., Amyl-N., Arg-N., Bell., Cact., Dig., Ferr-P.. Glon., Nat-M., Sang., Verat-V.*).

Headache, from least mental exertion (*Calc-A., Nat-M., Nux-V., Phos-Ac.*) (A.).

Fatty degeneration of the heart (*Phos.*) (A.).

Cardiac hypertrophy (*Rhus-T.*) (B.).

Sensation as if the heart stood still ; as though it ceased to beat and then suddenly gave one hard thump (*Sep.*) (A.).

Falling of the hair, especially in syphilis and mercurial affections (*Lyc., Nit-Ac.*) (A.).

Urine like butter-milk, with mucous sediment (*Phos-Ac.*) (G.).

Frequent nightly erections and pollutions (G.).

Tensive pain in the right testicle, as if bruised (R.).

Swelling of the right testicle, with aching when touched or rubbed (*Clem., Rhod.*) (R.).

Chronic orchitis (*Calc-F., Puls., Sil.*) (B.).

Testes swollen and hard (*Puls.*) (R.).

Sweat about genitals (B.).

Testes mere pendant shreds (R.).

Increased sexual desire (*Calc., Phos., Plat., Sulph.*) (Bt.).

Induration of the os uteri (Bt.).

Menstrual and uterine affections, with great melancholy ; worse at menstrual period (A.).

PROLAPSED AND INDURATED UTERUS :

FROM OVER-REACHING OR STRAINING (*Pod.*, *Rhus-T.*) ; OR FROM HYPERTROPHY (*Con.*) (A.).

Crushing weight under the sternum (*Bry.*, *Phos.*) (B.).

Angina pectoris (*Acon.*, *Lat-M.*, *Puls.*) (B.).

Craves nothing but sour things (Bt.).

Much difficulty of breathing ; frequently taking a deep breath (*Bry.*, *Ign.*, *Phos.*) (G.).

Sleeplessness : frightful dreams ; sobbing during sleep (G.).

Constipation : stools hard and knotty (C.).

Cirrhosis of the liver (*Mur-Ac.*, *Nit-Ac.*, *Phos.*) (P.).

The liver is swollen consecutive to cardiac disease (F.).

Hemiopia, the upper half of the field of visions seem covered by a black body, lower visible (N.).

Desire for open air (*Apis*, *Arg-N.*, *Calc.*, *Carb-V.*, *Lach.*, *Sep.*, *Sulph.*).

Syphilitic iritis (*Merc-C.*) ; *especially after abuse of mercury* (D.).

DEEP ULCERS AFFECTING THE BONES ; AFTER ABUSE OF MERCURY, OR WITH SYPHILITIC TAINT (N.).

Exostosis of skull and other bones, with boring pains, which drive to despair, especially when syphilitic, or after abuse of mercury (N.).

Double vision (*Bell.*, *Gels.*, *Stram.*) (D.).

Red, knobby nose (B.).

OFFENSIVE BREATH (*Ars.*, *Bapt.*, *Carb-V.*, *Hep.*, *Kali-A.*, *Lach.*, *Merc.*, *Nit-Ac.*, *Sulph.*).

Foul breath : in girls at puberty (A.).

NOSE INFLAMED ; FEELING OF SORENESS, ESPECIALLY WHEN TOUCHED ; CARIES OF BONES ; FETID DISCHARGE ; PAIN WORSE AT NIGHT (SYPHILITIC) (N.).

Oversensitiveness to all pain (*Coff.*) *and to the cold air* (*Hep.*, *Sil.*).

Inflammation of the bones (*Calc.*, *Calc-A.*, *Hep.*, *Merc.*, *Nit-Ac.*).

CARIES OF THE PALATE AND NASAL BONES (*Ars-I.*, *Kali-B.*, *Kali-I.*, *Merc.*, *Nit-Ac.*, *Sil.*).

Pain in the bones at night (*Merc.*, *Nit-Ac.*, *Syph.*).

Ulcerated, agglutinated, painful nostrils ; cannot breathe through the nose (*Lyc.*, *Nux-V.*, *Op.*) ; crusts. (N.).

Paralytic drawing in the limbs in the morning, when awakening and on getting cold.

Disposed to constipation (*Bry.*, *Nux-V.*, *Op.*, *Sep.*, *Sil.*, *Sulph.*) (A.).

Anxiety, with congestion of blood to the head and chest after exertion (A.).

Hysterical spasms, with laughing and crying alternately (*Ign.*, *Mosch.*, *Plat.*, *Puls.*).

Awakened by bone pains ; suffering so great he despairs, does not want to live (N.).

AGGRAVATION : In the morning ; on getting cold ;

while reposing ; in the cold air ; while lying down ; from mental exertion ; and in winter.

AMELIORATION : From moving ; while walking ; on getting warm ; in warm air ; and during summer.

RELATIONSHIP. *Aurum* follows and is followed well by *Syphilinum. Similar to* : *Asaf., Calc., Calc-F., Hep., Merc., Nit-Ac., Plat., Sep., Thuj.* and *Verat-V.*

Baptisia Tinctoria.

COMMON NAME : WILD INDIGO.

BAPTISIA is suitable to all stages of typhoid—early or late (F.).

Typhoid diseases, with stupor, delirium ; face dark red and a besotted expression ; eyes injected ; tongue coated brown, dry, particularly in the centre ; very offensive breath ; sordes on the teeth ; diarrhœa, with great fœtor of the stools and urine (Sm.).

Great prostration, with disposition to decomposition of fluids (*Ars., Lach., Pyrog., Sec.*) (A.).

Ulceration of mucous membranes (*Ars., Bor., Calc., Nit-Ac., Sulph.*) (A.).

DULL, STUPEFYING HEADACHE (*Bry., Nux-V., Stram.*) (Bt.).

Sinking feeling at stomach (*Sep.*) (Br.).

Stupor and delirium at night (Bt.).

Excitement of the brain, especially at night (Bt.).

ALL EXHALATIONS AND DISCHARGES FETID, ESPECIALLY IN TYPHOID OR OTHER

ACUTE DISEASE; BREATH, STOOL, URINE, PERS-PIRATION, ULCERS (*Psor.*, *Pyrog.*) (A.).

Head feels too heavy, with numbness (Bt.).

Skin of forehead feels tight ; seems drawn to back of head (Br.).

Head feels too large (*Agar.*, *Arg-N.*, *Arn.*, *Bell.*, *Bov.*, *Glon.*, *Nux-M.*, *Nux-V.*, *Ran-B.*) (Br.).

Dysentery of old people (*Aloe*, *Carb-V.*, *Merc.*, *Sulph.*).

Dysentery : stools scanty, of blood and mucus, with severe tenesmus and low fever (Bt.).

Puerperal fever (*Arn.*, *Ars.*, *Bry.*, *Hyos.*) (Br.).

Aversion to mental exertion ; indisposed, or want of power to think (A.).

WHILE ANSWERING A QUESTION, FALLS INTO A DEEP SLEEP IN THE MIDDLE OF A SENTENCE (Bt.).

Perfect indifference ; don't care to do anything ; inability to fix the mind or work (A.).

Wandering of the mind, whenever the eyes are closed (Bt.).

Insensible to pain (*Op.*) (B.).

Confusion of ideas (*Bell.*, *Bry.*, *Calc.*) (Bt.).

Sense of duality (*Anac.*, *Cann-I.*, *Lach.*, *Nux-M.*, *Petr.*, *Stram.*) (B.).

CONFUSION, AS IF INTOXICATED (*Bell.*, *Carb-S.*, *Glon.*, *Nux-M.*, *Nux-V.*, *Sil.*) (K.).

Slides down in bed (*Mur-Ac.*) (B.).

IMAGINES HE IS IN PIECES, AND SCATTE-

RED ABOUT THE BED, VAINLY ATTEMPTING TO GET HIMSELF TOGETHER (G.).

Can swallow liquids only (*Bar-C.*) ; *least solid food gags* (can swallow liquids only, but has aversion to them—*Sil.*) (A.).

Fœtor oris (*Ars.*, *Carb-Ac.*, *Kali-P.*, *Lach.*) (B.).

Can't swallow solids (B.).

Fetid lochia, with much prostration (*Sec.*) (G.).

SHE CANNOT GO TO SLEEP, BECAUSE SHE CANNOT GET HERSELF TOGETHER ; HER HEAD FEELS AS THOUGH SCATTERED ABOUT, AND SHE TOSSES ABOUT THE BED TO GET THE PIECES TOGETHER (Be.).

Diarrhœa : horribly foul, mushy, painless ; dark or slaty (B.).

Distension and rumbling in the abdomen (*Aloe, Nat-S.*, *Podo.*, *Sulph.*) (R.).

Abdomen sensitive in the right iliac region, with rumbling (N.).

Tongue ; at first coated white with red papillæ ; dry and yellow-brown in centre ; later dry, cracked, and ulcerated (A.).

Soreness of the eyeballs ; they feel as if they would be pressed into the head (Bt.).

Heavy feeling in the head, as if he could not sit up, causing a wild feeling (G.).

Dullness of hearing (*Phos.*, *Puls.*) (G.).

Decubitus in typhoid (*Arn.*, *Kali-P.*, *Mur-Ac.*, *Pyrog.*) (A.).

Putrid ulceration of the buccal mucous membrane, with salivation (Ha.).

Head, back and limbs ache fearfully, with low adynamic fever (Bt.).

IN WHATEVER POSITION THE PATIENT LIES, THE PARTS RESTED UPON FEEL SORE AND BRUISED (Ba.).

Limbs tremble and are very weak (*Hyos., Kali-P., Zinc.*) (Dg.).

Chilliness, with bruised pains and soreness over the entire body (R.).

Awakes with oppressed feeling, must have fresh air (*Sulph.*) (N.).

Nightmare and frightful dreams (Br.).

He dreams that he is chained to the bed, or that he is swimming a river (*Rhus-T.*), or undergoing some such ordeal as makes a great demand on his strength (F.).

Livid spots all over the body and limbs (*Lach.*) (Br.).

Frontal headache, with pressure at the root of the nose (*Stict.*) (C.).

Dark redness of tonsils and soft palate (Br.).

Tonsils and parotids are swollen (C.).

AGGRAVATION : From mental exertion ; from swallowing solids ; in a closed room ; and during sleep.

AMELIORATION : From drinking liquids ; in the open air ; and from motion.

RELATIONSHIP. Similar to : *Apis, Arn., Ars., Bry., Gels., Kali-P.,* and *Rhus-T.* in the earlier stages of fever with malaise, muscular soreness and nervousness.

It should be thought of in cases of typhoid where *Ars.* has been improperly given, or too often repeated.

After *Baptisia* : *Crot-H., Ham., Nit-Ac., Phos.,* and *Tereb.* act well in hæmorrhages of typhoid or typhus.

Baryta Carbonica.

COMMON NAME : BARIUM CARBONATE.

This is one of the leading so-called anti-scrofulous remedies (N.).

Great weakness of mind and body of old men (Anac., Lyc., Sil.).

LOSS OF MEMORY (*Anac., Calc., Kali-P., Lyc., Nat-M., Phos., Sep., Sil.*) (N.).

Mistrust (Acon., Ars., Bry., Cann-I., Kali-A., Lach., Lyc., Puls., Rhus-T., Sec., Stram., Sulph.).

WANT OF SELF-CONFIDENCE (*Anac., Aur., Bry., Chin., Gels., Kali-C., Lyc., Puls.*).

AVERSION TO STRANGERS (*Anac., Carb-An., Cham., Cic., Gels., Ign., Nat-M., Nux-V.*).

CHILDISH AND THOUGHTLESS (IN OLD AGE).

ALMOST IMBECILE (*Aloe, Ambr., Anac., Bar-M., Carb-S., Con., Hyos., Lyc., Nux-M., Op., Phos-Ac., Stram., Sulph., Verat.*).

Grief over trifles (*Nat-M.*)(Br.).

Vertigo (*Con., Ferr., Gels., Kali-C., Phos.*) (Br).

Brain feels as if loose (*Carb-An., Chin.*) (Br.).

Heaviness of the body (*Bry., Gels., Nux V.*).

Tension and shortening of muscles (*Amm-M., Caust.*).

Pain in the joints and bones (*Calc., Calc-F., Rhus-T., Ruta*).

Tearing in the limbs, with chilliness (*Nux-V., Puls., Rhus-T.*).

MENTAL AND PHYSICAL WEAKNESS ; BOTH ENDS OF LIFE ; DON'T GROW (N.).

Headache of aged people (*Ambr., Amm-C., Iod.*) (A.).

Hardness of hearing (*Bell., Calc., Carb-V., Caust., Graph., Lyc., Nit-Ac., Phos., Sil., Sulph., Verb.*) (Br.).

It removes predisposition to tonsilitis, and cures chronic enlargement of tonsils (D.).

Reverberation in the ear on blowing the nose (Br.).

Swelled and indurated glands (*Carb-An., Calc., Calc-F., Merc-I., Phyt.*).

TONSILS INFLAME, SWELL AND SUPPURATE REPEATEDLY, ON EVERY COLD EXPOSURE (*Hep., Merc., Sil.*) ; CHRONIC HYPERTROPHY AFTERWARDS (N.).

EMACIATION, WITH BLOATED FACE, SWELLED ABDOMEN AND DIFFICULT LEARNING IN CHILDREN (*Calc., Nat-M., Sil.*).

Glands swell, infiltrate, hypertrophy ; neck. parotids, sub-maxillary, groin, lymphatics, in the abdomen ; hypertrophy, sometimes suppuration (N.).

GREAT LIABILITY TO CATCH COLD (SORETHROAT, STIFFNESS OF THE NECK AND DIARRHŒA) (*Psor., Sulph.*).

Complaints of dwarfish children ; mind and body weak ; don't grow ; inclined to glandular swellings (N.).

Hemiplegia following cerebral hæmorrhage (Bl.).

PARALYSIS AND PALSY OF AGED PERSONS (*Alum., Arg-N., Kali-P., Nux-V., Op., Plb., Sil.*).

Offensive foot-sweats ; toes and soles get sore ; throat affections after checked foot-sweat (*Sil.*).

Infantilism : the memory is weak ; the child seems inattentive and stupid ; does not learn to play or walk ; and may approach a state bordering on idiocy (Bl.).

Prematurely old, thin and wrinkled children ; they look like a dwarf and show a condition of malnutrition, and appear stunted both physically and mentally (Bl.).

Toothache before and during menses (*Amm-C., Ars., Nat-M., Phos., Puls.*) (K.).

Arterio-sclerosis (*Calc., Calc-F., Sil.*) (B.).

Hæmorrhoids protrude every time he urinates (*Bar-M., Kali-C., Mur-Ac., Nit-Ac.*) (A.).

Throat affections after suppressed foot sweat (N.).

HYPERTROPHY OF THE PROSTATE (*Calc., Con., Dig., Puls., Sel.*) (Bl.).

Burning in the urethra on urinating (Br.).

TESTICLES ARE INDURATED (*Clem., Con., Graph., Kali-I., Med., Merc., Puls., Rhod., Sil., Spong.*) (Bl.).

Premature impotency (*Agn., Con., Graph., Kali-P., Lyc., Nat-M., Phos., Sulph.*) (Bl.).

Cough, worse in the evening, with a sensation as if the lungs were full of smoke (Bt.).

Cough after getting the feet wet, or the least exposure to cold air (Bt.).

Paralysis of the tongue (*Caust.*, *Gels.*, *Lyc.*, *Op.*, *Plb.*, *Rhus-T.*) (Br.).

Suffocative cough ; chest full of mucus, but lacking strength to expectorate (Br.).

Spasm of the œsophagus when food enters (*Bapt.*, *Hyos.*, *Merc-C.*, *Phos.*, *Sulph.*, *Zinc.*) (Br.).

Abdomen distended and hard in children (N.).

Complaints of old drunkards (*Carb·V.*) (A.).

AGGRAVATION : When sitting or lying on the painful side ; after slight exposure to cold ; from checked footsweat ; after meals ; washing the affected parts ; and when thinking of his complaint.

AMELIORATION : In warm atmosphere ; from warm covering ; and from walking.

RELATIONSHIP. *Similar to* : *Alum.*, *Bar-M.*, *Calc.*, *Calc-I.*, *Dulc.*, *Fluor-Ac.*, *Iod.*, *Lyc.*, *Sil.* and *Sulph.*

Frequently useful before or after *Hep.*, *Psor.*, *Sulph.* and *Tub.*

After *Bar-C.*, *Psor.* will often eradicate the constitutional tendency to quinsy.

Belladonna.

COMMON NAME : DEADLY NIGHTSHADE.

Adapted to persons who are lively and entertaining when well, but violent and often delirious when sick (A.).

Bad effects of fear and chagrin (*Ign.*).

Loss of consciousness (*Acon., Bar-C., Cann-I., Cocc., Hell., Hydr-Ac., Hyos., Ign., Lach., Mosch., Nux-M., Op., Phos-Ac., Puls.*).

FANTASTIC ILLUSIONS AND BITING RAGE (*Hyos., Stram.*).

FURIOUS DELIRIUM (*Bapt., Bry., Hyos., Lach., Stram., Verat.*).

FURIOUS DELIRIUM, WITH A WILD LOOK ; WISHES TO STRIKE, BITE OR QUARREL ; FACE FLUSHED AND EYES RED (Bt.).

Hallucinations : sees monstrous, hideous faces (*Hyos., Lach., Stram.*) (Br.).

ALMOST CONSTANT MOANING (*Acon., Apis, Ars., Bry., Cann-I., Cham., Cina, Hyos., Ign., Ipec., Kali-Br., Kali-C., Mur-Ac., Nux-V., Phos., Puls., Stram., Zinc.*) (Bt.).

BREAKS INTO FITS OF LAUGHTER AND GNASHES THE TEETH (A.).

The child cries out suddenly, and ceases just as suddenly (Bt.).

Desire to escape, with restlessness and anxiety (*Acon.,*

Agar., Ars., Bry., Cupr., Glon., Hyos., Lach., Nux-V.,
Op., Stram., Verat.) (Bt.).

Imagines he sees ghosts, hideous faces, and various
insects (Stram.) ; *black animals, dogs, wolves, etc.* (A.).

Crying, laughing, dancing, or muttering delirium,
with phantasms (Bt.).

Headache from suppressed catarrhal flow (*Bry., Kali-*
B., Lach., Nat-M., Stict.) (Br.).

OVERSENSITIVENESS OF ALL THE SENSES
(*Coff., Nux-V., Stram., Strych.*).

Plethora (*Acon., Ferr-P , Glon., Verat-V.*).

Burning in inner parts (*Apis, Ars., Camph., Lach.,*
Phos., Sec., Sulph.).

Sensation, as if inner organs were distended, or as if
they would burst.

Tearing in inner parts (from below upwards).

CONGESTION OF THE HEAD (*Acon., Amyl-N.,*
Bry., Ferr-P., Gels., Lach., Meli., Nat-M., Op., Sulph.,
Verat-V.).

SWELLING AND PULSATION IN THE BLOOD-
VESSELS (*Glon., Nat-M., Stram.*).

Carotids throb violently ; *jugulars swollen* ; *face*
bloated and red (Bt.).

Light and noise are intolerable (*Coff., Nux-V., Sulph.*)
(Bt.).

Vertigo, with vanishing of sight, stupefaction and
debility (*Chin.*).

Squinting (*Apis, Cic., Cycl., Gels., Stram.*) (D.).

Things look red ; sees sparks of fire (Bt.).

Diplopia (*Gels., Hyos., Nat-M., Puls., Sep., Stram.*) (Br.).

BLEEDING FROM INNER PARTS (*Acon., Chin., Ferr-P., Mill., Sab.*).

Pricking on the muscles or bones.

Pressing and tearing rheumatic pains, which wander from one place to the other.

Sensation as if a mouse was running in the muscles (Illusion of a mouse running from under her chair—*Act-R., Æth., Lac-C.*).

VERY ACUTE HEARING (*Coff., Nux-V., Op.*) (Br.).

OTITIS MEDIA (*Calc., Hep., Merc., Sil.*) (Br.).

Severe, boring pains in the ears, which come on suddenly and shoot from one ear into the other (D.).

CONTORTION OF THE LIMBS (*Acon., Ars., Cupr., Mag-P., Sec., Stram.*).

SPASMS OF SINGLE LIMBS, OR OF THE WHOLE BODY (*Æth., Apis, Hell., Lach., Lyc., Nux-V., Stram., Strych., Verat.*).

Loss of sensation and motion of one side of the body (*Caust., Cocc., Phos., Plb., Rhus-T., Zinc.*).

Grinding of teeth during sleep (*Acon., Ars., Bry., Calc., Cann-I., Cina, Merc., Plb., Podo., Sant., Stram.*) (K.).

THROAT : DRY, AS IF GLAZED ; ANGRY LOOKING CONGESTION ; RED, WORSE ON RIGHT SIDE (Br.).

The child bores its head into the pillow, and rolls it from side to side (*Stram.*) (D.).

Inflammation of inner parts (mucous membranes) with a tendency to suppuration or with nervous symptoms (Asaf., Hep., Sil.).

Indurations after inflammations (Graph., Merc., Sil., Sulph.).

Parotid glands hard, red and swollen (*Brom., Phyt., Stram.*) (Bt.).

A white tongue with the papillæ showing through it ; the so-called "strawberry tongue" (D.).

SLEEPINESS, BUT CANNOT SLEEP (G.).

The child remains in a drowsy, sleepy state, with starting and jumping while sleeping (Bt.).

PULSE FULL AND HARD (*Acon., Ferr-P., Verat-V.*).

NERVOUS FEVERS, WITH LOSS OF CONSCIOUSNESS OR DELIRIUM (*Hyos., Kali-P., Op., Phos-Ac.*).

INFLAMMATION OF THE BRAIN (*Apis, Hell., Hyos., Lach., Mur-Ac., Op., Phos., Stram.*).

Sleeplessness with drowsiness, or sleep which is stuporlike (*Gels., Hyos., Lach.*).

Pain in the stomach, worse during a meal (*Calc-P., Nux-M., Nux-V.*) (D.).

Gastralgia, pains go to the spine (D.).

Swelling and induration of the glands (Calc., Calc-F., Carb-An., Merc-I., Sil.).

Summer complaints of children, with crying and screaming and suddenly bending backwards (D.).

Diarrhœa from cold, with slimy, bloody discharges and some tenesmus (D.).

PUPILS DILATED (*Arg-N.*, *Calc.*, *Chin.*, *Gels.*, *Hyos.*, *Mang.*, *Sec.*, *Stram.*).

AVERSION TO LIGHT (*Acon.*, *Arg-N.*, *Ars.*, *Bar-C.*, *Calc.*, *Carb-S.*, *Chin.*, *Con.*, *Euphr.*, *Graph.*, *Lac-C.*, *Lyc.*, *Merc.*, *Nat-M.*, *Nat-S.*, *Nux-V.*, *Op.*, *Rhus-T.*, *Sulph.*).

Loss of sight (*Acon.*, *Aur-M.*, *Bov.*, *Chin.*, *Gels.*, *Hyos.*, *Merc.*, *Puls.*, *Sil.*, *Stram.*).

Is indicated in fever when there are present symptoms of delirium and cerebral excitement, and a pungent heat of the skin (D.).

Colour of the face is bluish-red (*Lach.*).

Pressure as though all the contents of the abdomen would issue through the female genital organs ; this is particularly felt early in the morning (Bt.).

Os uteri rigid, hot and dry (G.).

Profuse flooding, with a feeling as if everything would issue from the vagina (*Sep.*) (Bt.).

Spasmodic contraction of the uterus (Bt.).

Alternate redness and paleness of the skin.

EXANTHEMATA OF SCARLET COLOUR (*Stram.*).

Erysipelas : with bright red, rapid swelling of the skin ; the skin is smooth, shining and tense ; the pains are sharp, lancinating, stinging and throbbing (D.).

CONVULSIONS AND SPASMS IN TEETHING CHILDREN (D.).

Liability to take cold with great sensitiveness to draft of air (*Calc.*, *Hep.*, *Kali-C.*, *Sil.*).

BREASTS FEEL HEAVY, ARE VERY HARD AND REDNESS RUNS IN RADII (STREAKS FROM A CENTRE) (Bt.).

Indurated mammæ (*Bry.*, *Phyt.*, *Puls.*, *Sil.*).

NEURALGIC PAINS COME ON SUDDENLY AND DISAPPEAR SUDDENLY (pains increase gradually and decrease gradually—*Stann.*) (D.).

It will be demanded in puerperal fever, and during the early stages of variola, and in scarlatina when the skin is uniformly smooth, shining, and of a scarlet redness (Bt.).

Pain in the right ileo-cœcal region, worse by the slightest touch, even of the bed-cover (A.).

SPASM OF THE GLOTTIS (*Brom.*, *Lach.*, *Stram.*) (C.).

Head hot and painful ; face flushed ; eyes wild, staring ; pupils dilated ; pulse full and bounding, globular, like buckshot striking the finger ; mucous membrane of the mouth dry ; stool tardy and urine suppressed ; sleepy, but cannot sleep (A.).

Involuntary micturition ; constant dribbling ; paralysis of sphincter vesicæ (N.).

Pain in the small of back, as if it would break ; also pain in the lumbar and sacral region (N.).

FRIGHTFUL DREAMS. DREAMS OF QUARRELS, FIRE, ETC. (B.).

HOT HEAD WITH COLD LIMBS (*Carb-An.*, *Kali-Ars.*, *Sep.*, *Stram.*) (B.).

Perspiration : hot ; during sleep ; profuse ; and in covered parts (K.).

Colicky pain (*in the abdomen*) *comes quickly and goes quickly* ; *better from bending double or bending backward* ; *also better from lying on the abdomen* (K.).

BARKING COUGH (*Dros.*, *Spong.*, *Verb.*) ; AWAKING AFTER MIDNIGHT, WITH PAIN IN THE LARYNX AND THREATENED SUFFOCATION (C.).

AGGRAVATION : In the afternoon ; at night ; from touching the parts affected even softly ; while swallowing liquids ; from motion ; from noise ; from draught of air ; while looking at bright, shining objects ; after 3 P. M. ; from uncovering the head ; and in summer sun.

AMELIORATION : While reposing ; while standing ; while leaning the head against something ; and in a warm room.

RELATIONSHIP. *Complementary* : *Calc.*

Bell. is the acute of *Calc.*, which is often required to complete a cure.

Similar to : *Acon.*, *Amyl-N.*, *Bry.*, *Cic.*, *Ferr-P.*, *Gels.*, *Glon.*, *Hyos.*, *Melil.*, *Op.*, *Stram.*, and *Verat-V.*

Benzoic Acid.

COMMON NAME : BENZOIC ACID.

May be indicated in any form of disease characterized by the peculiar urine.

The urine in the clothing scents the whole room (N.).

URINE DARK BROWN, AND THE URINOUS ODOUR HIGHLY INTENSIFIED (*Nit-Ac.*) (A.).

Offensive or pungent smell in the urine (*Calc.*, *Merc.* *Nit-Ac.*, *Sulph.*) (C.).

Urine offensive and of a deep red colour (*Berb.*, *Lyc.*, *Stram.*) (A.).

Vesical catarrh from suppressed gonorrhœa (*Puls.*, *Sep.*) (C.).

Cough, with expectoration of green mucus (*Nat-S.*) (A.).

Cracking of the joints when moving (*Caps.*, *Led.*, *Nit-Ac.*, *Petr.*, *Rhus-T.*) (G.).

Gout, worse at night (*Colch.*, *Nit-Ac.*) (A.).

Extreme weakness or lassitude (A.).

Redness and swelling of joints (*Apis*, *Bell.*, *Colch.* *Led.*, *Merc.*, *Stram.*) (A.).

Tearing or stitching pains in large joints of big toe (*Nit-Ac.*) (A.).

Enuresis nocturna of delicate children ; dribbling urine of old men, with enlarged prostate ; strong characteristic odour ; excess of uric acid (A.).

Inclination to dwell on unpleasant subjects.

Often omits words while writing (*Bar-C.*, *Lyc.*, *Phos-Ac.*).

Perspiration while eating (*Carb-An.*, *Carb-S.*, *Carb-V.*, *Kali-C.*, *Merc.*, *Nit-Ac.*, *Sep.*).

Sensation as of a lump in the pit of the throat (*Bell.*, *Phyt.*).

Diarrhœa : white, very offensive and exhausting stools, running right through the diaper (*Calc-P.*, *Crot-T.*, *Podo.*) (A.).

Chilliness before stool (*Ars., Merc., Phos., Verat.*).

Gouty concretions (*Calc., Lyc., Sep., Sil.*) (A.).

Affects all the joints, especially the knees (A.).

Gouty nodosities (*Berb., Lith-C., Lyc.*) (A.).

Heart troubles of rheumatic origin (N.).

Pain in the region of the heart (C.).

Pains suddenly change their locality (*Kali-B., Led., Puls.*) (C.).

Symptoms go from left to right, and from below upward (C.).

Circumscribed redness of the cheeks (*Chin., Ferr., Lyc., Phos., Sulph., Tub.*) (C.).

Night sweats (*Calc., Merc., Nit-Ac.*) (B.).

Profuse sweat, without relief (*Merc.*) (B.).

Angina faucicum and tonsilitis with exceedingly offensive and high coloured urine (N.).

Valvular deposits in the heart (*Kalm., Led., Lith-C.*) (F.).

Nodular swellings in the joints (*Amm-P., Calc., Lyc.*) (F.).

AGGRAVATION : From motion ; and at night.

AMELIORATION : From rest ; and in the day time.

RELATIONSHIP. *Similar to* : *Berb., Cop., Ferr., Lith-C., Nit-Ac., Sep., Thuj.*, and *Viol-T.*

Useful after *Colch.* fails in gout ; after abuse of *Cop.* in suppression of gonorrhœa.

Berberis Vulgaris.

COMMON NAME : BARBERRY.

Cold feeling in the prepuce and scrotum (*Brom.*, *Dios.*, *Merc.*).

Acts principally upon the kidneys, bladder and liver (D.).

It is called for when the renal and vesical symptoms are prominent (D.).

Cutting in the bladder, extending down the urethra (D.).

Stitch from the urethra into the bladder (G.).

Tearing pains in the bladder (D.).

Sensation as if some urine remained after urinating (*Alum.*, *Ars.*, *Calc.*, *Caust.*, *Clem.*, *Gels.*, *Hep.*, *Kali-C.*, *Mag-M.*, *Nux-V.*) (Br.).

SHORT COUGH AND CHEST COMPLAINTS, ESPECIALLY AFTER OPERATIONS FOR FISTULÆ (*Calc-P.*, *Sil.*) (A.).

Crawling, burning and itching in and about the anus (R.).

Neuralgia of spermatic cords and testicles (*Clem.*, *Dios.*, *Ox-Ac.*, *Puls.*) (Br.).

Stitch from the urethra into the bladder (G.).

Is useful in liver troubles when there are sticking pains in he region of the gall-bladder ; these may simulate gall-stone colic, and are followed by jaundice (*Chel.*, *Lyc.*) and clay-coloured stool (Bl.).

Sticking pains under the ribs (D.).

Pressure or sticking pain in the region of the liver (N.).

Pains go from the liver to the abdomen (*Chel.*) (D.).

Fatigued, worn-out expression of the countenance ; sunken cheeks ; deep-seated eyes, surrounded with bluish borders (G.).

ARTHRITIC AND RHEUMATIC AFFECTIONS, PARTICULARLY WITH URINARY COMPLICATIONS (*Benz-Ac.*, *Calc.*, *Colch.*, *Graph.*, *Led.*, *Lyc.*, *Nit-Ac.*, *Sep.*, *Sulph.*) (N.).

Empty or bilious eructations (*Nux-V.*, *Puls.*, *Sep.*) (G.).

FISTULA IN ANO, WITH STICKING IN THE PARTS, PARTICULARLY IF COMPLICATED WITH COUGH (N.).

Frequent or constant desire for stool (*Nux-V.*) (F.).

Hard stools like sheep dung ; or soft, easy stools, with burning in anus (G.).

Burning pain in the urethra before, during and after urination (*Cann-I.*, *Canth.*, *Merc.*, *Nit.Ac.*, *Puls.*) (K.).

Burning pain in the urethra, ameliorated after urination (*Bry.*, *Cocc.*).

URETHRA BURNS WHEN NOT URINATING (*Asaf.*, *Bry.*, *Clem.*, *Graph.*, *Merc.*, *Staph.*, *Sulph.*, *Thuj.*) (Br.).

URINE : THICK, TURBID, YELLOW ; RED, MEALY, SANDY OR SLIMY SEDIMENT (B.).

RENAL COLIC (*Lyc.*, *Nux-V.*, *Ocim.*, *Puls.*, *Sars.*, *Thuj.*) (K.).

PAINS EXTEND DOWN THE BACK, AND DOWN THE URETERS INTO THE BLADDER (D.).

BUBBLING SENSATION IN THE RENAL REGION (N.).

STICKING, TEARING PAINS IN THE RENAL REGION ; WORSE FROM DEEP PRESSURE (D.).

LUMBAGO (*Calc.*, *Calc-F.*, *Kali-P.*, *Lyc.*, *Nat-M.*, *Nux-V.*, *Rhus-T.*, *Sulph.*) (B.).

The lumbar region is very painful ; pain radiates in all directions (D.).

THE BACK FEELS STIFF AND NUMB, AND THE PAINS RADIATE FROM THE KIDNEYS TO IT (D.).

PAINS RADIATING FROM THE RENAL REGION AND EXTENDING TO THE THIGHS (N.).

BRUISED PAIN, WITH STIFFNESS AND LAME-NESS IN SMALL OF BACK ; RISES FROM SEAT WITH DIFFICULTY (N.).

Backache in the region of the kidneys ; worse while sitting or lying, and in the morning in bed (*Calc.*, *Lyc.*, *Sars.*) (N.).

Backache, extending to the pelvis and posterior portion of the thighs (N.).

BERBERIS is one of the great remedies for patients who suffer from what is known as the "lithic acid diathesis" (R.).

Movement brings on or increases the urinary complaints (A.).

Renal colic, worse in the left side (*Tab.* ; either side, with urging and strangury—*Canth.* ; worse in the right side—*Lyc.*) (A.).

Burning and soreness in the vagina (*Apis, Canth., Kreos., Merc-C., Nit-Ac., Sulph.*) (Br.).

VAGINISMUS (*Acon., Bell., Cact., Canth., Ferr-P., Ham., Ign., Lyc., Mag-P., Nat-M., Nux-V., Plat., Plb., Puls., Sil.*) (Br.).

Cutting pain in the vagina, during coition (*Ferr-M.*) (Br.).

SEXUAL DESIRE DIMINISHED IN FEMALES (*Agn., Bar-C., Caust., Ferr., Graph., Helon., Lyc., Nat-M.*) (Br.).

Menses scanty, with pain preceding the flow (*Caul., Puls., Sep.*).

Headache, aggravated by movement, and relieved in the open air.

Melancholy, inclination to weep (*Ign., Nat-M., Puls., Stann.*).

Inflammation of the tonsils and pharynx, with swelling and fiery redness, and a sensation as if a lump were lodged in the side of the throat.

Unrefreshing sleep (*Nux-V.*).

Perspires easily from the least exertion (*Agar., Calc., Chin., Ferr., Graph., Iod., Kali-C., Kali-P., Lyc., Nat-C., Psor.*).

AGGRAVATION : From motion ; while walking ;

from carriage-riding ; from any sudden, jarring movement ; from lying down ; and from deep pressure.

AMELIORATION : After urination.

RELATIONSHIP. *Similar to* : *Canth.*, *Dios.*, *Lyc.*, *Nux-V.*, *Ocim.*, *Puls.*, *Sars.*, and *Tab.*, in renal colic.

Acts well after *Arn.*, *Bry.*, *Kali-B.*, *Rhus-T.*, and *Sulph.*, in rheumatic affections.

Bismuth.

COMMON NAME : HYDRATED OXIDE
OF BISMUTH.

Gastralgia alternating with headache (Bl.).

Dull, heavy headache (*Bry.*, *Cocc.*, *Nux-V.*, *Phos-Ac.*, *Sil.*) (Bt.).

Sensation of heaviness in inner parts (*Bry.*, *Calc.*, *Nux-V.*, *Phos.*).

Flushes of heat, especially upon the head and chest.

ANGUISH. HE SITS, THEN WALKS, THEN LIES, —NEVER LONG IN ONE PLACE (*Ars.*, *Kali-Br.*, *Phos.*) (A.).

Screwing pains.

Pressing, tearing in the bones of the hands and of the feet.

Cramping pains in the extremities (*Coloc.*, *Cupr.*, *Mag-P.*, *Plb.*, *Sec.*) (Bl.).

Morose, discontented and complaining about his condition (C.).

SOLITUDE IS UNBEARABLE (*Stram.*).

The child holds on to its mother's hand for company (*Kali-C.*, *Lil-T.*, *Lyc.*) (A.).

Pressing pain in the eyes, head, abdomen and testicles.

Catarrhal inflammation and irritation of the alimentary canal (Bl.).

Nausea after every meal (*Bry.*, *Cocc.*, *Colch.*, *Ipec.*, *Nux-V.*, *Puls.*, *Sep.*) (Bt.).

BURNING IN THE STOMACH, WITH VOMITING (*Ars.*, *Canth.*, *Phos.*, *Sec.*) (Bt.).

Lancinating, burning or griping pain in the epigastrium, causing him to bend backward (*Bell.*, *Caust.*, *Dios.*, *Kali-C.*) (Bl.).

Vomiting of all fluids (*in children*) ; *spasmodic vomiting* ; *food is ejected from the stomach with great force, as soon as it is partaken of* (*Ars.*) (Bl.).

Intense pressure, as of a load, in the stomach (Bt.).

Craves cold drink (*Apis*, *Ars.*, *Phos.*) (B.).

Face : deathly pale ; blue rings around the eyes (*Cina*, *Staph.*) (A).

Bitter or metallic taste in the mouth (*Merc.*) (C.).

Painless diarrhœa, accompanied with great thirst and vomiting (Bl.).

Frequent waking at night as from fright (*Bell.*, *Hyos.*, *Stram*) (C.).

10

Lascivious dreams, with seminal emissions (*Nux-V.,* *Phos., Sulph.*) (C.).

Headache returning every winter (A.).

Headache alternating with, or attended by gastralgia (A.).

VOMITING OF WATER, AS SOON AS IT REACHES THE STOMACH (*Ars., Bry., Cadm., Crot-T., Eup-P., Nux-V., Sep., Zinc.*) ; FOOD RETAINED LONGER (vomits food and water—*Ars.*) (A.).

Cardialgia and pyrosis (Nux-V., Puls.) (A.).

Toothache : ameliorated by holding cold water in the mouth (*Bry., Coff., Puls.*) (A.).

VOMITING OF ENORMOUS QUANTITIES, AT INTERVALS OF SEVERAL DAYS, WHEN FOOD HAS FILLED THE STOMACH (A.).

Convulsive gagging and inexpressible pain after laparotomy (*Nux-V., Staph.*).

Slow digestion, with fetid eructations (Br.).

Vomiting and purging, with great prostration, flatulence, white tongue and cadaverous stools (G.).

Cholera morbus and summer complaint, when vomiting predominates (*Ant-C., Ars., Podo.*) (A.).

Stools : foul, papescent, watery, offensive, and very prostrating (*Ars., Kali-P., Verat.*) (A.).

Eructations of wind after drinking water (C.).

Black ulcers (*Ars., Carb Ac., Lach., Sec.*). (B.).

Angina pectoris : Pain around heart, left arm to fingers (*Acon., Ars., Cact., Mag-P., Nux-V.*) (Br.).

Bismuth is one of our best remedies for cholera infantum—genuine cholera infantum—where the disease is sudden in its onset, and rapid in its course (N.).

Frequent and copious micturition (*Apis, Merc., Phos-Ac.*).

Surface covered with warm sweat (*Bell.*) (N.).

Cancer of the stomach (*Ars., Con., Kali-B., Kreos., Lach., Lyc., Nit-Ac., Phos., Sec.*) (G.).

AGGRAVATION : When alone ; during summer ; during winter ; from eating and drinking.

AMELIORATION : From cold drinks ; from holding cold water in the mouth (toothache) ; from remaining in company ; and while in motion.

RELATIONSHIP. *Similar to* : *Ars., Nux-V., Kreos., Phos., Sec.* and *Verat.*

Antidotes : *Calc., Caps.,* and *Nux-V.*

Blatta Orientalis.

COMMON NAME : INDIAN COCKROACH.

It appears to be most serviceable in corpulent individuals (*Amm-M., Calc., Graph., Kali-B., Kali-C., Phos.*) (Bl.).

ASTHMA, ESPECIALLY WHEN ASSOCIATED WITH BRONCHITIS (*Bry., Calc-S., Kali-M., Lyc., Merc., Nat-M., Phos., Sep., Sulph., Tab.*) (Br.).

Severe attacks of coughing, with dyspnœa (*Ant-T., Ars., Carb-V., Kali-Ars., Lach., Lyc., Nat-S.*) (Bl.).

Phthisis, with much pus-like mucus (*Ars., Calc., Hep., Kali-C., Kreos., Phos., Sep., Sil., Sulph.*) (Br.).

AGGRAVATION : During night ; and from lying down.

AMELIORATION : From expectoration.

RELATIONSHIP. It has cured bad cases of general dropsy, after *Apis*, *Apoc.*, and *Dig.* failed.

In asthma it is indicated after *Ars.*, when this is insufficient.

Borax.

COMMON NAME : BIBORATE OF SODA.

Anxious expression of face during the downward motions (Br.).

Nausea and giddiness from exertions of the mind (*Cocc.*, *Ferr-P.*, *Nux-V.*, *Puls.*, *Sep.*).

The whole buccal cavity covered with a white fungous growth (Bt.).

SORE MOUTH OF NURSING CHILDREN (*Bry.*, *Calc.*, *Kali-M.*, *Merc.*, *Rhus-T.*, *Sil.*) (D.).

APHTHÆ OF THE MOUTH AND TONGUE, WHICH BLEED EASILY (*Ars.*, *Carb-V.*, *Kreos.*, *Nat-M.*, *Nit-Ac.*, *Phos.*, *Sulph.*).

Mouth hot and tender (Br.).

Painful gum-boil (*Hep.*, *Merc.*, *Sil.*) (Br.).

Crying when nursing (Br.).

SENSITIVE TO SUDDEN NOISES. VIOLENT FRIGHT FROM REPORT OF A GUN, EVEN AT A DISTANCE (Br.).

FEAR OF THUNDER (*Phos.*) (Br.).

Excessively nervous, easily frightened (*Gels.*, *Kali-C.*, *Puls.*) (Br.).

Extreme anxiety, especially from motions which have a downward direction, rocking, being carried downstairs, or being laid down (Br.).

THERE IS DREAD OF DOWNWARD MOTION (D.).

FEAR OF FALLING IN CHILDREN, WHEN THEY ARE CARRIED DOWNSTAIRS (*Gels.*).

Starts and throws up hands on laying patient down, as if afraid of falling (Br.).

Acne in plethoric, young females (Bt.).

Parts which are usually red, turn white (*Ferr.*).

VERTIGO WHEN GOING DOWNSTAIRS (*Carb-Ac.*, *Chrom-Ac.*, *Con.*, *Gins.*, *Merl.*, *Merc.*, *Phys.*, *Plat.*, *Tarant.*) (N.).

Stinging or drawing, stitching pains (*Apis*, *Nit-Ac.*).

Pleurisy-like pain in the right pectoral region ; so that the patient can't move or breathe without a stitching pain (*Bry.*, *Kali-C.*, *Phos.*) (G.).

Salivation, especially during dentition (A.).

Weakness in the joints (*Caust.*, *Nat M.*, *Sil.*).

Stoppage of the right nostril, or first the right and then the left, with constant blowing of the nose (*Amm-C.*, *Lac-C.*, *Mag-M.*) (A.).

Unhealthy, easily suppurating skin (*Hep.*, *Sil.*, *Sulph.*)

The hair is rough and frowsy ; can't be combed smooth, gets into all kinds of snarls ; splits ; sticks together (G.).

Scabs and thick crusts in the nose (G.).

Granular eyelids (*Arg-N.*, *Caust.*, *Graph.*, *Nat-M.*, *Sep.*, *Sulph.*, *Thuj.*) (G.).

Blepharitis, with much soreness of the eyelids and agglutination after sleep (R.).

DESIRE TO RUB THE EYES (*All-C.*, *Apis*, *Carb-Ac.*, *Caust.*, *Con. Croc.*, *Fluor-Ac.*, *Kali-B.*, *Mezer.*) (K.).

LASHES TURN INWARD (*Graph.*, *Nat M.*, *Sep.*) Br.).

INVERSION OF EYELIDS (*Anan.*, *Calc.*, *Graph.*, *Merc.*, *Nat-M.*, *Nit-Ac.*, *Sulph.*, *Zinc.*) (K.).

REDNESS OF THE MARGINS OF THE EYELIDS (*Arg-N.*, *Ars.*, *Calc.*, *Carb-S.*, *Eup-P.*, *Euphr.*, *Graph.*, *Merc-C.*, *Nat M.*, *Rhus-T.*, *Sulph.*, *Zinc.*) (K.).

Anxious expression, when mother goes to lay the child down out of her arms (N.).

Menses too soon and too profuse, and attended with colic (Bt.).

Membranous dysmenorrhœa (*Brom.*, *Cham.*, *Lac-C.*) (Bl.).

COPIOUS, CLEAR AND ALBUMINOUS LEUCOR-RHŒA (*Alum.*, *Bov.*, *Nat-M.*, *Sep.*) (D.).

LEUCORRHŒA OF TRANSPARENT MUCUS AFTER MENSES ; FEELS AS IF WARM WATER WERE FLOWING (G.).

Sterility, with concomitant symptoms (G.).

Pruritus pudendi (*Ambr.*, *Calad.*, *Calc.*, *Kreos.*, *Merc.*, *Nat-M.*, *Nit-Ac.*) (Bl.).

Eczema of the vulva (*Ars.*, *Calc.*, *Dulc.*, *Graph.*, *Kreos.*, *Petr.*, *Rhus-T.*) (Bl.)

CHILD SCREAMS BEFORE URINATING (*Lach.,
Lyc., Nux-V., Sars.,* weeps before stool—*Phos., Puls.,
Rhus-T.*) (Br.).

Child weeps during stool (*Æth., Cham., Cina, Phos.,
Sil., Sulph.*) (K.),

Mucous stools, with aphthous sore mouth (*Ars., Ipec.,
Merc., Nux-V.*) (Br.).

Diarrhœa : stools loose, pappy and offensive ; preceded
by colic (Br.).

Brown, watery or green stools in infants (G.).

Smoking may bring on diarrhœa (*Brom., Cham.*) (A.).

The urine is hot and emits a pungent odour (*Benz-Ac.,
Nit-Ac.*) (R.).

Is obliged every few minutes to take a deep breath
(*Bry., Ign., Phos.*) (C.).

AGGRAVATION : From descending ; from laughing :
after menstruation ; from downward motion ; from sudden
noises ; before urinating ; and during cold weather.

AMELIORATION : From pressure ; holding painful
side with the hand.

RELATIONSHIP. *Borax* follows : *Calc., Psor.,
Sanic.* and *Sulph.*

Is followed by : *Ars., Bry., Lyc., Phos., Sil.*

Incompatible : Should not be used before or after
Acetic Acid, vinegar and wine.

Bovista.

COMMON NAME : PUFF BALL.

Headache (deep in the brain), with a feeling as though the head were enormously large or swollen (F.).

Discharge from the nose and all mucous membranes very tough, stringy and tenacious (Kali-B.) (A.).

Pale swelling of the upper lip.

Found it useful in epistaxis. Whether the hæmorrhage be associated with menstrual irregularity, or whether it arises from traumatism, *Bovista* may be the remedy (F.).

Bleeding of the nose early in the morning (during Sleep).

Bad effects of inhalation of charcoal vapours (*Arn., Op.*) (F.).

Ebullitions, with much thirst (Acon., Bell., Ferr-P., Sulph.).

Colic : the patient finds relief from bending double after eating (F.).

Intolerance of tight clothing around the waist (Calc., Carb-V., Lach., Lyc., Nux-V., Sulph.) (A.).

Sweat in axilla, smells like onions (*Petr.*) (A.).

Bleeding of the gums when sucking them (*Amm-C., Carb-V., Kali-B., Nit-Ac., Rat., Zinc.*).

Great weakness in the joints (Calc., Caust., Kali-C., Nat-M.).

Hæmorrhage : after extraction of teeth (*Arn.*, *Ham.*, *Kreos.*, *Mill.*, *Trill.*) (A.).

Hæmorrhages from relaxation of the capillary system ; epistaxis or menstrual hæmorrhages, where the blood flows with very little exertion ; the flow occurs more at night or in the morning (D.).

Diarrhœa : the stools are followed by tenesmus and burning (*Sulph.*) (F.).

Ineffectual urging to stool (*Nux-V.*). Diarrhœa before and during menses (*Amm-C.*) (A.).

Red urine (*Bell.*, *Lyc.*, *Sars.*) (F.).

Frequent desire to urinate, even immediately after urination.

Chilliness predominating during the pain (*Ars* , *Caust.*, *Puls.*, *Sep.*).

Awkwardness (*Æth.*, *Apis*, *Ign.*, *Lach.*, *Nat-M.*, *Nux-V.*) (F.).

AWKWARD IN SPEECH AND ACTION (B.).

Inclined to drop things from hands (*Apis*) (A.).

STUTTERING OR STAMMERING (*Bell.*, *Lach.*, *Stram.*) (F.).

Sad, depressed, and desponding (*Aur.*, *Ign.*, *Nat-M.*, *Puls.*, *Stann.*, *Sep.*).

Weak memory (*Agn.*, *Kali-P.*, *Phos.*).

Dull instruments produce deep impressions on the flesh ; for instance, the scissors on the fingers in using them.

FLOW BETWEEN THE PERIODS (*Calc.*, *Cham.*, *Ipec.*, *Phos.*, *Rhus-T.*, *Sabin.*, *Sil.*) (B.).

MENSES : FLOW ONLY AT NIGHT ; NOT IN THE DAY TIME (*Mag-C.* ; only during day, ceases lying —*Cact.*, *Caust.*, *Lil-T.*) (A.).

Thick slimy, tenacious, acrid or corrosive leucorrhœa (*Kreos.*, *Nat-M.*, *Sep.*). Voluptuous sensation in the female genitalia (Br.).

It produces an eruption much resembling herpes, which bleeds readily (F.).

MOIST   TETTER   (*Graph.*,   *Nat-M.*,   *Rhus-T.*). Urticaria, when attended with diarrhœa (F.).

Eruptions in the corners of the mouth. Eczema in back of the hand (*Graph.*, *Merc.*, *Sil.*) (Br.).

ITCHING COCCYX (*Agar.*, *Alum.*, *Bar C.*, *Bor.*, *Con.*, *Fluor-Ac.*, *Graph.*, *Lyc.*, *Petr.*, *Spig.*) (B.).

ITCHING ERUPTIONS : OOZING ; FORMING THICK CRUSTS OR SCABS, WITH PUS BENEATH (*Mezer.*) (B.).

Intolerable itching at tip of coccyx ; must scratch till parts become raw and sore (A.).

Acne on the face, worse in summer ; due to use of cosmetics (Br.).

The symptoms of asphyxia caused by this remedy are very much like those produced by the fumes of charcoal (*Arn.*) (F.).

Sleepiness after dinner, and early in the morning (*Nux-V.*).

The heart feels enormously large, with oppression of the chest and palpitation (F.).

Palpitation after a meal (Abies-C., *Calc.*, *Lyc.*, *Puls.*) *and also during menstruation* (F.).

Great weariness of hands and feet (*Gels.*, *Kali-P.*, *Phos.*, *Plb.*, *Rhus-T.*) (A.).

Objects fall from powerless hands (A.).

Tremor of the hands, with palpitation of the heart and

oppressive anxiety.

Objects seem to be too near the eye (*Phys., Rhus-T. Stram.*).

Dim eyes, without lustre (*Camph., Lyc., Verat.*).

Vertigo and feeling of stupidity in the head on rising (C.).

Vertigo ; falls over ; momentarily unconscious in the morning (C.).

Discharge of fetid pus from the ears (*Asaf., Calc., Hep., Merc., Sil., Tell.*).

Itching in the ears (*Rhus-T., Sulph.*).

Sensation as of a lump of ice in the stomach (*Colch.* ; sensation as of a burning ball—*Bell.*) (G.).

Nausea (in the morning) before breakfast (*Alum., Berb., Calc., Lyc., Nit-Ac., Petr., Sep., Tub.*) (K.).

Darting pain from perineum to rectum (G.).

Intermittent fever : chill every day from 7 to 10 P.M. (C.).

Chill, after going to bed at night.

Morning sweat, especially on the chest.

Chilliness and heat, with thirst.

Sensation in the wrist-joint, as if sprained.

In the urethra, stinging, itching, burning ; the orifice is inflamed, and feels as if glued up (*Graph.*).

Itching in the rectum, as from worms. Flatulency or rumbling, with constipation.

AGGRAVATION : At night ; during morning ; before and during menses ; after eating ; and when blowing the nose.

AMELIORATION : In the day-time ; from taking meals ; and from bending double.

RELATIONSHIP. Has been used as an antidote to the effects of charcoal fumes (**A.**).

It also antidotes effects of local applications of tar.

In chronic urticaria use *Bovista*, when *Rhus-T.* seemed indicated, but failed to cure.

Compare : *Amm-C.*, *Bell.*, *Calc.*, *Mag-S.*, and *Sep.* in menstrual irregularities.

ANTIDOTE : *Camphor.*

Bromium.

COMMON NAME: BROMINE.

An important remedy in laryngeal affections ; also in scrofulous and tubercular affections of the glands (N.).

Has done some wonderful work in diphtheria. The membrane first forms in the bronchi, trachea or larynx running upward (just opposite of *Lyc.*, which often forms first in the nose and runs downward) (N.).

Faucial angina and very troublesome sorethroat.

Complaints on the left side of the body (*Lach.*).

General trembling (*Arg N.*, *Kali-Br.*, *Phos.*, *Plb.*, *Zinc.*).

MEMBRANOUS CROUP : GREAT RATTLING OF MUCUS (*Ant-T.*, *Hep.*, *Nat-S.*, *Phos.*, *Sil.*, *Sulph.*). BUT NO EXPECTORATION. THERE SEEMS TO BE GREAT DANGER OF SUFFOCATION FROM ACCUMULATION OF MUCUS IN THE LARYNX (in bronchi—*Ant-T.*) (N.).

A sensation of something being alive in the skin, principally in the arms and legs.

Sensation of cobweb in the face (*Bor., Graph.*) (N.).

He perspires freely when exercising a little (*Bry., Chin., Nat-M.*).

SAILORS SUFFER FROM ASTHMA "ON SEA-SHORE" (A.).

Fan-like motion of alæ nasi (*Ant-T., Lycop.*) (N.).

DIZZINESS WHEN LYING DOWN, WITH HEAD ACHE, ESPECIALLY IN THE EVENING. DIZZINESS WHEN GOING OVER A RUNNING WATER.

Chest pains running upward (A.).

Hypertrophy of the heart from gymnastics (*Arn., Caust., Phos., Rhus-T.*) (N.).

Stony hard, scrofulous or tuberculous swelling of glands, especially on lower jaw and throat (thyroid, submaxillary, parotid, testes) (A.).

Croupy symptoms with hoarseness during whooping cough ; gasping for breath (A.).

Membranous dysmenorrhœa (*Bor., Lac-C., Merc-C.*) (N.).

Physometra : *loud emission of flatus from the vagina* (*Lyc.*) (A.).

Tumour in breasts, with stitching pains (*Con., Phyt., Sil.*) (Br.).

Chronic ovaritis (*Apis, Lach., Lyc., Merc., Puls.*) (R.).

Menses too early and too profuse (*Calc., Chin., Phos.*) (R.).

Cannot bear pressure on the mammæ ; stitching pain from the mammæ to the axillæ (R.).

SWELLING AND INDURATION OF THE (LEFT) TESTICLE, WITH SORE PAIN, OR SENSATION OF COLDNESS.

Great watchfulness in the evening. He has much trouble in getting to sleep at night.

Anguish in sleep, and sleep full of dreams.

Constant dreaming in sleep (Nat-C., Nux-V., Op., Phos., Staph.).

Jerking and starting whilst in sleep (Bell., Cina, Hyos., Stram.).

When getting awake at night trembling and sensation as if she could not rise for weakness.

Fantasy and illusions when asleep (Coff., Op., Phys. Piper-M.).

He cannot sleep enough in the morning.

He feels unrefreshed in the morning (*Cocc., Coff., Nux-V.*).

Colic, as if the abdomen would burst (*Arg-N., Cham., Lyc.*) (G.).

Diarrhœa, after taking oysters (*Aloe, Lyc., Podo., Sulph-Ac.*) (K.).

Excellent for patients in very bad humour (Bry. Cham., Cina, Nux-V., Sulph.). Quarrelsomeness (Aur. Bell., Nux-V., Stram., Sulph.).

Delusion that strange persons are looking over patient's shoulder, and that she would see some one on turning (Br.).

Desire for mental labour (G.).

Weakness of memory (*Ambr., Bar-C., Caust., Med., Nux-M. Phos-Ac., Sep., Verat.*) (K.).

Low spirited before menses (Br.).

Deep hoarse voice (Carb-V., Caust., Phos.) (D.).

Inspiration produces coughing (Acon., Bell., Calc., Camph., Hep., Kali-B., Meny., Puls., Rumx., Squil., Stict., Verb.) (D.).

SUFFOCATIVE FITS ; HE STARTS UP CHOKED WITH CROUPY OR WHEEZING COUGH (B.).

Spasm of the glottis (Chlor., Cupr., Phos.). (B.).

Extensive hepatization of the lower lobes of the lungs (Bt.).

Dyspnœa : cannot inspire deep enough ; as if breathing through a sponge or the air passages were full of smoke or vapour of sulphur ; rattling, sawing ; voice inaudible ; danger of suffocation from mucus in larynx (in bronchi—*Ant-T.*) (A.).

Thick, white expectoration (*Kali-M.*) (B.).

Cold sensation in larynx on· inspiration (*Rhus-T., Sulph.*) ; better after shaving (worse after shaving— *Carb An.*) (A.).

It should be remembered in fluent coryza, when there is long continued sneezing ; the margin of the nose and parts under the nose are corroded, painful and bleeding when wiped (Bl.).

AGGRAVATION : In the evening ; before midnight ; when at rest ; when lying down ; in warm, damp weather.

AMELIORATION : When moving about during exercise ; and when at sea.

RELATIONSHIP. *Compare* : in croup and croupy affections : *Chlor., Hep., Iod.,* and *Spong.*

Hard goitre cured after *Iod.* failed. *Brom.* has cured in croup after failure of *Hep., Iod., Phos.,* and *Spong.* ; especially in relapses after *Iod.*

Bryonia Alba.

COMMON NAMES : WHITE BRYONY ;
WILD HOP.

Rheumatic pains in the limbs with tension ; aggravated by motion and contact.

Stiffness in the joints (Amm-M., Bell., Caust., Colch., Rhus-T.).

Oversensitiveness of the senses to external impressions (Bell., Coff., Nux-V.).

AN IRRITABLE MOOD AND INCLINED TO BE ANGRY (*Nat-M., Nux-V., Sulph.*).

Ailments from chagrin, mortification or anger (Coloc., Ign., Staph.) (A.).

Desires things immediately which are not to be had, or which when offered are refused *(Cham.)* (A.).

THE CHILD DISLIKES TO BE CARRIED OR TO BE RAISED (A.).

During delirium the patient expresses a continual "desire to go home". He imagines that he is not at home and longs to be taken there in order to be properly cared for (F.).

Diarrhœa : bilious, acrid stools, with soreness of the anus ; stools like dirty water (leucorrhœa like blackish water—*Rhus-T.*) ; stools of undigested food (A.).

Diarrhœa ; from cold drinks when overheated, from fruit, or sour kraut ; worse in the morning, on moving even a hand or foot (A.).

DIARRHŒA : from cold drinks when over-heated, from fruit, or sour kraut ; worse in the morning, or on moving, even a hand or foot (A.).

Eyes very sore, and feel as if they would be pressed out of the head (Bt.).

During colic, must keep very still (G.).

Peritonitis : with stinging, burning pains (*Apis, Ars., Bell., Lach., Phos., Sulph.*) ; *abdomen very sore to the touch, with constipation* (Bt.).

Inflammation of the liver, with stitching pains, aggravated by motion (Bt.).

Tensive, burning pains in the region of the liver, which is swollen and sore (Hm.).

FREQUENT BLEEDING OF THE NOSE, WHEN THE MENSES SHOULD APPEAR (G.).

Swelling and stiffness of the affected parts (*Apis, Bell., Colch., Kali-C.*).

PRICKING, DARTING AND STINGING IN THE JOINTS, MUSCLES AND INNER PARTS.

Inflammations of the inner parts (*lungs and liver*).

Pain in the bones, as if the flesh had been beaten off

COLOUR OF THE FACE BLUISH-RED.

HEADACHE FROM IRONING (*Sep.*) (A.).

HEADACHE : AS IF THE HEAD WOULD SPLIT OPEN ; GREATLY AGGRAVATED BY MOTION, OPENING THE EYES, OR STOOPING ; RELIEVED BY PRESSURE AND CLOSING THE EYES (Bt.).

Headache from constipation (*Nux-V.*) (A.).

Congestive headache, as if forehead would burst open, *with epistaxis* (*Lach., Sep.*) (Bt.).

Nausea while drinking (K.).

CANNOT SIT UP FROM NAUSEA AND FAINTNESS (G.).

VOMITING OF BITTER SUBSTANCE (BILE) (*Cadm-S , Eup-P., Ipec., Nat-S., Nux-V., Podo.*).

THIRST ; HE DRINKS NOT OFTEN, BUT MUCH AT A TIME.

The taste is bitter and the tongue is dry and has *a yellowish coat.*

Dry, cracked lips (*Nat-M.*) (G.).

The mouth is unusually dry, with thirst (*Ars.,* *Nat-M., Sulph.*) (Bt.).

EVERYTHING TASTES BITTER (EVERYTHING TASTES BITTER EXCEPT WATER— *Acon., Stann.*) (Bt.)

Food is thrown up immediately after eating (*Ars.*) (G.).

PRESSURE IN THE PIT OF THE STOMACH, AS IF THERE WAS A STONE IN IT ; GOES OFF WITH MUCH ERUCTATION (*Carb-V., Nux-V.,* *Puls.*) (Bt.).

CONSTIPATION : FROM INDURATION OF THE STOOLS, OR BECAUSE THE FÆCES ARE TOO LARGE IN SIZE (*Op., Plb., Sel., Sulph.*).

Diarrhœa in the morning, as soon as she moves (*Nat-S.*) (Bt.).

Diarrhœa brought on by cold drinks in **warm** weather (diarrhœa) from drinking impure **water—** *Zingib.* (Bt.).

Diarrhœa after castor oil (K.).

CONSTIPATION, STOOLS DRY AND HARD, AS IF BURNT (Bt.).

Constipation, from inactivity of the rectum (*Alum., Op., Sulph.*); *no inclination* (*Plat., Sep., Sil.*); *stools large, hard, dark and dry* (A.).

Constipation of emigrants (from carriage-riding— *Ign., Plat.*).

Constipation on going to sea (*Plat.* ; constipation at sea-shore—*Mag-M.*) (A.).

RESPIRATION OPPRESSED AND DEEP (*Ant-T., Ars., Phos.*).

Cough : dry, spasmodic, with gagging and vomiting (*Kali-C.*); with stitches in the side of the chest ; with headache, as if the head would fly to pieces ; worse after eating, drinking, entering a warm room, and a deep inspiration.

Dry, hard racking cough, with scanty expectoration (*Nux-V.*) (A.).

Blood spitting or hæmoptysis (*Acon., Ars., Bell., Cact., Ferr., Lach., Mill., Nit-Ac., Phos., Puls., Rhus-T., Sep.*) (A.).

COMPLAINTS FROM SUPPRESSED DISCHARGES (SUCH AS MENSES, MILK, ETC.) OR ERUPTION OF AN ACUTE EXANTHEMATA (A.).

Chilliness after anger (*Acon., Ars., Cham., Nux-V., Teucr.*) (A.).

The pulse is hard and hurried (*Acon., Bell., Ferr-P., Stram., Verat-V.*).

REPERCUSSION OF ERUPTIONS (*Apis, Ars., Cupr., Hell., Phos., Sulph., Zinc.*).

Undeveloped measles (*Apis, Gels., Zinc.*) (B.).

Urine : hot, red, and diminished in quantity (Bt.).

Dark and scanty urine (A.).

Menses : too early, too profuse, and worse on motion (G.).

Frequent bleeding of the nose when the menses should appear (G.).

Vicarious menses (*Lach., Phos., Puls.*) (A.).

During menses, tearing pains in the legs, worse on motion (G.).

MAMMÆ : HEAVY ; OF A STONY HARD-NESS ; PALE BUT HARD ; HOT AND PAINFUL (*Bell*) ; MUST SUPPORT THE BREASTS (*Phyt.*) (A.).

Milk fever (*Ferr P., Puls., Rhus-T*) (F.).

Suppressed lochia (*Bell., Cham., Hyos., Nux-V., Op., Puls., Pyrog., Sec., Stram., Sulph., Verat., Zinc.*) (K.).

CHEWING MOTION OF THE JAW (*Acon., Bell., Calc., Cham., Hell., Ign., Merc., Phos.*) (K.).

DELIRIUM : TALKS CONSTANTLY ABOUT HIS BUSINESS (*Ars., Canth , Hyos., Stram.*), OR IN HIS DELIRIUM DESIRES TO GET OUT OF BED AND GO HOME (*Cimic., Hyos.*). (A.).

A sovereign remedy or all inflammations that have advanced to the stage of serous effusion (*Apis, Sulph.*) (Bt.).

Sour or oily sweat (*Calc., Mag-C., Merc., Nux-V., Sumb., Thuj.*) (B.).

Complains of heavy pressure just over the sternum (*Phos.*) (F.).

Pleurisy with effusion (*Apis, Kali-C., Phos., Sulph.*) (F.).

Pleuro-pneumonia ; *after croupous exudation* (F.).

Synovitis ; the affected joint is pale-red and tense ; there are sharp, stitching pains, aggravated by any motion (F.).

In intermittent fever the chills commences at the lips, or from the tips of the fingers and toes (Bl.).

In typhoid fever it is frequently of service when the mucous membranes are dry, the lips and tongue are parched and cracked, and the stools are dry, as if burnt. The patient is drowsy, or sleeps during the day, but is delirious at night, and desires to remain perfectly quiet.

AGGRAVATION : At 9 P. M. ; by motion ; from moving the affected parts ; during inspiration ; while lying on the painless side ; f om touch ; from warmth ; and during summer

AMELIORATION : While exhaling ; while lying on the painful side ; by tightly bandaging the affected parts ; from pressure ; during rest ; and from taking cold things

RELATIONSHIP. *Complementary* : *Alum.* and *Rhus-T*.

Similar to : *Apis, Bell, Hep, Kali-C., Merc., Phos, Puls., Ran-B., Sep.* and *Sulph.*

Cactus Grandiflorus.

COMMON NAME : NIGHT BLOOMING CEREUS.

In diseases that call for the use of *Cactus*, there will always be found more or less derangement of the heart (Bt.).

Sanguineous congestions in persons of plethoric habit (*Acon*, *Bell.*, *Ferr-P.*), often resulting in hæmorrhage A.).

HÆMORRHAGE : FROM NOSE, LUNGS, STOMACH, RECTUM OR BLADDER (*Arn.*, *Crot-H.*, *Ferr-P.*, *Mill.*, *Nit-Ac.*, *Phos.*) (A.).

Constriction of œsophagus (Br.).

Fear of death (*Acon.*, *Ars.*, *Calc.*, *Cimic.*, *Gels.*, *Lac-C.*, *Nit-Ac.*, *Phos.*, *Plat.*) **(A.).**

Believes the disease incurable (*Ars.*) **(A.).**

Melancholic, taciturn, sad and ill-humoured (Br.).

Angina pectoris (*Acon.*, *Ars.*, *Lach.*, *Lat-M.*, *Spig.*, *Verat.*) (Br.).

Pain in the apex of the heart, shooting down the left arm (Br.).

Adapted to hypertrophy of the heart ; palpitation of the heart ; rheumatism of the heart ; and acute and chronic carditis with rheumatism (Bt.).

Constriction : of throat, chest, heart, bladder, rectum, uterus and vagina ; often caused or brought on by the slightest contact (*Bell.*) (A.).

FEELING AS THOUGH AN IRON HAND WAS AROUND THE HEART, PREVENTING ITS NORMAL MOTION (Bt.).

Oppression of the chest, as from a great weight (*Ars., Bry., Phos.*) (A.).

Palpitation of the heart in debilitated patients ; worse when lying on the left side, when walking, and at night, with melancholy (Bt.).

Sensation of a cord tightly tied around lower part of chest, marking attachment of diaphragm (A.).

Acute rheumatism of the diaphragm (F.).

Heart feels as if clasped and unclasped rapidly by an iron hand ; as if bound ; "had no room to beat" (A.).

Chronic bronchitis, with profuse rattling of mucus in the lungs (*Ant-T , Carb-V., Hep., Lyc., Nat-S.*) (Bt.).

Hæmoptysis, with cardiac affections (*Lach., Naja, Phos.*) (D.).

Difficulty of breathing (Apis, Ars., Bry., Calc., Dig., Ferr-P., Gels., Hep., Ipec., Kali C., Lach., Mosch., Nux-V., Op.) (Bt.).

Arterial pulsation in the scrobiculus (Bt.).

THE WHOLE BODY FEELS AS IF CAGED, EACH WIRE BEING TWISTED TIGHTER AND TIGHTER (A.).

Rheumatism of all joints, beginning in upper extremities (beginning in lower extremities—*Led.*) (N.).

Right-sided prosopalgia ; constricting pains ; returns at the same hour daily (*Cedr.*) (Br.).

Headache : pressing like a heavy weight on the vertex ; during climacteric ; congestive ; periodic ; right-sided ; severe, throbbing, pulsating pain (A.).

Feels as if head were compressed in a vise (Br.).

Profuse nose-bleed with organic heart-disease (N.).

Menstrual flow ceases while lying down (Bov., Caust.) (A.).

Palpitation at approach of menses (A.).

Menses too early, dark, pitch-like (*Cocc., Kali-N., Mag-C.* (Br.).

Periodical attacks of suffocation, with fainting, cold perspiration on face and loss of pulse (N.).

Œdema of hands and feet (*Apis, Ars., Aur., Dig., Lach., Lyc., Nat-M., Phos., Puls., Rhus-T., Sep, Sulph.*) (Br.)

Quotidian intermittent fever (C.).

Fever paroxysm returns at 11 A. M. and 11 P. M. (A.).

Chilliness and chattering of the teeth not relieved by covering (R.).

Coldness predominates (*Camph., Kali-I., Verat.* (C.).

Burning heat with shortness of breath (R.).

Scorching heat at night with headache following a chill and terminating in perspiration (R.).

Constant irritation in urethra (*Apis, Canth., Merc-C.*) (C.).

Urine reddish, turbid and straw-coloured (Lyc., Sep., Tereb.) (C.).

Hæmaturia ; urination prevented by clots (C.).

AGGRAVATION : From slight contact ; when lying down ; when walking ; lying on the left side ; at 11 A. M. and 11 P. M. ; and going upstairs.

AMELIORATION : In the open air ; when sitting ; and from rest.

RELATIONSHIP. Compare : *Acon.*, *Ars.*, *Bell.*, *Conv.*, *Dig.*, *Gels.*, *Kalm.*, *Lach.*, *Naja*, *Nat-M.*, *Phos.*, *Spig.*, and *Tab.*

Antidotes : *Acon.*, *Camph.* and *Chin.*

Caladium Seguinum.

COMMON NAME : AMERICAN ARUM.

Very sensitive to noise ; slightest noise startles him from sleep (*Asar.*, *Bell.*, *Hyos.*, *Kali-C.*, *Nux V.*, *Stram.*, *Tarant.*) (A.).

Red, dry stripe down centre of the tongue widening toward tip (B.).

Hard cough with asthma, relieved from expectoration (*Caust.*, *Guai.*, *Hep*, *Iod.*, *Ipec.*, *Lach.*, *Phos.*, *Sang.*, *Sep.*) (B.).

Inclination to rest, and aversion to move.

Breathing impeded (*Bry.*, *Kali M.*, *Lach.*, *Lyc.*, *Puls.*, *Sulph.*) (Br.).

Face, head and hands hot ; legs and feet cold (C.).

Catarrhal asthma ; mucus not readily raised (*Amm-C.*, *Hep.*, *Nat-S.*) (Br.).

Coldness of single parts (*Calc.*, *Camph.*, *Carb V.*, *Dig.*, *Ipec.*, *Lach.*, *Nat-M.*).

HEAT DURING SLEEP, CEASES ON WAKING (*Mezer.*, *Op.*, *Samb.*) (B.).

FALLS ASLEEP DURING EVENING FEVER AND WAKES WHEN IT STOPS (A.).

Respiratory symptoms alternating with skin symptoms (*Ars.*) (B.).

Soft, pasty, clay coloured stools, passed with difficulty (*Alum.*, *Hep.*, *Sep.*) (C.).

Limbs feel tired and weak (*Bapt.*, *Bry.*, *Cimic.*, *Kali-P.*, *Rhus-T.*) (C.).

Burning in the stomach and skin (*Ars.*, *Phos.*, *Sulph.*).

Eructations : frequent, of very little wind, as if stomach was full of dry food (A.).

Food eaten seems too dry ; must drink to swallow (B.).

It is to be remembered in spermatorrhœa or in seminal weakness, particularly in nocturnal emissions, when there is complete relaxation of the organ ; so that emissions occur without any dreams, or if there be a dream, it is entirely forei n to sexual subjects (F.).

Perspiration, which very much attracts the flies.

Effects of sexual excesses ; there are emissions without any excitement (*Con* , *Nux-V* , *Sel.*) (D.).

Confused ; cannot concentrate the mind (C.).

Forgetfulness (*Ambr.*, *Anac.*, *Kali P.*, *Lyc.*) (C.).

Vertigo, with nausea in the morning (*Bry.*, *Cocc.*, *Nux-V.*, *Sep.*) (C.).

Dull pressive or cutting pain in the temples (C.).

Very irritable and depressed   (C.).

IMPOTEN E : WITH MENTAL DEPRESSION, RELAXED PENIS, WITH SEXUAL DESIRE AND EXCITEMENT (*Agn.*, *Con.*, *Lyc.*, *Nux-V.*, *Sel.*, *Sulph.*)   (A.).

Flaccid, sweaty genitals ; *glans like a rag* (B.).

IMPOTENCY AFTER GONORRHŒA (*Agn.* ; impotency after syphilis—*Merc.*)   (B.).

Erections when half asleep ; cease when fully awake (Br.).

Coldness of the sexual parts (*Agn.*, *Camph.*) (G.)

NO ERECTION, EVEN AFTER CA ESS ; NO EMISSION, NO ORGASM DURING AN EMBRACE (*Calc.*, *Graph.*, *Sel.*, *Sep.*)   (A.).

Pruritus vulvæ, with burning ; from pin worms (B.).

Pruritus, during pregnancy (*Bor.*) ; *with mucous discharge* (A. *)*.

PRURITUS VAGINÆ ; INDUCES ONANISM (*Nux-V.*, *Orig.*, *Plat.*, *Zinc.*)   (A.).

Crampy pains in the uterus at night   (Br.)

When nymphomania occurs as the result of worms escaping into the vagina and there exciting irritation *Calad.* is the remedy   (F.)

AGGRAVATION : From motion ; lying on painful parts ; inside a room ; and from 3 or 4 P. M. till midnight.

AMELIORATION : After a short sleep ; after perspiring ; from expectoration ; in the open air ; and from motion.

RELATIONSHIP. It destroys craving for tobacco (destroys craving for alcohol or liquor—*Sulphuric Acid*). It is also useful for mosquito and insect-bites (which burn and itch intensely).

Incompatible : Arum-T.

Compare ; A*n*., *Bry*., *Calc*., *Caust*., *Chin*., *Dig*., *Gels*., *Kali-P*., *Lyc*., *Nux-V*., *Op*., *Phos*., *Phos-Ac*., *Sel*., *Sulph* and *Zinc*.

Caladium antidotes *Nit-Ac*.

Calcarea Arsenica.

COMMON NAME :   ARSENITE OF LIME.

Great mental depression (*Aur*., *Bapt*., *Kali-P*., *Lach*., *Nat M*., *Puls*., *Sep*.) (A).

Desire for company (*Arg-N*., *Bism*., *Hyos*., *Kali-C*., *Lyc*., *Phos*. *Stram*.) (Br.).

Anger (*Ant-C*., *Bell*., *Bry*., *Nat-M*.) (Br.).

Violent backache (*Æsc*., *Cimic*., *Kali-C*., *Phos*., *Rhus-T* , *Sep*.) (Br.).

Nephritis : with frequent micturition ; burning and scanty urine that contains albumen. There is extreme sensitiveness over the region of the kidneys associated with dyspnœa and feeble action of the heart (Bl.)

Complaints of fleshy women when approaching the menopause (*Calc*., *Graph*., *Lyc*., *Sep*.) (A.).

Constriction and pain in the region of the heart (*Amyl-N*., *Cupr*., *Lach*.) (Br.).

Rush of blood to the head and left chest (Acon., Amyl-N., Glon., Lach.) (A.).

Dyspnœa with feeble heart (Br.).

Palpitation on the least exertion (Ars., Calc., Dig., Iod., Lach.) (Bl.).

THE SLIGHTEST EMOTION CAUSES PALPITATION OF THE HEART (Arg-N., Coff., Kali P., Naja, Nat M., Phos-Ac., Phos., Puls., Sep.) (A).

INFANTILE LIVER (Calc., Calc-I., Chel., Iod., Merc., Nit-Ac., Podo., Sep., Sil.) (Br.

Affections of mesenteric glands (Br.).

Feeling of suffocation (Acon., Ars., Carb-V., Ign., Lyc., Nux-V., Phos., Sulph) (Br.).

Burning pain in the uterus and vagina (Br.).

Offensive, bloody leucorrhœa (Calc., Kreos., Lach., Nit-Ac., Phos., Sulph.) (Br.).

Cancer of the uterus (Lach.) (Br.).

Pain in the upper limb before epileptic attack (K.).

Epilepsy, from valvular diseases of the heart (A.).

Aura felt in the region of the heart (Lach., Naja) (Br.).

Rush of blood to the head before an epileptic attack (Br.).

Pain in the left hand before epileptic fit (K.).

Chilliness (Kali-C., Nux-V., Puls., Sil.) (Br.).

Chronic malaria (Apis, Calc., Ipec., LyC., Nat-M., Puls , Tub.) (Br.).

Enlarged liver and spleen (Chel., Chin., Ferr., Nat-M., Sep.) (Br.).

Complaints of drunkards, after abstaining ; craving for alcohol (Asar., Nux-V., Sulph-Ac.) (A.).

AGGRAVATION : During climacteric ; while out of doors ; during cold weather ; and from least exertion.

AMELIORATION : During rest ; in the open air.

RELATIONSHIP. *Compare : Amyl-N., Ars., Asar., Bry., Calc., Con., Ferr-P., Glon., Lach., Lith-C., Lyc., Mosch., Naja, Nux-V., Phos., Puls., Sep., Sulph., Zinc.*

Follows well after : Con. in lymphatic, psoric or tuberculous persons.

Useful after abuse of quinine.

Calcarea Carbonica.

COMMON NAME : CARBONATE OF CALCIUM.

Often suitable during dentition of children (Bell., Merc., Podo., Sil.).

Nervous excitement, with debility and loss of strength (*Ars., Kali-P., Nux-V., Sep.*).

Sees objects on closing the eyes, which vanish when they are opened (Arg-N., Bell., Chin., Op., Sulph., Tarant.) (D.).

Apprehension of some future misfortune (Anac., Chin-S., Graph., Psor.).

Anxious shuddering and awe as soon as evening draws near (*Acon., Kali-C., Phos.*) (N.).

Low spirited and melancholic.

Despairing, hopeless of ever getting well again, with fear of death, tormenting all around him day and night (N.).

She fears she will lose her understanding, and that persons will observe her confusion of mind (*Act-R.*).

Palpitation : *at night, and after eating* (Br.)

Dry cough at night, which is apt to be loose during the day (*Hep., Puls.*) (D.).

SHORTNESS OF BREATH, ESPECIALLY ON GOING UPSTAIRS (*Ars., Bry., Phos.*) (D.).

Pain in the right side of the chest (D.),

Mucous rales are worse on the right side (D.).

PURULENT EXPECTORATION (*Hep., Merc.*) (D.).

Vertigo ; *when suddenly raising or turning the head* (*Con.*), *even when at rest* ; *or when going upstairs or up a hill* (N.).

Skin : unhealthy ; small wounds suppurate easily (D.).

Internal or external sensation of coldness on various parts of the head (N.).

It is useful for certain forms of eczema of the scalp with general *Calcarea* symptoms (D.).

Itching of the scalp ; children scratch their heads when their sleep is disturbed, or they are awakened.

HEAD TOO LARGE ; FONTANELLES NOT CLOSING, AND PROFUSE SWEAT (N.).

Great emaciation and swollen abdomen, the appetite being good (*Nat-M.*).

MALNUTRITION (*Abrot., Calc-P., Nat-M., Sanic, Sulph.*). (B.).

FOUL OR STRONG URINE (*Benz-Ac., Canth., Nit-Ac., Tereb., Viol-T.*) (B.).

White urinary sediment (*Cina, Nat-M., Phos-Ac.*) (B.)

SENSATION OF COLDNESS IN INNER PARTS (reverse of *Ars.* and *Sulph.*).

Aversion to the open air (*Hep., Nux-V., Psor., Sil.*).

Sensitiveness to cold and damp air, and inclination to catch cold (*Dulc., Nat-S., Rhod., Rhus-T.*).

Inflammation of conjunctiva or cornea caused by bathing, or getting wet, or . aggravated by damp weather (N.).

Lung diseases of tall, slender, rapidly growing youth (*Phos.*) ; upper third of right lung (*Ars.* ; upper third of left lung—*Myrt., Sulph.*) (A.).

Pupils dilated (*Bell., Hyos., Stram.*).

SCROFULOUS INFLAMMATION OF CORNEA OR CONJUNCTIVA, CHARACTERIZED BY PUSTULES, ULCERS, LACHRYMATION AND PHOTOPHOBIA. OPACITIES AFTER ACUTE INFLAMMATION (N.).

Dim-sightedness (*Phos., Sep.*) (G.).

Full habit and ebullitions (*Acon., Amyl-N., Bell., Ferr-P., Sang.*).

Extreme hunger, even when the stomach is full of food
(*Cina, Lyc., Nat-M., Phos.*) (G.).

GREAT DESIRE FOR TOBACCO (*Bell., Carb-Ac.,
Eug., Kreos., Nux-V., Plb., Tab., Thuj.*), AND BRANDY
(*Ars., Bry., Hep., Nux-V., Op., Petr., Phos., Sel., Sep.,
Spig., Sulph., Sulph-Ac.*).

Itching of the margin of the lids (*Bor., Graph., Merc.,
Sulph.*) (D.).

Styes (*Graph., Hep., Merc., Puls., Sil., Sulph., Thuj.*)
(D.).

Nodosities on the lids (*Sulph., Thuj.*) (D.).

CHALAZAE ON THE LIDS (*Calc., Graph., Sulph.,
Thuj.*) (D.).

Pain in the abdomen after every morsel of food or drink
(*Calc-P.*) (D.).

Sensation as if the stomach was hanging down, relaxed;
it seems to be flabby and weak (D.).

Dysentery, with pains worse after drinking water (*Nux-
V.*).

Constipation (*Bry., Ign., Nat-M., Op.*).

Pot-bellied children, with much colic and worms (**Ra.**).

Great inclination to perspire (*Bry., Calc., Chin.*), *even
whilst sitting* (*Ars., Calc., Con., Ferr., Kali-B., Rhus-T.*).

Intermittent fever consisting only of chilliness (*before
and after it hunger*).

In fever ravenous hunger for days before the attack (A.).

Croupy cough in winter alternating with sciatica in
summer (A₁).

RAVENOUS APPETITE DURING APYREXIA
(K.).

Cough only in the day time (*Am-C., Calc., Euphr., Ferr.,
Lach.*), *or only after dinner* (*Nux-V., Phos., Puls., Sulph.*);
particularly after eating meat (N.).

Cough excited by tobacco-smoke (*Spong.*) (A.).

The least motion makes the heart palpitate (*Carb-V.,
Con., Dig., Iber., Med., Merc., Nit-Ac., Phos., Spig.*) (N.).

Tight chest at close of coition (B.).

Gums spongy, and bleed easily (*Carb-V., Nat-M.*) (Bt.).

Mercurial affections of the teeth and gums; caries of the former, suppuration in the latter (Hr.).

The sound teeth, as well as those decayed, are very painful to the touch of food or drink (G.).

Premature decay and discoloration of teeth (*Kreos.*) (D.).

The teeth turn black and crumble as soon as they appear (*Plb., Thuj.*) (D.).

Hardness of hearing with swelling of the tonsils (*Bar-C.*), especially after abuse of mercury (N.).

Teeth show black streaks running over (N.).

Throat dry and rough, with soreness when talking and when swallowing (N.).

Sensation as of a round ball in the forehead; sitting firmly there even when shaking the head (N.).

The nervous system is worn out, exhausted (*Kali-P., Phos-Ac.*) (D.).

The patient is pale, the nose is peaked, the eyes are sunken and surrounded by dark rings (*Cina*) (D.).

Bad effects of chagrin (*Coloc., Ign., Nat-M.*) (G.).

Bad effects from thinking and brooding on sexual subjects (*Phos.*), *from anger* (*Bry., Coloc., Ign., Nux-V.*), *and from anxiety* (*Arg-N., Ars., Gels.*).

SAD AND IRRITABLE AND ESPECIALLY DEPRESSED AFTER A FIT OF ANGER, OR AFTER AN INSULT (D.).

Very peevish and gloomy (*Nux-V., Sulph.*) (D.).

Weakness of memory (*Arg-N., Caust., Hyos., Med., Nux-M., Phos-Ac.*) (D.).

The patient is moody, depressed, prefers solitude, is shy of the opposite sex (D.).

Throws things away indignantly, (*Cham., Cina*), or pushes them away on the table (N.).

Great indignation about things done by others or himself; grieving about consequences (N.).

Is very sensitive to the least impression; the least word that seems wrong, hurts her very much (*Ign.*) (G.).

Continually concerned about the future (*Bry., Calc., Chin-S., Cic., Ferr-P., Gels., Nat-C., Phos., Puls.*) (N.).

Hypochondriasis from sexual excess or by persistent dwelling of the mind on sexual subjects (N.).

PAIN IN THE ABDOMEN AFTER INDIGNA-TION (K.).

Flatulent colic (*Coloc., Lyc., Nux-V., Puls., Raph.*) (G.).

Colic after lithotomy or ovariotomy; attending abdominal section (*Bism., Hep.*) (A.)

Eczema with yellow, acrid moisture oozing from under the crusts; new vesicles form from contact of exudation (A.).

Dry, pediculated, cauliflower-like fig-warts, especially after abuse of mercury (*Nit-Ac., Sabin., Thuj.*) (A.).

Pain in small of the back, as if sprained; worse at rest at night, and in the morning, and when rising from a seat (N.).

Urging and pain after urinating in prostatic troubles of old men (*Sars.*) (A.).

BURNING OR SMARTING IN THE URETHRA WHEN NOT MICTURATING (*Berb., Bry., Graph., Merc., Nat-C., Sulph.*); CEASES WHILE URINE IS PASSING (N.).

Micturition too frequent; too sparing (*Bell., Canth., Merc.*) (G.).

Urinates in a slender stream (*Clem., Con., Thuj.*) (B.).

Prolapse of the bladder (A.).

Dysuria of brides, or in pregnancy (B.).

HAS TO SIT AT URINAL FOR HOURS (A.).

Voluptuous itching in the scrotum (*Crot-T., Sulph.*) (N.).

Priapism (*Canth., Phos., Pic-Ac.*) (B.).

Salpingitis (*Apis, Bell., Bry., Coloc.*) (B.).

Amorous dreams with emissions (*Nux-V., Phos., Sulph.*) (G.).

Itching or sensitive vulva (*Plat.*) (B.).

Pains from ovaries into thighs (B.).

Sleepy all day long; awake all night; body aches all over (N.).

Sweat smelling like rotten eggs (Sulph.) (C.).

AGGRAVATION: From anger; from indignation; from grief; from mortification; from loss of seminal fluids; from use of tobacco; after onanism; from sexual excesses; from the least touch on the affected parts; from cold drinks; at night; and in the morning.

AMELIORATION: From warmth; from rest; and after breakfast.

RELATIONSHIP: *Compare*: *Apis, Berb., Canth., Caust., Coloc., Con., Gels., Ign., Lyc., Merc., Nat-M., Phos., Plat., Puls., Rhus-T., Sab., Sep., Sil., Sulph* and *Thuj.....*

Complementary: *Caust.* and *Coloc.*

Staph. precedes or follows *Coloc.* well.

Antidote: *Camph.*

Staph. antidotes: *Merc.* and *Thuj.*

Stramonium.

COMMON NAME: THORN APPLE.

St. Vitus's dance (*Agar., Kali-Br., Merc., Nat-M., Sulph., Zinc.*)

Of use in certain forms of epilepsy (*Calc., Cupr., Hyos., Lach.*).

Tingling in the limbs (*Acon.*).

Trembling of the limbs (*in drunkards*) (*Hyos.*).

Increased and easy movability of the muscles subservient to the will (voluntary musculature), and slowness of the muscles not subject to the will (involuntary musculature).

Subsultus tendinum (*Hyos.*) (C.).

Twitching in the limbs (*Bell., Cupr., Gels., Hyos., Lach.*).

Twitching of single muscles, or groups of muscles, especially of upper part of the body (A.).

Carphology (*Hyos.*) (C.).

SPASM FROM FRIGHT (*Acon., Bufo, Calc., Cupr., Hyos., Ign., Indg., Op., Plat., Sec., Sulph., Verat., Zinc.*).

Chorea (*Agar., Cupr., Gels., Merc.*) (A.).

VIOLENT CONGESTIONS OF BLOOD TO THE HEAD (*Acon., Bell., Glon., Lach., Meli., Op., Sang., Sulph., Verat-V.*).

Spasmodic jerking of the head when up from the pillow (*Bell.*) (N.).

Abscesses, with violent pains driving one to madness (especially in the left hip) (N.).

Eyes bright, wild and suffused, with red face and wild delirium (*Bell.*) (D.).

Eyes wide open, prominent; pupils exceedingly dilated (*Bell., Hyos.*), *insensible* (*Op.*), *with injected conjunctiva* or total blindness (N.).

DIPLOPIA (*Aur., Bell., Gels., Hyos., Nat-M., Nit-Ac., Nux-V., Op., Plb.*) (K.).

Cannot walk in a dark room (A.).

Contortion of eyes and eyelids (A.).

Pupils dilate when the child is reprimanded (A.).

Suppression of all secretions and excretions (*Apis, Bell., Hyos.*).

EFFECTS FROM SUPPRESSED ERUPTIONS (*Ant-T., Apis, Bry., Cupr., Hyos., Lach., Op., Sulph.*).

Pain in loins (*Aesc., Bell., Calc., Kali-C., Lyc., Nux-V., Rhus-T., Sep., Sulph.*).

COLDNESS OF THE EXTREMITIES DURING FEVER (*Carb-An., Kali-Ars., Sep.*) (K.).

VIOLENT PERSPIRATION (*Bell., Camph., Merc., Sil., Verat.*).

Secretion of milk increased (*Asaf., Bell., Bry., Calc., Con., Iod., Phos., Puls., Rhus-T.*).

Dysmenorrhœa with excessive loquacity (N.).

Catamenia too profuse, the blood is clotted (*Croc., Sab., Ust.*).

Excessive loquacity during menses; face bloated with blood, with tears and prayers and earnest supplications (N.).

Urine turbid, brown and thick, which is very scanty (*Acon., Apis, Ars., Bell., Benz-Ac., Camph., Dig., Hep., Ipec., Merc-C., Phos., Plb., Sep., Sulph.*).

No force to the flow of the stream (of urine) (*Clem., Con., Hep., Sep.*).

The urine dribbles away very slowly and feebly (G.).

KIDNEYS SECRETE LESS OR NONE IN ACUTE DISEASES, ESPECIALLY IN CHILDREN (N.).

Grinding of teeth (*Apis, Bell., Hyos.*) (K.).

Circumscribed redness of cheeks (*Cham.*) (A.).

Stammering or entirely speechless (N.).

Dribbling of gluey saliva from the mouth (*Bell., Cinnb.*) (N.).

Voice suddenly gives out and takes a higher pitch (D.).

Risus sardonicus (*Bell., Hyos., Oena., Plb.*) (N.).

Oppression, with desire for open air (*Carb-V.*) (C.).

Nervous asthma (*Ars., Cupr., Phos.*) (D.).

Difficult, hurried respiration (*Ars., Kali-C.*) (C.).

FOREHEAD WRINKLED, IN BRAIN SYMPTOMS (*Hell.*), OR IN HEADACHE (*Caust., Hyos., Nat-M., Phos., Sulph.*) (K.).

Calls things by wrong names (C.).

Bright objects cause delirium, spasms and convulsions (D.).

SCREAMING OUT, TERRIFIED (*Bell.*) (D.).

Young men or women who pray, sing or talk so devoutly

or constantly as to excite the sympathy of all in the home (N.).

Cannot bear to be alone (*Bism.*) ; *wants hand to be held* (N.).

Awakens with a shrinking look, as if frightened at the first object seen (N.).

DESIRE TO ESCAPE, IN DELIRIUM (*Bell., Bry., Hyos., Op., Rhus-T.*) (A.).

Struggles to get out of bed (*Bell.*) (C.).

Imagines all sorts of things; that she is double, lying crosswise, etc. (*Petr.*) (A.).

Head feels as if scattered about (*Bapt.*) (A.).

Proud, haughty (*Lach., Plat.*) (C.).

Rapid changes from joy to sadness (*Ign.*) (Br.).

Child is delirious, does not know where it is; calls for papa and mamma, although they may be present trying to console it (G.).

FURIOUS DELIRIUM (*Bell., Lach.*) (Bt.).

Sensation as if the limbs were separated from the body (*Bapt.*).

Visions in delirium (*Bell., Hyos.*).

Mania with continuous phantastical illusions (*Bell., Hyos., Lach.*).

Mania, especially of drunkards (*Bell., Hyos., Lach.*).

PAINLESSNESS WITH MOST OF THE AILMENTS (*Op.*).

GREAT LOQUACITY, THE PATIENT TALKS ALL THE TIME (*Hyos., Lach.*). LAUGHS, PLAYS, SINGS AND PRAYS (*Verat*).

Fear of darkness (*Ars., Bell.*) (D.).

DESIRE FOR LIGHT AND COMPANY (*Bell., Calc., Gels., Lac-C.*).

Horrible hallucinations (*Bell.*) ; *objects start from every corner* (*Hyos.*) ; *animals spring up and terrify* (*Bell., Hyos.*) (D.).

Religious mania (*Aur., Sulph., Verat.*) (Br.).

VIOLENT RAGE (*Agar., Bell., Hyos.*).

Violent and lewd (*Phos.*) (Br.).

CONVULSIONS WITH CONSCIOUSNESS (*Nux-V.*) (A.).

Pangs of conscience; thinks he is not honest; does not know his friends; raves about his business (G.).

Mock laughter when looking at the picture of his father; face red; eyes wild; alternating with melancholy (G.).

One side paralysed, the other convulsed (*Hell.*) (N.).

THE CONVULSIONS ARE INDUCED BY CONTACT, AFTER EACH MOTION, FROM LIGHT AND FROM GLISTENING OBJECTS (*Lyss.*).

Stiff immovability of the body with consciousness (*Ign.*).

FACE HOT AND RED WITH COLD HANDS AND FEET (A.).

Hydrophobia; fear of water, with excessive aversion to liquids (*Bell., Lyss.*) (A.).

Screaming, biting, scratching (*Bell.*) (C.).

Spasmodic constriction of the throat (*Bell., Lach., Merc-C.*) (A.).

Convulsive hiccough (*Ars., Bell., Gels.*) (K.).

VIOLENT HICCOUGH (*Am-M., Calc-F., Cic., Cycl., Lob., Lyc., Mag-P., Nat-M., Nicc., Nux-V., Stront., Teucr., Verat.*) (K.).

Hiccough after hot drinks (*Verat.*) (F.).

Faintings with snoring (*Op.*).

Vertigo when walking in the dark, day or night; he staggers and falls down every time he attempts to walk (G.).

No desire for water, although the mouth is dry (*Puls.*) (Nd.).

Troublesome thirst even with much saliva (G.).

Saliva tastes salty (*Ant-C., Carb-An., Cycl., Hyos., Kali-I., Lyc., Merc., Merc-C., Nat-M., Phos., Sep., Sulph.*).

Sexual erethism, with indecent speech and action (*Hyos.*); hands constantly kept on the genital (Br.).

Violent thirst, especially for acid drinks (*Ant-T., Chin., Phos., Verat.*) (C.).

Nausea, with flow of very saltish tasting saliva (G.).

Diarrhœa of a cadaverous odour (*Ars., Bapt., Kali-P., Lach., Psor., Sulph.*) (G.).

Puerperal fever (*Bry., Hyos., Pyrog.*), and nymphomania (*Hyos., Verat.*) (Bt.).

Scarlet rash, with furious delirium (*Bell.*) (Bt.).

Spasm of larynx (*Brom., Lach., Phos.*) (B.).

Spasmodic cough (*Bell., Cupr., Dros.*) (B.).

Vertigo, as if he would fall forward and to the left (R.).

Throbbing in vertex and occiput (*Lach., Sulph.*) (R.).

Bores the head into the pillow (*Apis, Arn., Bell., Bry., Hell., Sulph., Tub.*) (R.).

Cerebro-spinal meningitis accompanied by a severe congestive headache, the pains being so severe that the patients are besides themselves (R.).

Delirium tremens (*Hyos., Lach.*) (Br.).

Gyratory and graceful motions (Br.).

Sees ghosts, hears voices, talks with spirits (*Hyos.*) (Br.).

Small objects look large (reverse of *Plat.*) (Br.).

Parts of the body seem enormously swollen (Br.).

All objects look black (all objects look red—*Phos.*) (Br.).

Juicy fruit tastes dry; food tastes like straw (A.).

Clean or whitish tongue, with red papillæ (A.).

Vomiting, as soon as he raises his head from pillow (*Ars., Bry., Colch.*); *or from a bright light* (A.).

Nausea and vomiting in the evening followed by violent, anxious heat (A.).

Dry, glowing heat over whole body, with redness of head and face, and coldness and paleness of the rest of the body (*Bell., Op.*) (A.).

Skin hot and burning, with sweat at the same time (*Bell., Sep.*) (A.).

During sweat, cannot bear to be uncovered (A.).

OILY SWEAT (*Phos.;* as if mixed with oil—*Chin.*) (A.).

Is beneficial in erysipelas, when the brain symptoms are pronounced (Bl.).

Children cry· out in sleep (*Apis, Bell.*) (A.).

Restless sleep, with tossing about (*Ars.*) (C.).

Sleepy, but cannot sleep (*Bell., Cham., Op.*) (A.).

AGGRAVATION: When alone; in the dark; from being touched; on looking at bright light or shining objects; on attempting to swallow, especially liquids; after sleep; from fright; from suppression of discharges; and from intemperance.

AMELIORATION: From bright light; from company; from warmth; and from cold water.

RELATIONSHIP: *Stram. often follows Bell., Cupr., Hyos.* and *Lyss.*

Antidotes: *Bell., Coff., Hyos., Nux-V.,* and *Tab.*

Stram. antidotes: *Merc.* and *Plb.*

Compare especially with Bell. and *Hyos.* It has less fever than *Bell.*, but more than *Hyos.* It causes more functional excitement of the brain, but never approaches the true inflammatory condition of *Bell.*

Strontiana Carbonica.

COMMON NAME: CARBONATE OF STRONTIAN.

Tearing pains in the joints, especially in the evening and at night (*Merc., Sil.*).

Chronic sprains of the ankle-joint with œdema (Bl.).

Most pains seem to be in the long bones and marrow (*Nit-Ac.*).

Swelling and caries of the bones, especially the femur (*Asaf., Aur., Flour-Ac., Nit-Ac.*) (D.).

Uncomfortable fullness and swelling of the abdomen (*Carb-V., Lyc., Nux-V.*).

Cramp about navel (B.).

The symptoms gradually become worse and decrease at the same ratio (*Stann.*).

Diarrhœa of a very violent and persistent kind (*Aloe, Podo., Sulph.*).

Diarrhœa worse at night (*Chin., Puls., Sulph.*) (D.).

There is a continuous urging; he is hardly off the vessel before he must return (Bl.).

Exhausting diarrhœa of yellow water (*Chin.*) (B.).

Pain in urinating (*Canth., Nux-V., Pareir.*).

Distress about or around the heart, as if pressed upon (*Cact.*).

Great restlessness at night because of smothering, actually preventing access of breath to lungs (*Ars., Kali-P., Samb.*).

Sensation as of a load on the chest (*Bry.*) (B.).

Threatened apoplexy; there is violent congestion of the head, with a red face while exercising (Bl.).

Headache: The pain comes up from the nape of the neck and spreads over the head (*Sil.*) (Bl.).

Constant, slight showing of the menses (*Sab., Sec.*).

Violent, involuntary starts of the body (*Bell., Stram.*) (G.).

Tension in inner or outer parts (G.).

Heat, with aversion to undress or uncover one's self (*Nux-V.*) (G.).

Violent perspiration at night (*Calc., Chin., Merc., Sil.*).

Fleeting pains, seemingly in bones (B.).

Sense of paralytic weakness (*Kali-P., Phos., Zinc.*) (B.).

Pale, ammoniacal urine (*Benz-Ac.*) (B.).

Burning in anus lasts a long time after stool (*Ratan., Sulph.*) (Br.).

Hard, knotty, difficult stool (*Plb., Sulph.*) (B.).

Shock after surgical operations (Br.).

Great sensitiveness to cold (*Hep., Psor., Sil.*) (Br.).

Rheumatic pain in the right shoulder (*Lyc.*) (Br.).

Cramp in calves and soles (*Cupr., Sec., Verat.*) (B.).

FLUSHES OF HEAT, DURING CLIMACTERIC (*Graph., Lach., Sep., Sulph.*) (B.).

Loss of appetite (*Kali-M., Nux-V., Puls., Sep., Sulph.*) (Br.).

Aversion to meat (*Graph.*) (Br.).

Craves bread (*Nat-M.*) and beer (*Bry.*) (Br.).

Cardialgia (*Mag-P., Nux-V., Puls.*) (Br.).

AGGRAVATION: In the evening; at night; while urinating; from cold; from undressing; in darkness; from rubbing; after lying down and rising again; while exercising; and from walking.

AMELIORATION: From light; from warmth; from wrapping up warmly; and from immersing in hot water.

RELATIONSHIP: Remedies following: *Bell., Caust., Kali-C., Puls., Rhus-T., Sep.* and *Sulph.*

Compare: *Arn., Bar-C., Bell., Carb-V., Chin., Ferr., Glon., Graph., Kali-M., Lach., Merc., Nit-Ac., Op., Puls., Ruta, Sep., Sil., Sulph., Thuj.* and *Verat.*

Antidote: *Camph.*

Strychninum.

COMMON NAME: AN ALKALOID OF NUX-VOMICA; STRYCHNINE.

STRYCHNINE is the principal alkaloid of *Nux Vomica* (as well *Ignatia*) Bean. It is so intensely bitter that 1 part in 600000 can be detected by the taste.

GENERAL ACTION OF STRYCHNINE.—The motor centres of the spinal cord are powerfully irritated, and hence their reflex excitability is enormously increased: the medulla is also stimulated and the respiratory centre is increased in activity, causing increased frequency and depth of movements of the chest; peristalsis is increased. It produces a condition very much like tetanus (D.).

TETANIC CONVULSIONS WITH OPISTHOTONOS (*Cupr., Ign., Nux-V.*) (Br.).

The muscles relax in between the paroxysms (Br.).

Trismus or lock-jaw (Cupr., Cur., Hydroc-Ac., Hyper., Ign., Nux-V.,Oenan., Phyost., Stram.) (Br.).

Vertigo, with roaring in the ears (*Calc., Chin., Kali-C., Nat-M., Puls.*) (Br.).

VIOLENT JERKING, TWITCHING AND TREMBLING OF THE EXTREMITIES (*Bell., Hyos., Ign., Nux-V., Stram.*) (Br.).

Spasms provoked by the slightest touch and attempt to move (Nux-V.) (Br.).

Violent jerks in spinal columns (Br.).

Icy sensation down the spine (Gels.) (Br.).

EXCESSIVE DYSPNOEA (*Ant-T., Arn., Ars., Cupr., Ferr-P., Lach., Laur., Lyc., Mosch., Nux-V., Phos., Sulph.*) (Br.).

Desire for coitus (*Canth., Lach., Phos., Plat.*) (Br.).

Any touch on the body excites a voluptuous sensation (*Plat.*) (Br.).

Fæces discharged involuntarily during spasms (*Oenan.*) (Br.).

Constant retching (Ant-T., Cupr., Ipec., Sec.); *violent vomiting (Ars., Cupr., Ipec., Verat.)* (Br.).

Deglutition impossible (*Bell., Lach., Phos.*) (Br.).

Spasm of the œsophagus (*Ign., Laur., Sec.*) (Br.).

AGGRAVATION: From the slightest touch, sound and odour; from motion; and after meals.

AMELIORATION: From lying on the back.

RELATIONSHIP: *Compare*: *Arn.*, *Bell.*, *Cic.*, *Cupr.*, *Cur.*, *Gels.*, *Hyos.*, *Ign.*, *Kali-P.*, *Lach.*, *Merc.*, *Nux-V.*, *Op.*, *Phos-Ac.*, *Rhus-T.*, *Sec.*, *Verat.*

Sulphur.

COMMON NAMES: BRIMSTONE; FLOWERS OF SULPHUR.

The king of remedies around which centres the whole Materia Medica (Bt.).

It acts upon every organ and tissue of the body (*Ars.*, *Calc.*, *Merc.*) (D.).

Is especially applicable to chronic diseases (*Sep.*) (D.).

IS THE LEADING ANTIPSORIC (N.).

Adapted to persons of a scrofulous diathesis (*Calc.*, *Phos.*, *Sil.*) (A.).

Dirty, filthy people, prone to skin affections (*Psor.*) (A.).

Great weakness; sallow, pale and yellow face; with marked anæmia (*Nat-M.*, *Sep.*).

Loss of vital strength (*Camph.*, *Chin.*, *Kali-P.*, *Phos-Ac.*, *Zinc.*).

WHEN OTHER REMEDIES FAIL TO ACT IT IS OF INESTIMABLE NEED IN RALLYING THE VITAL FORCES (*Op.*).

Is subject to venous congestion, especially of the portal system (*Aloe*, *Podo.*, *Sep.*) (A.).

PUSTULAR ECZEMA OF ANY PART (*Graph.*, *Merc.*, *Rhus-T.*).

The more the eruption is scratched the more it itches and burns (D.).

The skin is rough, coarse and measly (D.).

VOLUPTUOUS ITCHING, SOMETIMES RELIEVES; AFTER IT BURNING; SOMETIMES LITTLE VESICLES (N.).

Soreness in the folds of the skin (*Lyc.*) (D.).

After violent scratching, aching, numbness and swelling of the skin, even ulceration (N.).

ITCHING WORSE FROM HEAT OF BED (*Merc.*) (A.).

Child cannot bear to be washed or bathed (*Ant-C., Psor.*) (N.).

All the eruptions are greatly aggravated by washing and by being wet; wetting produces burning (D.).

Eruption of yellow crusts on the scalp (*Kali-S.*) (D.).

The troubles of the skin are apt to alternate with some internal trouble (*Graph., Rhus-T.*) (D.).

Defective osseous growth (*Calc.*) (D.).

Rickets and curvature of the spine (*Sil.*) (D.).

Burning of palms and soles (*Graph., Lach., Med., Sep.*) (D.).

PUTS THE FEET OUT OF BED AT NIGHT TO KEEP THEM COOL (D.).

Is used often for chronic diseases, that result from suppressed eruptions (*Caust., Psor.*) (A.).

Contracted pupils (*Aur., Bell., Calc., Euphr., Hyos., Merc-C., Op., Puls., Thuj.*).

Scurfy lids (*Graph., Nat-M., Sep.*).

Amblyopia in youthful girls with great loss of vigour, anorexia and costive state (*Puls., Sep.*).

Dimness of vision, as of a veil before the eyes (*Chin., Puls.*) (N.).

Aversion to light (*Con., Euphr., Nat-M.*) (G.).

Dark points or spots floating before the eyes (*Chin., Cocc., Nat-M., Phos., Physos., Sep., Sil., Tab.*) (N.).

Cataract (*Calc., Nat-M., Phos.*) (G.).

HALO OF COLOURS AROUND THE LIGHT (*Bell., Cycl., Kali-P., Lach., Nicc., Osm., Phos., Puls., Sep., Staph., Tub., Zinc.*) (K.)

Sharp darting pains like pins, needles, or splinters sticking into the eye (N.).

Scrofulous ophthalmia (*Calc.*) (Ma. & Ht.).

Hypertrophy of the lids, with itching and smarting and purulent exudations (*Sep.*) (Ma. & Ht.).

CANNOT BEAR TO HAVE THE EYES WASHED (N.).

Flushes in face (Graph., Sep.) (N.).

Very red lips, particularly with children (N.).

Deafness, with roaring, itching and dampness in the ear (Hm.).

*Purulent otorrhœa (Calc., Calc-S., Kali-S., Lyc., **Merc.**, Puls., Sil.*).

Stitches in the left ear (*Kali-B., Merc-C., Puls., Sabad., Staph.*) (N.).

Ears very red with children (N.).

Chronic, dry catarrh (Nux-V., Puls., Stict.) (D.).

Nose bleeds easily (Carb-V., Lach., Merc.) (D.).

There is a smell of old catarrh before the nose (D.).

Chronic local congestions in many parts, with burning sensation (*Sep.*) (N.).

Is often required to promote absorptions of effusions (*Kali-I.*). (N.).

Discharge from every outlet acrid, excoriating and reddening (Kreos., Nit-Ac.) (N.).

Bitter taste in the morning (*Puls.*) (D.).

Sour, clammy taste in the mouth (*Puls.*) (Bt.).

Tongue coated white, with red tip and edges, mostly in acute diseases (N.).

CANINE HUNGER (*Anac., Cina, Nat-M., **Phos.**, Staph.*).

Has to get up at night to eat (Phos., Psor.) (D.).

Eructations, with aversion to meat (Graph.), qualmishness (Nux-V., Puls.) and *nausea (Cycl., Ipec., Nat-M.*).

DRINKS MUCH, EATS LITTLE (N.).

Suffocative catarrh, with paralysis of the lungs (*Ant-T., Lycop., Phos.*) (Bt.).

Headache, with catarrhal affections (*Bry., Kali-B., Puls.*) (G.).

Sudden retrocession of eruptions, with cold skin and great prostration (*Ant-T., Apis, Carb-V., Phos., Sulph.*) (Bt.).

BAD EFFECTS OF SHOCK FROM INJURY; SURFACE OF THE BODY COLD; FACE PALE, BLUE; LIPS LIVID; PROFOUND PROSTRATION (A.).

Useful in cases of measles or scarlatina when eruption does not appear (*Ant-T., Bry., Cupr., Hell., Lach., Stram.*) (A.)

May be given in all sequelæ of measles (*Carb-V., Kali-C., Phos., Puls.*) (A.).

AGGRAVATION: During motion; at night; from contact; in cold air; and in the dark.

AMELIORATION; From warmth; when thinking of the existing complaint; in warm air; and from drinking cold water.

RELATIONSHIP: *Camphor* antidotes or modifies the action of nearly every vegetable medicine, such as tobacco, opium, etc.

Similar to: Acon., Ant-T., Ars., Carb-V., Cupr., Hydr-Ac., Laur., Nux-V., Phos., Sec. and Verat.

On account of its baneful influence *Camphor*

13

should not be allowed in the sick room in its crude form.

NOTE. A few large doses of *Camphor*, if given at the very start, will at once arrest many cases of diarrhœa during cholera epidemic.

Cannabis Indica.

COMMON NAME: INDIAN HEMP; HASHISCH.

Full of fun and mischief ; then perhaps moaning and crying (Puls.) (A.).

LAUGHS IMMODERATELY AT EVERY TRIF-LING WORD SPOKEN TO HIM (*Apis, Bell., Stram.*) (A.).

Anguish, with oppression (*Ars·, Lach.*) (R.).

Constantly theorizing (A.).

Imagines that he hears music (*Bell., Calc., Lyc., Merc., Nat-C., Stram.*) (R.).

VERY FORGETFUL ; FORGETS HIS LAST WORDS AND IDEAS ; BEGINS A SENTENCE, BUT FORGETS WHAT HE INTENDS TO SPEAK (A.).

Shuts his eyes and is lost in delicious thoughts (R.).

EXALTATION OF SPIRITS (*Coff., Phos., Stram.*) (R.)

Inability to recall any thought or event on account of other thoughts crowding his brain (*Anac.*, *Kali-P.*, *Lac-C.*) (A.).

Great apprehension of approaching death (*Acon.*, *Ars.*, *Calc.*, *Cimic.*, *Gels.*, *Lac-C.*, *Nit-Ac.*, *Phos.*, *Plat.*, *Verat.*) (A.).

Fixed ideas (*Anac.*) (R.).

DELIRIUM TREMENS (*Agar.*, *Ars.*, *Hyos.* *Kali-Br.*, *Lach.*, *Nat-M.*, *Nux-M.*, *Nux-V.*, *Op.*, *Stram.*, *Strych.*, *Verat.*) (A.).

EXCESSIVE LOQUACITY (*Bell.*, *Hyos.*, *Lach.*, *Stram.*, *Verat.*) (A.).

INCOHERENT TALK (*Lach.*, *Stram.*) (R.).

Double consciousness (*Anac.*, *Lach.*) (Bl.).

Mania of grandeur (*Con.*, *Phos.*) (B.).

EXAGGERATION OF TIME AND DISTANCE (A.).

TIME SEEMS TOO LONG (*Arg-N.*); A FEW SECONDS SEEM AGES (A.).

Produces the most remarkable hallucinations and imaginations (D.).

DISTANCE SEEMS IMMENSE; A FEW RODS SEEM MILES (*Glo१.*) (A.).

Delusion : head seems to be an inverted pendulum oscillating (K.).

Sees monstrous head on distant wall of the room (K.).

Clairvoyance (Anac., Crot-C., Hyos., Lach., Lyss., Nux-M., Op., Phos., Pyrus, Stram.) **(Br.).**

Unconscious every few minutes **(R.).**

SENSATION AS IF THE CALVARIUM WAS OPENING AND SHUTTING *(Act-R.)* **(A.).**

Stunning pain in the occiput **(R.).**

Shocks through the brain on regaining consciousness **(R.).**

Menses : very profuse ; painful ; too soon ; too long **(G.).**

Violent uterine colic (Bell., Caul., Cimic., Mag-P., Nux-V., Puls., Vib.) **(G.).**

Sensation of swelling in the perineum, or near the anus, as if sitting on a ball **(Sep.).**

Increased sexual desire and hysteria during the menstrual period **(Bl.).**

URETHRITIS, WITH PURULENT DISCHARGE, GREAT BURNING AND TENDERNESS ON URINATING *(Canth.)* ; GLANS PENIS DARK RED AND SWOLLEN **(D.).**

Urinary organs : Urging after micturition, with much straining ; dribbling after stream ceases (Thuj.) ; must wait a long time before the urine flows (Alum., Arn., Caust , Cop., Hep., Rhus-T., Sep.) ; stitching and burning in the urethra before, during and after urinating **(R.).**

Chordee (Canth., Cann-S., Nux-V., Pic-Ac.) **(D.).**

Oozing of white, glossy mucus on squeezing the glans (*Hep.*, *Kali-B.*, *Sil.*) (R.).

It is one of our great remedies in gonorrhœa (Bt.).

SPASMODIC CONTRACTION OF THE SPHINCTER VESICÆ ON URINATING (D.).

Dull pain in the region of the right kidney (Br.).

Nephritic colic (*Berb.*, *Lyc.*, *Ocim-C.*, *Puls.*) (B.).

Buzzing and ringing in the ear (*Bell.*, *Chin.*, *Puls.*) (R.).

Extreme sensitiveness to noise (*Bell.*, *Bor.*, *Coff.*, *Nux-V.*, *Stram.*, *Sulph.*) (Br.).

Hears noises like boiling water (R.).

Involuntary shaking of the head (*Agar.*, *Alum.*, *Caust.*, *Hell.*, *Lyc.*, *Merc.*, *Nat-M.*, *Zinc.*) (Br.).

RAVENOUS APPETITE (*Amm-C.*, *Arg-M.*, *Ars.*, *Calc-P.*, *Chin.*, *Cina*, *Ferr.*, *Graph.*, *Iod.*, *Lyc.*, *Nat-M.*, *Nux-V.*, *Petr.*, *Phos.*, *Sulph.*) (K.).

Weakness of the extremities, amounting to paralysis (*Gels.*, *Kali-P.*, *Plb.*, *Sil.*) (R.).

After sexual intercourse, backache (*Nit-Ac.*, *Sabal-Ser.*) (Br.).

Backache, worse from sitting (*Kobalt.*, *Sep.*, *Zinc.*) (F.).

Satyriasis (*Canth.*, *Phos.*, *Stram.*) (Br.).

Prolonged thrill during coition (Br.).

Dreams of the dead (*Anac.*, *Ars.*, *Calc*, *Sil.*, *Crot-H.*, *Graph.*, *Kali-C.*, *Mag-C.*, *Med.*, *Phos*, *Sulph.*, *Thuj.*' (K.).

Prophetic dreams (*Asaf.*, *Bor.*, *Mang.*, *Su lph.*).

In renal diseases, *Cannabis Ind.* is indicated when uræmia sets in, attended by severe he adache (F.).

Paralysis, with tingling in the affected parts (*Staph.*) (F.).

Stammering and stuttering (*Caust.*, *Stram.*) (C.).

Oppression of chest, with deep, laboured breathing. He feels as if suffocated, and has to be fanned (*Ant-T.*, *Apis*, *Ars.*, *Carb-V.*, *Chin.*, *Ferr.*, *Med.*, *Sulph.*)(C.).

AGGRAVATION : From coffee ; while eating ; from liquor and tobacco ; lying on right side ; and in the morning.

AMELIORATION : From fresh air ; from cold water ; and from rest.

RELATIONSHIP. *Compare* : *Anac.*, *Arg-N.*, *Bell.*, *Hyos.*, *Kali-P.*, *Lach.*, *Lyc.*, *Merc.*, *Nat-M.*, *Phos.*, *Stram.*, and *Zinc*.

In urinary diseases and gonorrhœa, *Canth.* has more tenesmus ; *Cann-I.* more burnıng and smarting.

Cannabis Sativa.

COMMON NAME : HEMP ; GALLOWS GRASS.

Cough, with green, viscid expectoration (*Kali-S.*, *Merc.*, *Nat-S.*, *Puls.*, *Sil.*).

ASTHMA OR DYSPNŒA : THE PATIENT CAN ONLY BREATHE BY STANDING UP (A.).

Choking in swallowing, things go down "the w rong way" (*Anac.*) (A.).

Rattling, wheezing, breathing (*Seneg.*) (Br.).

Fatigue, after bodily exercise (Ars., Bry., Calc., Con., Crot-H., Lach., Nat-C., Phos-Ac., Phos., Pic-Ac., Rhus-T., Sel., Spong.).

Great weakness after dinner (Amm-M., Bov., Carb-V., Dig., Graph., Iod., Lyc., Nat-M., Ox-Ac., Phos-Ac., Sil., Sulph., Thuj.) and when moving (Agar., Arg-M., Ars., Bry., Cocc., Hydr-Ac., Lach., Nux-V., Phos., Spong., Staph., Sulph., Tab.).

The mind is too active ; crowded with ideas (*Coff., Lach., Stram.*).

Sensation as if intoxicated (*Gels., Hyos , Nux-V., Op.,*).

Sadness (*Ign., Nat-M., Puls.*) (C.).

Tetanic spasms, especially of the upper extremities (Ars., Bry., Cham., Cic., Cocc., Crot-C., Cupr., Hyos., Ign., Ipec., Merc-C., Op., Plat., Sec., Sil., Stram., Strych., Sulph., Verat.).

Contraction of fingers after a sprain (A.).

PARALYTIC TEARING PAIN (*Caust., Rhus-T.*).

Deep tearing stitches (Bry., Kali-C., Nit-Ac.,). Rheumatic tearing, as if in the periosteum, especially while moving.

Sensation as from pinching with the fingers.

Dislocation of patella on going upstairs (A.).

It is the remedy par excellence with which to begin the treatment of gonorrhœa (N.).

Acute or inflammatory stage of gonorrhœa. (A.).

PAINFUL DISCHARGE OF MUCUS FROM THE URETHRA (*Canth.*) *Clem.*, *Dig.*, *Gels.*, *Hep.*, *Kali-B.*, *Kali-P.*, *Kali-S.*, *Lyc.*, *Merc.*, *Nat-M.*, *Nat-S.*, *Puls.*, *Sep.*).

URETHRA VERY SENSITIVE TO TOUCH OR PRESSURE ; CANNOT WALK WITH LEGS CLOSE TOGETHER ; IT HURTS THE URETHRA (A.).

THE URETHRA FEELS INFLAMED AND SORE TO TOUCH ALONG ITS WHOLE LENGTH DURING ERECTION TENSIVE PAIN (N.).

THE DISCHARGE OF URINE IS VERY PAINFUL AND ONLY BY DROPS (*Canth.*, *Con.*, *Hep.*, *Nux-V.*, *Puls.*, *Sars.*, *Sep.*, *Thuj.*). IT IS BLOODY AND BURNS (*Canth.*, *Merc-C.*, *Sars.*).

STINGING, BURNING AND SMARTING DURING AND AFTER MICTURITION (*Cann-I.*, *Canth.*, *Clem.*, *Merc-C.*, *Nit-Ac.*).

Great pain in the back in the region of the kidneys with urging to urinate, and bloody urine (N.).

Sensation of soreness in the renal area (*Berb.*, *Lyc.*).

Drawing pains from the region of the kidneys to the inguinal glands, with anxious nauseous sensation in the pit of the stomach (N.).

Pain extending from the orifice of the urethra backward, burning-biting, posteriorly more sticking, while urinating (A.).

Tearing pains along the urethra in a zigzag direction (A.).

The glans and prepuce are dark red (Bt.).

GREAT SWELLING OF THE PREPUCE, APPROACHING TO PHIMOSIS (*Apis, Canth., Merc., Rhus-T., Sulph.*) (Frn.).

OVER-SEXUAL EXCITEMENT IN EITHER SEX (*Canth., Phos., Plat.*) (G.).

Pressure, dragging sensation in the testicles when standing (*Berb.*) (C.).

IMPOTENCE FROM SEXUAL ABUSE (*Agn., Calad., Calc., Dig., Graph., Kali-P., Lyc., Nat-M., Phos., Sulph.*) (G.).

Painful jerks, as if something were moving about in the abdomen (*Croc.*) (C.).

Threatened abortion, on account of too frequent sexual intercourse (Bt.).

Threatened abortion, complicated with gonorrhœa (Bt.).

Great sexual excitement, with sterility (G.).

Gonorrhœal ophthalmia (*Arg-N., Hep., Merc., Nat-S., Sep.*) (Br.).

Opacity of cornea (*Calc., Merc., Nat-M., Sil.*) (Br.).

Dim-sightedness (*Caust., Chin., Merc., Phos., Sep., Sil.*) (G.).

Sensation as if drops of cold water were falling on the head.

Violent palpitation of the heart (*Ars.*, *Nat-M.*).

SENSATION AS OF DROPS FALLING FROM THE HEART (N.).

Dull stitches in the left side, just below the ribs, when breathing and when not breathing (C.).

Pericarditis (*Apis*, *Ars-I.*, *Bry.*, *Lach.*, *Phos.*, *Rhus-T.*, *Sulph.*) (Br.).

Shocks and beats in the region of the heart.

Obstinate constipation, causing retention of the urine (*Caust.*) (A.).

Constriction of anus (*Bell.*, *Lach.*) (A.).

Vertigo : when standing or walking ; with tendency to fall sideways (C.).

Epistaxis (*Acon.*, *Bell.*, *Carb-V.*, *Ferr.*, *Glon.*, *Ipec.*, *Kali-P.*, *Lach.*, *Merc.*, *Nit-Ac.*, *Puls.*) (G.).

Eructations of bitter or acrid fluid (*Ambr.*, *Dios.*, *Lyc.*, *Sep.*) (C.).

Affections of the ball of the foot or under part of the toes (G.).

AGGRAVATION : In the forenoon ; during the act of micturition ; after motion ; from talking ; on lying down ; from standing ; from going upstairs ; and after dinner.

AMELIORATION : From standing (dyspnœa) ; from expectoration ; and from remaining quietly.

RELATIONSHIP : *Similar to* : *Acon.*, *Apis*, *Ars.*, *Bell.*, *Canth.*, *Caps.*, *Gels.*, *Hep.*, *Kali-M.*, *Lach.*, *Merc.* and *Puls.* in early stage of specific urethritis.

CANNABIS SATIVA is very similar to CANTHARIS in its urethral phenomena. It has the same yellow discharge from the urethra. There seems to be more burning and smarting under *Cannabis*, while there is more tenesmus under *Cantharis*.

ANTIDOTES : *Camph.*; to large doses : lemon juice.

Cantharis.

COMMON NAME : SPANISH FLY.

The kind of suffering to which *Canth.* is best adapted, is of a violent, destructive character (G.).

The burning pain and intolerable urging to urinate are the red strands of *Canth.* in all inflammatory affections (A.).

Violent burning, with soreness in all parts of the body, especially in the cavities.

Throat and larynx painfully constricted and as if on fire (*Bell., Lach., Phyt.*) (B.).

Vesicles and canker in the mouth (J.).

Sensation of cutting in inner parts (*Bell., Merc., Nit-Ac.*).

Sensation of dryness in the joints (*Croc., Lyc., Nux-V., Phos-Ac., Puls.*).

Pricking in inner parts (*Bry.*, *Ign.*, *Kali-B.*, *Kali-C.*, *Phos.*, *Sil.*).

Burning thirst, but averse to liquids (*Ars.*) (B.).

Violent retching and vomiting (*Ars.*, *Cupr.*, *Nux-V.*, *Sec.*, *Tab.*, *Verat.*) (B.).

Tearing and stinging from without to within (*Bell.*, *Ign.*, *Ran-B.*).

Burning at the anus (*Aloe*, *Caps.*, *Lach.*, *Nux-V.*, *Sulph.*) (G.).

Tremendous burning pain through the whole intestinal canal (*Iris*) (Ra.).

Stools like the scrapings of the mucous membrane (*Merc-C.*), *mixed with blood, with burning and scanty urine* (Bt.).

Erysipelas, with blebs or large blisters filled with water and attended with burning pains (N.).

VESICULAR ERYSIPELAS (*Anac.*, *Apis*, *Crot-T.*, *Rhus-T.*, *Urt-U.*) (Frn.).

BURNS AND SCALDS, CAUSING VESICATION (Frn.).

TETANIC SPASMS, COMPELLING TO BEND FORWARD OR BACKWARD ; OFTEN AGGRAVATED BY THE SIGHT OF WATER (*Bell.*, *Hyos.*, *Lyss.*, *Stram.*).

Thoughts of drinking, sound of water, or touching the larynx, produce spasms (*Lyss.*) (Bt.).

Great desire to urinate, with complete strangury and

tenesmus of the cervix vesicæ (Bell., Caps., Con., Merc-C., Tereb.) (Bt.).

Violent cutting and burning pains in the bladder, before, during and after micturition (Merc-C.) (G.).

RETENTION OF URINE, WITH SPASMODIC PAIN IN THE BLADDER (Bell., Caust., Con., Gels., Lyc., Nux-V., Op., Pareir., Tarant., Tereb.).

NEPHRITIS (Apis, Ars., Merc-C., Tereb.) (G.).

CONSTANT DESIRE TO URINATE ; PASSING BUT A FEW DROPS AT A TIME ; SOMETIMES MIXED WITH BLOOD (Merc-C., Nux-V., Sars., Sulph. Thuj.,) (G.).

GREAT BURNING DISTRESS IN THE URETHRA (Apis, Cann-S., Merc-C., Nit-Ac., Tereb.) (Bt.).

The pains could not be worse if the urine were molten lead (F.).

Cutting, burning pains in the urethra, with ineffectual urging to urinate (Arg-N., Calc., Caps., Con., Eup-Pur., Ipec., Kali-C., Lyc., Merc., Nat-M., Nit-Ac., Nux-V., Op., Phos-Ac., Puls., Sars., Sep., Sulph., Thuj., Zinc.) (Bt.).

It produces and cures most violent cystitis (Merc-C., Tereb.) (R.).

Small, unsatisfactory quantity of urine passed at a time (N.).

Violent cutting or burning pains extend from the kidneys down either ureter to the bladder (F.).

Moaning or lamenting (*Bell.*, *Hyos.*, *Puls.*, *Stram.*) (G.).

Uncontrollable anguish, furious rage and frenzied delirium (*Bell.*, *Stram.*) (N.).

Barking (*Bell.*, *Calc.*, *Stram.*) (G.).

SATYRIASIS (*Bell.*, *Hyos.*, *Phos.*, *Stram.*).

AMOROUS FRENZY (*Phos.*, *Stram.*, *Verat.*) (B.).

THE PATIENT IS UNEASY, RESTLESS, DISTRESSED AND DISSATISFIED (G.).

SEXUAL DESIRE TOO STRONG ; EXCESSIVE DESIRE FOR SEXUAL CONGRESS (*Nux-V.*, *Phos.*, *Stram.*) (Bt.).

Debility bordering on paralysis (*Agar.*, *Con.*, *Gels.*, *Kali-P.*, *Lach.*, *Nux-V.*, *Op.*, *Phos.*, *Pic-Ac.*, *Rhus-T.*, *Sil.*).

Aching pains in the region of the kidneys (F.).

Voice low (*Arg-N.*, *Carb-V.*, *Phos.*).

Swelling of vulva, with irritation (*Rhus-T.*) (R.).

Menses too early and too profuse (*Calc.*, *Ferr.*, *Puls.*, *Sab.*) (G.).

Ovaries are extremely sensitive to touch (*Bell.*, *Lach.*) (R.).

Membraneous dysmemorrhœa (*Acet-Ac.*, *Bor.*, *Brom.*, *Cham.*, *Cycl.*, *Kali-B.*, *Lac-C.*, *Lach.*, *Phos.*, *Rhus-T.*, *Sab.*, *Ust.*, *Vib.*) (G.).

Sterility (*Alet.*, *Aur.*, *Bar-M.*, *Bor.*, *Con.*, *Graph.*, *Kreos.*, *Nat-C.*, *Nat-M.*, *Sep.*) (G.).

Puerperal convulsions (Apis, Bell., Cupr., Hyos., Stram.) (F.).

Nymphomania, with bladder symptoms (*Bell., Hyos., Stram.*) (D.).

Expels moles, dead fœtus and placenta ; promotes fecundity (G.).

Stringy and tenacious discharges from the mucous membranes (*Hydr., Kali-B.*) (N.).

Burning in the urethra, better lying quietly on the back, worse standing and walking (R.).

HYDROPHOBIA, WHEN ATTENDED WITH MOANING AND VIOLENT CRIES, INTERSPERSED WITH BARKING, AS OF A DOG (*Bell., Lyss., Stram.*) (G.).

Drawing pains in the spermatic cord while urinating (R.).

PRIAPISM : DESIRE ; DISTURBING SLEEP ; PAINFUL ERECTIONS MOST SEVERE AT NIGHT WITH CONTRACTION AND PAIN IN THE WHOLE OF THE URETHRA (R.).

Cutting pains extend along the spermatic cords to the testicles and down the penis, attended by drawing up of the testicles (F.).

Bloody, nocturnal emissions (*Led., Merc., Petr.*) (A.).

Pericarditis, with effusion (*Bry., Phos., Sulph.*) (C.).

The male child frequently pulls at the genital organ (*Bell., Bufo, Hyos., Merc., Stram.*) (F.).

It is a valuable remedy in the passage of renal calculi, especially when the pains are violent (F.).

Disgust for everything—drink, food, tobacco (Br.).

Drinking even small quantities of water increases pain in the bladder (A.).

Stitches in the chest (*Bry., Kali-C., Merc., Phos., Sulph.*) (C.).

Pleurisy, with exudation (*Apis, Bry., Kali-I., Nit-Ac., Phos., Sulph.*) (B.).

Grinding of teeth (*Ars., Bell., Calc.*) (C.).

Objects look yellow (*Aloe, Ars., Bell., Cann-I., Cina, Crot-H., Cycl., Dig., Kali-B., Plb., Sant., Sep., Sulph., Zinc.*) (D.).

Face : pale or yellowish, and bears on an expression of deep-seated suffering (F.).

Facial erysipelas : the erysipelatous inflammation begins on the nose, either with or without vesicles. It often spreads to one or the other cheek (F.).

Erythema, from exposure to sun's rays (sun-burn) (A.).

Fiery, sparkling, staring look (C.).

Thickly furred tongue (*Ant-C., Bry., Kali-M., Puls.*) (C.).

Pain in loins, with incessant desire to urinate (*Lyc.*) (C.).

The right side is mostly affected (*Lyc.*).

AGGRAVATION : From coffee ; before, during

and after micturition ; from sight of water ; from bright objects ; while drinking ; from touch or approach ; and at night.

AMELIORATION : From rubbing ; and from lying quietly on the back.

RELATIONSHIP. *Compare* : *Acon.*, *Apis*, *Ars.*, *Bell.*, *Bry.*, *Camph.*, *Cann-S.*, *Caps.*, *Cop.*, *Dig.*, *Equis.*, *Ferr-P.*, *Gels.*, *Hep.*, *Hyos.*, *Kali-B.*, *Lyc.*, *Merc.*, *Merc-C.*, *Nit-Ac.*, *Op.*, *Phos.*, *Puls.*, *Rhus-T.*, *Sab.*, *Sep.*, *Sulph.*, *Tereb.*, *Thuj.*, and *Urt-U.*

Antidotes : *Acon.*, *Camph.*, *Laur.*, and *Puls.*

COMPLEMENTARY : *Apis*, *Arg-N.*, *Merc-C.*, *Sep.*, and *Tereb.*

N. B.—It has been employed locally as well as internally in burns (locally 1 part to 40).

Capsicum.

COMMON NAME : CAYENNE PEPPER.

Phlegmatic temperament and laxness of the muscles (*Calc.*).

TENDENCY TO GET FAT (*Amm-M.*, *Ant-C.*, *Calc.*, *Calc-Ars.*, *Cupr.*, *Ferr.*, *Graph.*, *Kali-B.*, *Kali-C.*, *Lac-D.*, *Lyc.*, *Nat-C.*, *Sep.*).

Stiffness and painfulness of the joints, when beginning to move (*Rhus-T.*).

14

CRACKLING OF THE JOINTS (*Led., Nit-Ac., Petr., Rhus-T.*).

HOME SICKNESS (*Aur., Bell., Calc-P., Carb-An., Caust., Clem., Dros., Eup-Pur., Hyos., Ign., Kali-P., Lach., Mag-C., Merc., Nat-M., Phos-Ac., Puls., Sil., Staph., Verat.*), WITH REDNESS OF CHEEKS AND SLEEPLESSNESS.

Inclined to be jovial, yet gets angry at trifles (A.).

Taciturn and obstinate (*Ign., Nat-M., Sulph.*) (G.).

Peevish, easily offended (*Aur., Bry., Nux-V., Staph., Sulph.*).

Wants to be let alone (*Cham., Ign., Nat-M., Nux-V., Phos-Ac., Sep.*) (Br.).

Dreads any kind of exercise (*Bry., Nux-V., Phos-Ac.*).

Burning at the orifice of the urethra, before, during and after micturition (N.).

INTENSE BURNING ALONG THE URE-THRAL CANAL (*Canth., Merc-C., Sars., Sulph.*) (G.).

STRANGURY (*Bell., Canth., Merc-C.*) (Br.).

FREQUENT, BUT UNSUCCESSFUL DESIRE TO URINATE (*Apis, Bell., Canth., Ferr-P., Gels., Hyos., Nux-V., Puls., Sars., Sep., Sulph., Tereb., Thuj.*) (G.).

GONORRHŒA, WITH CHORDEE (*Arg-N., Canth., Merc., Nux-V., Phos.*) (Br.).

DISCHARGE FROM THE URETHRA PURU-LENT, BLOODY, CREAM-LIKE (N.).

Shrivelled spermatic cord (shrivelled genitalia—
Arg-N., Carb-S., Ign., Lyc., Merc.) (Hm.).

COLDNESS OF THE SCROTUM (*Aloe, Berb.,
Brom., Dios., Iris, Merc.*), WITH IMPOTENCE
(*Agn., Bar-C., Calad., Con., Graph., Lyc., Med.,
Phos., Sel., Sep., Sulph.*) (Hm.).

ATROPHY OF THE TESTES (*Ant-Ox., Aur.,
Bufo, Carb-An., Gels., Iod., Kali-I., Lyss., Staph.,
Zinc.*) (Hm.).

Fever, where chilliness predominates (*Nux-V.,
Rhus-T.*) (Bt.).

Influenza, with violent sneezing, and sorethroat(*All-C.,
Ars., Rhus-T., Sabad.*) (Bt.).

COUGH, WITH PAIN FAR FROM THE
CHEST.

Violent erections, only subdued by cold water
(G.).

Nervous spasmodic cough, in sudden paroxysms;
as if the head would fly to pieces (A.).

PAIN IN DISTANT PARTS (AS BLADDER,
KNEES, LEGS OR EARS) ON COUGHING (A.).

WITH EXPLOSIVE COUGH, (AND AT NO
OTHER TIME) THERE ESCAPES A VOLUME OF
PUNGENT, FETID AIR (A.).

*Very painful sensation in the throat when coughing,
with stitches in the neck of the bladder* (G.).

Constriction ; in fauces, throat, nares, chest,
bladder, urethra or rectum (*Bell., Lach.*) (A.).

BURNING AND SMARTING SENSATION, AS FROM CAYENNE PEPPER, IN THROAT AND OTHER PARTS, NOT RELIEVED BY HEAT (A.).

DIPHTHERIA (*Ars., Merc-Cy., Nit-Ac.*) (G.).

Tonsillitis : with burning, smarting pain ; intense soreness ; constriction of throat with burning ; inflamed, dark-red, swollen (A.).

Atonic dyspepsia (*Chin., Hep., Nux-V., Puls., Sep., Sulph.*) (Br.).

Intense craving for stimulants (*Ars., Asar., Crot-H., Hep., Lach., Nux-V., Sulph.*) (Br.).

THE BURNING, SPASMODIC CONSTRICTION AND OTHER PAINS, WORSE BETWEEN THE ACTS OF DEGLUTITION (*Ign.*) (A.).

Pain in the head as if it would burst ; cries out and grasps the head when coughing (*Bry.*).

LACK OF REACTION (*Ambr., Amm-C., Ars., Brom., Calc., Carb-V., Con., Gels., Hell., Laur.*), ESPECIALLY IN FAT PEOPLE (N.).

On the upper part of the legs cold perspiration.

Hæmorrhoids, with burning and tenesmus of rectum and pain in the small of the back (R.).

Catarrhal asthma, with red face and well-marked sibilant rales. He coughs, and a successful cough raises phlegm, which relieves the asthma (F.).

Every stool is followed by thirst and every drink by shuddering (A.).

Tearing drawing from above downward.

Burning and smarting, as though cayenne peppers were sprinkled upon the parts (*Ars.*) (Bt.).

Tenesmus of rectum and bladder at the same time (N.).

Increased acuteness of the senses (*Bell., Coff., Op.*) (G.).

Sensation of coldness in the stomach (*Ars., Camph., Carb-An., Chin., Hipp., Kali-B.*).

Much flatulent distention of the abdomen (*Arg-N., Carb-V., Chin., Nat-S., Podo., Puls., Sulph.*) (Bt.).

Diarrhœa : with severe burning in the lower part of the rectum, continued after stool (G.).

SORENESS OF THE ANUS (*Aloe, Ars., Hep., Nit-Ac., Sulph., Thuj.*) (D.).

STOOLS OF BLOODY MUCUS WITH TENES-MUS (*Aloe, Coloc., Merc., Nux-V., Rhus-T., Sulph.*) ; BURNING OF THE ANUS, WORSE AT NIGHT (*Ars., Iod., Nit-Ac., Sulph.*).

EXCESSIVE BURNING AND SORENESS IN THE MOUTH AND THROAT, WITH MUCH CONGESTION OF THE MUCOUS MEMBRANE. THROAT SMARTS AS IF FROM CAYENNE PEPPER, WITH SENSATION OF CONSTRICTION ON SWALLOWING (Bt.).

INFLAMMATION OF THE PETROUS (POR-TION OF THE TEMPORAL) BONE ; VERY TENDER TO THE TOUCH (*Hep., Lach.*) (G.).

CARIES OF THE MASTOID (*Aur.*, *Fluor-Ac.*, *Hep.*, *Sil.*) (N.).

Swelling and pain behind the ears (*Merc.*, *Sil.*) (Br.).

Fetid odour from the mouth (*Ars.*, *Aur.*, *Bry.*, *Carb-V.*, *Nux-V.*, *Puls.*) (Br.).

It should be studied in malarial fever when the liver and the spleen are enlarged, especially if the spleen is sensitive, swollen, indurated and large amount of quinine has been employed (Bl.).

INTERMITTENT FEVER CHILL PREDOMINANT ; THIRST IN THE CHILL, OR DURING THE CHILL AND HEAT, MUCH PAIN IN THE BACK AND LIMBS (Ma. & Ht.).

CHILL BEGINS BETWEEN THE SHOULDER-BLADES (N.).

Chill predominates in the back, and there is an inordinate desire for cold water (Bt.).

THE CHILL COMMENCES IN THE BACK WITH THIRST, BUT DRINKING CAUSES SHIVERING (D.).

During chill must have something hot to the back (Br.).

AS THE COLDNESS OF THE BODY INCREASES, SO ALSO DOES THE ILL-HUMOUR (A.).

AGGRAVATION : In the evening ; after eating ; after drinking ; when beginning to move ; in the open air ; and from uncovering.

AMELIORATION : After having moved about for some time ; and from heat.

RELATIONSHIP. *Compare* : *Apis, Arg-N., Ars., Bell., Bry., Calad., Canth., Cinch., Ign., Lach., Lyc., Merc., Nat-M., Nit-Ac., Nux-V., Phyt., Puls., Rhus-T., Sep., Sulph.* and *Thuj.*

Cina follows it well in intermittent fever.

ANTIDOTES : *Calad., Camph., Cina, Cinch.* and *Sulph.*

It antidotes : *Calad., Cinch.* and *Coff.*

Carbo Animalis.

COMMON NAME : ANIMAL CHARCOAL.

Diseases of elderly persons with marked venous plethora, blue cheeks, blue lips and great debility (A.).

Sensation of numbness, as if, in fact, the part had gone to sleep in many parts, especially the head (*Caust., Kali-Br., Nux-V., Phos., Rhus-T.*).

RHEUMATIC STIFFNESS OF THE JOINTS (*Agar., Ars., Bell., Calc., Caust., Colch., Form., Kali-C., Led., Lyc., Nat-M., Petr., Rhus-T., Sep., Sil., Staph., Sulph.*).

Pressing pain in the joints and muscles of the limbs (*Alum., Calc., Clem., Coloc., Kali-C., Led., Nat-S., Par.*).

Pain in the hip-joints at night (*Bell., Coloc., Ferr. Kali-B., Kali-C., Kali-I., Lach., Merc., Nat-S., Petr., Rhus-T., Sulph., Syph., Tarant.*).

Burning pains (*Apis, Ars., Caps., Carb-V., Lach.,*
Phos., Sep., Sulph.).

WEAKNESS AND EASY DISLOCATION OF THE JOINTS (*Calc., Caust., Coloc., Lyc., Puls., Rhus-T., Sulph., Thuj.*).

Tension and contraction of the parts (*Cupr.,*
Mag-P., Rhus-T., Sec.).

Earthy coloured face, with copper coloured spots
on both the face and body (Bt.).

GREAT SENSITIVENESS TO OPEN, COLD, DRY AIR (*Bell., Hep., Sil.*).

Often troubled with severe headache (*Bell., Bry.,*
Ferr., Gels., Kali-B., Lach., Nat-M., Nux-V., Puls.,
Rhus-T., Sep., Sil., Verat-V.) (Bt.).

Teeth very sensitive to the least cold air (*Acon., Bell.,*
Calc., Mag-P., Nat-M., Ox-Ac., Sin-N.) (Bt.).

Tearing pains in the teeth from salt food (Bt.).

Ankles turn when walking (A.).

Joints weak : easily sprained by slight exertion
(*Led.*) (A.).

Easily strained from lifting even small weights
(*Rhus-T.*) (A.).

Sour taste in the mouth (*Arg-N., Calc., Ign., Lyc.,*
Mag-C., Nat-Ars., Nat-C., Nux-V., Phos.) (K.).

LOOSENESS OF THE TEETH (*Amm-C., Bry., Carb-V., Caust., Hyos., Lyc., Merc., Merc-C., Nit-Ac., Phos., Sil., Staph.*), WITH BLEEDING GUMS (*Bar-C., Bov., Calc., Carb-V., Crot-H., Lach., Merc., Merc-C., Nat-M., Nit-Ac.*) (Bt.).

Great weakness of digestion (a very valuable remedy
for a host of digestive ailments).

WEAK, SORE, EMPTY FEELING AT THE PIT OF THE STOMACH (*Ant-C., Cocc., Dig., Hell., Hydr., Ign., Lac-C., Merc., Murx., Nux-V., Phos.*).

Glandular diseases of a scirrhous nature with fetid discharges, accompanied with great prostration and debility (Bt.).

PAINFUL INDURATION OF THE GLANDS OF THE MAMMÆ (*Aster., Bell., Bry., Calc., Caust., Cham., Con., Graph., Iod., Merc., Phyt., Sil., Sulph., Thuj., Ust.*).

HARD, PAINFUL NODES IN BREASTS (*Bell-P., Bufo, Calc-F., Carb-V., Con., Cund., Graph., Iod., Kreos., Lac-C., Lyc., Nit-Ac., Phyt., Sil.*) (B.).

SPONGY ULCERS AND EXCRESCENCES (*Lach., Phos., Thuj.*).

Great numbness and languor in the thighs, particularly during the menses (G.).

FOUL, EXHAUSTING SWEATS AT NIGHT, STAINING YELLOW (*Graph., Lach., Merc., Sil.*) (B.).

Copper coloured exanthemata (*Alum., Ars., Ars-I., Aur., Calc., Cor-R., Kali-I., Kreos., Lyc., Merc., Mezer., Nit-Ac., Psor., Syph.*).

In all the female diseases the patient is extremely prostrated ; can hardly stand up (*Cocc.,Sep., Stann.*) (Bt.).

THE MENSTRUAL FUNCTION SEEMS TO EXHAUST HER REMARKABLY, SO THAT SHE IS HARDLY ABLE TO SPEAK (*Alum., Cocc., Stann.,* (G).

Menses ; too soon ; last long, but not profuse ; feels

so exhausted during its continuance, she is hardly able to speak (G.).

Violent pressing in the loins, the small of the back, and the thighs, during the menses (*Kali-C., Nux-V., Sab., Vib-O.*) (G.).

WATERY, ACRID, BURNING LEUCORRHŒA (*Alum., Bor., Calc., Calc·S. Kreos., Puls., Sep., Sulph.*), PARTICULARLY WHEN WALKING (*Æsc., Alum., Aur., Bov., Calc., Graph., Kreos., Lac-C., Mag-M., Nat-M., Phos., Sars., Sep., Sulph., Tub.*); TURNS THE LINEN YELLOW (*Chel., Kreos., Prun.*). (G.).

Uterus hard and swollen (*Alum., Alumn., Aur., Aur-M., Bell., Chin., Con., Helon., Iod., Kali-Br., Lyss., Pall., Plat., Sep., Tarant.*). (Bt.).

MALIGNANT ULCERATIONS OF THE NECK OF THE WOMB, WITH FOUL DISCHARGES (*Ars., Ars-I., Con., Graph., Hydr., Kreos·, Lach., Lyc., Murx., Phos., Sep., Sil., Thuj.*) (G.).

Lochia too long continued, acrid, excoriating the parts, and very offensive (*Bapt·, Kreos., Pyrog., Rhus-T., Sep.*) (G.).

A stitching pain remains in the chest after recovery from pleurisy (*Bor., Kali-C., Ran-B.*) (A.).

All the glands may become more or less indurated (*Bad., Bar-M., Brom., Calc., Calc-F., Clem., Con., Iod., Phyt., Spong., Sulph.*) (Bt.).

GLANDS : INDURATED, SWOLLEN, PAINFUL ; IN NECK, AXILLÆ, GROIN, MAMMÆ; PAINS

LANCINATING, CUTTING, BURNING (*Ars-I., Con., Phyt.*) (A.).

Benign suppurations change into ichorous or malignant conditions (*Calc., Hep., Sil.*) (A.).

Hearing confused ; cannot tell from what direction a sound comes (*Phos., Puls.*) (A.).

Headache : as if a tornado in the head ; as if the head had been blown to pieces ; has to sit up at night and hold it together (*Syph.*) (A.).

Vertigo followed by nose-bleed (*Br.*).
Acne rosacea (*Aur-M., Calc-Sil., Carb-V., Caust., Eug., Lach., Psor., Rhus-T.*) (Br.).

Redness of the tip of the nose (*Aur., Bell., Calc., Crot-H., Lach., Nit-Ac., Sulph.*) (K.).

Buboes : indurated and mal-treated (*Bad.*) ; *refuse to heal* (*Sulph.*); *suppurating ; and accompanied by burning* (*Ars., Ars-I., Bell., Tarant.*) (K.).

Ichorous discharge from the ears, often accompanied by swelling of the parotid gland(*Amm-C., Ars., Carb-V., Lyc., Nit-Ac., Psor., Sep., Sil.*) (G.).

Ringing in the ears when blowing the nose (*Teucr.*) (K.).

Humming and singing in the ears (*Acon., Amm-M., Bell., Calc., Chin., Ferr., Graph., Hyos., Kali-C.*) (G.).

MAY BE INDICATED IN CONSTITUTIONAL OR TERTIARY SYPHILIS, AFTER ABUSE OF MERCURY (*Aur., Nit Ac.*) (F.).

While walking along the street objects seem to him to be far off (F.).

Dimness of sight on attempting to read, **relieved by** rubbing the eyes (*Sulph.*) (F

AGGRAVATION : Whi'e eating ; when lying on the side ; after shaving ; from slightest touch ; **after** midnight ; from loss of animal fluids ; in dry, cold air ; from lifting ; and during menses.

AMELIORATION : Laying hand on part ; and rubbing the eyes.

RELATIONSHIP. *Similar to* : *Bad., Brom., Carb-V., Iod.. Merc-I-F., Phos., Sep., Sulph.*

COMPLEMENTARY : *Calc-P.*

It is often useful after bad effects from spoiled fish and decayed vegetables.

Antidotes : *Ars., Camph., Nux-V.*

Carbo Vegetabilis.

COMMON NAME : VEGETABLE CHARCOAL.

Especially adapted to adynamic diseases with great prostration (*Ars.*) (Bt.).

Low, grave, depraved or cachectic state (*Ars., Chin., Phos., Sec.*) (B.).

Inflammation of parotid gland (*parotitis*) ; *with*

metastasis to the testes (Ars., Jab., Nat-M., Puls., Rhus-T. ; with metastasis to the mammæ—*Puls.*) (K.).

Burning pain in exterior parts, in ulcers and in bones (Ars.).

Pressing sensation in inner parts (*Bell., Coloc., Nux-V., Puls.*).

In the morning, when rising from the bed, the limbs feel as though broken (*Cocc., Eup-P., Plb.*).

Paralytic tearing in the limbs with flatulency and difficulty of breathing (Lyc., Nux-V.).

BAD EFFECTS FROM THE LOSS OF FLUIDS (*Carb-An., Cinch., Phos-Ac.*).

Great debility, much worse from the smallest exertion of body or mind, worse towards noon (Ars.).

Pricking from above downwards.

Pain with anxiety, heat, despairing hopelessness, and debility after the pain.

Pulsations here and there in the body (*Nat-M.*)

Trembling and twitching of the limbs through the day.

BAD EFFECTS FROM WINE INTOXICATION THE DAY PREVIOUS (*Cocc., Ipec., Nux-V., Puls.*).

Bad effects from cold drinking whilst overheated (*Ant-C., Bry., Puls.*).

Chronic, mal-treated cases of ague ; paroxysms irregular (*Ipec., Puls.*) (Bt.).

Intermittent fevers, with thirst only during the cold stage (*Apis, Arn., Ign., Nat-M.*).

Chill predominates in the hands and feet ; complexion very sallow ; great accumulation of flatus ; stomach bloated ; spleen swollen and painful ; with sour and profuse sweats (Bt.).

Frequent sneezing, with constant and violent crawling and tickling in the nose (*All-C., Ars., Sabad.*) (N.).

SEVERE NOSE-BLEED, LONG CONTINUED, OR SEVERAL TIMES DAILY FOR WEEKS (*Phos.*) (N.).

Ears too dry (*Calc., Graph., Lach., Nux-V.*) (N.).

Deafness : after acute exanthemata, or abuse of mercury (*Puls., Sil., Sulph.*) (N.).

Discharges from the ears : *bloody* ; *brownish* ; *excoriating* ; *fetid* ; *ichorous* ; *offensive* ; *purulent* ; *suppressed* ; *or watery* (K.).

OTORRHŒA AS A SEQUELA OF MEASLES OR SCARLET FEVER (*Bov., Crot-H., Lyc., Merc., Nit-Ac., Puls., Sulph.*) (K.).

FACE : VERY PALE, GRAYISH YELLOW OR HIPPOCRATIC (*Æth., Ant-T., Ars., Chin., Lach., Sec., Tab., Verat.*) (N.).

AFTER A FEW MOUTHFUL THERE IS A SENSE OF REPLETION (*Chin., Lyc., Plat., Sep., Sulph.*) (D.).

FLATULENCY : VERY FETID SMELL ; FLATU-

LENT COLIC (*Chin., Coloc., Dios., Mag-P., Nux-V., Puls.*).

Gastralgia: *stomach distended with flatulence; worse lying down* (*Dios., Nux-V., Puls.*) (N.).

COLIC FROM FLATULENCE (*Arg-N., Coloc., Dios., Nat-S., Nux-V., Sep.*) (N.).

ABDOMEN FULL TO BURSTING (*Arg-N., Chin., Lyc.. Nux-V., Puls., Raph.*) (N.).

Sensation as if the œsophagus was contracted (*Cact., Ign., Kali-C., Merc-C., Phos., Sulph-Ac.*) (Bt.).

The most innocent food disagrees (*Calc-P., Chin., Hep.. Lach., Lyc., Nux-M., Sep.*) (G.).

FREQUENT ERUCTATIONS, WHICH AFFORD ONLY TEMPORARY RELIEF (*Ant-T., Arg-N., Carb-S., Dios·, Graph., Ign., Kali-B., Kali-C., Lyc., Sang.*) (G.).

Neglected pneumonia, with expectoration of a dirty, yellow colour, and smelling badly (*Kali-C.*) (G.).

Has helped in a few desperate cases of pneumonia, last stage, with marked dyspnœa, cold breath, general coldness, weak pulse, and a tendency to collapse (R.).

Wheezing and rattling of mucus in the chest (*Ant-T.*) (Br.).

Great and long-lasting hoarseness (*Caust.*) (G.).

HOARSENESS IN THE EVENING (*Arg-M., Brom., Carb-An., Carb-S., Caust., Graph., Kali-B., Mang., Phos., Rumx., Sulph·*).

Indicated where the patient is troubled with occasional spells of long coughing attacks (*Ars., Con., Kali-B., Kali-C., Lach., Phos., Seneg.*).

Greenish and fetid expectoration (*Kali-I., Sil.*) **(**G.**)**.

AIR HUNGER (*Ars., Aur., Calc-I., Chin., Iod., Kali-I., Lach., Lyc., Puls., Sulph.*) (B.).

Bronchitis of the aged with profuse, yellow and fetid expectoration (Bl.).

WANTS TO BE FANNED (*Ant-T., Apis, Chin., Ferr., Med., Sulph.*). (K.).

DYSPNŒA : WORSE WHILE LYING ; WANTS DOORS AND WINDOWS OPEN ; BETTER FROM ERUCTATIONS (*Aur., Nux-V.*) (K.).

Profuse and constant salivation of stringy saliva (*Kali-B.*) (Be.).

Tongue painfully sensitive when chewing ; gums become loosened and retracted from the teeth (*Kali-P., Merc., Nit-Ac., Staph.*) (N.).

Burning in the chest as from glowing coals (*Ars., Phos.*) (R.).

Menstruation too early and too profuse (*Ars., Bell., Bov., Calc., Calc-P., Chin., Cocc., Cycl., Ferr., Ipec., Nat-M., Nux-M., Nux-V., Phos., Plat., Rat., Rhus-T., Sab.*).

Varicoseveins in the vulva and about the external genitals (*Ambr., Calc., Ham., Lyc., Nux-V., Thuj., Zinc.*) (N.).

Cough, with expectoration in the morning, greenish purulent, sometimes brownish (N.).

Great weakness or general prostration with cold knees at night in bed (N.).

Ulcers : secreting a foul, ichorous pus emitting an offensive odour (*Nit-Ac.*). (Bt.).

Frequent involuntary, putrid, cadaverous smelling stools, followed by burning in the anus (*Aloe*) (N.).

Large protruding, blue hæmorrhoids, sometimes suppurating, burning, and emitting a terrible odour (*Lach.*) (N.).

Dyspepsia : from over-eating or high living (*Ant-C. Kali-M., Nux-V., Puls.*) (D.).

Aversion to milk, which makes him flatulent (R.). MUCH BELCHING OF SOUR, RANCID FOOD. (*Alum., Bar-C., Calc., Cycl., Ferr-I., Graph., Kali-B., Laur., Merc., Phos., Puls., Sulph.*) (G.).

Craves acids, sweets, and salted things (*Arg-N., Calc., Calc-S., Med., Nat-M., Plb., Sulph.*) (K.).

Burning distress in the stomach (*Ars., Canth., Caps., Cic., Colch., Phos , Sec., Sulph.*) (Bt.).

Chronic dyspepsia of the aged (*Ant-C., Lyc., Sil.*) (D.). Cardialgia in nursing women (G.). Stomach troubles from abuse of alcohol (*Nux-V.*) (D.).

UNCEASING EMISSIONS OF FLATULENCE BY THE RECTUM (*Agar., Aloe, Arg-N., Carb-S., Chin., Coloc., Dios., Graph., Lyc., Nat-S., Olnd., Puls., Staph., Sulph.*) (G.).

15

CAN NOT BEAR TIGHT CLOTHING AROUND THE WAISTAND ABDOMEN (*Lach., Lyc., Nux-V.*). (Br.).

Humidity of the skin (moist exanthemata).

Blue colour of the body with terrible cardiac anxiety and icy coldness of the surface (*Dig., Lach., Phos.*).

Indented tongue (Ant-T., Ars., Chel., Dulc., Hydr., Ign., Iod., Kali-I., Merc., Plb., Podo., Rhus-T., Sep., Stram., Syph.) (K.).

Looseness of the teeth, with bleeding from the gums, which are very sensitive when chewing (Hep.) (N.).

Hæmorrhage from broken down condition of the mucous membranes anywhere, attended with great paleness of the skin (N.).

Vital powers low, venous system predominates (*Lach., Sec.*) (N.).

GUMS BLEED READILY AND ARE SPONGY (*Lach., Merc., Nit-Ac., Phos., Sulph.*) (Bt.).

Pure blood flows into mouth after sucking the teeth (*Amm-C., Bov., Kali-B., Nit-Ac., Rat., Zinc.*) (R.).

Induration of the glands, inguinal and axillary, particularly of syphilitic origin, when the induration is hard as a stone (Bad., Carb-An., Iod., Merc-IF, Sil.) (D.).

Weakness of memory and slowness of thought (*Bar-C., Calc., Con., Kali-P., Lyc., Nat-M., Phos., Sil.*) (A.).

IN THE LAST STAGES OF DISEASE, WITH COPIOUS COLD SWEAT, COLD BREATH, COLD TONGUE, AND LOSS OF VOICE, THE REMEDY MAY SAVE A LIFE. (A.).

Ailments : from quinine, abuse of mercury, salt, salted meats, spoiled fish, meats or fats, or from getting over-heated (*Ant-C.*) (A.).

PULSE IMPERCEPTIBLE, SMALL OR SOFT (*Camph., Verat.*) (G.).

Pulmonary hæmorrhage, with burning pains in the lungs, coldness of the skin and desire to be fanned (*Chin.*) (R.).

Anæmic, especially after acute diseases, which have greatly depleted the patients (N.).

Useful for persons who have never fully recovered from the exhausting effects of some previous illness ; has never recovered from the effects of typhoid, etc. (N.).

Want of susceptibility to well-selected remedies (*Ambr., Laur., Psor., Op., Sulph., Valer.*) (A.).

Dark, turbid urine (*Apis, Arn., Ars., Benz-Ac., Kali-C., Op., Tereb.*) (F.).

Is an excellent remedy for the terrible dyspnœa of chronic aortitis, especially when the patient has become very anæmic, dropsical, etc. (*Ars., Cupr., Lach.*) (F.).

May be administered in carbuncle, particularly when the affected parts are bluish or livid, and when the discharges are offensive and associated with burning pains. (F.).

Flatus : hot, moist and offensive. (Br.).

Acrid, corrosive moisture from the rectum (*Pæon.*) (Br.).

Discharge of blood from the rectum (*Ham., Ipec., Nit-Ac., Phos.*) (Br.).

Excoriation of anus (*Aloe, Merc., Sulph.*) (Br.).

Stools of foul blood and mucus (*Ham., Merc-C., Nit.-Ac., Sulph.*) (Bt.).

Lymphatic swellings, with suppurations and burning pains (*Ars-I., Lach.*).

Morning leucorrhœa, discharges very acrid, excoriating the parts (G.).

Aphthæ of the vulva, with much itching, heat and redness (*Calc., Kreos., Graph., Nit-Ac., Sulph.*) (G.).

Extraordinary rush of voluptuous thoughts (*Canth., Hyos., Phos., Plat.*) (G.).

Frequent emissions (*Dios., Kali-P., Nux-V., Phos-Ac., Sulph.*) (Bt.).

Onanism during sleep (*Camph., Plat., Thuj.*) (G.).

Icy coldness of the parts; they have a livid, purple look (gangrena senilis) (Bt.).

AGGRAVATION : In the morning ; at night ; before falling asleep ; from the abuse of quinine and mercury ; on rising from the bed ; while walking in the open air ; from butter, pork or fat food ; from singing or reading aloud ; and in warm, damp weather.

AMELIORATION : From eructations ; from being fanned ; in the open air ; from loosening the clothing around the waist ; and lying down.

RELATIONSHIP. *Complementary* : *China and Kali-C.*

Antidotes : *Ars., Camph., Coff., Lach.,* and *Sp-Nitr-D., Carb-V.,* itself antidotes ; *Chin., Lach.,* and *Merc.*

Compare : *Ant-T., Ars., Calc., Carbo-A., Chin., Ferr., Graph., Kali-C., Lach., Lyc., Merc., Nat-M., Nux-V., Phos., Phos-Ac., Sec., Sep., Sulph.,* and *Verat.*

Carbolic Acid.

COMMON NAME : CARBOLIC ACID.

Useful in cases of burns, when the affected parts ulcerate (*Ars., Canth., Nat-C.*) (F.).

Putrid discharges from the mouth, nose, throat, nostrils, rectum and vagina (*Anthr., Ars., Bapt., Carb-V., Lach., Merc., Nit-Ac., Psor., Pyrog., Sulph.*) (A.).

Headache, better from binding the head (*Arg-N., Bry., Mag-M., Puls., Sil.*) (K.).

HEADACHE, WITH A SENSATION AS IF A BAND WERE TIED AROUND THE FOREHEAD (*Ant-T., Gels., Merc., Sulph.*) (F.)

Dull, heavy frontal headache (*Bry., Nux-V., Sep.*) (A.).

Headache, worse from mental exertion, and *better from smoking* (*Am.-C., Aran., Calc.-P., Naja.*) or *strong tea* (*Glon.*) (K.).

Flatulence of the aged depending upon an imperfect digestion (*Anti-C., Carb-V., Lyc.*) (D.).

Acidity and burning in the stomach (*Ars., Calc., Carb-V., Nat-P., Sulph.*) (D.).

Menses too profuse and dark coloured (*Cycl., Kali-P., Lach., Sec.*) (C.).

Irritating leucorrhœa causing itching and burning (*Kreos., Nit-Ac., Sulph.*) (Br.).

BLACK URINE (*Colch., Dig., Nat-M.*) (F.).

ALKALINE URINE (*Bapt.*, *Ferr.*, *Fluor-Ac.*) (C.).

Leucorrhœa : *acrid, copious, fetid, green* (*Apis*, *Arg-N.*, *Bov.*, *Carb-V.*, *Cub.*, *Kali-P.*, *Lach.*, *Merc.*, *Nat-M.*, *Nit-Ac.*, *Puls.*, *Sep.*) (A.).

Erosions of cervix ; *fetid, acrid discharge* (*Aur.*, *Nit-Ac.*, *Rhus-T.*) (Br.).

Puerperal fever, with offensive discharge (*Arn.*, *Ars.*, *Bry.*, *Carb-V.*, *Kali-P.*, *Pyrog.*) (Br.).

Mental and bodily languor (*Ars.*, *Con.*, *Gels.*, *Kali-P.*, *Sil.*) (Br.).

Disinclination to study (*Aloe.*, *Bapt.*, *Chel.*, *Chin.*, *Lec.*, *Nux-V.*, *Phos.*) (Br.).

FŒTOR ORIS (*Ars.*, *Aur.*, *Bapt.*, *Carb-V.*, *Graph.*, *Hep.*, *Kali-P.*, *Lach.*, *Merc.*, *Nit-Ac.*, *Phos.*, *Sulph.*) (B.).

Constant belching of large quantities of wind (*Carb-V.*, *Lyc.*, *Puls.*) (C.).

Longing for whisky and tobacco (*Asar.*, *Carb-V.*) (A.).

Vomiting : of drunkards, in pregnancy, sea-sickness, or cancer ; of dark, olive-green fluid (*Pyrog.*) (A.).

Malignant scarlatina and variola (*Amm-C.*, *Ars.*, *Lach.*, *Phos.*, *Stram.*) (A.).

Vesicular eruptions all over the body, which itch excessively ; better after rubbing, but leaving a burning pain (*Sulph.*) (N.).

Itching of the scalp (*Caust.*, *Graph.*, *Sep.*, *Sil.*, *Sulph.*) (C.).

PAINS ARE TERRIBLE ; COME SUDDENLY, LAST

A SHORT TIME, AND DISAPPEAR SUDDENLY (*Arg-N., Bell., Ign., Kali-B., Mag-P., Nit-Ac., Phyt., Spig.*) (A.).

Physical exertion, even much walking, brings on abscess in some part, but generally in the right ear (Cp.).

Lacerated wounds from blunt instruments ; bones bare, crushed ; much sloughing of soft parts (*Calend.*) (A.).

PROFOUND PROSTRATION, COLLAPSE; SURFACE PALE AND BATHED IN COLD SWEAT (*Camph., Carb-V., Verat.*) (A.).

Dysentery : *fluid mucus, like scrapings of mucous membranes, and great tenesmus* (*Canth., Merc-C.,*) (A.).

Diarrhœa : *stool thin, involuntary, black, of an intolerable odour* (*Ars., Carb-V., Kali-P., Sulph.*) (A.).

Scarlet fever, with marked tendency to destruction of tissue internally, and fetid odour (*Ars., Bapt., Kali-P., Lach.*) (Br.).

CONSTIPATION, WITH HORRIBLY OFFENSIVE BREATH (*Aur., Carb-V., Nux-V., Op., Psor.*) (A.).

Ozœna, with fetor and ulceration (*Kali-B., Merc-C., Nit-Ac., Sil,, Thuj.*) (Br.).

Throat : *ulcerated patches on inside of lips and cheeks ; faces red and covered with exudation ; putrid discharge ; almost impossible to swallow* (*Lach., Mur-Ac., Nit-Ac.*) (Br.).

Cramps in the fore part of the leg, close to the tibia, during walking (Br.).

Easily fatigued by the least walk (C.).

Pain in the loin, worse when straightening himself and by jolting while riding (C.).

Sterterous respiration (*Amm-C*., *Ant-T*., *Apis*., *Ars*., *Camph*., *Chin*., *Cupr*., *Gels*., *Glon*., *Hyos*., *Lach*., *Laur*., *Lyc*., *Nit-Ac*., *Nux-V*., *Op*., *Phos*., *Puls*., *Spong*., *Stram*.) (K.).

Orbital neuralgia over the right eye (C.).

AGGRAVATION : While walking ; when straightening oneself ; by jolting ; and from mental exertion.

AMELIORATION : From smoking ; from strong tea ; from rubbing ; and by binding.

RELATIONSHIP. *Similar to* ; *Ars*., *Bapt*., *Carb-V*., *Gels*., *Hydr-Ac*., *Kali-P*., *Kreos*., *Lach*., *Merc-C*., *Mur-Ac*., *Nit-Ac*., *Petro*., *Phos*., *Pic-Ac*., *Rhus T*., *Sil*., *Sulph*., and *Thuj*

Compare : *Ars*., *Kreos*. and *Sulph*. in burns, and *Gels*., *Merc*., and *Sulph*. in ulcers with unhealthy, offensive discharges.

Carbolic Acid is antidoted by dilute cider vinegar, either externally or internally, when the said acid has been swallowed accidentally, or taken for suicidal purposes.

Carduus Marianus.

COMMON NAME : ST. MARY'S THISTLE.

Sad, depressed and hypochondriacal (*Ign*., *Nux-V*., *Sep*., *Staph*., *Sulph*.) (Bl.).

Dull frontal headache (*Bry.*, *Chin.*, *Kali-M.*, *Nux-V.*, *Puls.*, *Sep.*) (B.).

Dark or brown urine (*Benz-Ac.*, *Bry.*, *Chel.*, *Merc-C.*, *Phos.*, *Sep.*, *Sulph.*, *Zinc.*) (K.).

Want of appetite, with nausea and vomiting of a sour green fluid (*Calc.*) (Bl.).

TERRIBLE ATTACKS OF GALL-STONE COLIC (*Ars.*, *Bell.*, *Berb.*, *Chel.*, *Chin.*, *Dios.*, *Lyc.*, *Mag-P.*, *Nat-S.*, *Nux-V.*, *Podo.*, *Sep.*, *Verat.*) (A.).

Pain in the region of the liver, with dizziness, bad-tasting mouth, and jaundiced skin (*Chel.*, *Merc.*, *Nat-M.*, *Nat-S.*, *Podo.*) (N.).

The gall-bladder is enlarged and tender (*Chin.*, *Lach.*, *Merc.*, *Nat-S.*, *Sep.*) (Bl.).

CLAY-COLOURED STOOLS (*Aur-M-N.*, *Berb.*, *Chel.*, *Chin-Ars.*, *Chion.*, *Dig.*, *Gels.*, *Hep.*, *Iod.*, *Kali-B.*, *Lach.*, *Lept.*, *Merc.*, *Nat-S.*, *Podo.*, *Sep.*) (K.).

Jaundice : *with dull headache, bitter taste in the mouth, and white tongue* (*especially in the middle with red tips and edges*) ; *the stools are bilious, and the urine golden yellow* (F.).

CIRRHOSIS OF THE LIVER (*Chel.*, *Cupr.*, *Hep.*, *Hydr.*, *Mur-Ac.*, *Phos.*, *Plb.*, *Sulph.*) (A.).

Uncomfortable fulness in the region of the liver (*Chel.*, *Chin.*, *Lach.*, *Merc.*, *Nat-S.*, *Sep.*, *Sulph-Ac.*) (F.).

Vertigo, with tendency to fall forward (*Alum.*, *Calc-P.*,

*Ferr., Graph., Kali-P., Lach., Lyc., Nat-M., Nux-V ,
Podo., Rhus-T., Sil., Sulph.*) (K.).

Alternate diarrhœa and constipation (*Aloe., Ant-C.,
Bry., Dig., Lach., Lyc., Nat-M., Nit-Ac., Nux-V., Op ,
Podo., Sulph.*) (Br.).

Tension in the liver when lying on the right side
(*Aloe, Bry., Calc., Carb-V., Ferr., Mur-Ac., Nat-M.,
Nat-S., Nit-Ac., Sulph.*) (K.).

Stitches in the region of the seventh rib, when stooping ; afterwards the pain spreads all over front of the
chest, making movement of arms, walking and stooping
almost impossible *(Chel.)* (C.).

Severe spell of coughing, compelling him to sit up in
bed (*Hyos.*) Bl.).

AGGRAVATION : When lying on the right side ;
from stooping ; from motion ; and from pressure.

AMELIORATION : From sitting up in bed ; and from
lying on the unaffected side.

RELATIONSHIP. *Similar to :*   *Alum., Bry., Chel.,
Chin., Dig., Hep., Iod., Lach., Lyc., Merc., Nat-M.,
Nat-T., Nit-Ac., Plb., Podo., Sep., Sulph.* and *Zinc.*

Cascarilla.

COMMON NAME :   SWEET BARK.

Gnawing, pressing pain (*Caust., Puls., Sep., Sulph.*).

Pain in the stomach, as from a shock.

Pressing colic (*Bell.*, *Bry.*, *Chel.*, *Chin.*, *Dios.*, *Mag-P.*, *Nux-V.*, *Puls.*, *Sep.*, *Verat.*).

DESIRE FOR HOT DRINKS (*Ang.*, *Ars.*, *Bell.*, *Bry.*, *Calad.*, *Cedr.*, *Chel.*, *Eup-P.*, *Eup-Purp.*, *Graph,*, *Hyper.*, *Kreos.*, *Lac-C.*, *Lyc.*, *Merc-C.*, *Sabad.*, *Sulph.*) (A.).

DESIRE FOR HOT DRINKS, DURING FEVER (*Cedr.*, *Eup-P*, *Lyc.*) (K.).

As hungry after eating as before (*Calc.*, *Cina.*, *Lac-C.*, *Lyc.*, *Stront.*) (A.).

Stools difficult and hard (*Alum.*, *Bry.*, *Chel.*, *Graph.*, *Iod.*, *Kali-M.*, *Lyc.*, *Mur-Ac.*, *Nat-M.*, *Plb.*. *Sep.*, *Sulph.*)

Discharge of blood from the rectum (*Alum.*, *Alumn.*, *Ham.*, *Lept.*, *Lyc.*, *Nat-M.*, *Nit-Ac.*, *Phos.*, *Sulph.*).

Heat, with thirst for warm drinks (*Cedr.*).

Constipation : stool hard in pieces and covered with mucus (*Graph.*).

Alternate diarrhœa and constipation (*Ant-C.*, *Chel.*, *Lyc.*, *Nux-V.*, *Podo.*, *Sulph.*) (K.).

Burning heat of the inner and outer ear (*Sulph.*).

Flatulence and pain in the rectum (*Aloe*, *Nux-V.*, *Puls.*, *Sulph.*) (Bl.).

Empty eructations (*Arg-N.*, *Carb-V.*, *Iod.*, *Lyc.*) (K.).

AGGRAVATION : From cold and from eructations.

AMELIORATION : From hot drinks ; and from pressure.

RELATIONSHIP. Similar to : *Ars.*, *Bry.*, *Chel.*, *Eup-P.*, *Graph.*, *Hydr.*, *Lyc.*, *Merc.*, *Nat-M.*, *Sep.*, *Sulph.* and *Thuj.*

Castor Equi.

COMMON NAME : A red substance growing on the inside of the legs of the horse.

Acts on nails and bones (*Sil.*). (Br.).

Affects principally the female organs (*Carb-An., Lach., Phos.*) (Br.).

Swelling and violent itching of the breasts (Bl.).

SORE NIPPLES (*Graph., Nit-Ac., Sil.*). THEY ARE CRACKED AND RAGGED, AND ALMOST HANGING. (F.).

Bleeding and suppurating nipples (*Graph., Sil., Sulph.*).

Warts on the breast (Br.).

Pain in the right tibia and coccyx (Br.).

Chapped hands (*Calc., Calend., Graph., Hep., Petr., Rhus-T., Sars., Sep., Sulph.*) (Br.).

Warts on the forehead (Br.).

RELATIONSHIP. *Compare* : *Arn., Caust., Fluor-Ac., Graph., Phyt., Rat.,* and *Sil.*

Castoreum.

COMMON NAME : BEAVER.

Nervous, apprehensive and sad during menses (F.).

Predominant chilliness (*Ant-C., Aran., Arn., Bry., Camph., Chin., Meny., Nat-M., Nux-V., Sabad., Sec., Staph., Verat.*).

Is indicated in cases of nervous, hysterical woman, who are greatly prostrated as the result of some exhausting disease (Bl.),

Restless sleep, with frightful dreams and starting (*Ars., Bell., Cham., Hyos., Stram.*).

Constant yawning (*Brom., Chel., Cocc., Graph., Lyc., Nat-M., Sulph.*) (Bl.).

Attacks of chilliness with icy coldness in the back (*Amm-M., Cocc.*).

DYSPNŒA, WORSE FROM LYING ON THE BACK OR RIGHT SIDE, AND BETTER FROM LYING ON THE LEFT SIDE (K.).

Useful in some forms of chronic bronchitis (*Ant-T., Carb-V., Hep., Kali-B., Lyc., Nat-S., Phos., Sil., Sulph.*) (Bt.).

Menstrual colic, with pallor and cold sweat (*Verat.*) (N.).

The menstrual blood, owing to tenesmus, escapes only in drops (*Amm-C., Cycl., Graph., Sep.*) (F.).

Pains better from pressure (*Bry., Coloc., Mag-P., Rhus-T.*) (N.).

Lack of reaction (*Ambr., Amm-C., Caps., Laur., Op., Psor., Sulph.*) (K.).

Summer diarrhœa (*Bry., Camph., Chin.*) ; green mucous stools (B.).

Feels exhausted (*Carb-An., Carb-V., Chin., Cocc., Ferr., Kali-P., Lach., Mosch., Nat-M., Phos-Ac., Sep., Stann., Verat.*) (N.).

Exhausting sweats after fevers (*Bry.*, *Camph.*, *Carb-An.*, *Carb-V.*, *Chin.*, *Chin-S.*, *Ferr.*, *Iod.*, *Merc.*, *Phos.*, *Psor.*, *Samb.*, *Sep.*, *Tub.*) (B.).

Tearing pressure in different parts during menses (**F.**).

Inclination to stool during menses (*Amm.-M.*, *Bov.*, *Caust.*, *Nux-V.*, *Verat.*) (F.).

Abdomen distended with flatulence (*Carb-V.*, *Chin.*, *Lyc.*, *Nat-S.*, *Puls.*) (F.).

Cutting about the navel (*Aloe*, *Bell.*, *Coloc.*, *Dios.*, *Ipec.*, *Mag-C.*, *Nux-V.*, *Puls.*, *Stann.*) (F.).

Cutting colic before stool, better from pressure, or bending double (*Bell.*, *Coloc.*, *Nux-V.*, *Puls.*) (F.).

AGGRAVATION : During menses ; from lying on the back or right side ; and during hot weather.

AMELIORATION : From lying on left side ; from pressure ; and from bending double.

RELATIONSHIP : Compare : *Ambr.*, *Ign.*, *Mosch.*, *Mur-Ac.*, *Puls.*, *Sep.*, *Valer.*, and *Zinc.*

Antidote : *Colch.*

Caulophyllum.

COMMON NAME : BLUE COHOSH.

Especially suited to women, for their ailments during pregnancy, parturition and lactation (A.).

Is fretful and easily displeased (*Bell.*, *Cham.*, *Nux-V.*, *Sulph.*).

Leucorrhœa : acrid, exhausting ; preventing pregnancy (*Alum., Calc-C., Carb-A., Nat-C., Nit-Ac.*) (A.).

LEUCORRHŒA IN LITTLE GIRLS (*Calc., Cann-S., Cub., Merc., Merc-I-F., Puls., Senec,, Sep.*) (A.)

Sensation of fulness and tension in the hypo-gastric region (D.).

SHOULD BE USED DURING LABOUR, WHEN THE PAINS ARE INTERMITTENT, SHARP AND CRAMPY (*Bell., Cupr., Mag-P., Puls.*), AND APPEAR IN THE GROIN, BLADDER AND LOWER EXTREMITIES ; THEY ARE SPASMODIC AND FLY FROM ONE PLACE TO ANOTHER (D.).

May be called for false labour pains during the last months of pregnancy (*Gels., Mag-P., Nux-V., Puls., Sep.*) (D.).

Habitual abortion from uterine debility (*Alet., Gels., Helon., Sep.*) (A.).

Spasmodic rigid os delays labour (*Bell., Cupr., Sec.*) (A.).

Needle like pricking pains in the cervix (A.).

Uterine hæmorrhage, with a tremulous weakness felt over the entire body during the flow (G.).

LABOUR PAINS : SHORT, IRREGULAR, SPASMODIC ; TORMENTING, USELESS PAINS IN THE BEGINNING OF LABOUR (*Act-R., Bell., Cupr., Gels., Mag-P., Nux-V., Puls., Sec., Sep., Vib.*) (A.).

Will correct deranged vitality and produce efficient pains, if symptoms agree (A.).

After pains : after long, exhausting labour ; spasmodic, across the lower abdomen ; extend into the groins (A.).

Hæmorrhage, after hasty labour (*Arn., Chin., Sec.*) ; want of tonicity ; passive ; after abortion (*Sec., Thlaspi.*). (A.)

Sub-involution, after abortion or confinement (*Cimic., Kali-Br., Puls., Sep., Sulph.*) (C.).

Prolapsus uteri (*Abies-C., Alet., Calc-P., Helon., Lac-D., Nat-M., Sep.*) (F.).

RHEUMATISM OF THE SMALL JOINTS OF HANDS AND FEET, AND FLYING PAINS IN THE LIMBS.

Painful stiffness of affected joints (*Bell., Calc-F., Rhus-T.*) (A.).

Erratic pains changing place every few minutes (*Ign., Lac-C., Puls.*) (A.).

Severe pains and swelling in the joints of wrists and fingers ; shutting the hands produces severe pains (N.).

"Moth spots" on the forehead, with leucorrhœa (C.).

Frequent gulping up of sour, bitter fluid, with vertigo (*Iris, Nux-V., Puls., Sep.*) (C.).

Lochia : protracted ; great atony ; passive oozing for days from relaxed vessels (*Sec.*).

AGGRAVATION : During menses ; in open air ; from coffee ; and from motion.

AMELIORATION : From warmth.

RELATIONSHIP : *Compare* : *Act-S., Bell., Cimic.,*

Gels., Ign., Kali-B., Lil-T., Mag-P., Puls., Sec., Sep., Thlas., and *Vib.*

Caulophyllum is similar to *Gelsemium* in dys-menorrhœa and follows it well.

Incompatible : *Coffea.*

Causticum.

COMMON NAME: HAHNEMANN'S TINCTURA ACRIS SINE KALI.

Adapted to persons who are subject to affections of respiratory and urinary tracts (*Lyc., Merc., Nat-M.*) (A).

Useful for dark-haired persons with rigid fibres, psoric constitutions, suffering from long ago suppressions of skin diseases (N.).

Disturbed functional activity of brain and spinal cord, from exhausting disease or severe mental shock, resulting in paralysis.

Tension in the limbs with paralysis, especially of the extensor muscles (*Plb.*).

Rheumatic and gouty tearing in the limbs, relieved by warmth, especially by the heat of the bed.

Shortening of the flexor muscles.

Paralytic trembling, debility of the limbs when out of bed.

16

Numbness of the single parts, or of the right side of the body.

In children, soreness, swelling of the abdomen, easy falling, and late learning to walk (*Bar-C., Calc-P., Sil.*).

In the evening and while sitting, insupportable restlessness through the whole body and anxiety about the heart.

Burning of the exterior parts (ulcers) (Ars., Lach., Phos., Sulph.).

Warts of eye-brows and nose.

Dryness of the larynx (*Bell., Con., Lach.*) (D.)

MORNING HOARSENESS (*Calc., Calc-P., Carb-V., Kali-B., Mang., Phos., Sil., Sulph.*).

COMPLETE LOSS OF VOICE (*Am-Caust., Phos.*) (D.).

Weakness of voice from over-exertion (Hg.).

PARALYTIC APHONIA (*Alumn., Arg-M., Brom., Carb-V., Phos., Stram.*) (D.).

Cough, being obliged to swallow what has been raised (*Arn., Cann-S., Con., Dros., Gels., Kali-C., Kali-S., Lyc., Nux-M., Sep., Spong., Staph., Zinc.*).

COUGH, RELIEVED BY A DRINK OF WATER (D.)

Cough, worse when bending forward (N.).

COUGH, ACCOMPANIED BY A SPURT OF URINE (*Apis, Bry., Hyos., Nat-M., Nux-V., Phos-Ac., Phos., Puls., Rumx., Sep., Squil., Staph., Sulph., Thuj., Verat., Zinc.*) (D.).

Can not speak loud (Phos.) (D.)

Cough, with a sensation as if one could not cough deep enough to raise the mucus (N.).

Cough with pain in the hip (N.).

Phlegm in the throat that cannot be hawked up, which produces nausea (Bt.).

Sensation of tension and pain in the jaws, so that she could only with difficulty open the mouth, and also could not eat well because a tooth seemed too long (N.).

Can not keep the upper eyelids up, they are nearly paralyzed, and will fall down over the eyes (N.).

PARALYSIS OF THE EYELIDS (*Alum., Con., Dulc., Gels., Graph., Mag-P., Nat-C., Nit-Ac., Nux-M., Plb., Rhus-T., Sep., Spig., Stann., Zinc.*) (D.).

Heat, burning and feeling of sand in the eyes (*Arg-N., Ars., Sulph.*) (D.).

Double vision (*Alumn., Aur., Bell., Cann-I., Cycl., Dig., Gels., Hyos., Iod.*) (D.).

Constantly complains of shivering coldness (*Kali-I.*).

Frequent ineffectual efforts to stool (*Anac., Nux-V., Sulph.*), with much pain, anxiety and redness in the face (N.).

STOOL PASSES BETTER WHEN THE PATIENT IS STANDING (D.).

Hæmorrhoids : worse when preaching or straining the voice, or from standing (N.).

Fistula in ano (*Berb., Calc-P., Fluor-Ac., Phos., Sil.*), *and fistula dentalis* (*Fluor-Ac., Hep., Merc., Sil.*).

Obstinate constipation, with varices in the anus (G.).

Can not evacuate the stool sitting down, is obliged to stand (D.).

WORDS, SOUNDS AND THE PATIENT'S OWN VOICE RE-ECHO IN THE EARS (D.).

Fissures and other troubles in the anus or rectum rendering walking intolerably painful (*Nit-Ac.*, *Sulph.*) (N.).

Mucus collects in the throat, can not be raised, has to swallow it (N.).

Warts on the back of the tongue (N.).

Speechlessness from paralysis of the organs of speech (*Gels.*, *Plb.*) (N.).

Neuralgia, right side of cheek bone to mastoid process ; worse at night (Ra.).

FACIAL PARALYSIS (*Agar.*, *Anac.*, *Bar-C.*, *Cocc.*, *Cupr.*, *Cur.*, *Dulc.*, *Graph.*, *Kali-Chl.*, *Kali-P.*, *Nux-V.*, *Op.*, *Plb.*, *Strych.*, *Zinc.*), DUE TO EXPOSURE TO DRY, COLD WINDS (D.).

Burning itching in the face, discharging an acrid fluid, which forms crusts when drying (Ra.).

A white coating on both sides of the tongue (N.).

Paralysis of the tongue, lips and throat (*Gels.*, *Plb.*) (D.).

PARALYSIS OF THE BLADDER (*Alum.*, *Arn.*, *Ars.*, *Bell.*, *Camph.*, *Canth.*, *Cupr.*, *Dulc.*, *Gels.*, *Hyos.*, *Kali-P.*, *Lach.*, *Merc.*, *Nux-V.*, *Op.*) (D.).

INVOLUNTARY URINATION WHILE COUGHING (*Apis*, *Caps.*, *Ferr-P.*, *Kreos.*, *Lyc.*, *Nat-M.*) (D.).

Difficult, frequent, and painful urination (*Canth.*, *Dig.*, *Gels.*, *Lyc.*) (Hg.).

Urine loaded with lithic acid and lithates, with great debility (Hg.).

Nocturnal enuresis of children, during the first sleep (*Benz·Ac.*, *Cina*, *Kreos.*, *Phos Ac.*, *Sep.*) (D.).

INVOLUNTARY EMISSION OF URINE WHEN SNEEZING, BLOWING THE NOSE OR WALKING (N.).

Itching of the orifice of the urethra (*Petrosel.*, *Thuj.*) (N.).

Numbness or insensibility of the urethra ; can not tell when the urine is passing in the dark, only by the sense of touch (N.).

Sudden and frequent loss of sight, with a sensation of a film before the eyes (G.).

The parts upon which he lies become sore (*Arn.*, *Bapt.*, *Pyrog.*) (D.).

MENSES FLOW ONLY DURING THE DAY (*Cact.*, *Coff.*, *Cycl.*, *Ham.*, *Puls.* ; menses flow only during the night—*Bor.*, *Bov.*, *Coff.*, *Cycl.*, *Mag-C.*, *Nat-M.*) (D.).

Menses cease at night and flow during the day, while leucorrhœa flows at night, not during the day (N).

Spasms of the rectum, preventing walking (*Æsc.*, *Nit-Ac.*, *Thuj.*) (G.).

Very apt to have hæmorrhoids, which are made intolerable by walking (*Æsc.*, *Brom.*, *Carb-An.*, *Mur-Ac.*, *Sulph.* ; better from walking—*Ign.*).

Painful pustules near the anus, discharging pus, blood and serum (Ra.).

Ailments from long lasting grief (*Gels.*, *Nat-M.*, *Phos-Ac.*) (Br.).

Greasy taste in the mouth (*Asaf.*, *Cham.*) (Br.).

SENSATION AS IF LIME WERE BEING SLAKED IN THE STOMACH (N.).

Flatulence (*Chin.*, *Dios.*, *Lyc.*, *Nat-S.*, *Puls.*, *Sep.*, *Sulph.*) (Ra.)

Water-brash (*Ars.*, *Bar-C.*, *Bry.*, *Calc.*, *Carb-V.*, *Graph.*, *Lyc.*, *Mezer.*, *Nux-V.*, *Par.*, *Petr.*, *Puls.*, *Sabad.*, *Sang.*, *Sil.*, *Staph.*, *Sulph.*, *Verat.*) (Ra.).

Pressure and fullness in the abdomen, as if it would burst ; nourishment greatly increases the pain (G.).

Great melancholy ; looks on the dark side of everything ; especially during menstruation (G.).

Very suspicious and mistrustful (G.).

Excessive sympathy for others (G.).

Absent-minded (*Apis*, *Cann-I.*, *Lach.*) (G.).

Pains in the abdomen, causing her to bend double (*Bell.*, *Coloc.*, *Mag-P.*, *Nux-V.*, *Puls.*) ; greatly aggravated by the least nourishment (*Calc-P.*), or tightening her clothes (*Arg-N.*, *Lach.*, *Lyc.*, *Nux-V.*) (G.).

Menses too early and too abundant ; after it ceases, a little blood is passed from time to time, for many days, which smells badly (G.).

Old ulcers originating in a blister, with burning or itching (N.).

Burns that recover slowly, or remote effects of them (N.).

Dry, hollow cough, with soreness in the chest, caused by tickling and mucus in the throat, with expectoration only at night, of acrid tasting mucus, which he can not raise but has to swallow it again (J.).

Sensation of rawness or soreness of the scalp, throat, respiratory tract, rectum, anus, urethra, vagina, etc. (N.).

Sour perspiration (*Ars., Bry., Calc., Colch., Hep., Iod., Lyc., Mag-C., Merc., Nit-Ac., Psor., Sep., Sil., Sulph., Verat.*) (Bt.).

Glandular indurations (*Bad., Carb-An., Iod., Merc. Nit-Ac., Phyt., Rhus-T., Sil.*) (Bt.).

Cicatrices freshen up; old injuries reopen (*Graph.*) (Br.).

Aversion to sweets (*Ars., Graph., Merc., Nit-Ac., Phos., Sulph., Zinc.*) (Br.).

Fresh meat causes nausea ; smoked meat agrees.

Stitches in the liver (*Bell., Berb., Bry., Calc., Chel., Con., Lept., Mag-M., Merc , Nux-V., Ran-B., Sep.*).

Epileptic spasms (at night during sleep).

Left-sided sciatica (*Am-M., Cimic., Kali-B., Kali-C., Lach., Phos., Thuj.*), *with numbness* (*Coloc., Gnaph., Nux-V., Phyt., Rhus-T.*) (Br.).

Sciatic pains, worse from cold and coughing, and better from warmth or warmth of bed (K.).

Involuntary nodding of the head while writing (*Phos-Ac.*).

Dim-sightedness as if a thick fog were before the eyes (*Ars., Calc., Chin., Croc., Cycl., Gels., Merc., Phos., Puls., Sulph., Zinc.*).

Affects the right side most prominently (A.).

Vertigo : at night in bed, on rising and lying down again ; on looking fixedly at an object (*Cur., Kali-C., Lach., Nat-M., Phos., Sil., Spig., Sulph.*) ; and during menses (C.).

Photophobia, with constant necessity to wink (C.).

Leucorrhœa : profuse, flows like the menses, and has the same odour (C.).

May be used in spasmodic diseases, even in convulsions. When walking in the open air, the patient falls but soon recovers. During the unconscious stage, he passes urine. These attacks especially recur at the new moon (F.).

May be called for in colic after failure of *Colocynth*. The pains are of a griping, cutting character and are relieved by bending double (F.).

AGGRAVATION : In the evening ; in the open air ; after drinking coffee ; while perspiring ; in clear, fine weather ; during new moon ; from getting wet or bathing ; and from coming from the air into a warm room.

AMELIORATION : From warmth ; in damp, wet weather.

RELATIONSHIP. *Complementary* : *Carb-V., Petrosel.*

INCOMPATIBLE : *Phos.* Must not be used before or after *Phos.*, always disagrees ; *the Acids* ; *Coffea.*

Ceanothus Americanus.

COMMON NAME : NEW JERSEY TEA.

Leucorrhœa (*Arg-N., Calc., Kali-S., Lyc., Merc., Nat-M., Phos., Sep.*) (B.).

Periodical neuralgia (*Ars.. Bell., Cedro., Kali-B., Nat-M., Spig., Stann., Sulph.*) (B.).

ENORMOUS ENLARGEMENT OF THE SPLEEN (Br.).

DEEP-SEATED CUTTING PAINS AND FULLNESS IN THE REGION OF THE SPLEEN (N.).

Acute splenitis accompanied by severe pains and an increase in the area of flatness (Bl.).

Is also of service in chronic splenitis, dependent upon malaria and abuse of quinine (Bl.).

Feels worse during cold, damp weather. Is always chilly and dreads the cold (*Psor., Sil.*) (Bl.).

This remedy seems to possess a specific relation to the spleen (Br.).

Chronic bronchitis, with profuse expectoration (Br.).

Violent dyspnœa (*Ars., Kali-P., Lach., Phos.*) (Br.).

LEUCÆMIA(*Ars., Ferr., Nat-M., Sep., Sulph.*) (Br.).

Sore mouth (*Bor., Kali-M., Merc., Nat-M., Sulph.*) (Bl.).

PAIN IN THE LIVER AND BACK (*Chel.*, *Merc.*, *Nat-S.*, *Phos.*, *Podo.*, *Sep.*, *Sulph.*) (Br.).

GREEN URINE (*Ars.*, *Aur.*, *Berb.*, *Camph.*, *Carb-Ac.*, *Chel.*, *Colch.*, *Iod.*, *Merc-C.*, *Phos.*) (B.).

Constant urging to urinate (*Bell.*, *Canth.*, *Dig.*, *Ferr-P.*, *Nux-V.*, *Puls.*, *Sep.*, *Thuj.*) (Br.).

AGGRAVATION : From motion ; from lying on the left side ; and during damp weather.

AMELIORATION : In warm weather.

RELATIONSHIP. *Similar to* : *Ars*, *Berb.*, *Cedr.*, *Chin-S.*, *Dig.*, *Ferr.*, *Ferr-M.*, *Hep.*, *Iod.*, *Lach.*, *Merc-C.*, *Nat-M.*, *Phos.*, *Sep.*, and *Thuj.*

COMPLEMENTARY : *Nat-M.*

Chamomilla.

COMMON NAME : COMMON CHAMOMILLE.

Exceedingly irritable, fretful (*Nux-V.*) (A.).

"*Too ugly to live*" (A.).

Can not bear to be spoken to (*Ars.*, *Con.*, *Hyos.*, *Nit-Ac.*, *Nux-V.*, *Sep.*) (A.).

Aversion to talking (*Aur.*, *Carb-An.*, *Cocc.*, *Glon.*, *Phos-Ac.*, *Plat.*, *Sulph.*) (A.).

Can not endure any one near him (*Anac.*, *Ign.*, *Nat-M.*, *Nux-V.*) (A.).

Bad effects from wrath, from coffee and narcotic palliatives.

Snappish ; can not return a civil answer.

Cross and peevish, angry disposition (*Bell., Cina., Lyc., Nux-V., Sulph.*).

Unceasing crying and yelling (*Bell., Cina, Nat-M., Stram.*).

Anxious restlessness in mind and body with tossing about (*Ars.*).

THE CHILD WANTS TO BE CARRIED, AND IS THEN MORE QUIET (*Cina*).

THE CHILD *wants and cries for things and when it gets them it throws them away* (D.).

THE CHILD IS EXCESSIVELY FRETFUL ; MUST BE CARRIED UP AND DOWN THE ROOM ALL THE TIME ; IS ONLY QUIET THEN (G.).

Often gives vent to her ill humour, inspite of all restraint (G.).

Oversensitiveness to pain, and of the organs of sense to fresh air and wind (*Bell., Coff., Nux-V.*).

Pain : seems unendurable, drives to despair ; worse by heat ; worse in the evening before midnight ; with heat, thirst and fainting (A.).

Puts his feet out of bed ; soles burn (*Sulph.*). (Hr.).

TWITCHINGS AND CONVULSIONS OF CHILDREN DURING DENTITION (*Acon., Bell., Calc., Cupr., Hyos., Mag-P., Stram.*).

STOOLS LIKE CHOPPED EGGS AND SPINACH (G.).

HOT, DIARRHŒIC STOOLS, SMELLING LIKE ROTTEN EGGS (G.).

Pulsating pain, as from concealed suppuration (*Bell., Hep., Nat-M.*).

Bitter taste in the mouth with bilious vomiting (Bry., Ipec., Nat-S., Nux-V., Sep.) (Bt.).

Tongue coated yellow (*Chel., Nat-P., Nat-S.,* (Bt.).

Colic, with green diarrhœa and restlessness (*Acon., Ars., Colch., Coloc., Merc.*) (G.).

Severe colic ; abdomen distended like a drum ; wind passes off only in small quantities (G.).

Heat and redness of one cheek (*Cina, Ferr., Lachn.*).

Pains accompanied by thirst and heat (*Bell., Ferr-P., Stram.*).

Perspiration of the head, especially the borders of the hair (*Calc., Calc-P., Chin., Merc., Nat-M., Rhus-T., Sil.*).

Rheumatic pains drive the patient out of bed and compel him to walk about (D.).

The pain almost drives him crazy (*Acon., Ars., Coff*) (D.).

Drowsiness with moaning and starting (Bell., Gels., Hyos., Lyc., Podo., Stram.).

Sleepy, but cannot sleep (*Bell.*, *Caust.*, *Op.*) (A.).

Pain with numbness of the affected part (*Acon.*, *Ars.*, *Con.*, *Kali-N.*, *Plat.*, *Plb.*, *Puls.*) (A.).

A dry, teasing cough, keeping the child awake, or else a rattling cough, as if the bronchi were full of mucus (D.).

TOOTHACHE: IF ANY THING WARM IS TAKEN INTO THE MOUTH (*Bism.*, *Bry.*, *Coff.*, *Kali-C.*, *Lach.*, *Puls.*; *Sep.*), ON ENTERING WARM ROOM. (*Ant-C.*, *Bry.*, *Iris*, *Kali-S.*, *Mag-C.*, *Nux-V.*, *Phos-Ac.*, *Puls.*)., IN BED., FROM COFFEE., DURING MENSES OR PREGNANCY (*Acon.*, *Bell.*, *Calc.*, *Lyss.*, *Mag-C.*, *Merc.*, *Puls.*, *Sep.*) (A.).

Throbbing headache in one-half of the brain (*Bell.*, *Glon.*, *Lach.*, *Nat-M.*, *Verat-V.*) (Br.).

Flatulent colic, after anger, with red cheeks hot perspiration (Br.).

Abdomen distended like a drum (*Arg-N.*, *Ars.*, *Carb-V.*, *Chin.*, *Cocc.*, *Colch.*, *Hyos.*, *Lach.*, *Lyc.*, *Phos.*, *Tereb.*) (N.).

Diarrhœa: from cold, anger or chagrin; during dentition; after tobacco; in child-bed; from downward motion (*Bor.*, *Sanic.*) (A.).

Stool green, watery and corroding (*Merc.*, *Sulph.*) (A.).

Stitching, griping pains in the pit of the stomach and beneath the short ribs, impeding respiration (R.).

Vertigo after eating, or on rising from bed, with tendency to faint (C.).

Coldness of one part with heat of another (B.).

Eructations smelling of bad eggs (*Agar.*, *Ant-T.*, *Arn.*, *Psor.*, *Sep.*) (C.).

Great thirst for cold water (*Bry.*, *Nat-M.*, *Phos.*, *Sulph.*) (C.).

Profuse sweat on covered parts (*Bell.*, *Chin.*, *Ferr.*, *Nit-Ac.*, *Nux-V.*, *Sec.*, *Thuj.*) (C.).

High fever with sweating, especially on the head (*Bell.*) ; *thirsty* ; *one cheek red and hot, the other pale and cold* (N.).

Sweats with the pains (*Ant-T.*, *Bell.*, *Bry.*, *Chel.*, *Coloc.*, *Hep.*, *Lach.*, *Merc.*, *Nat-C.*, *Sep.*) (N.).

Face sweats after eating or drinking (N.).

Warm sweat on the head wetting the hair (*Bell.*) (N.).

Restless sleep ; moaning, starting up, crying, tossing about and talking while asleep (N.).

Frequent discharge of coagulated blood, with tearing pains and frequent desire to urinate (G.).

Violent labour-like pains in the uterus (*Bell.*, *Cimic.*, *Mag-P.*, *Puls.*, *Sec.*, *Sep.*, *Vib.*) (Bt.) .

HER LABOUR PAINS ARE SPASMODIC AND DISTRESSING ; CAN HARDLY BEAR THEM ; WANTS TO GET AWAY FROM THEM ; IS VERY IMPATIENT (G.).

Labour pains pass upward ; she is hot and thirsty, cross and inclined to scold (N.).

Burning in the vagina, as if excoriated (*Ars.*, *Kreos.*, *Sulph.*), with yellow, smarting leucorrhœa (*Calc.*, *Kreos.*, *Nat-S.*, *Sep.*) (G.).

CONVULSIONS OF CHILDREN FROM NUR-SING, AFTER A FIT OF ANGER IN MOTHER (*Nux-V.* ; after fright in mother—*Op.*) (A.).

AGGRAVATION : In the night ; after break-fast ; after suppressed perspiration ; on getting warm in bed ; in the evening ; from anger ; in open air ; in the wind ; and from eructations.

AMELIORATION : From being carried ; from fasting ; and in warm, wet weather.

RELATIONSHIP. *Complementary : Bell.*, in dis-eases of children, or cranial nerves.

Useful in cases spoiled by the use of *Opium* or *Morphine* in complaints of children.

Mental calmness contra-indicates *Chamomilla*.

COMPARE : *Bell.*, *Bor.*, *Bry.*, *Coff.*, *Puls.* and *Sulph.*

Chelidonium.

COMMON NAME : CELANDINE.

Often called for in affections of the liver, when there is a great deal of pain and soreness of that organ (N.).

Cough loose and rattling, difficult, associated with hepatic derangement (D.).

Disinclination to move, which he does very reluctantly (*Bry., Gels., Op.*).

Dyspnœa with oppression and constriction of the chest, worse on the right side (*Lyc.*) (D.).

Capillary bronchitis or pneumonia with hepatic or bilious symptoms (D.).

Paralytic drawing and lameness in single parts (*Plb., Rhus-T., Sil.*).

DISTRESSING PAIN UNDER THE RIGHT SCAPULA (*Bry., Card-M., Chen-A., Con., Lac-C., Lycps., Nat-M., Nux-V., Phos., Pic-Ac., Podo., Ruta., Sec.*) (D.).

Sleepiness and desire to lie down, without being able to sleep (*Gels., Nux-V., Puls.*).

Expectoration is not easily raised (*Ant-T., Bry., Caust. Kali-C., Phos., Sulph.*) (D.).

FAN-LIKE MOTION OF THE ALÆ NASI (*Am-C., Ant-T , Brom., Iod., Kreos., Lyc., Merc-I-F., Phos., Pryrog., Spong., Sulph-Ac., Zinc.*) (D.).

All complaints lessen after dinner (N.).

Yellow tongue, taking the imprints of teeth (*Ant-T., Ars., Carb-V., Dulc., Hydr., Iod., Merc., Plb., Podo., Rhus-T., Sep.*) (D.).

Chilliness predominating (*Anac., Bry., Calc., Camph., Caust., Colch., Ferr., Graph., Hep., Lyc., Mezer., Nux-V., Puls., Tarax.*).

Gastralgia relieved by eating (**Anac.**, **Graph.**, **Petros.**, **Sep.**) (D.).

Great debility and great lassitude in the morning when awakening and after eating.

Nothing but very hot drinks relieve the nausea and vomiting (N.).

ICTERUS (**Ars.**, **Bry.**, **Chin.**, **Dig.**, **Iod.**, **Lach.**, **Lyc.**, **Merc.**, **Nat-S.**, **Phos.**, **Podo.**, **Sep.**, **Sulph.**).

Pain in the hepatic region and across the umbilicus. as if the abdomen were constricted by a string (N.).

CONSTIPATION : STOOL HARD, ROUND BALLS LIKE SHEEP'S DUNG (**Alum.**, **Alumn.**, **Mag-M.**, **Merc.**, **Nat-M.**, **Nit-Ac.**, **Op.**, **Plb.**, **Sulph.**) (A.).

Alternate constipation and diarrhœa (**Ant-C.**, **Nit-Ac.**, **Nux-V.**, **Op.**, **Podo.**, **Sulph.**) (A.).

Burning and itching of the anus (**Æsc.**, **Carb-V.**, **Lyc.**, **Merc.**, **Sulph.**) (Br.)

Diarrhœa : at night ; slimy, light gray ; bright yellowish ; brown or white ; watery ; pastry ; involuntary.

GALL-STONES, WITH PAIN UNDER THE RIGHT SHOULDER-BLADE (**Card-M.**, **Chin.**, **Podo.**) (A.).

Retarded menstruation, but when the menses do come on they continue too long (Bt.).

Catamenia too late and too profuse (**Graph.**, **Puls.**, **Sep.**).

Large and flabby tongue (**Hydr.**, **Lyss.**, **Merc.**, **Nat-Ars.**, **Sep.**) (Br.).

17

Bad odour from the mouth (*Ars.*, *Bry.*, *Carb-Ac.*, *Merc.*, *Nux-V.*, *Puls.*, *Sil.*, *Sulph.*) (Br.).

Desire for very hot drinks (*Ars.*, *Bry.*, *Graph.*, *Kreos.*, *Lac-C.*, *Lyc.*, *Sabad.*) ; *unless almost boiling stomach will not retain them* (*Ars.*, *Casc.*) (A.).

PREFERS HOT FOOD AND DRINK (*Ang.*, *Ars.*, *Cupr.*, *Lyc.*, *Sabad.*) (Br.).

Longs for milk (*Apis.*, *Ars.*, *Aur.*, *Bry.*, *Calc.*, *Elaps*, *Lac-C.*, *Merc.*, *Nat-M.*, *Nux-V.*, *Phos-Ac.*, *Rhus-T.*, *Sabad.*, *Sil.*, *Sulph.*) (Bl.).

CONSTANT PAIN UNDER THE LOWER AND INNER ANGLE OF THE RIGHT SCAPULA (*Kali-C.*, *Merc.*, under the left scapula—*Chenop.*, *Sang.*) (N.).

JAUNDICE, WHEN THE SCLERA, FACE, URINE, AND STOOL ARE VERY YELLOW (N.).

Loathing of food (*Ant-C.*, *Puls.*, *Sep.*) (Bt.).

Urine : dark yellow ; turbid on passing ; dark brownish red ; staining linen or diaper dark yellow (N.).

Face, forehead, nose, cheeks remarkably yellow (*Sep.*) (A.).

Vertigo ; aggravated when rising from the bed or from sitting, or when closing the eyes (*Alum.*, *Arn.*, *Cycl.*, *Lach.*, *Sep.*, *Ther.*, *Thuj.*) (Br.).

Feels as though he were falling forward (Bl.).

AFFECTS RIGHT SIDE MOST ; RIGHT EYE, RIGHT LUNG, RIGHT HYPOCHONDRIUM AND ABDOMEN, RIGHT HIP AND LEG RIGHT FOOT COLD AS ICE, LEFT NATURAL (*Lyc.*) (A.).

Despondency (*Ars., Aur., Calc., Cimic., Crot-C., Ferr., Graph., Ign., Kali-P.,*) (B.).

Inclination to weep (*Gels., Ign., Puls., Stann.*).

Averse to mental exertion or conversation (*Aur., Bapt., Carb-An., Gels., Nux-V., Phos., Plat., Puls., Sulph., Verat., Zinc.*(B.).

Old, putrid, spreading ulcers, with a history of liver disease, or of a tubercular diathesis (A.).

Periodical orbital neuralgia (right side), with excessive lachrymation ; scars fairly gush out (*Rhus-T.*) (A.).

Acute and chronic hepatitis (*Aloe, Bry., Chin., Kali-M., Lach., Lyc., Merc., Nat-S., Podo., Sep., Sulph.*) (Bt.)

PNEUMONIA OF THE RIGHT LUNG, WITH LIVER COMPLICATIONS (*Ant-T., Iod., Merc., Sang.*) (A.).

Spasmus glottidis (*Ars., Bell., Brom., Chlor., Cupr., Gels., Ign., Iod., Lach., Mosch., Phos. Samb., Spong., Verat.*) (Bt.).

Spasmodic cough ; small lumps of mucus fly from the mouth when coughing (*Bad., Kali-C.*) (A.).

Loss of hearing during cough (*Puls ; better during cough—Sil.*).

Ears feel stopped (*Asar., Carb-V., Con., Lyc., Merc., Puls., Sil.*) (C.).

Heaviness in the occiput (*Bry., Cocc., Gels., Petrol., Sil.*) (C.).

ONE FOOT COLD, THE OTHER HOT (*Dig., Ipec. Lyc., Puls.*) (K.).

AGGRAVATION : From change of weather ; from motion ; from touch ; from lying on the right side ; early in the morning ; and 4 A.M. and 4 P.M.

AMELIORATION : After dinner ; from hot drinks ; from pressure ; from hot food ; during dinner : and bending backward.

RELATIONSHIP, COMPLEMENTARY : *Ars.*, *Lyc.*, *Merc-D.*, and *Sulph.*

ANTIDOTES : *Acon.*, *Cham.* and *Coff.*

CHEL. antidotes the abuse of *Bry.*, especially in hepatic complaints.

COMPARE : *Acon.*, *Bry.*, *Kali-B.*, *Lyc.*, *Merc.*, *Nux V.*, *Op.*, *Sang.*, *Sep.*, *Sulph.*

China.

COMMON NAME : PERUVIAN BARK.

Headache, aggravated by a draft of air, in the open air, and from the slightest contact, and relieved by hard pressure.

INTENSE THROBBING HEADACHE, AFTER EXCESSIVE HÆMORRHAGE (*Carb-V.*, *Ferr.*) (Bt.).

Over-sensitiveness, low-spirited with aversion to all noise (*Coff.*, *Nat-M.*, *Nux-V.*, *Sulph.*).

Long lasting congestive headache (*Bell.*, *Lach.*, *Nat-M.*, *Sang.*, *Verat-V.*), with deafness and noises in the ears (*Carb-V.*, *Lyc.*, *Nat-M.*, *Phos.*, *Sep.*, *Sulph.*) (Br.).

DEBILITY FROM LOSS OF FLUIDS (AN EXCELLENT INDICATION IN DEBILITATING PERSPIRATION.

Heaviness of the head, with loss of sight, fainting and ringing in the ears (*Puls.*, *Sep.*, *Sulph.*) (Hr.).

Unrefreshing sleep or constant sopor : worse after **3** A.M. ; wakens early (A.).

AILMENTS FROM LOSS OF VITAL FLUIDS, ESPECIALLY HÆMORRHAGES, EXCESSIVE LACTATION, DIARRHŒA, OR SUPPURATIONS (*Carb-V.*, *Ferr.*, *Phos.*) (A.).

Headache, worse from sitting or lying ; must stand or walk, after hæmorrhage or sexual excesses. (A.)

Headache : as if the skull would burst (*Bry.*) ; intense throbbing of head and carotids, with flashed face (*Bell.*) (A.).

Attacks of pain, caused by the slightest touch of the body and then increasing gradually and becoming very severe.

Sleeplessness at night ; he lies awake nearly all night, thinking, restless and uneasy, and miserable the next day (Hm.).

The parts on which one lies go to sleep (*Calc.*, *Graph.*, *Puls.*, *Rhus-T.*).

Restlessness of the affected parts.

One hand icy cold, the other warm (*Dig.*, *Ipec.*, *Puls.*) (A.).

Thick, dirty, yellow coating upon the tongue, with bitter taste (*Bry.*, *Chel.*, *Nat-P.*, *Nat-S.*) (Bt.).

Complete loss of appetite, especially in people suffering from malaria (*Carb-V.*, *Ferr.*, *Nat-S.*, *Puls.*, *Sep.*) (Bt.).

Much colic every afternoon (*Lyc.*) (Bt.).

Excessive flatulence of stomach and bowels : fermentation or borborygmus (A.).

Great longing for acids (*Ant-C.*, *Ars.*, *Calc.*, *Cor-R.*, *Hep.*, *Mag-C.*, *Phos.*, *Puls.*, *Sec.*, *Sep.*, *Sulph.*, *Thuj.*, *Verat.*) (Bt.).

Sour vomiting of water, mucus and food (*Nat P.*, *Nux-V.*, *Sulph-Ac.*) (J.).

CANINE HUNGER, ESPECIALLY AT NIGHT (*Aran.*, *Ign.*, *Lyc.*, *Phos.*, *Psor.*, *Sep.*, *Sulph.*, *Tarent.*) (Bt.)

Colic : at a certain hour each day ; periodical, from gall-stones (*Chel.*, *Card-M.*) ; worse at night and after eating : better from bending double (*Bell.*, *Coloc.*) (A.).

Enormous distension of the abdomen, feels packed full, not relieved by eructations or dejections. (Bt.)

Abdomen feels full and tight as if stuffed : eructations give no relief. (Bt.).

Diarrhœa of yellow, watery, undigested stools, with much flatulence and no pain (*Podo.*, *Puls.*, *Sulph.*) (Bt.)

After eating fruit, undigested stools, sometimes involuntary (Hr.).

Diarrhœa, of watery or undigested food, mostly at night (*Ferr.*, *Puls.*, *Sulph.*) (Bt.).

HÆMORRHAGES : OF MOUTH, NOSE, BOWELS OR UTERUS : LONG CONTINUED (*Carb-V.*, *Phos.*) (A.)

Dyspnœa : wants to be fanned (*Ant-T.*, *Apis*, *Carb-V.*, *Ferr.*, *Med.*, *Sulph.*) (K.).

DISPOSITION TO HÆMORRHAGES FROM EVERY ORIFICE OF THE BODY (*Carb-V.*, *Crot-H.*, *Ferr.*, *Lach.*, *Merc.*, *Nit-Ac.*, *Phos.*, *Sec.*), WITH RINGING IN THE EARS, FAINTING, LOSS OF SIGHT, GENERAL COLDNESS, SOMETIMES CONVULSIONS (*Ferr.*, *Phos.*, *Sec.*) (A.).

HÆMORRHAGE AFTER LABOUR (*Arn.*, *Ipec.*, *Sec.*) (N.),

AMAUROSIS (*Arg-M.*, *Bell.*, *Con.*, *Gels.*, *Kali-I.*, *Nat-M.*, *Phos.*, *Puls.*, *Sec.*, *Sil.*, *Stram.*, *Sulph.*) (Br.).

NIGHT BLINDNESS (*Bell.*, *Chels.*, *Hyos.*, *Lyc.*, *Merc.*, *Nit-Ac.*, *Puls.*, *Stram.*, *Verat.*, *Zinc.*) (Br.).

Spots before eyes (*Alum.*, *Caust.*, *Con.*, *Cycl.*, *Jab.*, *Kali-C.*, *Phos.*, *Sulph.*, *Verat-V.*) (Br.).

FREQUENT SEMINAL EMISSIONS, FOLLOWED BY GREAT WEAKNESS (*Gels.*, *Kali P.*, *Phos-Ac.*, *Sulph.*) (Br.).

Fever returns every seventh or fourteenth day (*Ars.*, *Sulph.*) (A.).

General shaking chill over whole body (N.).

Intermittent fever without thirst or thirst only between the cold and hot stage.

Weakening night-sweats till morning (*Ant-T.*, *Ars.*, *Carb-V.*, *Lach.*, *Lyc.*, *Nit-Ac.*, *Psor.*) (Hr.).

PAROXYSMS COME ON AN HOUR OR TWO EAR-
LIER, EVERY DAY, OR EVERY OTHER DAY. (*Ars.,
Ign., Nat-M., Nux-V.*) (Bt.).

*The three stages are sharply marked—chill, fever and
perspiration.*

The chill may be absent, but the fever and perspiration
must be present (Bt.).

THE SWEAT IS GENERALLY PROFUSE AND
EXHAUSTIVE (*Carb-V., Merc., Nat-M., Phos., Sulph.*)
(Bt.).

Recent intermittents, with gastro-bilious symptoms,
followed or accompanied by exhaustive perspiration (Bt.).

The malarial fever of China never returns at night
(an exception to the general rule of *China*) (A.).

Sweats profusely all over on being covered, or during
sleep (*Con.*) (A.).

Sees faces on closing the eyes (*Bell., Calc., Op.*) (K.).

Full of plans and projects, especially in the evening
and at night (*Coff.*) (Hm.).

She thinks she is very unfortunate, and constantly
harassed by enemies (G.).

Apathetic, indifferent, taciturn (*Aur., Ign.; Nat-M.,
Phos-Ac., Sep.*) (A.).

Despondent, gloomy ; has no desire to live, but lacks
courage to commit suicide (*Aur., Hep., Merc., Nit-Ac.,
Nux-V.*) (A.).

Face pale, hippocratic (*Carb-V., Sec., Verat.*) ; eyes

sunken and surrounded by blue margins (*Cina, Staph.*) ; pale, sickly expression, as after excesses(*Carb-V., Nat-M., Phos-Ac.*) (A.).

Toothache, while nursing the child (A.).

Toothache, better from pressing teeth firmly together and by warmth (Br.).

Is of service in intermittent fever, which may be often tertian or double tertian, quotidian or double quotidian type (Bl.).

Appetite wanting in foggy weather (K.).

Anorexia ; appetite returns after eating a mouthful (*Anac., Calc., Mag-C., Sabad.*) (K.).

The food is apt to lay a long time in the stomach and is finally vomited undigested (D.).

Liver and spleen swollen and enlarged (*Calc., Chel., Merc., Nat-M., Nux-V., Podo.*) (Br.).

Jaundice (*Chel., Iod., Nat-S., Nux-V., Sep., Sulph.*) (Br.).

Dropsy following excessive loss of fluids (N.).

Palpitation of the heart (*Carb-V., Ferr., Kali-C., Lach., Lyc., Nat-M., Puls.*) (G.).

Scalp sensitive to touch ; roots of hair hurt, when hair is moved (N.).

Salivation (years after having taken mercury) uninterrupted day and night (N.).

Consequences of onanism and excessive seminal losses (*Phos-Ac.*) (N.).

AGGRAVATION : At night ; from the least draught of air ; after drinking milk ; every other day ; from the slightest contact : from motion : after eating or drinking. from walking : from motion : and from loss of fluids.

AMELIORATION : From hard pressure from bending double ; and from lying down.

RELATIONSHIP. Compare : *Arn.*, *Ars.*, *Bell.*, *Calc.*, *Carb-V.*, *Cedr.*, *Coff.*, *Ferr.*, *Graph.*, *Lyc.*, *Merc.*, *Nat-M.*, *Nux-V.*, *Phos-Ae.*, *Phos.*, *Puls.*, *Sec.*, *Sep.*, *Sulph.*, and *Tarant.*

ANTIDOTES : *Arn.*, *Ars.*, *Carb-V.*, *Ferr.*, *Ipec.* *Lach.*, *Nat-M.*, *Nux-V.*, *Puls.*, *Sep.*, *Sulph.*, and *Verat.*

CHINA ANTIDOTES : *Ars.*, *Cupr.*, *Ipec.*, *Ferr.*, and *Merc.*,

Is useful in bad effects from excessive tea drinking. (*Puls.*).

COMPLEMENTARIES : *Calc-P.*, *Carb-V.*, and *Ferr*

Chininum Arsenicum

COMMON NAME : ARSENATE OF QUININE.

Mental dullness (*Gels.*, *Kali-P.*, *Lyc.*) (C.).

Wishes to be quiet and let alone (*Gels.*, *Ign.*, *Nat-M.*, *Phos-Ac.*) (C).

Depression of spirits (*Act-R.*; *Ign.*, *Kali-P.*, *Nat-M.*, *Sep.*) (C.).

Great irritability (*Aur.*, *Nat-M.*, *Nux-V.*) (Br.).

Pressure in "the solar plexus" with tender spine just back of it (F.).

Watery, fetid, pappy stools (*Aloe*, *Podo.*) (R.).

There is burning in the anus following stool (*Aloe, Carb-V., Iris, Lach., Sulph.*) (Bl.).

Diarrhœa, after eggs or fish (K.).

Intermittent fever : chill always in the forenoon, not at a regular hour : sometimes once every day, again , every other day ; sometimes paroxysms close with perspiration, sometimes without perspiration (C.).

Rapid, weak pulse (*Ars.*, *Carb-V.*, *Hydr-Ac.*, *Nat-M.*, *Phos.*, *Verat-A.*) (R.).

Headache, yawning and stretching before the attack of of fever (C.).

SUFFOCATIVE ATTACKS, OCCURRING IN PERIODICAL PAROXYSMS (*Ars.*, *Cact.*, *Calc-P.*, *Colch.*, *Plb.*, *Sulph.*) (Br.).

CARDIAC DYSPNŒA (*Ars.*, *Dig.*, *Lach.*, *Naja.*, *Phos.*, *Sulph.*) (Br.).

GREAT PROSTRATION (*Ars.*, *Carb-V.*, *Gels.*, *Phos.*, *Sep.*) (R.).

Angina pectoris, with dropsical symptoms, venous hyperæmia and cyanosis (*Carb-V.*, *Lach.*, *Verat.*) (C.).

PROFUSE SWEAT (*Carb-V.*, *Ferr.*, *Graph.*, *Hep.*, *Iod.*, *Kali-C.*, *Lyc.*, *Merc.*, *Nat-S.*, *Sep.*, *Sulph.*) (R.).

Must sit forward, and, if possible, at an open window during attack of suffocation (*Ars., Carb-V., Lach.*) (C.).

Vertigo, worse on looking up (*Calc., Caust., Cupr., Graph., Lach., Nux-V., Petr., Phos., Puls , Sang., Sep., Sil., Tab., Thuj.*) (Br.).

GUSHING OF HOT TEARS FROM THE EYES (*Apis, Ars., Chin., Euphr., Rhus-T., Sulph.*) (C.).

INTENSE PHOTOPHOBIA (*Arg-N., Bell., Con., Euphr., Graph., Nat-M., Nux-V., Rhus-T., Sulph.*) (Br.).

Ringing in the ears (*Bell., Calc., Chin., Chin-S., Kali-C., Kali-S., Petr., Puls., Sep.*) (C.).

Hyper-chlorhydria (*Calc., Iris, Lyc., Nat-P., Puls., Sulph-Ac.*) (Br.).

Hemicrania (*Arg-N., Coff., Kali-P., Plat., Puls., Spig.*) (C.).

Coldness of hands and feet (*Camph., Carb-V., Sec., Verat.*) (Br.)

AGGRAVATION : In the forenoon ; on looking up ; and from motion.

AMELIORATION : In the open air ; and on sitting up.

RELATIONSHIP : Compare : *Apis, Ars., Chin., Lach., Lyc., Nat-M , Phos., Puls., Sep., Sulph.*).

Complementary : *Ferr., Nat-M., Sep.*

Cicuta Virosa.

COMMON NAME : WATER HEMLOCK.

Pains as from contusions or blows on many parts of the body.

Chilliness and desire for heat (*Ign.*).

When reading, letters seem to turn, go up or down, or disappear (*Cocc.*) (A.).

Shocks of the brain, as from electricity through the head, arms and legs.

Eczema : no itching : exudation forms into a hard, lemon-coloured crust (A.).

Pustules run together, forming thick, yellow scabs on the head and face (A.).

Puerperal convulsions (eclampsia) : frequent suspension of breathing for a few moments, as if dead ; upper part of the body most affected ; continue after delivery (A.).

CONVULSIONS : VIOLENT, WITH FRIGHTFUL DISTORTIONS OF LIMBS AND WHOLE BODY : WITH LOSS OF CONSCIOUSNESS OR OPISTHOTO-NOS ; RENEWED FROM THE SLIGHTEST TOUCH, NOISE OR JAR (*Sulph.*) (A.).

CONTORTIONS OF THE LIMBS, BLUISH FACE, INTERRUPTED BREATHING, FOAMING AT THE MOUTH, FOLLOWED BY INSENSIBILITY (*Cupr.*, *Hyos.*, *Œna.*).

CONVULSIONS IN CHILDREN FROM WORMS (*Bell.*, *Calc.*, *Cupr.*, *Mag-P*, *Nat-P.*, *Op.*, *Sil.*).

Twitching, especially in the extremities (**Bell., Gels., Hyos., Ign., Lach., Plb., Stram.**).

Burning pains and burning, moist eruptions with yellow crusts.

Catalepsy : limbs hang down and patient appear lifeless (C.).

Trismus and tetanus from getting splinters into the flesh (**Hyper.**) (**A.**).

Sudden rigidity with jerks, afterward relaxation and weakness (C.).

Injurious chronic effects from concussions of the brain and spine (**Arn., Hyper., Nat-S.**), especially spasms (**A.**).

Epilepsy : with swelling of the stomach as from violent spasms of the diaphragm ; screaming ; red or bluish face ; lock-jaw : loss of consciousness and distortion of the limbs ; frequent during the night ; recurring, first at short, then at long intewals (**A.**).

Brain disease from suppressed eruptions (**Caust., Cupr., Zinc.**) (**A.**)

Grinding of teeth (**Ars., Bell., Bry., Calc., Cina, Merc., Nat-P., Sulph.**) (C.).

ABNORMAL APPETITE FOR CHALK, COAL OR CHARCOAL AND OTHER INDIGESTIBLE THINGS (**Alum., Calc., Ferr., Nat-M., Nit-Ac., Nux-V.**) (**A.**).

VIOLENT HICCOUGH (**Bell., Cupr., Hyos., Nat-M., Nicc., Nux-V., Sec., Stram.**) (C.).

LOUD HICCOUGH (K).

HICCOUGH WITH CONVULSIONS (*Bell.*, *Cupr.*, *Hyos.*, *Ran-B.*) (*K.*).

Rumbling and roaring in the abdomen (*Crot-T.*, *Nat-S.*, *Podo.*, *Verat.*) (C.).

Congestion to head with vomiting and purging (B.).

Insanity : does all sorts of absurd and foolish things ; confounds the present with the past ; thinks himself a young child.

Involuntary micturition (*Bell.*, *Calc.*, *Hyos.*, *Nat-M.*, *Puls.*, *Sep.*) (C.).

Spurting of urine (*Calc-P.*, *Helon.*, *Puls.*, *Spig.*) (C.).

Sadly affected by sad tales.

Objects appear double (*Aur.*, *Bell.*, *Caust.*, *Cycl.*, *Dig.*, *Gels.*, *Hyos.*, *Lyc.*, *Nat-M.*, *Nit-Ac.*, *Stram.*) (C.).

Violent vertigo, so that the patient falls down (*Ars.*, *Bell.*, *Carb-An.*, *Cocc.*, *Con.*, *Ferr.*, *Gels.*, *Kali-P.*, *Lyc.*, *Nux-V.*, *Rhus-T.*, *Stram.*, *Sulph.*, *Zinc.*) (Hm.).

Momentary loss of sight (*Chin.*, *Puls.*) (G.).

Unconsciousness (*Apis*, *Bell.*, *Cupr.*, *Hyos.*, *Gels.*, *Hydr-Ac.*, *Op.*, *Phos-Ac.*, *Verat.*) (C.).

Weeping, moaning and howling (*Bell.*, *Cina*, *Cupr.*, *Hyos.*, *Stram.*) (C.).

Excitement and apprehension about the future (*Bry.*, *Calc.*, *Chin-S.*, *Gels.*, *Lach.*, *Nat-M.*, *Phos.*, *Puls.*, *Staph.*, *Sulph.*) (C.).

Most important in many cases of cerebro-spinal meningitis (*Cocc.*, *Hyos.*, *Lach.*, *Nux-V.*, *Op.*, *Stram.*) (Tr.).

Biting the tongue during convulsions (*Art-V.*, *Bufo*, *Caust.*, *Cupr.*, *Œna.*, *Op.*, *Sec.*, *Tarent.*, *Valer.*) (F.).

Spasm of the œsophagus ; the patient can not swallow, and strangles when attempting it (*Nat-M.*,) (Bl.).

Spasmodic symptoms are followed by profound exhaustion (*Strych.*) (F.).

Bent backward like an arch (*Cup.*, *Nux-V.*, *Sec.*) (R.).

Stares persistently at an object (*Hyos.*) (Br.).

Colic with convulsions (Br.).

Burning eruptions on the hairy scalp, also on the face (milk-crust) (N.).

Repeated movements of the head, as twitching, jerking throwing the head backward, etc. (N.).

AGGRAVATION : From tobacco smoke ; from touch ; from draughts ; from concussion ; from worms ; from turning the head ; from suppressed eruptions ; from noise ; from jar ; and from cold.

AMELIORATION : From heat.

RELATIONSHIP. Compare : *Absinth.*, *Acon.*, *Apis*, *Bell.*, *Calc.*, *Con.*, *Cupr.*, *Gels.*, *Hydr-Ac.*, *Hyos.*, *Hyper.*, *Ign.*, *Kali-P.*, *Lach.*, *Lyc.*, *Mosch.*, *Nux-V.*, *Op.*, *Puls.*, *Rhus-T.*, *Sec.*, *Sil.*, *Stram.*, *Strych.*, *Sulph.*, *Verat.*, and *Verat-V.*

ANTIDOTES : *Arn.*, *Op* ; for large doses : *Tobacco*. *Cicuta antidotes* : *Opium*.

Cina.

COMMON NAME : WORM SEED.

Is principally a children's remedy, corresponding to many conditions that may be referred to intestinal irritation, such as worms, etc. (D.).

Worm complaints in children (*Bell., Calc., Calc-P., Ferr., Graph., Ipec., Kali-M., Kali-P., Lach., Lyc., Merc., Nat-M., Phos., Sep., Sil., Sulph., Zinc.*).

THERE IS GRINDING OF THE TEETH AND THE CHILD BORES WITH HIS FINGERS INTO THE NOSE.

Face pale (*cold, with cold perspiration*); (*Camph., Carb-V., Sec., Verat.*).

At night sleeplessness, with restlessness and tossing about (*Acon., Ars., Kali-P., Rhus-T.*).

Involuntary discharges (*urine and whitish diarrhœtic stool*).

THE CHILD DOES NOT WANT TO BE TOUCHED (*Ant-C., Arn., Cham., Kali-C.*).

Violent screaming attacks at night, the patient afflicted lying on the back and striking and kicking with the hands and feet (*Bell., Hyos., Lyc., Stram.*).

Sickly, pale face, with rings around the eyes (*Staph.*) ; gritting of the teeth at night ; canine hunger, or variable appetite ; the child picks its nose and cries out in its sleep ; jerking of hands and feet ; urine milky (D.).

18

The child wakes in a fright, screams, trembles and can not be quieted; they are proof against all caresses; they are cross, irritable, nervous and peevish; they want to be rocked (*Cham.*) (D.).

Ill-humored; wants to be carried, but carrying gives no relief (A.).

Disposition to be offended by trifling jest.

There is no child more contemptible than the *Cina.* He is easily excited; weak; screams, strikes and bites; is cross and obstinate. (R.).

Twitches and contortions of the limbs (*Bell., Cic., Cupr., Hyos., Ign., Nux-V., Op., Stram.*).

Desires many things, but rejects everything offered (*Cham.*) (A.).

Frequent swallowing, as if to swallow something down the throat (Bt.).

Tossing during sleep (Bt.).

One cheek red, the other pale (*Cham.*).

Sensation as if there is a ball rising in the throat (*Asaf., Ign., Mosch.*) (Bt.).

Rufuses mother's milk (*Ant-C., Lach., Merc., Sil., Stann., Stram.*) (A.).

Craving for sweets and different things (*Kreos., Phos.*) (A.).

CANINE HUNGER: HUNGRY SOON AFTER A FULL MEAL (*Chin-S., Iod., Lyc., Phos.*) (A.).

CANINE HUNGER, DURING OR BEFORE THE INTERMITTENT FEVER.

Belly hard and distended, with mucous stools (Bt.).

Alternate canine hunger, or no appetite at all (N.).

Weeping during coughing (*Ant-T.*, *Arn.*, *Bell.*, *Hep.*). (K.).

Stools mixed with lumbrici (*Calc.*, *Merc.*, *Nat-P.*, *Sulph.*). (Bt.).

Itching of the anus (*Aloe*, *Calc.*, *Caust.*, *Graph.*, *Lyc.*, *Merc.*, *Sulph.*) (Bt.).

Constantly digging and boring at the nose ; picks the nose all the time ; itching of the nose ; rubs the nose on the pillow, or on the shoulder of the nurse (*Merc-V.*) (A.).

Cough ends in a spasm (*Cupr.*, *Ipec.*) (Br.).

Diarrhœa always after drinking (*Arg-N.*, *Ars.*, *Crot-T.*, *Ferr.*, *Ferr-Ars.*, *Nux-V.*, *Podo.*, *Tromb.*, *Verat.*) (Bt.).

Pinching colic in the umbilical region (Bt.).

REGULARLY RECURRENT, CHOKING COUGH, THEN GURGLING DOWN THE THROAT (B.).

WHOOPING COUGH WITH STIFFNESS OF THE CHILD BEFORE IT AND WITH GREAT PALENESS OF THE FACE.

Child is afraid to speak or move for fear of bringing on a paroxysm of coughing (*Bry.*) (A.).

Lachrymation with cough (*Euphr.*, *Nat-M.*, *Puls.*, *Squil.*) (K.).

THE URINE TURNS MILKY AFTER STANDING A LITTLE (*Phos-Ac.*, *Stann.*) (G.).

Spasms of children resembling epilepsy (*Bell.*, *Calc.*, *Cupr.*, *Lach.*, *Stram.*, *Sulph.*) (Bt.).

Stiffens out during cough (B.).

Vision gets dim, can see more clearly for a while rubbing the eyes (N.).

Weak sight from masturbation (*Phos.*) (Br.).

Aversion to light (*Con., Nat-m., Nux-V.*).

Dilated pupils (*Arg-N., Bell., Calc., Chin., Gels., Hyos., Mang., Sec., Stram.*) (B.).

Coloured vision (*Agar., Bell., Bry., Calc., Cic., Cycl., Dig., Iod., Kali-B.; Mag-P., Merc., Nat-M., Phos., Puls., Sep., Stram., Sulph.*) (B.).

GREEN OR YELLOW VISION (*Cann-I. Canth., Cycl., Dig., Kali-Ars., Kali-C., Lac-C., Sep., Stront., Sulph., Zinc.*) (Br.).

Fever with pale face (*Ars., Cocc., Croc., Ipec., Lyc., Nat-M., Puls., Rhus-T., Sep., Spong., Thuj., Verat.*):(B.).

Cold sweat about the nose and forehead (B.).

PALE SICKLY LOOK ABOUT THE EYES OR WHITE AND BLUE ABOUT THE MOUTH (N.).

Frequent sudden attacks of very high fever, with glowing red hot face, with paleness around the mouth and lips, or sometimes alternates with pale face with dark, bluish rings around the eyes (N.).

Pain in the head when using the eyes (*Nat-M., Ruta*) (Br.).

Rising heat and glowing redness of the cheeks, without thirst ; after sleep ; with worm symptoms (N.).

MUCH FEVER, ASSOCIATED WITH CLEAN TONGUE (Br.).

Fever daily at the same hour (*Cact.*) (C.).

THIRST DURING CHILL (*Apis. Arn., Caps., Eup-P., Ign., Nat-M., Nux-V., Pyrog., Sep., Sil., Tub., Verat.*) (K.).

Worm complaints of children ; with convulsions (N.).

Frequent hiccough (*Am-M., Ars., Ars-I., Cic., Cycl., Hyos., Ign., Iod., Lyc., Mag-P., Merc., Nat-Ars., Nat-C., Nat-M., Nicc., Nux-M., Nux-V., Sec., Stram., Teucr.*).

Vomiting of lumbrici and ascarides ; of food and mucus.

Feeling of emptiness in the abdomen (*Carb-An., Ign., Sep., Sulph.*).

Sleeplessness with restlessness, crying and lamentations (*Bell., Hyos., Puls.*).

Child will sleep only when violently rocked (N.).

Child flops over on its belly ; sleeps better that way (N.).

AGGRAVATION : At night ; on locking fixedly at an object ; from external pressure ; in sun ; in summer ; from worms ; and when yawning.

AMELIORATION : From motion ; when lying on the abdomen ; and from wiping the eyes.

RELATIONSHIP. *Antidotes* : *Camph., Caps., Chin.,* and *Ipec.*

Compare : *Ant-C., Ant-T., Bell., Bry., Calc., Cham.,*

Kreos., *Nat-M.*, *Nux-V.*, *Sil.*, *Staph.* and *Sulph.* in irritability of children.

Useful in pertussis, after *Drosera* has relieved the severe symptoms. *Santonine* (the alkaloid of *Cina*) sometimes cures in worm affections when *Cina* seems indicated, but fails.

CINA ANTIDOTES : *Caps.*, *Chin.*, and *Merc.*

Cinnabaris.

COMMON NAME : MERCURIC SULPHIDE.

An excellent remedy when there is a combination of syphilis and sycosis (F.).

Pressure at the root of nose, as if heavy pair of spectacles were there (D.).

Congestions of blood to the head (*Aur.*, *Bell.*, *Cact.*, *Ferr.*, *Gels.*, *Glon.*, *Lach.*, *Meli.*, *Nat-M.*, *Op.*, *Sulph.*, *Verat-V.*).

Face purple red (*Bapt.*, *Bell.*, *Bry.*, *Gels.*, *Hyos.*, *Op.*, *Sang.*, *Sec.*, *Sulph.*, *Verat-V.*).

Coldness of the feet, day and night.

Coldness of the joints (*Camph.*, *Nat-M.*, *Petr.*, *Rhus-T.*, *Sumb.*).

Itching, especially about the joints (F.).

Leucorrhœa : *bloody*, *copious*, *purulent*, *or yellow* (K.).

BUBOES (*Ars.*, *Bad.*, *Bufo*, *Carb-An.*, *Hep.*, *Kali-M.*, *Lyc.*, *Merc.*, *Nit-Ac.*, *Sil.*) (Br.).

Testicles enlarged (*Arg-N.*, *Aur.*, *Bar-M.*, *Iod.*, *Puls.*, *Rhod.*, *Sulph.*) (Br.).

FIERY RED ULCERS (Bl.).

Violent itching of the corona glandis.

HARD CHANCRES (*Merc.*, *Merc-C.*, *Merc-I-F.*, *Merc-I-R.*) (K.).

SYPHILITIC ULCERS (*Ars.*, *Aur.*, *Hep.*, *Kali-B.*, *Lach.*, *Merc.*, *Merc-C.*, *Nit-Ac.*, *Sulph.*, *Thuj.*).

Redness and swelling or warts on the prepuce, itching, bleeding, and sensitive. (N.).

Small, shining, red points on the glans penis.

Squamous syphilides (*Ars.*, *Kali-Ars.*, *Kali-Chl.*, *Kreos.*, *Merc.*, *Nit-Ac.*, *Sil.*) (Bl.).

Easily bleeding condylomata (*Med.*, *Nit-Ac.*, *Sulph.*, *Thuj.*) (Br.).

Violent erections in the evening (*Alum.*, *Bar-C.*, *Cact.*, *Fago*, *Nat-S.*, *Phos.*).

The fig-warts are apt to be fan-shaped (F.).

Fretful, easily provoked (*Aur.*, *Nit-Ac.*, *Sulph.*).

Very sleepless during the night, but when he awakes in the morning he feels as if he needed no sleep.

Hoarseness in the evening (*Carb-V.*, *Caust.*, *Phos.*).

Swollen and dry throat, with swollen tonsils, and stringy mucus in the posterior nares, which passes into the throat (*Hydr.*, *Kali-B.*) (D.).

Naso-pharyngeal catarrh (*Calc-S.*, *Ferr-P.*, **Hep.**, *Kali-B.*, *Lyc.*, *Nat-C.*, *Nat-M.*, *Psor.*, *Sep.*, *Sil.*, *Thuj.*) (B.).

Ciliary neuralgia (*Merc-C.*) (D.).

Nodes on the shin bones (G.).

PAIN STARTS FROM ONE CANTHUS AND GOES AROUND THE BROW OF THE EYE TO THE OTHER CANTHUS (*Gels.*, *Ign.*, *Mag-M.*, *Merc-C.*, *Nit-Ac.*, *Phyt.*, *Spig.*) (D.).

Fiery looking ulcers in the mouth and throat (Br.).

Clematis Erecta.

COMMON NAME : VIRGIN'S BOWER.

Arthritic pains, as a sequel of suppressed gonorrhœa (*Med.*, *Puls.*, *Thuj.*) (A.).

Muscles relaxed (*Calc.*, *Caps.*, *Cocc.*, *Gels.*, *Kali-C.*, *Phos.*).

Twitching of the muscles (*Agar.*, *Asaf.*, *Cact.*, *Hyos.*, *Ign.*, *Iod.*, *Kali-C.*, *Mezer.*, *Nat-C.*, *Stram.*, *Zinc.*).

Great emaciation (*Abrot.*, *Ars.*, *Ars-I.*, *Bar-C.*, *Calc.*, *Calc-I.*, *Chin.*, *Ferr.*, *Graph.*, *Hell.*, *Iod.*, *Lyc.*, *Nat-H.*, *Nat-M.*, *Nit-Ac.*, *Nux-V.*, *Phos.*).

After eating, weakness in all the limbs and pulsation the arteries.

Toothache : worse at night and from tobacco (Br.).

TOOTHACHE, RELIEVED BY HOLDING COLD WATER IN THE MOUTH (*Bry., Coff., Puls.*) (N.).

Teeth feel too long (*Caust., Lach., Mag-C.*).

Dull pain in a hollow tooth, alleviated by cold water, or sucking the tooth (N.).

Painful swelling and induration of the glands (*Carb-An., Iod., Merc-I., Phyt., Rhus-T.*).

Aggravation of all skin symptoms by the heat of bed and from washing.

Eruptions red and moist during the increasing moon ; pale and dry during the decreasing moon.

Painful tettery skin, not itching, however, over the whole body.

Eruption on occiput at base of hair, moist, pustular, sensitive, itching (Br.).

Terrible itching, worse from washing in cold water (Br.).

Produces burning vesicles, which pustulate and discharge a yellowish, corrosive ichor (F.).

Intense pains along the urethra at the glans penis (F.).

Has to wait a long time before his efforts to urinate are successful (Y.).

The urine flows by fits and starts (F.).

Mucus in the urine (*Cop., Merc., Nat-M.*) (F.).

Inability to pass all the urine (*Caust., Con., Op.*) (Br.).

Has to strain to pass a few drops and dribbling after micturition (*Cann-I., Hep., Nat-M., Sep., Thuj.*) (R.).

CONSTRICTION OF THE URETHRA (*Canth., Cop., Dig., Nux-V., Petr., Puls., Verat.*).

SLOW OR INTERMITTENT FLOW OF URINE (*Agar , Arg-N., Con., Gels., Hep., Merc., Op.*) (N.).

INTERRUPTED FLOW OF URINE, WITH BURNING DURING, BUT MOST AT THE BEGINNING OF MICTURITION, OR DURING INTERRUPTIONS (C.).

The urethra is painful to pressure.

GONORRHŒAL ORCHITIS ; THE TESTICLE IS INDURATED AND HARD AS A STONE AND VERY PAINFUL. (D.).

PAIN ALONG THE SPERMATIC CORD (*Berb., Calc., Ham., Merc., Nux-V., Ol-An., Ox-Ac.; Phos., Puls., Sars., Spong., Thuj.*) (Br.).

RIGHT SPERMATIC CORD SENSITIVE, TESTICLE DRAWN UP (*Rhod.*) (C.).

Swelling and induration of the mammary gland (*Carb-An., Con., Phyt., Sil.*).

Violent long-continuing erections (*Canth., Pic-Ac.*).

Cancer of the breast (*Apis, Ars., Brom., Bufo, Carb-An., Cond., Con., Graph., Kreos., Lach., Merc., Nit-Ac., Phos., Phyt., Sil., Sulph., Thuj.*).

Sharp stitch in the heart, from within to without.

Chronic conjunctivitis (*Arg-N., Con., Kali-B., Lyc., Nat-M., Puls., Sep., Sil., Sulph., Thuj.*) (B.).

Epithelioma (*Ars., Con., Hydr.*) (F.).

Cancer of the lower lip (*Ars., Merc-I-F., Phos., Sep., Sil.*) (K.).

Sensation of a veil before the eyes (*Ars., Calc., Caust., Chin., Croc., Cycl., Gels., Merc., Phos., Puls., Sulph., Zinc.*) (C.).

Memory impaired (*Agn., Arg-M., Caust., Con., Kali-P., Lyc., Nat-M., Phos-Ac.*).

Aversion to talk (*Bry., Nat-M., Nux-V.*).

Low-spirited (*Caust., Gels., Med., Nat-M., Puls., Sep.*).

AGGRAVATION : From washing ; from heat of bed ; when moving the head ; from smoking tobacco ; at night ; and during increasing moon.

AMELIORATION : From scratching ; from holding cold water in the mouth ; in open air ; and from sweating.

RELATIONSHIP. *Compare* : *Ars., Berb., Brom., Bry., Calc., Carb-An., Cimic., Con., Graph., Merc., Nat-M., Nux-V., Petr., Phyt., Puls., Rhod., Rhus-T., Sars., Sep., Sil., Staph., Sulph.,* and *Thuj.*

Antidotes : *Bry., Camph.* and *Cham.*

Complementary : *Merc.*

Coca.

COMMON NAME : ERYTHROXYLON COCA.

Coca is used by the natives of South America as we use *Coffee, Tea* and *Tobacco* (C.).

Its principal alkaloid is *Cocaine.*

The mountaineer's remedy. Useful in a variety of complaints incidental to mountain climbing, such as palpitation, dyspnœa, anxiety and insomnia (Br.).

Generally called for persons who are wearing out under the physical and mental strain of a busy life, and who suffer from exhausted nerves and brain (Fluor-Ac., Kali-P., Nux-V.) (A.).

Sensation as if a band were stretched over the forehead, from temple to temple (C.).

EMPHYSEMA (*Am-C., Ant-Ars., Ant-T., Ars., Brom , Camph., Carb-V., Chlor., Dig., Hep., Lach., Lob., Phos., Sulph.*) (Br.).

SHORTNESS OF BREATH IN OLD PEOPLE (*Bar-C., China, Seneg.*) (A.).

Want of breath in those engaged in athletic sports (Ars., Calc., Lach., Lyc., Lycps., Nat-M.) (A.).

Loss of voice (*Am-Caust., Arg-N., Carb-V., Caust., Phos., Stann.*) (Br.).

Excited fancies ; wonderful visions (C.).

Melancholy, bashful, timid and ill at ease in society (A.).

Sad or irritable (*Ign.*, *Nat-M.*) (A.).

Delights in solitude and obscurity (*Ign.*) (Br.).

Sense of impending death (*Acon.*) (B.).

Headache with vertigo, preceded by flashes of light (*Bell.*, *Phos.*) (Br.).

Caries of teeth (*Calc-F.*, *Merc.*, *Sil.*) (Br.).

Faining fit from climbling mountains (*Agar.*) (Br.).

Longing for alcoholic liquors and tobacco; for the accustomed stimulants (A.).

Diplopia, while writing (*Graph.*) (K.).

Hæmoptysis, with oppression of the chest and dyspnœa (*Acon.*, *Bell.*, *Cact.*, *Ferr.*, *Ferr-P.*, *Ipec.*, *Kali-P.*, *Lach.*, *Nit-Ac.*, *Phos.*, *Sulph.*) (A.).

Diabetes (*Acet-Ac.*, *Berb.*, *Lyc.*, *Merc.*, *Phos-Ac.*, *Sep.*, *Sulph.*) (Br.).

Frequent urination (*Gels.*, *Kali-P.*, *Lyc.*, *Nat-M.* *Phos-Ac.*) (C.).

Seminal emissions, with voluptuous dreams (*Nux-V.* *Phos.*) (C.).

Bad effects from mountain climbing or balooning (*Ars.*); *of stimulants, alcohol and tobacco* (A.).

Singing, roaring and ringing in the ears (*Chin.*, *Merc.*, *Puls.*) (C.).

Incessant dyspnœa, with desire to take a deep breath (*Bry.*, *Phos.*) (C.).

Violent palpitation: from incarcerated flatus (*Arg-N.*, *Lyc.*, *Nux-V.*); from over-exertion (*Ars.*);

and from heart strain (*Arn.*, *Bor.*, *Caust.*, *Rhus-T.*) (A.).

Tympanitic distension of the abdomen (*Arg-N.*, *Carb-V.*, *Chin.*, *Lyc.*, *Tereb.*) (Br.).

Loss of appetite (*Alum.*, *Calc.*, *Kali-M.*, *Nux-V.*, *Puls.*, *Sep.*) (C.).

Crawling numbness in the arms (*Cocc.*, *Graph.*, *Rhus-T.*) (B.).

Awakes with a shock in the brain (B.).

Sleepy, but can find no rest anywhere (A.).

Nocturnal enuresis (*Kreos.*, *Merc.*, *Nat-P.*, *Puls.*, *Rhus-T.*, *Sep.*, *Sil.*) (Br.).

AGGRAVATION : From ascending ; in high altitudes.

AMELIORATION : From wine ; from riding ; in open air ; and after dinner.

RELATIONSHIP. *Complementary to* : *Fluor-Ac.*

Antidote : *Gels.*

Compare : *Arn.*, *Ars.*, *Bell.*, *Caust.*, *Ferr.*, *Flur-P.*, *Kali-P.*, *Lach.*, *Nux-V.*, *Phos.*, *Sep.*, *Sulph.*, *Verat.*, *Verat-V.*

Cocculus Indicus.

COMMON NAME : INDIAN COCKLE.

Within the sphere of action of *Cocculus* are many spasmodic and paretic affections, notably those affecting one-half of the body (Br.).

Often useful in those who nurse the sick (D.).

Bad effects from anger (*Bry.*, *Ign.* *Nux-V.*, *Staph.*) or from Chamomilla (*Coff.*, *Nux-V.*).

Aversion to the open air (warm and cold). (*Nux-V.*, *Psor.*, *Sil.*).

OF APPROVED VALUATION IN SEA-SICKNESS (*Colch.*, *Con.*, *Kreos.*, *Nux-V.*, *Petr.*, *Tab.*).

SWIMMING AND GIDDINESS WITH NAUSEA (*Acon.*, *Bry.*, *Camph.*, *Carb-V.*, *Chin-S.*, *Ferr.*, *Glon.*, *Lob.*, *Nat-M.*, *Petr.*, *Phos.*, *Sep.*).

Paroxysms of vertigo as from intoxication, with nausea (*Nux-V.*, *Tab.*) (N.).

Violent headache: is unable to lie on back of the head; is forced to lie on the side; unable to bear the least light; noise excites nausea and vomiting (N.).

Emptiness and sensation of hollowness in the abdomen (*Ign.*, *Sep.*, *Sulph.*) (N.).

Intermittent fever with lameness in the small of the back and colic.

Nausea while riding in a boat, cars, carriage, etc. (N.).

Has been of service in a low type of nervous fever, when there is severe occipital headache, vertigo and nausea present (Bl.).

Aversion to acids (*Bell., Ferr., Ign., Nux-V., Phos-Ac., Sabad., Sulph.*) (K.).

Hard, cold swelling of the glands with stinging pains (*Con., Iod., Sil.*).

AVERSION TO FOOD (*Ars., Bry., Colch., Lyc., Puls., Sep.*) (N.).

LOATHING WHEN MERELY LOOKING AT THE FOOD (*Ant-T., Colch., Kali-B, Kali-C., Lyc., Phos-Ac., Sil., Sulph., Xanth.*) (N.).

Desire for cold drinks, especially beer (C.).

Tearing and gnawing in the bones (*Am-M., Bell., Phos., Ruta, Staph.*).

Bones feel as if they were broken (*Aur., Bry., Cupr., Eup-P., Hep, Nat-M., Ruta, Verat., Vip.*).

From little exercise he becomes very much fatigued, even to fainting (*Ars., Carb-V., Sep., Verat.*).

Discharge of bloody mucus from the uterus during pregnancy (N.).

Hard and difficult evacuations (*Bry., Nux-V., Op. Plat.*) (C.).

Sensation as though worms were moving in the stomach (C.).

Black spots before the eyes (*Cycl., Puls., Sep.*).

Perspiration of the affected parts (*Ambr., Ant-T. Merc., Rhus-T., Sep.*) (K.).

SENSATION IN INNER ORGANS OF EMPTI-NESS (*Phos., Sep., Stann.*), OR CONSTRICTION (*Bell., Coloc., Lach., Plb., Sec.*).

Weakness of cervical muscles ; unable to support the head (*Nat-M.*) (N.).

Hysterical spasms in the chest, with sighing and moaning.

Paralytic pain in lower back, with weakness of hips, knees and legs (N.).

Stiffness and cracking of the joints (*Calc., Kali-B., Led., Petr., Rhus-T.*).

Disposition to tremble. (*Agar., Gels., Kali-Br., Kali-P., Lach.; Merc., Nux-V., Phos.*).
Paralysis from the small of the back downward (bladder, rectum and legs) (*Alum., Plb., Op.*).
ONE-SIDED PARALYSIS, WITH NUMBNESS OF THE LIMBS (*Caust., Nux-V.*).

Much paralytic pain in the small of the back, rendering ; walking puite difficult and sometimes impossible ; cumbing feet and hands (N.).

Should be remembered in diarrhœa, that is pro-duced by riding in cars and automobiles (Bl.).

Headache in the back part of the head and nape, with tendency to stretch the head backwards (D.).

Ill effects of loss of sleep from long continued watching (N.).

19

The sleep is frequently interrupted by waking and starting (*Bell., Hyos., Stram., Sulph.*) (Bl.).

Sensation as if the head were opening and shutting (*Cann-I., Cimic., Lyc.*) (D.).

Thirst without desire to drink (*Ang., Merc-C., Mezer., Nat-M., Nux-V.*) (K.).

Speaks hastily (*Bell., Hep., Hyos., Lach., Merc., Stram.* (A.).

Dullness and confusion (*Bar-C., Kali-P., Nux-V., Phos-Ac.*) (R.).

Must read a passage over several times in order to understand it (*Agar., Alum., Calc., Lyc., Nat-M., Nux-M., Phos-Ac.*) (R.).

Cannot bear contradiction (A.).

Profound sadness (*Ars., Aur., Caust., Gels., Ign., Nat-M., Puls., Sep.*) (Br.).

TIME PASSES TOO QUICKLY (*Atrop., Coca, Elaps, Op., Sulph., Ther., Thuj.*) (K.).

Abdomen distended with wind, and feeling as if full of sharp stones when moving (Br.).

Flatulent colic at midnight (Bt.).

She feels too weak to talk aloud (*Stann.*) (G.).

So weak during menstruation, scarcely able to stand (*Alum., Carb-An., Graph., Helon., Kali-C., Phos., Sep., Verat.*) (Br.).

Convulsion after loss of sleep (K.).

Menstrual colic ; *the pains are of a spasmodic, irregular character* (*Caul.*, *Mag-P.*, *Nux-V.*, *Sep.*) (G.).

Depleting menses ; worse from standing on tip toe ; replaced by gushes of leucorrhœa (B.).

WHIRLING VERTIGO ON RISING UP IN BED (*Bry.*, *Chel.*, *Ferr.*, *Nat-M.*, *Nux-V.*, *Phos.*, *Phyt.*, *Sep.*, *Sil.*, *Stram.*, *Sulph.*, *Verat-V.*) (N.).

Metallic taste in the mouth (*Merc.*, *Nat-C.*, *Rhus-T.*, *Seneg.*) (K.).

Leucorrhœa : in place of menses, or between the periods (*Iod.*, *Xanth.*) ; like the washings of meat (*Alum.*, *Kreos.*, *Lyc.*, *Nit-Ac.*) ; like serum, ichorous, bloody ; during pregnancy (*Kreos.*, *Murx.*, *Puls.*, *Sep.*) (A.).

Cannot sit up even one or two hours later than usual in the evening without feeling languid and exhausted throughout the entire day following (F.).

Umbilical hernia, with obstinate constipation (A.).

AGGRAVATION : From loss of sleep ; from talking ; on riding in a carriage ; from smoking tobacco ; from laughing ; from crying ; from walking ; from drinking coffee ; in the open air ; after drinking ; on board the ship ; on rising from bed ; from eating ; and from night-watching.

AMELIORATION : In a warm room ; when lying quiet.

RELATIONSHIP : *Antidotes* : *Camph.*, *Cham.*, *Cupr.*, *Ign.*, and *Nux-V.*

Cocculus antidotes: Alcohol, *Cham., Cupr., Ign.,*
Nux-V.

Compare: *Alum., Ars., Bell., Bry., Coff., Cupr.,*
Ferr., Gels., Ign., Ipec., Kali-P., Lyc., Nux-V., Petr.
Phos., Plb., Puls., Sep., Sil., Sulph., Tab., Ther., and
Verat.

Coffea Cruda.

COMMON NAME : COFFEE.

It produces a nervous erethism (over- sensitiveness).
All the senses are rendered more acute, and pains are
felt intensely (D.).

EXCITED AND OVER-SENSITIVE (*Bell., Hyos.,*
Lach., Nux-V., Stram.).

GREAT SENSITIVENESS TO PAIN (*Acon., Bell.,*
Cham., Hep., Lach., Plat., Stram.) ; DRIVING TO
DESPAIR WITH WEEPING (*Puls.*).

Great movability of the muscles.

Excessive activity of the vital powers (*Cann-I., Nux-*
V., Piper-M.).

Twitching of the limbs (*Bell., Hyos., Ign., Mygale,*
Tarant.).

HEADACHE : AS IF A NAIL HAD BEEN
DRIVEN INTO THE PARIETAL BONE ; WORSE IN
THE OPEN AIR (D.).

Hemicrania (*Bry.*, *Cimic.*, *Iris*, *Kali-B.*, *Lach.*, *Lyc.*, *Nat-M.*, *Puls.*, *Spig.*, *Tab.*) (D.).

BAD EFFECTS FROM OVER-JOY WITH EXALTA-TION, FROM DRINKING TOO MUCH WINE AND FROM COLD.

Sleepless after labour (G.).

Wide-awake condition ; impossible to close the eyes (A.).

Long and vivid dreams (C.).

Insomnia : berfore or after midnight ; from excessive joy ; from nursing the sick (*Cocc.*) ; *and from activity of the mind* (*Ars.*, *Calc.*, *Hep.*, *Nux-V.*, *Puls.*) (K.).

SLEEPLESSNESS ON ACCOUNT OF EXCES-SnIE EXCITABILITY OF THE MIND AND OF THE BODY.

AWAKES AT OR HEARS EVERY SOUND (B.).

THE MIND IS ACTIVE WITH PLANS AND FANCIES (D.).

Aversion to open air (*Nux-V.*, *Psor.*, *Sil.*).

Weeping from delight (*Lach.*, *Plat.*) (A.).

Buoyancy and exaltation of the mind (*Piper-M.*) (D.).

Now joyous, now gloomy (*Ign.*, *Puls.*) (B.).

Alternate laughing and weeping (*Puls.*) (A.).

Faints easily (*Ars.*, *Asaf.*, *Ign.*, *Lach.*, *Nat-C.*, *Verat.*) (B.).

ALL THE SENSES ARE MORE ACUTE—SIGHT, HEARING, SMELL, TASTE AND TOUCH (*Bell.*, *Cham.*, *Nux-V.*, *Op.*) (A.).

ACUTE HEARING ; OVERHEARS DISTANT SOUNDS (*Bell.*, *Chin.*, *Lach.*, *Nux-V.*, *Op.*) (B.).

Incessant cough, especially with measles (*Cop.*, *Eup-P.*, *Spong.*, *Squil.*) (B.).

Unusual activity of mind and body (A.).

Full of ideas ; quick to act ; no sleep on this account (A.).

BAD EFFECTS OF SUDDEN EMOTIONS OR PLEASURABLE SURPRISES (A.).

TOOTHACHE, RELIEVED BY ICE WATER (*Puls.*) (B.).

Intermittent or jerking toothache (A.).

Nightly toothache (*Merc.*) (Bt.).

Pains are felt intensely ; seem almost insupportable, driving the patient to despair (*Acon.*, *Cham.*) (A.).

Tossing about in anguish (*Acon.*, *Ars.*, *Cham.*) (A.).

Hasty eating and drinking (*Bell.*, *Hep.*) (A.).

Is in a complete state of ecstasy (G.).

Headache : from over-mental exertion, thinking, or talking (A.).

Sensation as if the brain were torn or dashed to pieces (A.).

Child cries easily ; while crying it suddenly laughs quite heartily, and finally cries again (G.).

Reads fine print easily (Hr.).

Burning, sour eructations (*Lyc.*, *Sulph.*, *Sulph-Ac.* (T.).

Violent spasmodic eructations, with rising of the ingesta (T.).

Colic so painful as to drive the patient mad (G.).

Stomach feels over-loaded (*Bry.*, *Chin.*, *Kali-C.*, *Lyc. Nux-M.*, *Nux-V.*, *Puls.*, *Sep.*) (B.).

Profuse flow of watery urine (*Acet-Ac.*, *Gels.*, *Phos-Ac.*) (Bt.).

NOCTURNAL EMISSIONS, FOLLOWED BY GREAT LANGUOR AND IRRITABILITY OF TEMPER (*Nux-V.*, *Staph.*, *Sulph.*) (Bt.).

EXCESSIVE EXCITABILITY OF THE SEXUAL DESIRE (*Anan.*, *Bar-M.*, *Calc.*, *Calc-P.*, *Cann-I.*, *Canth.*, *Con.*, *Lyc.*, *Lyss.*, *Nux-V.*, *Phos.*, *Pic-Ac.*, *Plat.*, *Puls.*, *Sil.*, *Staph.*, *Tub.*, *Zinc.*) (Bt.).

Great nervous agitation and restlessness (*Ars.*, *Phos.*) (Br.).

Neuralgia in various parts ; always with great nervous excitability and intolerance of pain (Br.).

Violent, irregular palpitation, especially after excessive joy or surprise (*Bad.*, *Puls.*) (Br.).

Cough and sleeplessness after measles (N.).

Sense of smell more acute (*Acon.*, *Agar.*, *Bell.*, *Colch.*, *Hep.*, *Lyc.*) (C.).

Feels exhausted after coughing (Bt.).

Spasmodic, dry, hacking cough (*Alum.*, *Bell.*, *Cimic.*, *Hyos.*) (C.).

Crural neuralgia : *worse from motion, in the afternoon and at night ; better by pressure* (Br.).

Chilliness increased by every movement (*Apis*, *Arn.*, *Bry.*, *Caps.*, *Merc-C.*, *Nux-V.*, *Rhus-T.*, *Sep.*, *Sil.*, *Squil.*) (C.).

Internal chilliness with external heat of the face and body.

Increased hunger, with rapid, hurried eating.

Genital organs itch voluptuously, and are very sensitive (*Plat.*) (G.).

Excessive sensitiveness about the vulva, with voluptuous itching ; would like to rub or scratch the part, but it is too sensitive (G.).

Labour pains insupportable to her feelings ; she feels them intensely ; weeps and laments fearfully (G.).

Menses too early and long lasting (*Calc.*, *Carb-An.*, *Carb-V.*, *Ferr.*, *Kali-C.*, *Nat-M.*, *Nux-V.*, *Plat.*, *Rat.*, *Rhus-T.*, *Sabin.*) (Br.).

Excessive excitability of the sexual organs (*Nux-V.*, *Phos.*, *Sulph.*) (Bt.).

Measly spots on the skin, with dry heat at night (N.).

Prosopalgia extending to molar teeth, ears, forehead, and scalp (Br.).

Convulsions after over-excitement (C.).

AGGRAVATION : In the open air ; from drinking wine ; from taking cold ; at night ; from strong odours ; from noise ; from sudden, pleasurable surprise ; from excessive exaltation ; and from narcotics.

AMELIORATION : From cold water ; and from lying down.

RELATIONSHIP. *Compare* : *Acon., Ars., Bell., Bry., Caust., Cham., Chin., Cocc., Hyos., Ign., Lyc., Mag-P., Nux-V., Op., Phos., Plat., Puls., Sep., Sulph., Zinc.*

ANTIDOTES : *Cham., Ign., Nux-V.,* and *Puls.*

Coffea antidotes : *Cham., Coloc.,* and *Nux-V.*

Colchicum.

COMMON NAME : MEADOW SAFFRON.

Affects markedly the muscular tissue, periosteum and synovial membranes of the joints.

Weakness and debility from night study and loss of sleep (*Nux-V.*).

Tearing in the limbs during warm weather, and stinging during cold weather.

Tingling in many parts of the body, as if frost-bitten whenever the weather changes.

Shocks as from electricity through one-half of the body, with sensation of paralysis.

Sensitiveness of the whole body, especially the affected parts, to contact and to motion.

Frequent startings (*Bell., Hyos., Kali-C., Stram., Sulph.*).

Tingling in the points of the fingers and toes.

General exhaustion of mind and body (*Gels., Kali-P., Phos.*) (D.).

Dropsy of the uterus, from suppression of the menses (Bt.).

Dropsical swelling and dropsy of the skin.

BROWN TONGUE (*Ars., Bapt., Bry., Chin-Ars., Hyos., Kali-P., Lach., Phos., Plb., Rhus-T., Sec.*) (D.).

Scanty discharge of dark-red urine, with tenesmus (*Canth., Lyc., Tereb.*).

Extreme aversion to food (*Bry., Kali-M., Puls.*) (D.).

NAUSEA FROM THE ODOUR OF FAT MEAT OR EGGS.

NAUSEA AND LOATHING AT THE THOUGHT OF FOOD (*Ars., Cocc., Graph., Sep.*) (D.).

HE GAGS FROM MERE MENTION OF FOOD (D.).

Loss of appetite (*Chin., Graph., Hep., Ipec., Lyc., Merc., Nat-S., Puls., Sep.*) (D.).

Abdomen is distended enormously, with urging to stool and passage of jelly-like mucus (D.).

DYSENTERY, WITH GASTRIC SYMPTOMS AND DISCHARGE OF WHITE MUCUS WITH MUCH TENESMUS (*Aloe, Merc-C., Nux-V., Sulph.*).

Spasm of the sphincter ani (*Caust.*, *Ferr.*, *Tab.*) (D.)

SUDDEN SINKING OF THE VITAL FORCES (*Ars.*, *Camph.*, *Hydr-Ac.*, *Kali-P.*, *Verat.*) (Ra.).

Bad effects from suppressed perspiration (*Sil.*).

METASTASIS OF GOUT TO HEART (*Benz-Ac.*, *Kalm.*, *Led Puls.*) (D.).

Cutting pains about the heart and oppression (*Ars.*, *Bry.*, *Cact.*, *Iod.*) (D.).

Rheumatic pericarditis (*Acon.*, *Bry.*, *Kalm.*, *Lach.*, *Lyc.*, *Merc.*, *Rhus-T.*) (Bt.).

Dry, hacking cough, with burning and feeling of constriction across the chest (Bt.).

Burning, or icy coldness in the stomach and abdomen (*Camph.*) (A.).

Cholera : *sero-mucous vomiting and rice-water stools, thrown off with great force, with cramps of the abdomina muscles, flexors of the arms and feet, and sunken features* (*Ars.*, *Bism.*, *Kali-P.*, *Verat.*) (Bt.).

Cold surface, tongue and breath, mottled skin and bluish nails (*Camph.*, *Carb-V.*, *Laur.*) (Bt.).

Œdematous swelling of the face (*Apis*, *Phos.*).

Intense boring or tensive pain in the ovary, causing her to draw up double, with great restlessness (N.).

Affected parts very sensitive to contact and motion (*Apis*, *Arn.*, *Bry.*, *Hep.*, *Lach.*) (A.).

ARTHRITIC PAINS IN THE JOINTS ; PATIENT SCREAMS WITH PAIN ON TOUCHING A JOINT, OR STUBBING A TOE (A.).

REDNESS, HEAT AND SWELLING OF THE AFFECTED PARTS (*Apis, Led., Rhus-T.*) (G.).

Whitish sediment in the urine (*Calc., Phos-Ac.*) (C.).

Ailments from grief or misdeeds of others (*Staph.*) (A.).

Pulse ; small, weak, irregular ; at times rapid, at times slow, intermittent, scarcely perceptible (R.).

Every motion excites or renews the vomiting ; canno| sit erect (*Bry., Verat-V.*) (C.).

Salivation (*Merc., Nit-Ac., Sep.*). (K.).

SMELL PAINFULLY ACUTE ; NAUSEA AND FAINTNESS FROM THE ODOUR OF COOKING FOOD, ESPECIALLY FISH, EGGS OR FAT MEAT (*Ars., Sep.*) (A.).

Peevish, nothing satisfies him (*Sulph.*) (C.).

The small joints are most affected (Bl.).

Hydrothorax ;   with marked dyspnœa and œdema of the extremities (*Merc-Sulph.*) (Bl.).

Swelling of joints moving from one place to another (*Kali-S., Puls., Spig.*) (N.).

FALL DYSENTERIES, WHEN THE DAYS ARE WARM AND NIGHTS ARE COLD ; STOOLS SHREDDY AND BLOODY, LIKE SCRAPINGS (*Canth., Merc-C.*) (N.).

AGGRAVATION : In the evening ; in the night ; during an expiration ; from exertion ; from motion ; while drawing breath ; from touching the parts ; during walking; from odour of cooking ; food from mental emotion ; and from loss of sleep.

AMELIORATION : While stooping ; after evacuation ; while reposing ; when sitting ; from lying quietly ; and in the open air.

RELATIONSHIP : *Compare.* : *Arn.*, *Ars.*, *Benz-Ac.*, *Berb.*, *Bry.*, *Carb-V.*, *Cocc.*, *Ipec.*, *Kali-B.*, *Merc.* *Nat-M.*, *Nux-V.*, *Phos.*, *Puls.*, *Rhod.*, *Rhus-T.*, *Tereb.*, *Thuj.*, *Urt-U.*, *Verat.*

Antidotes : *Camph.*, *Cocc.*, *Nux-V.*, *Puls.*, and *Thuj.*

COMPLEMENTARY : *Ars.* and *Spig.*

Collinsonia.

COMMON NAME : STONE ROOT.

Pelvic and portal congestion, resulting in dysmenorrhœa and hæmorrhoids (*Aloe*, *Podo.*, *Sulph.*) (A.).

Flushes of heat, with oppressed breathing (*Amyl-N.*, *Arg-N.*, *Ferr-P.*, *Graph.*, *Sang.*, *Sep.*, *Sulph.*) (Br.).

Bitter taste in the mouth (*Bry.*, *Carb-V.*, *Chel.*, *Chin.*, *Coloc.*, *Merc.*, *Nat-M.*, *Nat-S.*, *Nux-V.*, *Puls.*, *Sulph.*) (Br.).

CONGESTION OF PELVIC VISCERA, WITH HÆMORRHOIDS, ESPECIALLY IN THE LATTER MONTHS OF PREGNANCY (*Æsc.*, *Am-M.*, *Caps.*, *Lach.*, *Nat-M.*, *Nux-V.*, *Sep.*) (A.).

Itching of the anus (*Æsc.*, *Aloe*, *Am-C.*, *Calc.*, *Caust.*, *Fluor-Ac.*, *Graph.*, *Lyc.*, *Nit-Ac.*, *Nux-V.*, *Sulph.*) (Br.).

The bowels are more apt to move in the evening (F.).

CHRONIC, PAINFUL, BLEEDING PILES (*Æsc.*, *Aloe.*, *Carb-V.*, *Graph.*, *Ham.*, *Lach.*, *Lyc.*, *Mur-Ac.*, *Nat-M.*, *Nit-Ac.*, *Rat.*, *Sep.*, *Sulph.*, *Thuj.*) (A.).

Hæmorrhoidal dysentery, with tenesmus (*Aloe*, *Caps.*, *Coloc.*, *Merc-V.*, *Nux-V.*, *Rhus-T.*, *Sulph.*) (A.).

Constipation with prolapsus uteri and hæmorrhoids (*Nat-M.*, *Sep.*) (D.) .

Stools lumpy and light coloured, with straining and dull pain in the anus (Bt.).

SENSATION AS IF STICKS, SAND OR GRAVEL HAD LODGED IN THE RECTUM (*Æsc.*, *Caust.*, *Graph.*, *Iris*, *Nux-V.*, *Sulph.*) (A.).

Sense of weight in the rectum (*Aloe*, *Cact.*, *Caust.*, *Hep.*, *Sep.*, *Sil.*, *Thuj.*) (C.).

Stools in form of balls (*Alum.*, *Alumn.*, *Mag-M.*, *Nat-M.*, *Op.*, *Plb.*) (C.).

Alternate diarrhœa and constipation (*Ant-C.*, *Chel.*, *Hep.*, *Ign.*, *Kali-B.*, *Lach.*, *Nit-Ac.*, *Nux-V.*, *Op.*, *Podo.*, *Sulph.*) (A.).

Stools are preceded and followed by severe pains in the hypogastrium (Bt.).

Congestive inertia of lower bowels ; stools sluggish and hard, with pain and great flatulence (A.).

Headache from suppressed hæmorrhoids (*Aloe*, *Lach.*, *Sep.*, *Sulph.*) (C.).

Membranous dysmenorrhœa (*Bor.*, *Brom.*, *Cycl.*, *Kali-B.*, *Lac-C.*) (Br.).

Pruritus in pregnancy (*Ambr.*, *Fluor-Ac.*, *Helon.*, *Merc.*, *Sep.*), *with hæmorrhoids ; unable to lie down* (A.).

Dropsy from cardiac disease (*Apis*, *Ars.*, *Aur.*, *Dig.*, *Lach.*, *Lyc.*, *Merc.*, *Naja*, *Phos.*, *Rhus-T.*) (A.).

Palpitation in patients subject to piles and indigestion (*Carb-V.*, *Dios.*, *Lach.*, *Lyc.*, *Nux-V.*, *Sep.*) (A.).

Heart's action persistently rapid but weak (*Dig.*, *Lach.*, *Phos.*, *Sep.*) (A.).

After heart is relieved old piles reappear, suppressed menses return (A.).

Cough from excessive use of voice (*Arg-N.*, *Arum-T.*, *Caust.*, *Rhus-T.*) (Br.).

Yellow coating along the centre or base of the tongue (*Ant-C.*, *Calc-S.*, *Chin.*, *Kali-S.*, *Merc.*, *Merc-I-F.*, *Nat-P.*, *Nux-V.*) (C.).

Functional paralysis, coming from fatigue or from mental emotions (*Cocc.*, *Ign.*, *Nat-M.*, *Phos.*, *Stann.*) (F.).

AGGRAVATION : From mental emotion ; from mental excitement ; from cold ; at night ; and during pregnancy.

AMELIORATION : From heat.

RELATIONSHIP. *Compare* : *Æsc.*, *Aloe*, *Caps.*, *Carb-V.*, *Dios.*, *Ham.*, *Lach.*, *Lyc.*, *Lycps.*, *Merc.*, *Mur-Ac.*, *Nat-M.*, *Nit-Ac.*, *Op.*, *Plb.*, *Rat.*, *Sep.*, *Sil.*, *Sulph.*
Antidote : *Nux-V.*

Has cured colic after *Coloc.* and *Nux-V.* failed.

In heart disease complicated with hæmorrhoids, consult *Coll.*, when *Cact.*, *Dig.*, and other remedies f i

Colocynth.

COMMON NAME : BITTER CUCUMBER.

Colocynth develops most of its symptoms in the abdomen and head, causing neuralgias. The nerves around the hip-joint are also a marked centre of action (D.).

All the limbs are drawn together.

Shortening of the muscles (*Am-M.*, *Cup.*, *Mag-P.*, *Rhus-T.*).

Twitching of the muscles (*Bell.*, *Cupr.*, *Hyos.*, *Ign.*, *Mag-P.*, *Stram.*).

Stiffness of the joints (*Calc.*, *Calc-F.*, *Caust.*, *Kali-C* ,*Lach.*, *Nat-S.*, *Rhus-T.*).

Tearing pains longitudinally.

Constrictions and contraction of internal and external parts.

Pain in the hip, and when walking a sensation as if the psoas muscle was too short.

Affections of the right upper extremity ; also right lower extremity, right eye, right side of the chest, etc. (G.).

Inclination to become angry and indignant (*Cham.*, *Ign.*, *Nux-V.*, *Staph.*).

Bad effects, either from mortification caused by an offence, or else from anger with indignation (*Staph.*).

Does not like to talk, to answer, or to see friends, or anybody (*Bry.*, *Ign.*, *Staph.*) (N.).

Extremely irritable ; becomes angry when questioned (*Bry.*) (Br.).

Irritable ; *throws things out of his hands* (*Ars., Bry., Cham., Cina, Kreos., Staph., Stram.*) (A.).

Sleeplessness after anger (*Nux-V.*).

It is to be remembered for articular rheumatism, when the joints remain stiff and unwieldly, and the pains in the affected parts are of a boring character (F.).

COLICKY PAINS IN THE ABDOMEN COM-PELLING ONE TO BEND DOUBLE (*Caust., Cham., Mag-P., Plb., Puls., Sep.*), WITH GREAT ANGUISH AND RESTLESS CONSTRICTION IN THE BOWELS, OR PAIN AS IF CUTTING WITH KNIVES, OR PAIN AS THOUGH THE BOWEL WAS PRESSED BETWEEN TWO STONES (*Cocc.*).

A VIOLENT, AGONIZING ABDOMINAL COLIC, RELIEVED BY BENDING DOUBLE AND BY PRESSING SOMETHING HARD INTO THE ABDOMEN (D.).

COLIC, BETTER FROM LYING ON THE ABDO-MEN (*Aloe, Am-C., Bell., Bry., Ind., Phos., Plb., Rhus-T., Stann.*) (K.).

Vomiting and diarrhœa, with colic (*Acon., Cupr., Nux-V., Sec.*) ; doubling up ; from anger with indignation (N.).

Colic so distressing, that they seek relief by pressing corners of tables or heads of bed-posts against the abdomen (Hr.).

20

Severe colicky pains, mostly around the navel ; has to bend double, being worse in any other posture ; with great restlessness and loud screaming on changing position ; worse at intervals of five or ten minutes (N.).

Colicky pain, worse after eating or drinking the least amount (G.).

Rumbling in the bowels (*Podo.*).

Dysentery-like diarrhœa, renewed each time after taking the least food or drink (*Arg-N., Colch., Crot-T., Ferr., Sulph.*) (N.).

It has been of service in mucous colitis when there were griping and cutting pains that caused the patient to writhe and bend double, press upon the abdomen and ask for hot applications.

Chronic watery diarrhœa in the morning, with pain in the sides of the abdomen (Ra.).

Ovarian neuralgia : sharp pain in the ovarian regions, relieved by bending double and by pressure (*Mag-P.*) (D.).

Sciatica : Sharp, spasmodic attacks of pain shoot down the sciatic nerve to the feet ; crampy pains, as if the parts were screwed in a vise ; it is worse on the right side and tends to be paroxysmal ; relieved by warmth and rest (D.).

Crampy pain in the hip-joint, as though the parts were screwed in a vise ; lies on the painful side with knees bent up (N.).

Vertigo when turning the head to the left (*Calc-P.*) (Br.).

Frequent urging to urinate (*Nux-V.*), *with scanty urine, and sometimes thick, fetid, viscid, or jelly-like urine* (N.).

Persistent bitter taste in the mouth (*Bry., Chin., Nat-S., Nux-V., Sep.*) (B).

Dysuria : straining ineffectual ; worse before, during and after urination, which is scanty (Hm.).

It cures diarrhœa caused from anger, from eating fruit, from drinking ice-water or lemonade (R.).

Griping in the epigastrium after each meal ; worse towards evening (C.).

AGGRAVATION: In the evening ; from anger ; after eating ; in repose ; and from motion.

AMELIORATION: From bending double ; from hard pressure ; from coffee ; from heat ; from discharge of flatus ; and from lying upon the abdomen.

RELATIONSHIP : *Complementary* : *Merc.* in dysentery, with great tenesmus, and *Caust.* in colic, etc.

Compare : GNAPH. in intense pain along the right sciatic nerve ; darting, cutting, from the right hip-joint down to the foot, alternating with numbness.

Compare also *Staph.* in abdominal pains, etc., from anger, reserved indignation or silent grief.

Antidotes : *Camph., Coff., Op.* and *Staph.*

Conium Maculatum.

COMMON NAME: POISON HEMLOCK.

Suitable for old men, old maids, women with tight, rigid fibre ; scrofulous and cancerous people ; children prematurely old (N.).

Ailments and weakness of old men (*ecchymosis*).

SWELLING AND INDURATION OF THE GLANDS, WITH STINGING AND TINGLING, AFTER BRUISES AND CONTUSIONS.

Great sensation of debility in the morning in bed (*Ambr., Carb-V., Lach., Nat-M., Phos., Puls., Sil., Staph.*).

Induration after contusion and bruises.

Obscuration of the cornea (*Calc., Caust., Merc., Sil.*).

MUCH TROUBLED WITH VERTIGO, WHICH IS WORSE WHEN TURNING THE HEAD, TURNING IN BED, OR LYING DOWN (N.).

Easily intoxicated (Bt.).

Paralysis and apoplexy of old persons (*Bar-C., Gels., Glon., Op.*).

Useful in paresis and paralysis that extend from below upward (Bl.).

VERTIGO, AS THOUGH THE BED AND THINGS IN THE ROOM WERE TURNING IN A CIRCLE (*Alum.*, *Bry.*, *Calc.*, *Cycl.*, *Ferr.*, *Lyc.*, *Mosch.*, *Nat-M.*, *Phos.*, *Puls.*) (N.).

Hysterical and hypochondriacal attacks after excessive sexual indulgence, or after entire abstinence.

Weakness of the lower limbs, staggering; worse by turning the head, or looking around sidewise (N.).

Unable to sustain any mental effort (A.).

Great concern about little things (Bt.).

Dreads being alone, but avoids society.

Very easily excited (*Nux-V.*, *Phos.*) (Bt.).

Convulsive twitching of the limbs (*Acon.*, *Bell.*, *Cocc.*, *Cupr.*, *Glon.*, *Hyos.*, *Lach.*, *Merc.*, *Nat-M.*, *Puls.*).

GREAT SENSITIVENESS TO LIGHT, WITHOUT CORRESPONDING INFLAMMATION OF THE EYES (*Nux-V.*, *Sulph.*) (N.).

No inclination for business or study (A.).

On opening the lids, tears squirt out (Apis, Ipec., Merc-C., Rhus-T.) (N.).

Lips and teeth have black crusts on them (Bt.).

Frequent, sour eructations, with hardness and distension of the abdomen (G.).

SWEAT DAY AND NIGHT, AS SOON AS

ONE SLEEPS, ON EVEN CLOSING THE EYES
(*Calc.*, *Carb-An.*, *Lach.*, *Thuj.*) (N.).

Vomiting, that looks like black coffee-grounds (*Ars.*, *Cadm-S.*, *Lyc.*, *Merc-C.*, *Nat-M.*, *Phos.*) (G.).

Cough ; in spasmodic paroxysms caused by a dry spot in the larynx (A.).

Cough during pregnancy (*Puls.*) (A.).

HACKING, ALMOST CONTINUAL COUGH, WORSE AT NIGHT WHEN LYING DOWN (*Hyos.*, *Kali-Br.*, *Puls.*, *Sulph.*) (N.).

MUCH DIFFICULTY IN VOIDING URINE ; THE FLOW SUDDENLY STOPS, THEN FLOWS AGAIN, SEVERAL TIMES, AT EACH EMISSION (N.).

Urine flows better when standing (can only pass urine while standing—*Hyper.*, *Sars.*) (K.).

Emission of prostatic fluid while passing flatus, from fondling a woman, during lascivious thoughts and with stool (K.).

BAD EFFECTS FROM SUPPRESSED SEXUAL DESIRE, OR FROM EXCESSIVE INDULGENCE (N.).

Enfeebled state of the sexual organs from masturbation (*Nux-V.*, *Phos.*) (D.).

Induration of the testicles (*Brom.*, *Rhod.*) (Bt.).

Incomplete erection, during coition (*Camph.*, *Graph.*, *Lyc.*, *Phos.*, *Sulph.*) (K.).

SEMINAL EMISSIONS, WHILE FROLICKING WITH A WOMAN (*Phos.*, *Sars.*) (K.).

Acrid, corrosive leucorrhœa (*Ars.*, *Calc.*, *Nit-Ac.*, *Sulph.*) (Bt.).

Leucorrhœa ten days after menses (A.).

Induration and enlargement of the ovary (*Iod.*, *Merc.*, *Sep.*, *Thuj.*) (G.).

Swelling and soreness of the breasts preceding the menses (*Calc.*, *Kali-C.*, *Kali-S.*, *Lac-C.*, *Murx.*, *Tub.*) (N).

Dysmenorrhœa, with aching about the heart (N.).

Indurations of the breast, hard as a stone, especially after a blow or injury (N.).

STINGING, LANCINATING PAINS IN THE NECK OF THE UTERUS, WITH INDURATIONS AND SCIRRHOSIS. (N.).

Constipation, with constant and ineffectual urging to stool (*Nux-V.*, *Sulph.*)(Bt.).

Constipation on alternate days (*Alum.*, *Bry.*, *Caust.*, *Nat-M*, *Nux-V.*, *Sep.*, *Sulph*, (B.).

Palpitation, worse after drinking, from exertion and after stool (*Ars.*, *Caust.*) (K.).

Objects seem red (*Bell.*, *Hyos.*, *Iod.*, *Nux-M.*, *Phos.*, *Stront.*) (K.).

Paralysis of the optic nerve (*Bell.*, *Gels.*, *Kali-I.*, *Nat-M.*, *Phos.*, *Puls.*, *Sil.*) (G.).

Nasal polypus (*All-C., Calc., Graph., Kali-B., Merc., Nit-Ac., Sang., Teucr., Thuj.*) (B.).

Expectoration only after long coughing (*Caust., Nux-V., Puls.*) (*Br*).

Mucus can not be expectorated —must be swallowed (*Arn., Cann-S., Caust., Kali-C., Kali-S., Sep., Spong., Staph., Zinc.*) (D.).

Blood-red ear-wax (C.).

Ears feel as if stopped up on blowing the nose (*Alum., Calc., Mang., Spig., Sulph*; stopped feeling in the ear, better from blowing the nose —*Merc., Stann.*) (C.).

AGGRAVATION : In the night ; while eating ; from light ; from milk ; in snow-air ; while standing ; while lying down ; from sexual excesses ; from masturbation ; when lifting the affected part ; and from turning in bed.

AMELIORATION : While fasting ; in the dark ; from letting the limbs hang down ; from motion ; from walking ; from pressure ; and on sitting down.

RELATIONSHIP : Similar to : *Bar-C., Carb-An., Caust., Curare, Gels, Hydr., Hyos., Kali-P., Lyc., Nat-M., Nux-V., Phos., Puls., Rhus-T., Sep., Sil., Sulph., Thuj.,* and *Zinc.*

Compare : *Arn., Ham.,* and *Rhus-T.* in contusions ; *Ars., Ast-R., Bar-C., Brom., Carb-An., Iod., Phos., Phyt.* and *Sil.* in cancer : and *Brom., Calc., Calc-I., Merc-I., Phyt.* and *Psor.* in glandular swellings.

Corallium Rubrum.

COMMON NAME : RED CORAL.

Is useful in a combination of syphilis and psora (F.).

Congestion of blood to the face and head (after dinner).

Dry coryza ; nose feels stopped up (*Ars., Nux-V., Stict.*) (Br.).

Painful ulcers in nostrils (*Bor., Calc-S., Hep., Merc., Nit-Ac.*) (Br.).

INSPIRED AIR FEELS COLD : (*Æsc., Ant-C., Ars., Brom., Cist., Hydr., Kali-B.*) (N.).

Profuse discharge of thick, yellow, and stringy mucus from nasal passages (*Hydr., Kali-B., Nat-S.*) (A.).

Epistaxis, especially at night (*Bell., Carb-V., Merc., Nit-Ac., Puls.*) (C.).

Profuse secretion of mucus through the posterior nares, obliging one to hawk frequently.

Is useful for cough like whooping cough. The night paroxysms are very severe (N.).

"MINUTE GUN COUGH" DURING THE DAY, AND WHOOPING COUGH AT NIGHT (A.).

May be used in any kind of cough, when the attack comes on with a very rapid cough, and the attacks follow so closely as to almost run into each other (G.).

Feels suffocated and greatly exhausted after whooping cough (Br.).

Laryngismus stridulus (Brom., Chlor., Iod., Phos., Samb.) (Bl.).

Paroxysms of violent, spasmodic cough, commencing with gasping for breath, and continuing with repeated crowing inspirations, until the patient grows purple or black in the face (Dn.).

REDDISH ULCERS ON THE PENIS, VERY SENSITIVE TO CONTACT (*Hep.*).

Chancroids or soft chancres (Merc., Nux-V.) may find a swift and sure cure in Cor-R. (N.).

Has also been found useful in chancre. The ulcer is red (coral red), flat and exceedingly sensitive. Sometimes painful (N.).

Chancres on any part of penis or scrotum (N.).

Sexual power weakened (*Calad., Nux-V., Sel., Sulph.*),

Profuse perspiration on the genitals (*Aur., Calad., Fluor-Ac., Hydr., Lyc., Merc., Petr., Sel., Sep., Sil., Thuj.*) (Br.).

Short, quick-and ringing cough (D.).

Cough as soon as he eats (*Ant-T., Ars., Bry., Carb-V., Coc-C., Ipec., Kali-B., Nux-V., Phos., Rumx., Sep.*) (B.).

Difficult and oppressed respiration (*Brom., Carb-V., Lach., Phos., Sulph.*) (C.).

Psoriasis of palms and soles (*Ars., Ars-I., Graph., Kali-Ars., Merc., Petr., Sep.,* (Br.).

Copper-coloured spots on the skin (*Carb-An., Merc., Kali-I.,Nit-Ac., Syph., Thuj.*) (Br.).

Too hot if covered, but chilled by uncovering (B.).

There are smooth spots on the surface of the body mostly on the palms of the hands. At first they are of a coral-red hue, but they finally become darker, and assume the well-known copper colour, characteristic of syphilis (F.).

LONGING FOR ACIDS AND SALT FOOD (*Arg-N., Calc., Calc-S., Carb-V., Con., Med., Merc-I-F., Nat-M., Phos., Plb., Sulph., Thuj., Verat.*).

Head feels too large (*Arg-N., Bell., Glon., Nux-M., Nux-V., Ran-B.*)

Very violent headache, as if the parietal bones were forced asunder ; aggravated by stooping (C.).

AGGRAVATION : From deep inspiration ; at night ; from stooping ; after dinner ; from touch ; from uncovering ; and in open air.

AMELIORATION : From covering.

RELATIONSHIP : *Compare* : *Ant-T., Bell., Brom., Chlor., Coc-C., Cupr., Hyos., Dros., Kali-B., Merc., Meph., Nit-Ac., Phos., Rumx., Sep., Sil.,* and *Sulph.*
Complementary : *Sulph.*

Crataegus Oxyacantha.

COMMON NAME : HAWTHORN BERRIES.

The few provings that have been made show conclusively that its action is directly upon the heart, which, primarily, it excites moderately, but to such a degree that it becomes quite evident that the long-continued use of the drug would result in lowering the tone of the heart and enfeebling its action.

Great pallor of the skin, with rush of blood to the head (Bl.).

Urine : diminished ; contains traces of albumen and an excess of phosphates (Bl.).

Giddiness (*Calc.*, *Dig.*, *Ferr-P.*, *Kalv-P.*) (*Br.*).

Apprehensive and despondent (*Ars.*, *Aur.*, *Dig.*, *Lach.*, *Nit-Ac.*) (*C.*).

Pain in the back of head and neck (*Coc-C.*, *Petr.*, *Rhus-T.*, *Sil.*) (*Br.*).

Extremities are cold and œdematous (*Ars.*, *Carb-V.*, *Phos.*) (*Bl.*).

General anasarca (*Apis*, *Blatta*, *Dig.*, *Merc-Sulph.*, *Nat-S.*, *Phos.*) (*C.*).

CARDIAC DILATATION (*Ars.*, *Aur.*, *Cact.*, *Dig.*, *Lach.*, *Mur-Ac.*, *Phos.*) (*B.*).

Weak and exhausted (*Gels.*, *Kali-P.*, *Phos.*, *Sep.*) (B.),

EXTREME DYSPNŒA ON LEAST EXERTION (*Ars.*, *Calc.*, *Coca*, *Ipec.*, *Lach.*, *Lob.*, *Lyc.*, *Lycps.*, *Nat-M.*, *Spong.*) (*C.*).

Irregular respiration (*Ail., Ang., Bell., Cupr., Dig., Morph., Op.*) (C.).

Useful in the beginning of heart mischief after rheumatism (*Colch., Kalm., Led., Lyc., Phos.*) (Br.).

Pain in the region of the heart (*Acon., Ars., Aur., Bry., Cact., Dig., Lat-M., Rhus-T., Spig., Verat-V*). (C.).

Angina pectoris (*Arg-N., Glon., Naja, Tab.*) (B.).

Palpitation and tachycardia, dependent upon anæmia (*Carb-V., Chin., Ferr., Phos., Sep.*) (Bl.).

Failing compensation (*Ars.*) (Br.).

Pulse irregular and intermittent (*Gels, Lach., Nat-M., Phos., Verat.*) (C.).

Insomnia of aortic patients (Br.).

Excessive perspiration (*Calc., Camph., Carb-V., Chin., Merc., Nat-M., Sulph., Verat.*) (Br.).

AGGRAVATION : In a warm room ; from least exertion ; during night ; and from rheumatic affections.

AMELIORATION : From fresh air ; from remaining quiet ; and from taking rest.

RELATIONSHIP : Compare : *Apis, Ars., Bry., Conva., Dig., Ferr-P., Gels., Ipec., Kali-Ars., Kali-C., Lach., Lat-M., Lyc., Merc-Sulph., Nat-S., Phos., Rhus-T., Stroph., Sulph.* and *Verat-V.*

Crocus Sativus.

COMMON NAME: SAFFRON.

Sore burning in the eyes after reading; also dimness; must wink frequently and wipe the eyes, as though a film were before the eyes (N.).

Feeling in the eyes as though she had wept violently, as though water were constantly coming into the eyes (N.).

VERY CHANGEABLE TEMPERAMENT (*Ign., Mosch., Puls.*).

Epistaxis of very thick blood, with cold sweat on the forehead, yellowish face, and fainting (N.).

METRORRHAGIA, WHEN THE DISCHARGE IS DARK, BLACK, VISCID AND STRINGY; IT SMELLS BADLY, AND IS WORSE ON MOTION (N.).

Stitches in the abdomen arresting respiration (Bt.).
Sensation of hopping and jumping, as from something alive in the abdomen and in the chest.

Tingling in various parts of the body (*Acon., Alum., Kali-P., Nux-V., Phos., Plat., Plb., Rhus-T., Zinc.*).

BLEEDING FROM VARIOUS ORGANS OF THE BODY (*Acaly., Calc., Carb-V., Chin., Ferr-P., Ham., Merc., Nit-Ac.*); THE BLOOD IS BLACK AND TOUGH.

Skin scarlet-red (*Bell.·, Ferr-P., Stram., Verat-V.*)
St. Vitus's dance (*Agar.·, Tarant.*).

These attacks are of a recurrent nature—are
evening attacks—and associated with singing,
laughing and dancing spells.

Sings during sleep (**Bell., Phos-Ac.**) (**Bt.**).

*She is worse every evening, with alternations of
excessive, happy, affectionate tenderness and rage* (G.).

JUMPING, DANCING, LAUGHING, AND
WHISTLING (*Bell.·, Stram.*) (G.).

WANTS TO KISS EVERYBODY (G.),

DARK, FOUL, STRINGY MENSES (*Plat., Ust.*)
(B.).

Great debility and palpitation of the heart on going
up-stairs (*Ars., Calc., Phos.*) (G.).

*The patient is alternately cheerful or depressed.
In the former state she will sing, dance, jump, laugh
and whistle, love and want to kiss everybody. In
the latter, she will cry, get into a rage, abuse her
friends, and then repent it* (N.).

Headache, worse during menses (*Bell., Glon.,
Graph., Kreos., Lyc.·, Nat-M., Sep.*) (Br.).

Spasmodic contractions and twitchings of single
sets of muscles (*Agar., Ign.·, Zinc.*) (**A.**).

Giddiness with fainting (*Chin., Kali-P., Phos-Ac.*).

Sensation of coldness in the back (*Bol.*, *Cact.*, *Caps.*, *Eup-P.*, *Eup-Purp.*, *Lach.*, *Nat-M.*, *Nat-S.*, *Puls.*, *Sil.*, *Sulph.*, *Verat.*).

Eyes dry on reading (*Arg-N.*) (T.).

Music affects her. Hearing one sing, she begs involuntarily to join in; but there is not the subsequent relief from music (F.).

AGGRAVATION : In the morning ; from fasting ; in a warm room ; before breakfast ; during pregnancy ; looking fixedly at an object ; and from lying down.

AMELIORATION : In the open air; and after breakfast.

RELATIONSHIP : *Compare* : *Acon.*, *Bell.*, *Calc.*, *Chin.*, *Ham.*, *Ign.*, *Ipec.*, *Kali-B.*, *Lach.*, *Merc.*, *Nat-M.*, *Plat.*, *Phos.*, *Sab.*, *Sep.*, *Thuj.*, *Tril.*, and *Ust.*

Complements : *Nux-V.*, *Puls.* and *Sulph.*
Antidote : *Acon.*, *Bell.* and *Opium.*

Crotalus Horridus.

COMMON NAME : RATTLE-SNAKE POISON.

Is indicated in adynamic conditions that are characterized by a hæmorrhagic tendency (Bl.).

Apoplectic convulsions in inebriates, hæmorrhagic or broken down constitutions (A.).

HÆMORRHAGES FROM EVERY ORIFICE OF THE BODY, EVEN FROM THE PORES OF THE SKIN. (Ra.).

Mouldy smell from the mouth (Nd.).

Is indicated in yellow fever, in the stage of black vomit, when there is low delirium, yellow skin, and oozing of blood from every orifice of the body (D.).

BLOOD EXUDES FROM THE EYES (*Arn., Both., Carb-V., Lach., Nux-V., Phos.*) (N.).

Retinal hæmorrhage (*Arn., Bell., Glon., Ham., Lach., Merc-C., Phos., Prun., Sulph.*) (K.)

Tendency to carbuncles or blood boils (*Anthr.*) (A.).

Stuffed feeling in the ears, worse in the right, associated with a feeling as if hot ear-wax was trickling out (F.).

HÆMORRHAGE FROM THE GUMS, NOSE, STOMACH, LUNGS, URETHRA, WOMB AND BOWELS (Nd.).

BLOODY SWEAT (*Cur., Lach., Lyc., Nux-V., Petr.*) (A.).

Yellow colour of the conjunctiva (*Nux-V., Phos., Sep.*) (A.).

Sudden and great prostration of the vital forces (*Ars., Camph., Carb-V., Phos., Sec.*) (Bt.).

MALIGNANT JAUNDICE (*Ars., Bry., Chel., Chin., Dig., Hep., Iod., Lach., Merc., Nat-S., Phos., Sep.*) (A.).

Fever always assumes the low typhoid form (*Ars.*, *Bapt.*, *Hyos.*, *Kali-P.*, *Lach.*) (Bt.).

Purpura hæmorrhagica : *Blood comes on suddenly from all orifices, skin, nails and gums* (A.).

Dark, besotted face (*Bapt.*, *Gels.*, *Stram.*) (B.).

Most of the symptoms appear on the right side (*left side—Lach.*) (Bt.).

Tongue : *scarlet-red, or brown and swollen* (Hr.).
Very foul breath, with swollen face (Hr.).

Malignant diphtheria or scarlatina ; œdema or gangrene of the fauces or tonsils ; pain worse from empty swallowing ; if vomiting or diarrhœa come on (A.).

Severe frontal headache, with coma and delirium (*Bapt.*, *Nat-M.*, *Stram.*) (Bt.).

Cerebro-spinal-meningitis (*Bell.*, *Gels.*, *Hyos.*, *Lach.*, *Op.*, *Rhus-T.*, *Stram.*, *Verat-V.*) (Bt.).

Fetid diarrhœa (*Ars.*, *Bapt.*, *Chin.*, *Graph.*, *Lach.*, *Merc.*, *Nat-S.*, *Podo.*, *Sulph.*) (Bt.).

Anxious, laboured breathing (*Ant-T.*, *Ars.*, *Lyc.*, *Phos.*, *Verat.*) (Bt.).

Yellow colour of the whole body (C.).

Vertigo and trembling of the whole body (*Agar.*, *Kali-Br.*, *Kali-P.*, *Lach.*, *Nux-V.*, *Phos.*, *Sep.*) (Bt.).

Vomiting : *bilious, with anxiety and weak pulse ; every month after menstruation ; cannot lie on the right side or back without instantly producing dark, green vomiting* (A.).

Sore pain from the pit of the stomach to the region of the liver, with qualmishness, nausea and vomiting of green, bilious matter (Nd.).

Diarrhœa : *stools black, thin, like coffee-grounds ; offensive ; during yellow fever, cholera, typhoid or typhus* (A.).

Bad effects of vaccination, insect-stings or dissecting wounds (*Ars.*) (A.).

Extremities inflamed, swollen and gangrenous (*Ars., Carb-V., Lach., Sec.*) (C.).

Easily tired by slight exertion (*Ars.*) (C.).

INTESTINAL HÆMORRHAGE : BLOOD DARK, FLUID, NON-COAGULABLE (*Carb-V., Lach., Nit-Ac., Phos.*) (A.).

Weeping mood (*Nat-M., Puls.*) (Br.).

Clouded perception and memory (*Bapt., Kali-P., Lyc., Op.*) (Br.).

Vicarious menstruation (*Bry., Ferr., Lach., Phos., Puls.*) (A.).

Malignant diseases of the uterus ; great tendency to hæmorrhage; blood dark, fluid and offensive (*Lach., Sec.*) (A.).

Loquacious, with desire to escape (*Hyos., Stram.*)
(Br.).

Impatient (*Cham., Ign., Nux-V., Sep., Sulph.*) (Br.).

Headache : must walk on tip-toe to avoid
jarring (Br.).

Smothering sensation when awaking (*Grind., Lach.,
Sulph.*) (Br.).

Grinding teeth, during sleep (*Ars., Bell., Cann-I.,
Cina, Tub.*) (K.).

Delirium, especially at night (*Ars., Bapt., Bell.,
Canth., Lach., Plb., Stram.*) (C.).

AGGRAVATION : From lying on right side ;
from falling to sleep ; in warm weather ; during
spring ; from alcohol ; on awaking ; and from jar.

AMELIORATION : From motion.

RELATIONSHIP : *Compare : Ars., Bapt., Canth.,
Carb-V., Elaps, Lach., Naja, Nit-Ac., Phos., Pyrog.,
Sep. and Tarant.*

Antidotes : Alcohol, Am-M., Camph. and *Lach.*

Croton Tiglium.

COMMON NAME : CROTON OIL SEEDS.

Can't inhale deeply enough (B.).

Œdematous swelling of the eyelids (eyelids look
puffed).

Eruptions around the eyes (Br.).

Asthma with cough (*Ant-T., Lyc., Nat-S.*) (Br.).

Pressing headache in the forehead, especially in the orbits (*Sang., Spig.*).

As soon as the head touches the pillow a spasmodic paroxysm of cough sets in (*Caps., Con., Dros.*) (A.).

Feels suffocated from coughing ; must walk about the room or sleep in a chair (for fear of coughing) (A.).

Colic, relieved by hot milk (*Chel., Op.*).

NAUSEA (*Ant-C., Bry., Cina, Ipec., Nux-V., Podo., Tab., Verat.*).

BURNING IN THE ŒSOPHAGUS (*Alumn., Ars., Camph., Carb-Ac., Cycl., Euph., Hep., Kreos., Lyc., Merc-C., Nit-Ac., Phos., Sang.*).

Drawing pain through the chest from breast to scapula, of same side, every time the child nurses (A.).

Nodes in the mammæ (*Carb-An.*) (B.).

Very sore nipple (*Arn., Bapt., Caust., Cham., Fluor-Ac., Lach., Nit-Ac., Phel., Sil.*) (A.).

Copious lachrymation (*Euphr., Merc., Nat-M., Sulph.*) (C.).

Opacity of the cornea (*Arg-N., Calc., Caust., Con., Kali-B., Merc-C., Sil.*) (K.).

Conjunctiva full of dark vessels (*Apis, Bell., Con.. Euphr., Graph., Kali-B., Merc-C., Nat-M., Sep., Sulph.*) (K.).

Photophobia (*Euphr., Graph., Lyc., Merc., Nat-M.. Nux-V., Rhus-T., Sulph.*) (K.).

Pustular conjunctivitis (*Apis, Calc., Clem., Graph., Kali-Chl., Petr., Puls., Sep., Sulph.*) (K.).

The bowels are moved as if by spasmodic jerks— "coming out like a shot" (*Gamb.*) (A.).

PASSAGE OF STOOLS AS SOON AS THE PATIENT EATS, DRINKS, OR EVEN WHILE EAITNG (*Arg-N., Ars., Chin., Ferr., Sanic.*) (A.).

YELLOW, WATERY STOOLS (*Aloe, Dulc., Gamb., Nat-S., Olnd., Pic-Ac., Podo.*) (A.).

STOOLS POURING OUT LIKE WATER FROM A HYDRANT (*Gamb., Olnd., Podo.*) (D.).

Diarrhœa associated with nausea and vomiting (*Ars., Camph., Ipec., Verat.*) (D.).

Watery stools that escape suddenly from the bowels, with great prostration (*Ars., Bism., Camph., Phos.,*) (Bt.).

Intense itching of genitals of both sexes (*Petr., Rhus-T., Sulph.*) ; vesicular eruption on the male genital organs ; so sensitive and sore is unable to scratch (A.).

VESICULAR ERUPTION ON THE SCROTUM AND PENIS, WITH FREQUENT, CORROSIVE ITCHING (*Rhus-T.*) (N.).

Vesicles on the skin, with a yellow, plastic exudation, that burns like a fire (Bt.).

Urticaria of the skin of the abdomen (Bt.).

Vesico-pustular eruptions (*Canth., Rhus-T., Sep., Sulph.*) (B.).

Vesicular erysipelas (*Apis, Canth., Rhus-T.*) (Br.).

Herpes zoster (*Ars., Clem., Graph., Iris, Merc., Mezer., Ran-B., Rhus-T.*) (Br.).

SCARLET-RED SKIN (*Agar., Am-C., Apis, Bell., Graph., Merc., Rhus-T., Stram.*).

INTENSE ITCHING OF THE SKIN, BUT SO TENDER IS UNABLE TO SCRATCH ; RELIEVED BY GENTLE RUBBING (*Rhus-T.*) (A.).

ECZEMA OVER THE WHOLE BODY (*Ars., Graph., Mezer., Petr., Psor., Rhus-T., Sulph.*) (A.).

Coldness of the feet, extending as far up as the calves (C.).

Perspiration on the forehead (*Verat.*).

Stitches in the region of the heart during an expiration.

Palpitation prevents him from going to sleep.

Burning in the urethra when urinating (*Canth., Merc., Nat-M., Sep., Sulph., Tereb., Thuj.*).

CONSTANT URGING TO STOOL FOLLOWED BY SUDDEN EVACUATION, WHICH IS SHOT OUT OF THE RECTUM (*Gamb., Grat., Podo., Thuj.*) (A.).

Colic and diarrhœa immediately after nursing (G.).

Cholera infantum: excessive nausea and frequent discharges of greenish or yellowish stools (Sm.).

Colicky pain in the transverse colon before every stool.

SWASHING SENSATION IN THE INTESTINES AS FROM WATER, BEFORE STOOL (*Aloe, Kali-C., Merc., Nat-M., Phos-Ac.*) (A.).

Stools with burning at the anus (*Aloe, Ars., Sulph.*).

AGGRAVATION : From every motion ; after drinking ; while eating or nursing ; during summer ; from fruit and sweetmeats ; the least food or drink ; from scratching ; and from lying down.

AMELIORATION : From gentle rubbing ; and after sleep.

RELATIONSHIP : Compare : *Aloe, Arg-N., Ars., Chin., Ferr., Kali-Br., Phos.,* and *Sulph.* in chronic infantile diarrhœa ; and *Sil.,* in pain from the nipple through to the back when nursing.

Antidote : Ant-T.

Croton Tig. antidotes : *Rhus* poisoning.

Cuprum Arsenicosum.

COMMON NAME : ARSENITE OF COPPER.

Icy coldness of the whole body, with cramps (R.).

Haggard face (*Carb-V., Sec., Verat.*) (R.).

Vomiting and diarrhœa (*Acon., Ars., Cupr., Kali-P., Nux-V., Verat.*) (B.).

Terrible enteralgia or abdominal neuralgia, with great restlessness (*Acon., Ars., Bell., Coloc., Cupr., Dios., Mag-P., Plb., Staph., Verat.*) (D.).

Sharp, shooting abdominal pains (B.).

Violent cramps and colics (*Cupr., Mag-P., Sec., Verat.*) (B.).

Rice-water stool (*Ars., Camph., Cupr., Kali-P., Phos-Ac., Phos., Sec., Verat.*) (B.).

Periodical colic (*Ars., Cham., Chin., Cupr., Ipec., Nux-V., Sulph.*) (K.).

Cold, clammy, intermittent sweat (*Calc., Camph., Carb-V., Phos., Verat.*) (B.).

Obstinate hiccough (*Ars., Cic., Cupr., Cycl., Hyos., Ign., Mag-P., Nicc., Nux-V., Sec., Stram., Verat.*) (B.).

Intense thirst (*Acon., Ars., Bry., Phos., Sec., Sulph., Verat.*) (R.).

Burning along œsophagus from stomach to mouth (*Iris*) (R.).

Vomiting and purging, with cramps and collapse (*Cupr.*, *Phos.*, *Sec.*, *Verat.*) (R.).

Bronchial asthma and emphysema (*Carb-V.*, *Lyc.*, *Sulph.*) (Br.).

URÆMIC CONVULSIONS (*Canth.*, *Crot-H.*, *Cupr.*, *Hydr-Ac.*, *Kali-S.*, *Mosch.*, *Plb.*, *Tereb.*) (K.).

Nephritis of pregnancy (*Apis*, *Canth.*, *Merc-C.*, *Phos.*, *Sep.*) (Br.).

Renal inefficiency and uræmia (*Apis*, *Ars.*, *Bell.*, *Camph.*, *Canth.*, *Kali-P.*, *Lach.*, *Lyc.*, *Op.*, *Phos.*, *Plb.*, *Sec.*, *Verat.*) (Br.).

AGGRAVATION : After eating and drinking at a fixed time ; and during diarrhœa.

AMELIORATION : From hard pressure.

RELATIONSHIP : *Compare* : *Acon.*, *Ars.*, *Bell.*, *Camph.*, *Cupr.*, *Dios.*, *Kali-P.*, *Lach.*, *Lyc.*, *Merc-C.*, *Nux-V.*, *Op.*, *Phos.*, *Plb.*, *Sec.*, *Sulph.*, *Verat.*

Cuprum Metallicum.

COMMON NAME : COPPER.

Contact renews and aggravates the ailment (*Nux-V.*)

Giddiness accompanying almost all ailments, the head falling forward and on the chest.

Metastasis to the brain from the other organs (N.).

Coldness and blueness of the surface of the body (*Lach.*) (D.).

Mania in attacks followed by perspiration (*Bell.,* *Canth., Hyos., Stram., Verat.*).

Delirium, with biting in the bed-clothes, their own hands, or the hands of others (*Bell.*) (N.).

After-pains : severe, distressing, in calves and soles (A.).

Imperfect, stammering speech (A.).

Constant prostration and retraction of the tongue like a snake (*Lach.*) (A.).

CONVULSIONS WITH BLUE FACE AND CLENCHED THUMBS (A.).

Spasm of the glottis (*Brom.,* *Chlor., Lach., Phos.,* *Samb.*) (Br.).

Intussusception (*Alum., Op., Plb., Verat.*) (Br.).

Hiccough preceding the spasms (Br.).

There is frothing at the mouth during convulsion (*Art-V., Bufo, Cina, Hyos.*) (D.).

The eyeballs are distorted (D.).

There is blueness of the face and lips (*Carb-V.,* *Lach., Verat.*) (D.).

Delirium in attacks, with incessant, disconnected talking (R.).

Bellowing (*Bell.*, *Canth.*) (K.).

Convulsions following cholera (*Canth.*) (D.).

VIOLENT CONVULSIONS, WITH PIERCING CRIES (*Apis*, *Bell.*, *Glon.*, *Hyos.*, *Plb.*, *Stram.*, *Verat-V.*).

Twitching at night (*Ars.*, *Bell.*, *Kali-C.*, *Strych.*, *Sulph.*).

Spasms or convulsions beginning in fingers and toes and spreading from thence (N.).

Affections arising from repercussed eruptions, brain affections, convulsions, etc. (N.).

Convulsions during pregnancy (*Apis*, *Cedr.*, *Cham.*, *Cic.*, *Hyos.*, *Lyc.*) (G.).

Puerperal convulsions (*Bell.*, *Cic.*, *Hyos.*, *Stram.*) (G.).

Spasmodic movements of the abdominal muscles (cramps) (N.).

What he drinks descends with a gurgling noise (*Ars.*, *Cina*, *Hydr-Ac.*, *Laur.*).

SEVERE SPASMODIC PAIN IN THE ABDOMEN WITH CONVULSIONS (*Plb.*).

ICY COLDNESS OF THE WHOLE BODY (*Camph.*, *Carb-V.*, *Kali-P.*, *Laur.*, *Phos.*, *Sec.*, *Verat.*).

Vomiting, 'which is flaky, with colic and spasms (Acon., Æth., Ipec., Verat.).

Flaky diarrhœa (Acon., Colch., Ipec., Merc-C., Sulph.).

CHOLERA (Acon., Ant-T., Ars., Carb-V., Kali-P., Phos., Ricin., •Verat.).

The pulse is slow and scarcely perceptible (Acon., Ars., Camph., Carb-V , Hydr-Ac., Laur., Op., Sec., Verat.).

Painful, spasmodic contractions of the chest (Ant-T., Arg-N., Hydr-Ac., Laur., Naja, Phos., Sec., Verat.).

Metallic taste in the mouth (Cocc., Merc., Nat-C., Rhus-T., Seneg.) (B.).

CkAMPS OF THE MUSCLES, THOSE OF THE CALVES AND THIGHS ARE DRAWN UP INTO KNOTS (D.).

There is distress in the pit of the stomach and great dyspnœa (D.).

Knife-like, violent pains in the abdomen, which are better from pressure, but are not better from heat (D.).

Cough relieved by a drink of cold water (Am-Caust., Caust., Coc-C., Iod., Kali-C., Op., Sulph., Verat.) (D.).

Cold water also relieves vomiting (Phos., Puls.) (D.).

Whooping cough : the attacks come on in quick succession, accompanied perhaps by spasms, threatening suffocation (*Ipec.*) (D.).

Symptoms disposed to appear periodically and in groups (A.).

Epilepsy : aura begins in the knees and ascends ; worse at night during sleep (*Bufo*) ; about new moon ; at regular intervals (menses) ; from a fall or blow upon the head ; from getting wet (A.).

Mental or bodily exhaustion from over-exertion of mind, or loss of sleep (*Nux-V.*) (N.).

Head drawn backward (*Cic., Hyos., Stram.*) (R.).

Uræmic convulsions attended with loquacious delirium and followed by apathy, cold tongue, cold breath and collapse (*Sec.*) (Bl.).

Bores the head into the pillow (*Apis, Bell., Hell., Stram., Tarant., Tub.*) (B.).

Grinds teeth (*Apis, Ars., Bell., Cina*) (B.).

Scantiness or entire suppression of urine (*Apis, Camph., Op., Sec., Verat.*) (C.).

Dyspnœa : cannot bear anything near mouth (B.).

Cataleptic when coughing (Bt.).

AGGRAVATION : At night ; from contact ; from repercussed eruptions ; during pregnancy ; about new moon; from loss of sleep; in cold air; from cold wind; from suppressed foot-sweat; and before menses.

AMELIORATION: From pressure; by a cold drink; and during perspiration.

RELATIONSHIP; *Complementary*: *Calc-C.*, *Compare*: *Ars.*, *Bell.*, *Camph.*, *Canth.*, *Carb-V.*, *Dig.*, *Ipec.*, *Kali-P.*, *Lach.*, *Laur.*, *Naja*, *Op.*, *Phos.*, *Sec.*, *Stram.*, *Tereb.*, and *Verat.*

Verat. follows it well in whooping cough ,and cholera; and *Apis* and *Zinc.* in convulsions, from suppressed exanthema.

Cyclamen.

COMMON NAME: SOW BREAD.

It has many things in common with *Pulsatilla* (Bl.).

Best suited for leuco-phlegmatic 'persons with anæmic or chlorotic conditions (A.).

Easily fatigued, and in consequence not inclined to any kind of labour (A.).

Pale, chlorotic, with deranged menses, and accompanied by vertigo, headache and dim vision (A.).

Satiety after a few mouthful (Lyc.); food then becomes repugnant, causes nausea in throat and palate (A.).

THIRSTLESSNESS (*Ant-T., Apis, Chin., Colch., Gels., Hell., Ipec., Meny., Nux-M., Phos-Ac., Puls., Sabad.*).

BAD EFFECTS FROM EATING MUCH FAT FOOD (PORK) (*Puls.*).

Saliva and all food has a salty taste (A.).

Desire for lemonade (*Bell., Calc., Eup-Per*) (K.).

Hiccough during pregnancy (*Op.*) (B.).

Aversion to bread and butter (*Mag-C.*) (C.).

Chilly all over (*Nux-V., Puls.*) (B.).

CATAMENIA TOO PROFUSE (*Bov., Calc., Chin., Cocc., Erig., Ferr., Helon., Ipec., Mill., Murx., Nat-M, Phos., Sabin.*).

MENSES : TOO EARLY ; TOO PROFUSE ; BLACK AND CLOTTED ; MEMBRANOUS ; FEELS BETTER DURING THE FLOW (*Lach., Zinc.*) (A.).

Post-partum hæmorrhages, with colicky, bearing-down pains, which are relieved after a gush of blood (Bl.).

Milk in virgin breasts (*Asaf., Merc., Puls., Tub., Urt-U.*) (B.).

Sensation of something alive in the abdomen (*Croc., Hyos., Sep., Thuj.*) (K.).

Inclined to weep (Gels., Ign., Puls.) (A.).

Irritable, morose, ill-humoured (A.).

Great sadness and peevishness (*Nat-M.*) (A.).

Ailments : from suppressed grief and terrors of conscience from duty not done, or bad act committed (A.).

Desire for solitude (*Anac., Gels., Ign., Nat-M., Nux-V.*) (A.).

Pressing, drawing and tearing pain, principally in the periosteum.

Chilblains of the feet (*Agar., Anac., Carb-An., Lyc., Merc., Petr., Puls., Zinc.*).

As long as he walks about, he feels well with the exception of languor, but as soon as he sits down, especially in the evening, he suffers various inconveniences.

Burning, sore pain in the heels, when sitting, standing or walking in open air (*Agar., Caust., Phyt., Valer.*) (A).

Aversion to open air (reverse of *Puls.*) (A.).

Acne in young women (*Calc-P.*) (Br.).

Palpitation in the evening (*Puls.*) (C.).

Headache in anæmic patients (*Calc-P., Ferr., Nat-M.*) with flickering before eyes or dim vision, on rising in the morning (A.).

Flickering before eyes (*Bell., Carb-S., Graph., Lach., Nat-M., Phos., Sep., Sulph.*) (A.).

Sees fiery sparks, as of various colours, and glittering needles (A.).

22

Dim vision of fog or smoke (*Ars.*, *Calc.*, *Chin.*, *Croc.*, *Gels.*, *Phos.*, *Puls.*, *Sulph.*, *Zinc*) (A.).

Sees countless stars (*Aur.*, *Calc.*, *Con.*, *Hyos.*, *Kali-C.*, *Puls.*) (Br.).

The catarrhal discharges are thick and bland (*Kali-M.*, *Puls.*, *Stann.*) (Bl.).

Nasal catarrh, with loss of taste and smell (*Puls.*) (F.).

Periodical, semilateral headache, with dizziness (Bt.).

Frequent sneezing (*Am-M.*, *Ars.*, *Carb-.*, *Coc-C.*, *Merc.*, *Nux-V.*, *Sulph.*) (K.).

Spasmodic sneezing (*Ars.*, *Gels.*, *Kali-I.*, *Rhus-T.*, *Sabad.*).

AGGRAVATION : In the evening ; while at rest ; in open air ; from cold water ; from cold bathing ; before menses ; from fat food ; when sitting ; and when standing.

AMELIORATION : Whilst walking ; during menses ; in a warm room ; from moving about.

RELATIONSHIP : *Antidote* : *Camph.*, *Coff.*, and *Puls.*

Compare : *Ambr.*, *Chin.*, *Ferr.*, *Kali-P.*, *Lach.*, *Merc.*, *Nux-V.*, *Puls.*, *Rhus-T.*, *Sep.*, *Sil.* and *Sulph.*

Compare, especially *Chin.*, *Ferr.* and *Puls.* in chlorosis, and anæmic affections.

Cinnabaris.

(Continued from P, 280)

Profuse perspiration between the thighs (Aur., Hep., Nux-V.), which is offensive and corrosive.

Chest oppressed, feels contracted ; relieved by stretching himself.

Salivation (Chin., Kali-I., Merc., Nit-Ac., Puls., Rhus-T.)

Intense headache ; he cannot raise his head from the pillow ; relieved by external pressure.

AGGRAVATION ; In the evening ; at night (except of the perspiration, which is worse at midday) ; after sleeping ; from lying on the right side ; from touch ; from light ; and from dampness.

AMELIORATION : In the open air ; after dinner ; and in sunshine.

RELATIONSHIP : *Compare* : *Carb-An.*, *Hep.*, *Kali-B.*, *Kali-M.*, *Merc.*, *Merc-C.*, *Nit-Ac.*, *Sep.*, and *Thuj.*

Antidotes : *Hep.*, and *Sulph.*

Complementary : *Thuj.*

Cinnamonum.

COMMON NAME: CINNAMON.

Menses : early, profuse, prolonged and bright red (*Calc.*, *Ipec.*, *Phos.*) (Br.).

Bearing down sensation (*Bell., Nux-V., Sep.,*)(Br.).

Sexual desire is increased (*Nux-V., Phos., Sulph.*).

PROFUSE HÆMORRHAGE FROM A STRAIN OR MIS-STEP (F.).

METRORRHAGIA AFTER DELIVERY ; THE BLOOD IS THIN AND PALE (*Carb-V., Chin., Ferr., Sabin., Sec., Ust.*).

The flow is profuse, the extremities are cold and the surface of the body is pallid (*Carb-V., Chin., Sec.*) (Bl.).

POST-PARTUM HÆMORRHAGE (*Arn., Caul., Chin., Erig., Ferr., Ham., Ipec., Sec.*) ; IT INCREASES LABOUR-PAINS AND CONTROLS PROFUSE OR DANGEROUS FLOODING (A.).

Post-partum hæmorrhages, or those hæmorrhages caused by over-lifting ; flow sudden, profuse and of a bright red colour (N.).

Nose-bleed (*Acon., Bell., Carb-V., Ferr-P., Lach., Merc.. Nit-Ac.. Phos., Sep.*) (Br.).

Hæmoptysis (*Acaly., Bry., Ferr., Lach., Phos., Sec., Sulph.*) (Br.).

Feeb'e patients, with languid circulation (*Carb-V., Chin., Ferr., Nat-M.*) (Br.).

AGGRAVATION : After labour ; from a strain or mis-step ; and from overlifting.

AMELIORATION : From rest.

RELATIONSHIP : *Compare* : *Acon.*, *Bell.*, *Carb-V.*, *Chin.*, *Ferr.*, *Ham.*, *Ipec.*, *Lach.*, *Merc.*, *Nit-Ac.*, *Phos.*, *Sabin.*, *Sec.*, *Sep.*, *Sulph.*, *Trill.*, *Ust.*

Antidote : *Acon.*

Digitalis Purpurea.

COMMON NAME: FOX-GLOVE.

Pulse : *Full, irregular* ; *very slow and weak* ; *intermiting every third, fifth or seventh beat* (A.).

Stinging pain in the muscles of the upper and lower extremities (*Apis*, *Bry.*, *Dulc.*, *Guai.*, *Kali-C.*, *Kali-S.*, *Rhus-T.*, *Valer.*).

The fingers "go to sleep" frequently and easily (A.).

Constant desire to breathe deeply, but it seemed as if the chest could be only half-filled because of some impediment in the chest (R.).

Great weakness of the chest ; *cannot bear to talk* (*Stann.*) (A.).

Faintish debility with perspiration (*Ars.*,*Chin.*, *Cocc.*, *Kali-P.*, *Verat.*).

Attacks of excessive debility, especially after break-fast and dinner (*Carb-V.*, *Phos-Ac.*, *Sil.*).

FEELING OF WEAKNESS, EMPTINESS OR GONENESS IN THE ABDOMEN (*Carb-An.*, *Cocc,.* *Kali-P.*, *Olnd.*, *Petr.*, *Phos.*, *Podo.*, *Puls.*, *Sep.*, *Stann.*, *Sulph.*, *Tab.*).

Nausea and vomiting (Ars., Ipec., Nux-V., Tab., Verat.).

A clean tongue with gastric and other derangements. (N.).

Is often beneficial in nocturnal emissions when there is great weakness and mental despondency (Bl.).

Excessive desire to be alone (*Ign., Nat-M., Phos-Ac.*) (Bt.).

Gloomy and apprehensive (*Ars., Kali-P., Nat-M.*) (D.).

Great weakness of the genitals after coitus (*Calad., Ccn., Gels., Lyc., Nux-V., Phos., Sulph.*) (A.).

Violent erections even chordee (*Canth., Pic-Ac., Sulph.*).

Dropsy of external and internal parts (Apis, Apoc., Ars., Blatta., Chin., Ferr., Lyc., Nux-V., Phos., Sulph.).

THE URINARY DISCHARGE IS TOO SCANTY Apis, Berb., Lach., Lyc., Merc-C., Phos., Tereb.),

Cyanosis (Carb-V., Lach., Verat.).

Blue tongue (Ant-T., Ars., Carb-V., Cupr-S., Iris, Mur-Ac., Op., Tab.).

SLOW PULSE (AN EXCELLENT INDICATION).

Frequent desire to urinate with small discharges (Apis, Canth., Gels., Kali-C., Lyc., Merc., Nux-V., Thuj.).

Urinary secretion increased (Apis, Kali-C., Lyc., Merc., Phos-Ac., Sulph.).

Cough after eating with vomiting of food (*Ant-T.,
Bry., Coc-C., Dros., Ferr., Ipec., Kali-C., Laur., Nat-M.,
Puls., Sep.* (**N.**)

Enlarged prostate (*Con., Gels., Lyc., Puls., Sep.*) (Br.).
Thick, yellow discharge from the urethra (*Alum.,
Arg-M., Cann-S., Caps., Cub., Hep., Hydr., Med., Merc.,
Psor., Puls., Sil., Sulph.*) (D.).

VIOLENT AND AUDIBLE PALPITATION OF THE HEART (*Aesc., Agar., Am-C., Apis, Ars., Bell., Calc., Colch., Iod., Nat-M., Sep., Spig , Thuj.*).

Heart slow, weak or irregular (*Gels., Kalm., Op.,
Sep., Stram.*) (B.).

Blue lips (*Ars., Asaf., Bapt., Bell., Bry., Camph.,
Cann-I., Carb-V., Cupr., Hyos., Ipec., Lach., Morph., Op.,
Verat., Verat-V.*).

When going to sleep the breath fades away and
seems to be gone, and the heart slows or stops ; then
awakens with a gasp to catch it. (N.).

Enlarged, sore and painful liver (*Chel., Chin., Hyos.,
Merc., Nat-S., Sep.*) (Br.).

Breathing irregular, difficult, deep or sighing (Br.).

Cardiac dropsy (*Apis, Ars., Cact., Lach., Lyc.,
Nat-M., Spig.*) (Br.).

SENSATION AS IF THE HEART WOULD STOP BEATING IF SHE MOVED (Ha.).

*The least movement produces violent palpitation of the
heart* (*Carb-V., Con , Phos., Spig.*) (Bt.).

The stools are gray, ash-coloured or white (*Ars. Calc.*, *Chel.*, *Hydr.*, *Kali-C.*, *Merc.*, *Nat-M.*, *Op.*, *Phos-Ac.*, *Phos.*, *Sep.*).

Dropsical swelling of the genitals (*Apis*, *Ars.*, *Sulph.*) (Br.).

Œdematous infiltration of the penis and scrotum (C.).

Pneumonia of old people, with prune-juice like expectoration, symptoms of collapse and heart-failure (C.).

Objects appear of various colours, as blue or green (F.).

AGGRAVATION : When sitting, especially when sitting erect ; from motion ; after meals ; from music ; from exertion ; from lying on the left side ; and from sexual excesses.

AMELIORATION : From lying on back ; in the open air ; when the stomach is empty ; and from rest.

RELATIONSHIP : *Antidotes* ; *Camph.* and *Chin.*

Digitalis antidotes ; *Wine.*

Compare : *Ant-C.*, *Apis*, *Apoc.*, *Ars.*, *Bell.*, *Bry.*, *Calc.*, *Con.*, *Ferr-P.*, *Hell.*, *Ipec.*, *Kali-P.*, *Lach.*, *Lob.*, *Lyc.*, *Merc.*, *Nux-V.*, *Op.*, *Phos.*, *Puls.*, *Rhus-T.*, *Sep.*, *Spig.*, *Sulph.*, *Tab.*, *Verat.*, and *Zinc.*

Dioscorea Villosa.

COMMON NAME : WILD FARN.

Calls things by wrong names (C.). Irritability and restlessness (*Ars.*, *Phos.*).

Persons of feeble digestive powers, old or young (*Ant-C., Carb-V., Lyc., Nux-V , Puls., Sep.*) (A.).

Belching of large quantities of offensive gas (*Asaf., Carb-V., Lyc., Nat-S.*) (Br.).

Burning in the stomach (*Ars., Carb-V., Iris, Lach., Lyc., Nat-P., Phos., Sulph,*) (G.).

Mouth very dry, bitter and clammy in the morning (N.).

Pains shoot from liver to right nipple (*Chel*) (B.).

Griping pains in the abdomen about the umbilicus (*Coloc., Nux-V.*) (A.).

Hurried desire for stool (*Aloe, Sulph.*) (B.).

Flatulence after meals or after eating, especially of tea-drinkers (*Chin., Lach., Puls., Thuj.*) (A.).

Distressing pyrosis (*Nux-V., Puls.*) (Hlm.).

VIOLENT TWISTING COLIC OCCURRING IN REGULAR PAROXYSMS, AS IF THE INTESTINES WERE GRASPED AND TWISTED BY A POWERFUL HAND (A.).

Dull, hard, grinding pain in liver or in region of gall-bladder (N.).

COLICKY PAINS WORSE FROM BENDING FORWARD AND WHILE LYING ; BETTER ON STANDING ERECT OR BENDING BACKWARDS (reverse of *Coloc.*) (A.).

Colic with rumbling and passing of much flatus (*Carb-V., Lyc.*) (N.).

Colic pain begins at umbilicus and radiates to all parts of the body even extremities (N.).

Seminal emissions during sleep ; vivid dreams of women all night (*Staph.*) ; knees weak ; genitals cold ; great despondency (*Phos., Staph.*) (A.).

Stong-smelling sweat on the scrotum and pubes (Br.) Hæmorrhoidal tumours like red cherries, with pain. and distress in the anus (C.).

Diarrhoea early in the morning, driving out of bed (*Aloe, Sulph.*) (C.).

Very profuse, thin, yellow stool in the morning (*Aloe*) (C.).

Sciatica ; right side ; only felt when moving the limb or when sitting ; better when lying perfectly quiet (C.).

Violent dysmemorrhoea (*Bell., Coloc., Mag-P., Nux-V., Puls., Sen.,* (B.).

Dysentery with violent lancinating pains in the bowels (Rg.).

Spasmodic stricture of the urethra (*Apis, Berb., Canth., Clem., Gels., Hep., Kali-B., Lyc., Merc., Nat-M., Petr., Sep., Sil., Thuj.*) (Bt.).

Renal colic (*Berb., Lyc., Nux-V., Ocimum, Puls.*). Pain particularly in the right ureter (*Lyc.*).

Pain from the ureter extending to the penis and testes (*Nux-V.*).

Constant desire to pass urine.

Disposition to paronychia (*Hep., Sil.*) (A.).

Felons : *early when pains are sharp and agonizing* ; *when pricking is first felt* (A.).

Nails brittle (*Ant-C., Graph., Thuj.*) (A.).

AGGRAVATION : From lying down ; from sitting : from bending double ; in the evening ; at night ; from seminal emissions.

AMELIORATION : From motion ; from bending backwards ; from standing erect ; from pressure ; from walking ; and from riding.

RELATIONSHIP : *Compare* : *Bell., Bry., Cham., Coloc., Gels., Kali-C., Lyc., Mag-C., Nux-V., Phos., Podo., Rhus-T., Sil., Staph., Thuj.*

Antidotes : *Camph., Cham.*

Diphtherinum.

COMMON NAME : DIPHTHERITIC VIRUS (OR THE TOXIN PRODUCED BY THE KLEBS— LOEFFLER BACILLUS).

The attack from the onset tends to malignancy (*Lac-C., Merc-Cy.*) (A.).

Weak and restless, but without pain (B.).

Yellow, thick, nasal discharge (B.).

Talks in sleep with open eyes (B.).

Jerking of single parts (B.).

Dark-red swelling of the tonsils and palatine arches ; *parotid and cervical glands greatly swollen* ; *breath and discharges from the throat, nose and mouth very offensive* ; *tongue swollen, very red, little coating.* (A.).

Breath horribly offensive (*Ars., Carb-V., Merc.,*
Mur-Ac., Nit-Ac., Phos., Sulph.) (A.).

Diphtheritic membrane, thick, dark gray or brownish black ; temperature low or sub-normal ; pulse weak
and rapid ; extremities cold and marked debility ;
patient lies in a semi-stupid condition ; eyes dull,
besotted (*Apis, Bapt.*) (A.).

Swallows without pain but, fluids are vomited or
returned by the nose (*Gels., Kali-P., Lach.*) (A.).

Epistaxis or profound prostration from very onset
of attack (*All-C., Apis, Carb-Ac.*) (A.).

Laryngeal diphtheria (*Chlor., Kali-B., Lac-C.*).

Sopor or stupor, but easily aroused when spoken
to (*Bapt., Sulph.*) (A.).

Post-diphtheritic paralysis (*Gels., Lach., Mur-Ac.*)(B.).
Fluids are returned by the nose.

When the patient from the first seems doomed, and the
most carefully selected remedies fail to relieve or perma-
nently improve.

RELATIONSHIP : Similar to *Ars., Bapt., Brom.,*
Carb-Ac., Caust., Chlor., Gels., Lach., Mur-Ae., Phos.,
Sulph.

Drosera.

COMMON NAME : SUNDEW.

Painful sneezing (*Ars., Carb-An., Cina, Kali-P.*)(B).

WHOOPING COUGH, WITH BLEEDING

FROM THE NOSE AND MOUTH WITH A NIGHTLY AGGRAVATION.

Barking-cough coming so frequently that the patient cannot get his breath (D.).

Constant, titillating cough in children, begins as soon as the head touches the pillow at night (*Bell.*, *Hyos.*, *Puls.*, *Rumx.*) (A.).

Severe bronchitis (*Ant-T* , *Bry.*, *Kali-M.*. *Phos.*, *Sulph.*)

Spasmodic cough, coming on in the evening; efforts to raise the phlegm end in retching and vomiting (D.).

Constriction and crawling in the larynx ; hoarseness and yellow or green sputa (*Phos.*) (A.).

Constriction of chest (*Ars.*, *Cact.*) (B.).

Phthisis (*Calc.*, *Merc.*, *Nit-Ac.*, *Phos.*, *Puls.*, *Sep.*, *Sil.*, *Sulph.*, *Tub.*) (D.).

Sensation of feather in the larynx, exciting cough (A.).

Laryngeal phthisis following whooping cough (following bronchial catarrh—*Coc-C.*) (A.).

Deep-sounding, hoarse, barking cough, worse after midnight, during or after measles (A).

DURING COUGH VOMITING OF WATER, MUCUS, AND OFTEN BLEEDING AT THE NOSE AND MOUTH (*Cupr.*) (A.).

Twitching attacks in the limbs, and after the attack becomes drowsy and sleepy.

Gnawing, stinging pain in the joints.

The limbs on which he lies fee. sore, as if the bed was too hard (*Arn.*, *Bapt.*, *Pyrog.*).

Gnawing, stinging pain through all the long bones, worse during rest.

Clergyman's sore-throat ; with rough, scraping, dry sensation deep in the fauces ; voice hoarse, deept, one-less, cracked, requires exertion to speak (*Arum-T.*, *Caust.*) (A.).

Intermittent fever with angina and nausea.

Constant chilliness, cannot get warm (*Aran.*) (A.).

Profuse discharge of watery saliva during the febrile tages (Hn.).

Aversion to and bad effects from acids.
Food has no taste ; bread tastes bitter (A.).
Putrid taste (*Puls.*) (B.).

PROLONGED PERIODICAL FITS OF RAPID, INCESSANT, DEEP BARKING OR CHOKING COUGH (B).

Rigors or shuddering spells (G.).

Constrictive pain in the both hypochondria, which impedes coughing ; must support with the hands when coughing (C.).

Cough, with purulent or bloody expectoration (*Chin.*, *Ferr-P.*, *Lyc.*, *Merc.*, *Phos.*, *Plb.*, *Sep.*, *Sil.*) (C.).

Anxious, depressed mood, with gloomy fore-bodings (C.).

Frequent desire to urinate, with scanty urine—frequently only a few drops.

Pressing headache (temples) with stupefaction and nausea (morning) ; worse when stooping and from heat, better from motion and in the cold air.

AGGRAVATION : Towards morning ; from heat ; during rest ; from warmth ; from drinking ; from singing ; from laughing ; from weeping ; from lying down and after midnight.

AMELIORATION : From motion ; in the cold air ; from sitting up in bed ; and from remaining quiet.

RELATIONSHIP : *Complementary to* : *Nux-V.* and *Sulph.*

Follows well : *after Samb., Sulph., and Veral.*

Is followed by ; *Calc., Puls., and Sulph.*

Compare : *Ant-T., Bell., Cina, Coc-C., Coral., Cup., Hep., Ipec , Kali-C., Meph., Naph., Puls., Rumx., Sil., and Sulph.*

Antidote : *Camph,*

Dulcamara,

COMMON NAME : BITTER SWEET.

TEERING IN THE LIMBS AND OTHER DIS-ORDERS FROM CATCHING COLD.

PARALYSIS OF SINGLE PARTS (*Caust., Phos., Zinc.*)

PARALYSIS FROM LYING ON THE DAMP GROUND (D.).

Dropsical swellings (*Apis, Dig., Rush-T., Sulph.*).

Anasarca ; after ague, rheumatism or scarlet fever (A).

Dropsy : *after suppressed sweat, suppressed eruptions or exposure to cold.* (A.).

Swelling and induration of the glands (*Bad., Carb-An., Con., Merc-I-F., Sil.*).

One-sided spasms with speechlessness (*Zinc.*).

Great emaciation (*Abrot., Calc-P., Nat-M., Sars.*)

A rooting-up and digging painfulness.

Excessive secretions of the mucous membranes (*Hydr., Puls., Rhus-T.*).

TINEA CAPITIS (*Caust., Graph., Kali-S., Psor.*).

CRUSTA LACTEA (*Ars., Calc., Clem., Graph.*).

TETTERY ERUPTIONS (*Merc., Mez., Nat-M.*).

Twitching of the eyes in the cold air.

Urticaria over the whole body, no fever; itching burns after scratching; worse in warmth, better in cold (A.).

Herpes on the male genitals (C.).

Dryness of the skin and itching blotches (*Apis, Bry., Clem., Graph., Lyc., Sulph.*).

EXANTHEMA LIKE NETTLE-RASH (*Apis, Ars., Bov., Calc., Puls., Rhus-T., Sulph.*).

ERUPTIONS BEFORE AND DURING THE CAT AMENIA (*Aur-M.*).

Thick brown-yellow crusts on the scalp, face, forehead, temples, chin; with reddish borders, bleeding when scratched (A.).

SUPPRESSED MENSES.

Colic as if diarrhœa would occur, from taking cold (N.).

Diarrhœa from repelled eruptions (D.).

Mucous diarrhœa in summer, during the cool days (*Acon., Rhus-T., Sulph.*).

Mucous, green or changeable stools of sour odour (D.).

Yellow watery diarrhœa in damp weather (*Nat-S.*) (D.)

CUTTING AT THE NAVEL THEN PAINFUL, GREEN, SLIMY STOOLS (B.).

Perspiration of the palms of the hands (*Calc., Carb-V., Cham., Con., Fl-Ac., Hep., Ign., Iod., Kali-C., Nux-V., Sep., Sil., Sulph.*).

Paralysis of the bladder or any part of the body brought on or made worse by damp weather (*Rhus-T.*)(D.)

Catarrhal ischuria in grown-up children, with milky urine; from wading with bare feet in cold weather; involuntary urination (A.).

Frequent urination (*Phos-Ac., Sep.*) (B.).

For the bad effects or abuse of Mercury (A.).

FROM TAKING COLD, THE NECK STIFF; THE BACK PAINFUL; THE BONES ACHE (Hr.).

Cough with expectoration of bright blood (*Acon., Bell., Ferr-P.*).

Oppression of the chest from mucus (*Ant-T., Phos., Sulph.*).

They have to cough a long time to expel phlegm, especially in infants and old people, from threatened paralysis in the vagi (Hg.).

After the disappearance of tetters in the face, face-ache and violent asthma (Hr.).

Tenacious, soapy saliva (*Berb., Merc., Phos.*) (B.).

DIFFICULT SPEECH (*Bell., Crot-C., Gels., Lach., Nat-M., Op., Stann., Stram.*) (K.).

Offensive sweat, night and morning, over the whole body (A.).

AGGRAVATION: From cold air; from wet weather; whilst reposing; whilst sitting; at night; during rest; from suppressed menstruation: from suppressed eruptions; from suppressed sweat.

AMELIORATION: From motion; when moving the affected part; when walking; from warmth; and in dry weather.

RELATIONSHIP: *Complementary to*: *Bar-C., Kali-S.* and *Nat-S.*

Incompatible with: *Acet-Ac., Bell.* and *Lach.* (should not be used before or after).

Follows well after: *Calc., Bry., Lyc., Rhus-T.* and *Sep.*

Antidote: *Camph.*

23

Echinacea Angustifolia.

COMMON NAME: PURPLE CONE FLOWER.

Is indicated in cases of blood-poisoning and septic conditions (Bl.).

WEAK, TIRED AND ACHY (*Arn., Bapt., Gels., Nux-V., Rhus-T.*) (B.).

Sharp pain deep in the brain (*Apis, Bell., Glon., Nux-V.*) (B.).

CAN'T EXERT MIND (*Kali-P., Phos-Ac., Sil.*) (B.).

Depressed, or cross and out of sorts (*Bry., Cham., Nux-V., Sulph.*) (B.).

Slow: speech, gait, replies, etc. (B.).

Flashes of heat and chilliness over the back (Bl.).

Is profoundly prostrated (*Ars., Kali-P., Lach., Mur-Ac., Phos., Zinc.*) (Bl.).

The urine is scanty and contains albumen (*Apis, Kali-C., Rhus-T.*) (Bl.).

Aphthæ (*Bor., Kali-M., Merc., Nat-M., Nux-V., Sil., Sulph.*) (B.).

The brain seems too large (*Arg-N., Arn., Bell., Glon., Nux-M., Nux-V., Ran-B., Spig.*) (B.).

SEVERE HEADACHE (*Bell., Bry.*) (Bl.).

Blood follows stool (*Am-C., Carb-V., Lach., Phos., Sulph.*) (B.).

Bed sores (*Arn., Ars., Bapt., Lach., Mur-Ac., Sil.*) (Bl.).

Increasing, but variable pulse (B.).

Gums recede and bleed easily (*Merc., Nit-Ac., Phos.*) (C.).

Sordes (*Ars., Bapt., Carb-Ac., Chin., Hyos., Kali-P., Merc., Mur-Ac., Phos-Ac., Phos., Pyrog., Rhus-T., Sulph-Ac.*) (C.).

Puerperal septicæmia; discharges suppressed; abdomen sensitive and tympanitic (*Bry., Chin., Kali-P., Lach., Lyc., Puls., Rhus-T., Sec.*) (C.).

White coating of tongue with red edges (*Ars., Bry., Merc., Nux-V., Phos., Rhus-T., Sulph.*) (C.).

Foul-smelling discharges from any source (*Arn., Ars., Bapt., Carb-Ac., Graph., Hep., Kali-P., Lach., Merc., Nit-Ac., Pyrog., Sec.*) (C.).

RELATIONSHIP: *Similar to: Ars., Bapt., Calc-S., Hep., Kali-P., Lach., Mur-Ac.* and *Rhus-T.*

Valuable as a local cleansing and anti-septic wash.

Equisetum Hyemale.

COMMON NAME: SCOURING BUSH.

Dull pain in the region of the right kidney, with urgent desire to urinate (C.).

Burning in the urethra when urinating (Canth., Merc., Sulph.) (N.).

CYSTIC IRRITATION WITH TENESMUS (*Apis, Bell., Canth., Dulc., Ferr-P., Merc-C., Nux-V., Puls., Sep., Thuj.*) (Bl.).

Pain in the bladder, as if distended, not relieved by micturition (C.).

Much inclination to. urinate (*Canth., Merc., Tereb., Thuj.*) (N.).

Nocturnal enuresis (Apis, Benz-Ac., Caust., Ferr., Graph., Kreos., Lac-C., Mag-P., Nat-M., Puls., Sep., Sil., Sulph.) (Bl.).

PAIN AND TENDERNESS IN THE REGION OF THE BLADDER (*Bell., Canth., Lach., Merc-C., Tereb.*) (C.).

Dysuria following confinement and during pregnancy (*Arn., Canth., Lyc., Nux-V., Puls.*) (Bl.).

CYSTITIS (*Bell., Canth., Con., Gels., Staph., Thuj.*) (D.).

Sharp, burning, cutting pain in the urethra while urinating (*Canth., Merc-C., Tereb.*) (A.).

Urine shows great excess of mucus after standing a short time (C.).

Paralysis of the bladder in old women (*Con., Gels., Kali-P.*) (Bl.).

FREQUENT AND INTOLERABLE URGING TO URINATE (A.).

Constant urging, with scanty discharge (C.).

Severe pain at the close of urination (*Berb., Nat-M., Sars., Thuj.*) (N.).

URINE HIGH-COLOURED AND SCANTY (*Acon., Apis, Berb., Lyc., Sep., Tereb.*) (C.).

Dribbling urine (*Canth., Clem., Lil-T., Merc.. Merc-C., Nux-V., Plb., Puls., Sulph., Tereb.*) (B.).

Much blood and mucus in the urine (*Canth., Merc-C., Tereb.*) (C.).

RELATIONSHIP: *Complementary: Sil.*

Similar to: Apis, Berb., Canth., Dig., Ferr-P., Gels., Hep., Kali-B., Lyc., Merc., Merc-C.. Nat-M., Puls., Sep., Tereb. and *Thuj.*

Erigeron Canadense.

COMMON NAMES: HORSEWEED; BUTTER-WEED; CANADA FLEABANE.

Hæmorrhages from all orifices of the body (*Crot-II., Ipec., Mill., Phos.*) (A.).

HAEMORRHAGE: BRIGHT AND GUSHING (*Bell., Ipec., Phos., Sab.*) (B.).

VESICO-RECTAL TENESMUS (*Canth., Merc-C., Nux-V., Sulph.*) (B.).

Hæmorrhage increased by every motion (D.).

Epistaxis, with congestion to the head (N.).

DYSURIA (*Bel., Canth., Nux-V., Staph.*) (B.).

Hæmaturia, with stone in the bladrer (*Berb., Canth., Lyc., Sep.*) (N.).

Stool small, streaked with blood; tormina; burning in the bowels and rectum (*Sulph.*) (C.).

Urination painful or suppressèd (*Apis, Bell., Canth., Stram.*) (C.).

UTERINE HAEMORRHAGE (*Arn., Calc., Kali-P., Lach., Nit-Ac., Phos., Sab., Sec., Sulph.*) (N.).

Metrorrhagia, with prolapsus of the uterus (Bl.).

Post-partum hæmorrhages (*Arn., Chin., Ferr., Kali-P., Lach., Sec.*) (Bl.).

Leucorrhœa: the discharges consist of much mucus mixed with blood (Bl.).

Pallor and weakness (*Calc-P., Carb-V., Chin., Ferr., Graph., Kali-C., Nat-M., Sep.*) (C.).

Hæmatemesis, with violent retching and burning in the stomach (*Crot-H., Lach., Phos., Sec.*) (N.).

Hæmoptysis and blood-spitting (*Bry., Chin., Ferr., Ham., Ipec., Kali-P., Mill., Nux-V., Phos., Puls., Sep.*) (N.).

Incipient phthisis (*Calc-P., Ferr-P., Phos., Sep.*) (C.).

Bloody lochia returns after the least motion (C.).

Bleeding from the hæmorrhoids, with burning (*Caps., Lach., Sulph.*) (N.).

AGGRAVATION: From every motion.

AMELIORATION: From lying quietly.

RELATIONSHIP: *Similar to: Acon., Bell., Canth., Chin., Cinnamon., Ferr-P., Ipec., Nux-V., Sab., Sec., Tereb.* and *Trill.*

Eupatorium Perfoliatum.

COMMON NAME: BONE-SET.

Cachexia, from prolonged or frequent attacks of bilious or intermittent fevers (*Ars., Chin., Ferr., Lach., Lyc., Nat-M., Puls., Sep.*) (A.).

Painful soreness of eyeballs (*Arn., Bell.*) (N.).

ACHING PAINS AS IF IN THE BONES, WITH MOANING (N.).

Intense backache, as if beaten (*Rhus-T.*) (B.).

BONE-PAINS AFFECTING BACK, HEAD, CHEST, LIMBS, ESPECIALLY THE WRISTS (A.).

Calves of the legs feel as if they had been beaten (N.).

Soreness and aching of the arms and forearms (N.).

Excruciating headache, with soreness of the scalp and eye-balls, redness of the face, nausea, etc. (Bl.).

BRUISED FEELING, AS IF BROKEN, ALL OVER THE BODY (*Arn., Bapt., Bellis, Nux-V., Pyrog.*) (A.).

Thirst a long time before the chill, continues during the chill and heat, absent during sweat (N.).

Intense thirst, but drinking cold water causes shuddering and vomiting of bile (N.).

INTERMITTENT FEVER: THE CHILL COMMENCES ABOUT 7 OR 9 IN THE MORNING IN THE BACK, ACCOMPANIED BY THIRST, AND THERE IS INTENSE ACHING IN ALL THE BONES, AS IF THEY WERE BROKEN; THIS IS FOLLOWED BY HEAT AND AN INCREASE OF THE ACHING, AND THIS BY A SCANTY OR PROFUSE SWEAT (D.).

Canine hunger (after quinine) (A.).

VOMITS WATER OR FOOD THAT HAS BEEN TAKEN, OR BILE AS THE CHILL PASSES OFF (D.).

Chill at 7 to 9 A.M. one day, and at noon the next day (A.)

Insatiable thirst before and during chill and fever; knows the chill is coming, because he cannot drink enough.

Desire for ice-cream (Calc., Phos., Tub., Verat.) (A.).

Influenza (or La Grippe): Great soreness and aching of the entire body; hoarseness and cough, with great sore-

ness of the larynx and chest; a great coryza and thirst, and drinking causes vomiting; the cough hurts the head and chest and the patient holds the chest with the hands (Bry.) (B.).

Prostration in epidemic influenza (La Grippe) (*Ars., Phos.*) (N.).

Cough decreased by getting on hands and knees (N.).

Cough: chronic; loose with hectic; chest sore, must support it with hands (*Bry., Nat-C., Phos.*); worse at night; following measles or suppressed intermittents (A.).

VERY RESTLESS, CAN'T KEEP STILL, ALTHOUGH THERE IS A GREAT DESIRE TO DO SO, AND IS NOT RELIEVD BY MOTION (Dr. Kl.).

Bilious effects; yellow eyes, face, vomit, etc. (Bry., Chel., Chin., Nat-S.) (B.).

Soreness and swelling of the feet (*Dn.*).

Tongue coated thickly yellow (*Ant-C., Chel., Merc., Nux-M., Rhus-T., Spig., Sulph.*) (Bt.).

Vertigo; sways to the left (Calc., Lach., Nat-M., Stram., Sulph., Zinc.) (B.).

Urine scanty, dark mahogany colour (Ha.).

Great weakness during the fever (Ant-T., Ars., Bapt., Bry., Carb-V., Ign., Mur-Ac., Nat-M., Phos-Ac., Phos., Puls., Rob., Rhus-T., Sulph.) (Dg.).

Yellow, jaundiced skin (*Chel., Chin., Merc., Nat-M., Nat-S., Sep.*) (R.).

Soreness in the region of the liver on moving or coughing (R.).

Scanty urine, depositing a whitish, clay-like deposit (R.).

RELATIONSHIP: *Compare: Chel., Lyc., Nat-S., Podo.,* and *Sep.,* in jaundiced conditions.

Is followed well by: Nat-M. and *Sep.*

Bry. is the nearest analogue, having free sweat, but pains keep the patient quiet; while *Eup-P.* has scanty sweat and pains make the patient restless.

Euphorbium.

COMMON NAMES: WOLF'S MILK; GUM EUPHORBIUM; GOPHER PLANT.

Rheumatic pains of a tearing, pressing, and stinging character, but only during rest.

Paralytic weakness in the joints and mostly when beginning to move.

Burning pain in internal parts (Ars., Carb-V., Phos., Sec., Sulph.).

Diseases of mucous membranes.

VESICULAR ERYSIPELATOUS ERUPTION UPON THE FACE (*Anac., Canth., Rhus-T.*).

Stinging exanthemata (*Apis*).

Yellowish exanthemata (*Ant-C.*).

Stinging in the skin (*Apis, Nit-A.*).

Coryza with swelling; much abortive sneezing (B.).

Burning in the throat, extending to the stomach (*Ars., Canth., Caps., Merc-C.*) (C.).

Sensation of burning heat on either cheek, generally left side (G.).

Erysipelas bulbosa; vesicles as large as peas, filled with yellow liquid (A.).

Stitches from the epigastrium into the sides of the chest on coughing (B.).

TERRIBLE BURNING PAIN, AS IF A LIVE COAL WERE ON OR IN THE PARTS, OF CANCER, CARBUNCLE OR ERYSIPELAS (when *Ars.* or *Anthr.* fails to relieve) (A.).

Profuse diarrhœa and vomiting (*Crot-T., Podo., Verat.*) (C.).

STOOLS: PROFUSE, DIARRHOEIC, DYSENTERIC, FERMENTED AND THIN, LIKE WATER (C.).

Gangrene or blood-boils of old person (*Ars., Carb-V., Sec.*) (A.).

Thirst for cold drinks (*Acon., Ars., Bry., Nat-M., Phos., Puls., Verat.*) (C.).

Frequent hic-cough (*Mag-P.*) (C.).

Burning in caries and necrosis of bone (A.).

Toothache, as if screwed in, with jerking and throbbing (C.).

Much rumbling in the abdomen, followed by emission of flatus (C.).

Old, torpid, indolent ulcers, with biting, lancinating, and lacerating pains (A.).

AGGRAVATION: During rest, especially while sitting; from contact with the affected part; and when beginning to move.

AMELIORATION: During motion; and from continued moving when walking.

RELATIONSHIP: *Similar to: Apis, Ars., Canth., Graph., Iris, Kreos., Lach., Nat-S., Petr., Phos., Rhus-T., Sec., Sep., Sulph.* and *Verat.*

Euphrasia.

COMMON NAME: EYE-BRIGHT.

Pains, as from cramp.

Like *Arnica Montana,* is of approved valuation in nullifying the bad effects of contusions and other mechanical injuries subsequent to trauma (*Arn., Ham.*).

During the whole night wandering itching stitches, here and there, with great restlessness.

Amenorrhœa, with catarrhal symptoms of the eyes and nose (A.).

MENSES: PAINFUL, NOW LASTING ONLY ONE HOUR (*Psor.*); OR LATE, SCANTY, SHORT,

LASTING ONLY ONE DAY (*Alum., Apis, Bar-C., Nux-V., Psor., Sep., Thuj.*) (A.).

Sycotic excrescences in association with the costive state.

CATARRHAL AFFECTIONS OF THE MUCOUS MEMBRANES, ESPECIALLY OF THE EYES AND NOSE (*All-C., Calc., Kali-M., Merc., Nat-M., Puls.*) (A.).

Inflammations of the eye of paramount importance (acute and burning lachrymation most in evidence).

Cornea bluish.

THE EYES WATER ALL THE TIME AND ARE AGGLUTINATED IN THE MORNING; MARGINS OF LIDS RED, SWOLLEN, BURNING (*All-C.*) (A.).

AVERSION TO LIGHT (*Bell., Calc., Con., Graph., Merc., Nat-M., Phos., Sep., Sulph., Zinc.*) (A.).

Blepharitis; injected eyes; discharge thick and excoriating, the tears scald and irritate the cheeks; photophobia, worse in the artificial light. Traumatic conjunctivitis (D.).

Feeling as though the cornea were covered with much mucus; it obscures his vision and obliges him to frequently close and press the lids together (N.).

FLUENT CORYZA (*All-C., Am-C., Arg-M., Ars., Bell., Calc., Dulc., Kali-Ars., Kali-I., Lac-C., Merc., Merc-C., Nat-C., Nat-M., Nit-Ac., Nux-V., Puls., Sabad., Sulph., Tell., Thuj.*).

Profuse, fluent coryza in the morning, with violent cough and abundant expectoration; worse from exposure to warm south wind (A.).

When attempting to clear the throat of an offensive mucus in the morning, gagging until he vomits the breakfast just eaten (*Bry.*) (A.).

PROFUSE, ACRID LACHRYMATION, WITH PROFUSE, BLAND CORYZA (reverse of *All-C.*) (A.).

Profuse expectoration of mucus by voluntary hawking, worse on rising in the morning (A.).

PERTUSSIS: EXCESSIVE LACHRYMATION DURING COUGH; COUGH ONLY IN DAY-TIME (*Am-C.*, *Arg-M.*, *Calc.*, *Ferr.*, *Lach.*, *Mang.*, *Nat-M.*, *Phos.*, *Staph.*, *Thuj.*, *Viol-O.*) (A.).

In measles with watery eyes and fluent coryza it is sometimes the best remedy (N.).

Chemosis (*Apis*, *Arg-N.*, *Hep.*, *Kali-I.*, *Lach.*, *Nat-M.*, *Rhus-T.*, *Vesp.*) (B.).

Cataract (when the eyes water a great deal) (G.).

Dim-sightedness (*Agar.*, *Bell.*, *Calc.*, *Caust.*, *Con.*, *Gels.*, *Lach.*, *Nit-Ac.*, *Phos.*, *Puls.*, *Ruta*, *Sep.*, *Sil.*, *Sulph.*) (B.).

Sensation as though a hair is hung over the eye, and must be wiped away (C.).

Spots, vesicles and ulcers on the cornea (*Hep.*, *Merc.*, *Sil.*) (C.).

Smarting in the eyes, as from sand.

AGGRAVATION: In the evening; during the night; whilst lying down; from the glare of the day-light and the sun; in bed; indoors; from warmth; after exposure to south wind; and when touched (*Hep.*).

AMELIORATION: In the dark; in the open air; and from wiping the eyes.

RELATIONSHIP: *Similar to*: *Puls.* in affections of the eyes; reverse of *All-C.* in lachrymation and coryza.

Antidotes: *Camph.*, *Puls.*

Ferrum Metallicum.

COMMON NAME: IRON.

Great emaciation (*Ars.*, *Bar-C.*, *Calc.*, *Chin.*, *Graph.*, *Iod.*, *Lyc.*, *Nat-M.*, *Nit-Ac.*, *Phos.*, *Sil.*, *Sulph.*, *Tub.*)

Weakness amounting to paralysis (*Ars.*, *Caust.*, *Gels.*, *Kali-P.*, *Nux-V.*, *Phos.*, *Plb.*, *Sep.*).

Restlessness in the affected limbs (*Rhus-T.*, *Zinc.*).

Cracking in the joints (*Calc., Caps., Kali-B., Led., Nat-C., Nit-Ac., Petr., Rhus-T., Sep., Thuj.*).

Disposition to languor and rest on account of internal weakness (*Bry., Calc-P., Gels., Kali-P., Phos-Ac., Sep., Sil., Zinc.*).

Walking in the open air greatly affects him.

Produces a false plethora: an irregular distribution of blood, with headache, nose-bleed, dyspnœa, etc. (D.).

Chill with red face and thirst (D.).

Fever mal-treated by quinine (A.).

Profuse, long-lasting debilitating sweat; clammy and cold at night (A.).

During the day-time, sudden spasms of the limbs are complained of.

Vomiting of ingesta after every cough (*Bry., Ipec., Nux-V.*) (N.).

RHEUMATIC COMPLAINTS (*Bry., Calc., Kali-M., Rhus-T., Ruta, Sil.*).

RHEUMATIC PAIN IN THE LEFT DELTOID MUSCLES (*Rhus-T.*) (D.).

Nightly emission with backache (B.).

Contortion of the limbs (*Cupr., Mag-P., Sec.*).

EXTREME PALENESS OF THE FACE, WHICH BECOMES RED AND FLUSHED ON THE LEAST PAIN, MOTION OR EXERTION (*Amyl-N.*) (A.).

Varices (*Calc-F., Ham., Nat-M., Sep.*).

Vertigo: on going down hill, or on crossing water, even though the water be smooth (D.).

BLUSHING (*Amyl-N., Coca*) (A.).

CHLOROSIS (*Alum., Ars., Calc-P., Cycl., Ferr-Ars., Graph., Lyc., Mang., Nat-M., Nit-Ac., Phos., Puls., Sep.*).

COLOUR OF THE FACE YELLOW, OR ELSE EARTHY (*Calc., Nat-M., Puls., Sep.*).

Circumscribed red area on the cheeks (*Lachn., Phos., Sulph.*).

RED PARTS BECOME WHITE—LIPS, FACE, TONGUE (A.).

Congestions (not limited to any part of the body, but useful throughout).

Swelling and distension of blood-vessels (Glon., Nat-M., Verat-V.) (G.).

METRORRHAGIA WITH RED FACE AND SWELLED VEINS *(Bell., Glon., Sang.).*

Menses intermit for a few days *(Puls., Sep.)* (Bl.).

CATAMENIA: TOO EARLY AND TOO PROFUSE *(Ars., Bell., Bov., Calc., Cocc., Cycl., Ipec., Nat-M., Nux-V., Phos., Plat., Rat., Sab.).*

Milky, corrosive leucorrhœa *(Calc.)* (R.).

Constipation: from intestinal atony *(Alum., Bry., Op.)* ; ineffectual urging; stools hard and difficult, followed by backache or cramping pain in the rectum (A.).

HAEMORRHAGIC DIATHESIS; BLOOD BRIGHT RED; COAGULATES EASILY *(Ferr-P., Ipec., Phos.)* (A.).

SPITTING BLOOD, WITH FLYING PAINS IN THE CHEST, RELIEVED BY SLOWLY WALKING ABOUT (N.).

Hæmorrhages in debilitated or anæmic subjects (N.).

Headache: hammering, beating pulsating pains; must lie down; with aversion to eating and drinking (A.).

Headache after the menses (C.).

PALPITATION WITH FEAR, AMELIORATED BY SLOWLY WALKING ABOUT (N.).

Impotence (Agn., Bar-C., Calad., Con., Graph., Kali-P., Lyc., Med., Nat-M., Nux-V., Phos., Sel., Sep., Sulph.).

Pettish, quarrelsome, disputative, easily excited; least contradiction angers *(Anac., Nux-V., Sulph.)* (A.).

Desire for solitude *(Ign., Phos-Ac., Sep.)* (R.).

Anxiety from slight cause (R.).

Bellows-sound of the heart, and anæmic murmur of the arteries and veins (Bt.).

Aversion to fat food and vomiting of what has been eaten (*Cycl., Phos., Puls.*).

Bad effects from the abuse of tea and from the abuse of quinine (*Puls.*).

Ravenous appetite (*Iod., Nat-M., Phos., Tub.*) (D.).

Alternate canine hunger and anorexia (N.).

Regurgitation and eructation of food in mouthfuls (*Alum.*), without nausea (A.).

Averse to meat (B.).

Dropsy: after loss of vital fluids (*Chin.*); abuse of quinine (*Ars., Nat-M., Puls., Sep.*); suppressed intermittent (*Carb-V., Chin.*) (A.).

Diarrhœa: undigested, painless, sometimes involuntary stools; desire to go to stool as soon as anything touches his stomach (D.).

Diarrhœa, worse after mid-night (D.).

AGGRAVATION : At night, towards morning; while at rest; when sitting quietly; and during menses.

AMELIORATION : By slow motion; from walking slowly about; and in summer.

RELATIONSHIP : *Complementary to* : *Alum.* and *Chin.*

Chin. its vegetable analogue follows well in nearly all diseases, acute or chronic.

Antidotes : *Chin., Puls.* and *Thea.*

Fluoric Acid.

COMMON NAME : HYDRO-FLUORIC ACID.

Complaints of old age, or of premature old age; in syphilitic mercurial dyscrasia (A.).

YOUNG PEOPLE LOOK OLD (*Agn., Ambr., Bar-C., Bufo, Kali-C., Lyc., Sel.*) (A.).

Pale, miserable, cachectic, flabby and broken down (B.).

DISEASES OF THE BONES, ESPECIALLY OF LONG BONES (*Calc-F., Calc-P., Kali-I., Merc., Mezer., Nit-Ac., Phos., Sil.*), BETTER FROM COLD (relieved by warmth—*Sil.*) (N.).

Caries and necrosis, especially of long bones, in psoric or syphilitic subjects; or after abuse of mercury or silica (A.).

Aversion to all about him, even his own family (*Sep.*); sensation as if danger menaced him.

Increased ability to exercise without danger (*Coca*) (A.).

Forgetfulness of dates and of his common employment.

FISTULA DENTALIS OR LACHRYMALIS (*Merc., Sil., Sulph.*) (A.).

Roughness and harshness of the skin, with great itching in spots; worse from warmth and better from cold (D.).

Nævus or birth-marks on children (N.).

Capillary aneurism (*Calc-F.*) (A.).

Is of service when the liver is engorged or indurated; hepatic cirrhosis, with ascites (Bl.).

RAPID CARIES OF TEETH (*Calc., Calc-F., Kreos., Merc., Phos., Staph.*) (A.).

Old cicatrices become inflamed around the edges and itch violently (Graph.) (N.).

Ulcers: red edges and vesicles; decubitus; copious discharge; worse from warmth, and better from cold; violent pains, like streaks of lightning, confined to a small spot (A.).

Cannot bear the extremes of heat and cold in summer and winter (N.).

Always too hot; wants to bathe in cold water (B.).

Exostoses of bones of face (*Aur., Calc., Calc-F., Hecla, Merc., Sil.*) (A.).

Alopecia (Calc., Graph., Phos-Ac.) (Bl.)

Brittle, tousy hair (*Bor., Kali-C.*) (B.).

Varicose veins and ulcers (*Ham., Nat-M., Sep.*) (A.).

ONYCHIA (*Ant-C., Graph., Merc., Sil., Thuj.*) (Bl.).

FELON (*Apis, Ars., Dios., Hep., Lach., Merc., Sil.*) (B.).

Offensive or pungent perspiration on the male sexual organs (K.).

Sweat on the hands and feet (B.).

Stunning headache, ameliorated by urination (B.).

Severe pressing pain in the temples, from within outward (C.).

A short sleep suffices and refreshes him (C.).

Pain along the cranial sutures (C.).

Gnawing hunger; for pungent or cold things (B.).

Acrid leucorrhœa (*Bor., Nit-Ac.*) (C.).

Impaired hearing, ameliorated by bending the head backward (K.).

Bed-sores (*Arn., Ars., Bapt., Carb-V., Lach., Lyc., Merc., Nit-Ac., Phos., Sec.*) (B.).

RELATIONSHIP: *Complementary*: Coca, Sil.

Follows well: after *Ars.* in ascites of drunkards; after *Kali-C.* in hip-joint disease; after *Coff., Staph.* in sensitive teeth; after *Phos-Ac.* in diabetes; after *Sil., Symph.* in bone diseases; and after *Spong.* in goitre.

Is especially useful after the abuse of *Sil.* in suppurations.

Gelsemium.

COMMON NAME: YELLOW JASMINE.

Adapted for children and young people, especially women of a nervous, hysterical temperament (*Croc., Ign., Lyc., Nat-M.*) (A.).

CONFUSION OF THE MIND (*Calc., Cann-I., Carb-V., Glon., Lach., Merc., Nat-M., Nux-M., Op., Petr., Rhus-T., Sep., Strych.*) (Bt.).

Mental faculties dull, cannot think; drowsy, with dull red face (N.).

UTTER LACK OF COURAGE (*Acon., Bar-C., Chin., Graph., Lyc.*) (A.).

FEAR OF FALLING (*Bor., Cupr., Lac-C.*); THE CHILD GRASPS THE CRIB OR SEIZES THE NURSE (*Bor., Sanic.*) (A.).

Bad effects from fright, fear, exciting news and sudden emotions (*Ign., Puls.*) (A.).

DESIRE TO BE QUIET, TO BE ALONE; DOES NOT WISH TO SPEAK OR HAVE ANY ONE NEAR HER, EVEN IF THE PERSON BE SILENT (*Ign., Nat-M.*) (A.).

Great depression of spirits in onanists, accompanied with excessive languor (Bt.).

Amaurosis from masturbation (*Con., Nat-M., Phos., Puls., Sulph.*) (Bt.).

STAGE-FRIGHT, NERVOUS DREAD OF AP-PEARING IN PUBLIC (*Arg-N.*) (A.).

THE ANTICIPATION OF ANY UNUSUAL ORDEAL, PREPARING FOR CHURCH, THEATRE, OR TO MEET AN ENGAGEMENT, BRINGS ON DIARRHOEA (A.).

Hysteria, with spasms, palpitation of the heart, and great nervous excitability (*Kali-P.*) (Bt.).

Fears that unless on the move the heart will cease beating (fears it would cease beating if she moved—*Dig.*) (A.).

Headache, principally in the occiput, ameliorated by reclining the head and shoulders on a high pillow (N.).

HEADACHE, P R E C E D E D BY· BLINDNESS (*Hyos., Iris, Kali-B., Lac-D., Nat-M., Podo., Psor., Sep.*) (A.).

Intense congestion of the brain (*Acon., Bell., Glon., Verat-V.*) (Bt.).

Headache: worse from mental exertion, smoking, heat of sun and lying with head low (A.).

Heaviness of the head (or headache) relieved by profuse flow of urine (Ferr-P., Ign., Kalm., Meli., Sang., Sil.) (N.).

Nervous headache: the pain commences in the cervical portion of the spinal cord, and then spreads over the whole head (Bry., Sang., Sil.) (Bt.).

Sensation of band around the head above the eyes (*Carb-Ac., Sulph.*) (A.).

Scalp sore to touch (*Bell., Chin.*) (A.).

COMPLETE RELAXATION AND PROSTRATION OF THE WHOLE MUSCULAR SYSTEM, WITH MOTOR PARALYSIS (A.).

Weakness and trembling: of tongue, hands, legs; or of the entire body (A.).

Hysterical spasms, with great excitement and numb feeling in the extremities (Bt.).

LACK OF MUSCULAR CO-ORDINATION; CONFUSED; MUSCLES REFUSE TO OBEY THE WILL (A.).

Catarrhal deafness with pain from the throat into the middle ear (N.).

Progressive loco-motor ataxy (Bt.).

General depression from the heat of sun or summer (A.).

Inspiration long, with crowing sound; expiration sudden and forcible (N.).

Slow, weak pulse of old age (N.).

Numbness of the tongue; feels so thick that he can hardly speak; partial paralysis (N.).

VERTIGO: SPREADING FROM THE OCCIPUT (*Sil.*); WITH DIPLOPIA, DIM VISION, LOSS OF SIGHT; SEEMS INTOXICATED WHEN TRYING TO MOVE (A.).

Great heaviness of the eyelids; cannot keep them open (*Caust., Graph., Sep.*) (A.).

Dimness of vision (*Calc., Cycl., Kali-C., Lyc., Puls., Sep.*) (Bt.).

Beginning typhoid; headache, drowsy, stupid, wants to lie still; great prostration; tongue trembles when protruding it; eyelids droop; trembles all over when trying to move (N.).

Sleep: languid and drowsy; but cannot compose the mind for sleep (N.).

Nocturnal emission and sexual dreams, followed the next day by great languor and irritability (*Phos-Ac.*) (Bt.).

Genitals cold and relaxed (*Calad.*).

Involuntary emissions without erections (*Chin., Cob., Dios., Graph., Ham., Nat-C., Nuph., Phos-Ac., Sel., Sulph.*) (N.).

Spasmodic labour-pains (*Bell., Caul., Mag-P., Puls.*).

Rigidity of the neck of the uterus (*Bell., Sec.*).

Chill: without thirst, especially along the spine; running up and down the back in rapid, wave-like succession; from the sacrum to the occiput (A.).

Nervous chill: violent shaking with no sense of coldness (N.).

Desire to quiet; too weak to move (*Bry., Kali-C., Phos-Ac.*) (N.).

WANTS TO BE HELD THAT HE MAY NOT SHAKE SO MUCH (*Lach.*) (A.).

General deep-seated muscular pain with prostration (la grippe) (N.).

Could tell when the chill was about to return, as incontinence of urine would set in (A.).

Catarrh with violent paroxysms of sneezing; worse in the morning, with tingling in the nose (hay fever) (N.).

AGGRAVATION: In damp weather; before a thunder-storm; from emotion or excitement; from bad news; from tobacco-smoking; when thinking of his ailments; and when spoken to of his loss.

AMELIORATION: From profuse urination; from remaining quiet.

RELATIONSHIP: *Compare*: *Bapt.* in threatening typhoid fever; *Ipec.* in dumb ague, after suppression by quinine; and *Arg-N.* in neurasthenia.

Glonoine.

COMMON NAME: NITRO-GLYCERINE.

The symptoms calling for it are violent and appear suddenly (*Amyl-N., Bell., Ferr-P.*) (Bl.).

Head troubles from working under gas-light, when heat falls on the head; cannot bear heat about the head, heat of stove or walking in the sun (*Lach., Nat-C.*) (A.).

HEADACHE FROM BELOW UPWARDS; BRAIN AS IF MOVING IN WAVES (N.).

Headache: worse from bending the head backwards; is relieved in the open air; cannot keep still; must walk about (D.).

CEREBRAL CONGESTION, OR ALTERNATE CONGESTION OF THE HEAD AND THE HEART (A.).

Headache from recent exposure to the sun (N.).

Over-heating in the sun, or sun-stroke (*Acon., Gels., Nat-M., Verat-V.*) (N.).

Can't bear anything on the head especially hat; or pressure as of a hat (N.).

Sudden local congestion, especially to the head and chest; bursting headache, rising up from the neck, with great throbbing and sense of expansion as if to burst; cannot bear the least jar (N.).

Fullness of the head; distinct feeling of a pulse in the head; throbbing with or without pain (N.).

Can't bear any heat about the head; can't walk in the sun; must walk in the shade or carry an umbrella (G.).

IS AFRAID TO SHAKE THE HEAD; IT INCREASES THE ACHE AND SEEMS AS THOUGH THE HEAD WOULD DROP IN PIECES (N.).

Sun-stroke: face pale; full round pulse; laboured respiration; eyes fixed; cerebral vomiting; white tongue; sinking at the pit of the stomach (D.).

Tinnitus aurium (Chin.) (Bl.).

Throbbing in the head synchronous with contraction of the heart (Bl.).

Sun headache: increases and decreases every day with the sun (*Kalm., Nat-C., Nat-M., Spig.*) (A.).

Eyes injected, protruding, look wild; pupils dilated; objects dance before them with every pulsation (N.).

Sparks and flashes before the eyes (*Bell.*) (C.).

Great vertigo on assuming an up-right posture from rising up in bed; rising from a seat, etc.

" Meniere's disease " (*Ther.*) (Bl.).

Frequently congestion in the head is attended with convulsions (*Acon., Bell.. Verat-V.*) (Bl.).

Is useful in puerperal convulsions.

The face is red, the pulse is full and hard; the urine contains albumen; the patient is unconscious and froths at the mouth (Bl.).

VIOLENT ACTION OF THE HEART; DISTINCT PULSATION OVER THE WHOLE BODY, ESPECIALLY IN THE BACK OF NECK AND HEAD (N.).

Heart's action laboured, oppressed; blood seems to rush to heart, and rapidly to head (*Amyl-N.*) (A.).

Has exalted ideas; thinks she is the Almighty and every one her inferior (*Plat.*) (R.).

CONFUSION, CANNOT TELL WHERE HE IS; WELL-KNOWN STREETS SEEM STRANGE; FORGETS ON WHICH SIDE OF THE STREET HE LIVES (N.).

The chin feels too long.

Unusually bright and loquacious, with great flow of ideas (*Cann-I., Coff., Lach., Stram.*).

Acute and chronic interstitial nephritis with high arterial tension (Bl.).

Bad effects of mental excitement, fright, fear, mechanical injuries and their consequences; from having the hair cut (*Acon., Bell.*) (A.).

SHOULD BE REMEMBERED IN CASES OF INCREASED VASCULAR TENSION (BLOOD-PRESSURE) OF THE AGED (Bl.).

Desire to take a long, deep inspiration.

Children get sick in the evening when sitting before an open coal fire, or falling asleep there (A.).

Convulsions of children from cerebral congestion (A.).

Meningitis (*Apis, Bell., Bry., Hell., Hyos., Lach., Nat-M., Op., Sulph., Verat-V.*) (A.).

Flushes of heat: at the climacteric (*Amyl-N., Bell., Graph., Lach., Sang.*); *also with the catamenia* (*Ferr., Sep., Sang., Sulph.*) (A.).

Headache occurring after profuse uterine hæmorrhage (*Chin., Ferr.*) (A.).

Rush of blood to the head in pregnant women (A.).

Intense congestion of brain from delayed or suppressed menses (A.).

HEADACHE IN PLACE OF MENSES (A.).

Intense throbbing pains in the epigastrium (*Acon., Chin., Ferr., Sep.*) (Bt.).

Cardiac pains radiate to all parts—towards arms (B.).

Awakes fearing apoplexy (B.).

Heat, with hot sweat (*Bell.*) (B.).

Unsteady gait (*Alum., Nux-V., Pic-Ac., Zinc.*).

AGGRAVATION: In the sun; from exposure to sun's rays; from gaslight; from over-heat; from jar; from stooping; on ascending; from touch of hat; from having the hair cut; and from wine.

AMELIORATION: From cold applications; in cold air; and from pressure.

RELATIONSHIP: *Compare*: *Acon., Amyl-N., Bell., Ferr., Ferr-P., Gels., Melil., Strom.* and *Verat-V.*
Is of service in the cerebral congestion of children, when *Bell.* does not afford the desired relief.

Antidotes: *Acon., Camph., Coff.* and *Nux-V.*

Gnaphalium.

COMMON NAMES: EVER-LASTING; INDIAN POSY.

Offensive diarrhœa with colic, worse in the morning (*Nat-S., Podo., Sulph.*) (B.).

Cholera morbus: colic with vomiting and purging (*Ars., Bism., Crot-T., Nux-V., Sec., Verat.*) (Bl.).

INTENSE PAIN ALONG THE RIGHT SCIATIC NERVE, DARTING, CUTTING, FROM THE RIGHT HIP-JOINT DOWN TO THE FOOT; WORSE FROM LYING DOWN, MOTION, AND STEPPING, AND AMELIORATED BY SITTING (A.).

Intense sciatic pains, alternating with numbness or formication (B.).

Lumbago, with sensation of weight in the region of the pelvis.

Gouty pains in the big toes.

Exercise on foot is excessively fatiguing.

Dysmenorrhœa: menses are scanty and very painful the first day (*Calc-P., Caust., Graph., Kali-C., Lap-A., Vib.*) (Bl.).

Sensation of weight and fulness in the pelvis (*Aloe, Podo., Sep.*) (Bl.).

Dysmenorrhœa, with scanty, chocolate-brown discharges and distress in the pelvic region (C.).

AGGRAVATION: At night; from lying down; from motion; when stepping; during menses; and on walking.

AMELIORATION: From sitting; and from flexing the limbs.

RELATIONSHIP: *Similar to*: *Cham., Coloc., Mag-P.* and *Xanth.*

Gossypium.

COMMON NAME: COTTON PLANT.

Gossypium is a powerful emmenagogue. It has a wide reputation as an abortifacient. It produces firm, regular and strong uterine contractions, resembling *Cimicifuga* in its action (C.).

Flow of saliva (*Am-C., Arum-T., Bar-C., Bor., Fluor-Ac., Iod., Ipec., Kali-C., Lyso., Merc., Merc-C., Nat-M., Nit-Ac., Nux-V., Puls., Sep., Sulph., Verat.*) (B.).

Nausea on awaking (*Alum., Asar., Bor., Con., Lac-Ac., Petr.*) (B.).

Vomits on motion or rising up (*Bry., Cocc., Sulph.*).

HYPEREMESIS GRAVIDARUM (*Ars., Asar., Colch., Cup-Ars., Kreos., Lac-Ac., Nux-V., Petr., Phos., Puls., Sep., Sil., Symphori., Tab., Verat.*) (B.).

NAUSEA, WITH INCLINATION TO VOMIT BEFORE BREAKFAST (*Alum., Arg-N., Berb., Bov., Calc., Fago, Lyc., Nit-Ac., Petr., Sep., Tub.*) (C.).

Intermittent pains in the ovarian region, worse from motion and better from rest (Bl.).

SUPPRESSED MENSTRUATION (*Bry., Cycl., Ferr., Graph., Kali-C., Lach., Nat-M., Puls., Sep.*) (C.).

Menses: late, scanty and watery (*Alum., Calc-P., Nat-M.*) (B.).

Sensation that the flow is about to start, but it does not (C.).

Backache, and weight and dragging in the pelvis (*Nat-M., Rhus-T., Sep.*) (C.).

Uterine fibroids (*Calc., Calc-F., Lyc., Nux-V., Puls., Sep.*) (Bl.).

Tumour of the breast (*Carb-An., Con., Sil.*), with swelling of the axillary glands (C.).

Uterine sub-involution (*Calc., Cimic., Kali-Br., Kali-C., Puls., Sec., Sep., Sulph., Ust.*) (Bl.).

Sensitive womb (*Apis, Bell., Lach.*) (B.).

Labia swollen and itching (C.).

AGGRAVATION: From motion; from pressure; and before breakfast.

AMELIORATION: From rest.

RELATIONSHIP: *Similar to*: *Alum., Bry., Cimic., Kreos., Lac-Ac., Lil-T., Nat-M., Puls., Sab., Senec., Sep., Symphori.* and *Ust.*

Graphites.

COMMON NAME: BLACK LEAD.

Suited to women, inclined to obesity, who suffer from habitual constipation; with a history of delayed menstruation (A.).

Sexual desire diminished (*Agn., Bar-C., Caust., Ferr., Helon., Hep., Lyc., Mag-C., Nat-M., Phos-Ac., Rhod., Sep., Sulph.*) (K.).

"What *Pulsatilla* is at puberty, *Graphites* is at the climacteric" (A.).

CATAMENIA IS TOO SCANT AND TOO PALE (*Alum., Cycl., Ferr., Kali-C., Nat-M., Puls., Sep.*).

Soreness of the nipples (*Arn., Bapt., Caust., Crot-T., Fluor-Ac., Lach., Lyc., Merc., Nit-Ac., Phel., Phyt., Sep., Sil., Sulph.*).

Menses: too scanty, pale, late with violent colic; irregular; delayed from getting the feet wet (*Puls.*) (A.).

Morning sickness during menstruation (*Am-C., Apoc., Calc., Cupr., Kali-C., Lach., Lyc., Phos., Puls., Sep., Sulph., Verat.*) (G.).

Very weak and prostrated during menses (*Alum., Ars., Bov., Carb-An., Caust., Cocc., Helon., Iod., Kali-C., Mag-C., Murx., Nux-V., Phos., Sec., Sep., Sulph., Uran., Verat.*) (A.).

VERY PROFUSE LEUCORRHOEA; OCCURS IN GUSHES, DAY AND NIGHT, AND IS OFTEN EXCORIATING (G.).

The ovaries are very apt to be affected (*Apis, Bell., Lach., Lyc., Merc., Nit-Ac., Puls., Sep.*) (Hg.).

LEUCORRHOEA BEFORE AND AFTER THE MENSES (Before—*Sep.*; after—*Kreos.*).

Feeling as if the womb would press out of the vagina, with obstinate constipation, in fleshy women (Bt.).

Hard cicatrices remaining after mammary abscess, retarding the flow of milk; cancer of the breast, from old scars and repeated abscesses (A.).

DEEP CRACKS IN THE NIPPLES (*Cast-Eq., Caust., Fluor-Ac., Hydr., Lyc., Merc-C., Phyt., Rat., Sep., Sil., Sulph.*) (Bt.).

INDURATION OF THE OVARIES (*Apis, Arg-M., Ars-I., Aur., Bar-I., Brom., Con., Iod., Lach., Pall., Sep., Ust.*) (K.).

ITCHING OF THE FEMALE GENITALIA BEFORE MENSES (*Merc., Sulph., Tarant., Zinc.*) (K.).

DECIDED AVERSION TO COITION (in BOTH SEXES) (*Agn., Caust., Kali-C., Lyc.; Nat-M., Petr., Phos., Psor., Rhod., Sulph.*) (A.).

WEAKNESS OF THE SEXUAL POWERS (*Agn., Calad., Con., Dig., Gels., Kali-P., Lyc., Nux-V., Phos., Phos-Ac., Sep., Sulph., Zinc.*).

INCOMPLETE ERECTIONS DURING COITION (*Camph., Con., Lyc., Phos-Ac., Phos., Sep., Sulph., Ther.*) (K.).

Enjoyment absent during coition (*Agar., Anac., Calad., Lyc., Nat-M., Plat., Sep.*) (K.).

Sexual desire very strong (*Anan., Bar-M., Calc., Calc-P., Cann-I., Canth., Con., Lyc., Lyss., Nux-V., Phos., Pic-Ac., Plat., Puls., Staph., Tub., Zinc.*).

Moist eruptions on the male genitalia (*Carb-V., Hep., Rhus-T.*) (K.).

GLEET, WITH GLUEY DISCHARGE FROM THE URETHRA (K.).

Twitching and contortions of the limbs (*Bell., Cupr., Kali-Br., Lach., Mag-P., Phos., Plb., Puls., Sep., Zinc.*).

Drawing through the whole body with disposition to stretch the limbs.

Stiffness of the limbs (*Bell., Cupr., Nux-V., Plb., Rhus-T.*).

Sensation of trembling in the whole body with twitches in all the limbs (*Gels., Kali-Br., Tarant., Zinc.*).

The limbs go to sleep (*Agar., Con., Gels., Kali-P., Nux-V., Phos.*).

Contraction of the muscles (*Am-C., Bell., Cupr., Nux-V., Sec.*).

Rheumatic tearing, especially in such limbs as are affected with ulcers.

When walking in the open air many pains cease.

Disposition to catch cold and aggravation from getting cold (*Hep., Kali-C., Sil.*).

Pulsations in all the arteries from every motion.

Great debility without pain which induces to sigh.

Pains which are felt during sleep.

Pain during change of weather (*Nat-S., Rhod., Rhus-T.*).

Varices, with stinging tension and itching.

Swelling and induration of the glands (*Calc., Iod., Merc., Sil.*).

Hard swelling with stinging.

SUFFOCATION, AFTER MIDNIGHT, AMELIO-RATED BY EATING (B.).

Rushes of blood to the head (*Lach.*) (B.).

Flatulency (Carb-V., Lyc., Nux-M., Nux-V., Puls.).

Incarcerated flatulency (Carb-V., Lyc., Mag-P., Sulph.).

SOUR ERUCTATIONS (*Calc., Carb-V., Chin., Ign., Iris, Kali-B., Kali-S., Lith., Lyc., Mag-C., Nat-C., Nat-M., Nat-P., Nux-V., Phos., Rob., Sulph., Sulph-Ac.*).

AVERSION TO FISH, MEAT, SWEETS, WARM AND SALT FOOD (K.).

NAUSEA FROM TAKING SWEETS (*Arg-N., Ipec.*) (K.).

PAIN IN THE STOMACH AMELIORATED AFTER EATING (*Anac., Brom., Chel., Cina, Ign., Iod., Kali-B., Mag-M., Nat-C., Petr., Phos., Raph., Verat.*) (K.).

Gastric ulcers (Arg-N., Ars., Hydr., Kali-B., Kreos., Lyc., Merc-C., Phos.).

CONSTIPATION (*Alum., Bry., Chel., Mag-M., Nat-M., Nux-V., Op., Phos., Sep., Sil., Sulph.*)

Diarrhœa, often caused by suppressed eruptions (*Psor.*) (A.).

The stool has a sour odour (Calc., Hep., Mag-C., Merc., Rheum, Sulph.).

LUMPY STOOLS, UNITED BY MUCOUS THREADS (C.).

Stools: dark-coloured, half-digested, of an intolerable odour (C.).

Mucus remaining in the anus after stool (Ant-C.) (C.).

CONSTIPATION: LARGE, DIFFICULT, KNOT-TY STOOLS (G.).

Itching in the anus (Alum., Ars., Calc., Cina, Merc., Sulph.) (C.).

ANAL FISSURE (*Nit-Ac.*) (C.).

Urinary discharge too scanty (*Apis, Bell., Canth., Merc., Sep.*).

Urine has also a sour smell (*Ambr., Benz-Ac., Calc., Chel., Hep., Merc., Nat-C., Petr., Sep.*).

HUMMING IN THE EARS (*Chin., Puls., Sep.*).

HEARS BETTER WHEN IN A NOISE, WHEN RIDING IN A CAR OR CARRIAGE OR WHEN THERE IS A RUMBLING SOUND (*Nit-Ac.*) (A.).

Eruptions upon the ears (*Tell.*).

Eczema of eyelids; eruption moist and fissured; eyelids red and margins covered with scales or crusts (*Alum., Bor., Nat-M., Sulph.*) (A.).

Dryness of the skin, with crippled nails.

Every injury suppurates (*Hep., Sulph.*) (A.).

Old cicatrices break open again (A.).

ERYSIPELAS (*Apis, Ars., Bor., Canth., Hep., Rhus-T., Sulph.*).

Wandering or recurrent erysipelas (B.).

ECZEMATOUS ERUPTIONS WITH GLUTINOUS DISCHARGE (*Calc., Carb-S., Nat-M., Sulph.*) (K.).

Eczematous affections markedly benefitted.

Offensive perspiration (*Ars., Merc., Petr., Sil., Sulph.*).

Rhagades (*Ant-C., Calc., Carb-S., Kreos., Nat-M., Nit-Ac., Petr., Sars., Sep., Sulph.*).

Cracks or fissures in ends of fingers, nipples, labial commissures; between the toes (A.).

NAILS GROW THICK, CRACKED, OUT OF SHAPE (N.):

Sad and despondent; inclined to weep; thinks of nothing but death (*Aur., Nit-Ac.*) (N.).

Music makes her weep (A.).

Excessive cautiousness; timid, hesitates; unable to decide about anything (*Puls.*) (A.).

Anxiety about the future.

Forgetfulness; chooses wrong words in speaking or writing.

AGGRAVATION: At night; during and after menstruation; from music; from day-light; from suppressed menstruation; and from becoming cold.

AMELIORATION: When riding in a carriage; when in a noise; after eating; in the dark; and from eructation.

RELATIONSHIP: *Complementary: Caust., Hep.* and *Lyc.*

Graphites follows well after: Lyc. and *Puls.;* and after *Calc.* in obesity of women; follows *Sulph.* well in cutaneous diseases; and after *Sep.* in gushing leucorrhœa.

Similar to: Lyc. and *Puls.* in menstrual troubles.

Guaiacum.

COMMON NAME: LIGNUM VITAE.

Gouty nodosities (Am-M., Caust., Benz-Ac., Lyc., Sars.) (D.).

The affected parts are very sensitive to contact (*Arn., Kali-C., Lach.*).

Rheumatic affections, with contraction of the flexors and stiffness of the joints (Am-M., Caust., Cimex, Nat-M.) (A.).

JOINTS BECOME DISTORTED BY CONCRETIONS (*Apis, Benz-Ac., Calc., Calc-F., Colch., Form., Graph., Led., Lith., Lyc., Sil.*) (D.).

The limbs go to sleep.

Great weakness and debility in the legs with disinclination to move (*Cocc., Con., Kali-C., Nat-S., Nux-M., Nux-V., Phos-Ac., Plb., Rhus-T., Sep., Thuj.*).

Stiffness of the contracted parts (Am-M., Caust., Lyc.).

Tearing and stinging pain in the muscles of the upper and lower extremities, with heat of the parts.

Swelling and softening of the bones (*Calc., Calc-P., Sil.*).

Caries (*Calc., Calc-P., Merc., Nit-Ac., Phos., Sil.*).

Small pulse (*Ars., Camph., Carb-V., Cupr., Dig., Laur., Sec., Sil., Stram., Verat.*) (G.).

Sensation of protruding and swelling of the eyes; the lids seem too short to cover them (N.).

THROAT: BURNING, DRY, PAINFUL TO THE TOUCH (*Ars., Phyt., Sulph.*) (B.).

One-sided complaints.

Uncomfortable feeling in the body.

Painful duglutition (*Bell., Merc.*) (Bl.).

Follicular tonsillitis (*Kali-C.*) (Bl.).

Sweats profuse, on single parts, face, etc. (B.).

Night-sweats (*Hep., Kali-C., Merc., Nit-Ac., Phos., Sil., Sulph., Thuj.*) (B.).

Dry cough, with sharp, pleuritic pains (*Bry., Con., Phos.*) (Bl.).

COUGH WITH EXPECTORATION OF FETID PUS (*Ars., Calc., Caps., Kali-C., Merc., Nit-Ac., Phos., Sil.*) (N.).

Recurrent pleurisy (*Calc., Carb-An., Kali-C., Phos., Sil., Tub.*) (B.).

Constipation (*Alum., Bry., Sulph.*).

Hard and crumbling stools (*Am-M.*).

AGGRAVATION: From motion; in the evening; in the morning; while sitting; in the open air; in the fore-noon; from pressure; and from heat.

AMELIORATION: In the room.

RELATIONSHIP: *Similar to: Am-M., Bry., Caust., Hep., Merc., Nit-Ac., Phos., Sil.* and *Tub.*

Hamamelis.

COMMON NAME: WITCH HAZEL.

Adapted to venous hæmorrhage from every orifice of the body: nose, lungs, bowels, uterus and bladder (*Crot-H.. Ipec., Lach., Nit-Ac., Phos.*) (A.).

Small loss of blood causes great amount of prostration (*Phos.*) ʼ(G.).

Much weariness; easily gets tired (*Carb-An., Chin., Kali-P., Stann.*) (G.).

EPISTAXIS, EITHER ACTIVE OR PASSIVE; LONG-LASTING (*Carb-V., Lach., Phos.*) (Pr.).

HAEMOPTYSIS: ACTIVE OR PASSIVE, BLOOD VENOUS, AND COMES UP INTO THE MOUTH WITHOUT COUGHING, OR SCARCELY ANY EFFORT (*Ferr.*) (Py.).

Tickling cough, with taste of blood or Sulphur (A.).

Long-lasting hæmorrhage from extracting the teeth (*Carb-V., Lach., Phos., Sec.*) (Bt.).

Nose-bleed, ameliorates headache (*Ferr-P., Kali-B., Meli., Mill., Petr., Psor.*) (A.).

Hæmatemesis, with vomiting of large quantities of dark-coloured blood (*Con., Crot-H., Lach.*) (Pr.).

HAEMORRHOIDS BLEED VERY PROFUSELY, WITH SENSATION OF SORENESS, WEIGHT AND BURNING IN THE RECTUM; THEY PROTRUDE, AND ANUS FEELS SORE AS IF RAW (*Aloe, Lach., Mur-Ac., Sep., Sulph.*) (G.)

Dysenteric stools, loaded with dark, black blood (*Carb-V., Lach., Sulph.*) (Du.).

Discharge of blood per ani, in large quantities, of a tar-like consistency (*Lept.*); hence a specific in typhoid fever, with a bloody crisis (G.).

Uterine hæmorrhage; occurring at any time, where the flow is steady and slow (*Carb-V., Ferr., Sep.*); *the blood is dark-coloured; no uterine pains; profuse discharge of dark blood (Sab., Sec., Sep., Ust.)* (G.).

VICARIOUS MENSTRUATION (*Bry., Lach., Phos., Puls., Sulph.*) (A.).

HAEMATURIA OF DARK, BLACK BLOOD (*Ars., Crot-H., Lach.*) (Pr.).

Hæmaturia from passive congestion of the kidneys; dull pain in the renal region (Berb., Lyc., Sep.) (N.).

All sufferings worse at the menstrual period (Caul., Cimic., Graph., Puls., Sep) (A.).

Metrorrhagia: from jolting while riding over rough roads; or after a fall (A.).

Dysmenorrhœa, from ovarian irritation (Kn.).

Leucorrhœa, with much relaxation of the uterine walls (*Calc-P., Helon., Sep.*) (Ha.).

Cutting, tearing pains in the ovary, which is swollen and very tender (Apis, Lach.) (Bt.).

Traumatic conjunctivitis (*Arn., Ferr-P.*) (A.).

Intense soreness of the eyeballs (Arn., Calend., Led.) (A.).

Sugillations or extravasations into the chambers of the eyes from severe coughing (Arn.).

Blood-shot eyes (Bell., Stram.) (B.).

VARICOSE VEINS: HARD, KNOTTY, SWOLLEN, AND PAINFUL (*Calc-F., Ferr-P., Flour-Ac., Nat-M., Puls., Sep.*) (G.).

Articular and muscular rheumatism (*Arn., Bry., Caul., Ferr., Kali-B., Lyc., Merc., Nat-S., Petr., Rhus-T., Sep., Sil.*) (A.).

BRUISED SORENESS OF THE AFFECTED PARTS (*Arn., Bapt., Eup-P., Rhus-T.*) (A.).

Back feels as if it would break (Nat-M., Rhus-T., Sep., Sulph.) (G.).

Chronic effects of mechanical injuries (*Arn., Con., Sulph-Ac.*) (A.).

ORCHITIS, WITH MUCH PAIN, AND GREAT TUMEFACTION OF THE TESTICLES (*Arg-M., Clem., Puls., Spong.*) (Bt.).

VARICOSIS OF THE SPERMATIC VEINS; TESTICLES MUCH SWOLLEN, WITH DRAWING PAINS IN THE SPERMATIC CORDS (*Clem., Puls., Thuj.*) (Pr.).

Ecchymoses (*Arn., Sulph-Ac.*) (B.).

HAMMERING HEADACHE (*Bell., Chin., Nat-M.*) (B.).

Phlegmasia alba dolens (*Apis, Ars., Dig., Kali-C., Phos., Sep.*) (C.).

Great lassitude and weariness in the limbs and elsewhere (C.).

Scapular pains (*Chel., Kali-C., Phos., Sulph.*) (B.).

Takes cold easily from every exposure, especially in warm, moist air (A.).

Incised, lacerated or contused wounds (*Calend.*) (A.).

INJURIES FROM FALLS (*Arn.*) (A.).

AGGRAVATION: From pressure; from exposure to cold air; from jar; from motion; from touch; from riding in a carriage; and at night.

AMELIORATION: From taking rest; and lying quietly.

RELATIONSHIP: *Complementary*: *Ferrum*, in hæmorrhages and hæmorrhagic diathehis; and *Fluor-Ac.* in varicosis.

Compare: *Arn.* and *Calend.* for traumatic, and to hasten absorption of intra-ocular, hæmorrhage.

ANTIDOTES: *Puls.*

Like *Arn.* and *Calend., Hamamelis* has often seemed to act well as a local application.

Helleborus Niger.

COMMON NAMES: SNOW ROSE; CHRISTMAS ROSE.

Dropsy after scarlatina (*Apis, Ars., Calc., Dig., Kali-C., Lach., Lyc., Phos., Sulph.*).

Desquamation of the skin (*Ars., Kali-Ars., Sars., Sulph.*).

Vesicular eruption between the fingers and toes (*Rhus-T.*).

A falling off of both nails and hair (*Graph.*).

In the open air, he feels better, but has the sensation of having been ill for a long time.

Boring, stinging pains in such parts as cover the bones.

Stinging pain in the joints (Apis, Bell., Berb., Kali-C., Nit-Ac., Sil.).

When inattentive, the muscles refuse their office; in a word, whilst inattentively walking, there is a staggering in evidence (Con., Gels.).

CONVULSIVE TWITCHING OF THE MUSCLES, ESPECIALLY DURING SLEEP.

The pains, of a stinging, pressing or tearing character, often run across the affected parts.

Dullness of the internal senses (*Gels., Op., Phos-Ac.*).

STUPOR (*Arn., Bapt., Cupr., Gels., Kali-P., Lach., Lyc., Nux-V., Op., Phos-Ac., Sulph., Zinc.*).

HYDROCEPHALUS (*Apis, Bell., Bry., Canth., Gels., Hyos., Lach., Lyc., Op., Podo., Sulph., Zinc.*) (Bt.).

Slow comprehension (Gels., Op., Phos-Ac., Zinc.) (Ra.).

Coma: the patient cannot be roused (Op.) (Bl.).

HEAD ROLLS FROM SIDE TO SIDE ON THE PILLOW, OR IS DRAWN BACKWARD (*Apis, Bell., Cic., Cupr., Hyos., Lyc., Op., Podo., Stram., Tub., Zinc.*) (Bl.)

Beating the head with hands (A.).

Shocks pass through the brain like electricity (Ra.).

CHILD SUDDENLY SCREAMS AND BORES ITS HEAD INTO THE PILLOW (*Apis*) (D.).

FOREHEAD DRAWN IN FOLDS, AND COVERED WITH COLD PERSPIRATION (G.).

Brain symptoms during dentition (*Apis, Bell., Pod.*) (A.).

Eye-balls are distorted (D.).

Eyes are wide open and staring, but insensible to light (*Op.*) (Bl.).

Squinting; pupils dilated (G.).

BLUNTED SENSES AND SLUGGISH RESPONSES (*Arn., Bapt., Hyos.*) (B.).

Eyes half-open (*Lyc., Op.*) (A.).

Nostrils dirty and dry (Ra.).

Frequent rubbing of the nose (*Arum-T., Caust., Cina, Lyc., Merc., Nux-V., Phos-Ac., Sulph., Teucr.*) (G.).

Face pale and puffed (*Apis, Bry., Ferr., Nat-M., Puls., Sep.*) (G.).

Fœtor oris (*Carb-Ac., Kali-P., Merc., Nit-Ac., Sulph.*) (B.).

CHEWING MOTION OF THE MOUTH (*Acon., Bell., Bry., Calc., Cham., Gels., Lach., Merc., Phos., Sep. Stram.*) (Ra.).

DRINKS GREEDILY (*Ars., Bry., Sulph.*) (D.).

Bites spoon, but remains unconscious (A.).

Ptyalism (*Kali-B., Merc., Rhus-T.*) (B.).

Rumbling and rolling in the bowels (*Lyc., Podo., Sulph.*) (G.).

Diarrhœa (*Apis, Bapt., Kali-P.*).

Diarrhœa of jelly-like mucus (*Kali-B.*) (Ra.).

Diarrhœa during acute hydrocephalus, dentition or or pregnancy (A.).

Stools: *watery, clear, tenacious, colourless, mucous; like frog spawn (Phos.)* ; *involuntary* (A.).

Urine, after settling, looks like coffee-grounds (G.).

Dropsy: of brain, chest, abdomen; after scarlatina, intermittents; with fever, debility, suppressed urine; from suppressed exanthemata (*Apis, Rhus-T., Zinc.*) (A.).

Suppressed sexual desire (*Con., Phos.*).

Amenorrhœa from cold (*Puls.*) (B.).

Dreams: confused, unremembered; and anxious (C.).

SOPOROUS SLEEP, WITH SCREAMING AND STARTING (*Apis, Bell., Hyos., Stram.*) (G.).

Lies on the back with knees drawn up (B.).

Roaring and ringing in the ears (*Chin., Phos., Puls.*) (C.).

Aphthæ in the mouth (*Bor., Hep., Kali-M., Merc., Nat-M.*) (C.).

Nausea and vomiting of food (*Bry., Nux-V., Puls.*) (C.).

Chilliness and coldness predominating when the remedy cures.

Rigidity of the muscles of the neck, and limbs, one or both (Ra.).

AUTOMATIC MOTION OF ONE ARM AND ONE LEG (Ra.).

Convulsions with extreme coldness of the body, except head or occiput, which may be hot (*Arn.*) (A.).

Slow, small pulse (*Apis, Dig., Mur-Ac., Op., Phos., Verat-Alb.*).

Difficult breathing (*Ant-T., Carb-V., Lyc., Phos., Sulph*). (R.).

Chest constricted (*Ars., Cact., Lach., Sulph.*) (C.).

Gasps for breath (*Ipec., Phos.*) (C.).

Want of reaction (Ambr., Camph., Laur., Op., Sulph., Zinc.) (R.).

AGGRAVATION: In the cool air; during sleep; in the evening; from exertion; during dentition; and from suppressed eruptions.

AMELIORATION: In the open air; and from strong attention.

RELATIONSHIP: Compare *Apis, Apoc., Ars., Bell., Bry., Canth., Dig., Ferr., Gels., Kali-P., Lach., Lyc., Sulph., Tub.* and *Zinc.* in brain or meningeal affections.

Complementary: *Zinc.*

Antidotes: *Camph., China.*

Helonias Dioica.

COMMON NAME: UNICORN PLANT.

Generally called for women worn out with hard work, mental or physical, or enervated by luxury and indolence (A.).

Tendency to prolapsus and mal-positions of the uterus following confinement (*Nat-M., Sep.*) (Bl.).

So tired cannot sleep (A.).

Over-taxed muscles burn and ache (A.).

Tired, aching feeling in the back and limbs, with impaired nutrition (*Nat-M.*) (D.).

BAD EFFECTS OF ABORTIONS AND MISCARRIAGE (*Caul., Kali-C., Sec., Sep.*) (A.).

Great soreness and weight in the womb (D.).

A CONSCIOUSNESS OF A WOMB (D.).

Feels the womb move when she moves; it is so sore and tender (*Lyss.*) (A.).

Breast swollen, nipples painful and tender (*Con., Lac-C., Puls.*) (A.).

MENSES: TOO EARLY, TOO PROFUSE, FROM UTERINE ATONY IN WOMEN ENFEEBLED BY

LOSS OF BLOOD (*Chin., Sab., Sec.*); WHEN PATIENT LOSE MORE BLOOD THAN IS MADE IN THE INTER-MENSTRUAL PERIOD (A.).

Foul, lumpy or curdled leucorrhœa (*Calc.*) (B.).

PRURITUS VULVAE (*Calc., Kreos., Sep., Sulph.*) (Ha.).

Intense irritation of the external labia, which are puffed, hot, red, itch, and burn terribly (*Kreos.*) (Ha.).

Passive menorrhagia (*Ham., Puls., Sep.*) (Ha.).

Amenorrhœa, from anæmia, and general atonic condition of the system (Ha.).

Saccharine urine (*Lyc., Sep., Sulph.*) (A.).

EXCESSIVE URINE (*Apis, Gels., Kali-C., Lyc., Merc., Phos-Ac.*) (B.).

Acute or chronic albuminuria (*Apis, Ars., Kali-C., Phos., Sep.*) (A.).

NEPHRITIS OF PREGNANCY (*Apis, Merc-C., Phos.*) (B.)

Burning in the region of the kidneys (D.).

Deep gloom; melancholy (*Aur., Ign., Nat-M., Puls., Sep., Stann.*) (B.).

Irritable (*Bry., Nat-M., Nux-V., Sulph.*) (B.).

Wants to be let alone (*Ign., Nat-M., Sep.*) (B.).

Fault finding (*Nux-V., Sulph.*) (A.).

Cannot endure least contradiction, or receive least suggestion (*Anac., Aur., Cham., Nat-M.*) (A.).

ALWAYS BETTER WHEN OCCUPIED—WHEN NOT THINKING OF THE AILMENT (*Calc-P., Ox-Ac.*) (A.).

Restless; must be continually moving about (*Ars., Phos., Rhus-T.*) (A.).

AGGRAVATION: From motion; during and after menses and from contradiction.

AMELIORATION: When not thinking of her ailment.

RELATIONSHIP: *Compare*: *Alet., Chin., Ferr., Lil-T., Phos-Ac., Senec.* and *Sep.*

Similar to: *Alet.* in debility from prolapsus, protracted illness, and defective nutrition.

Hepar Sulphur.

COMMON NAMES: HAHNEMANN'S CALCIUM SULPHIDE; SULPHURET OF LIME.

Bad effects from the abuse of mercury (*Fluor-Ac., Nit-Ac., Sil.*).

Rheumatic swellings with heat and redness and a sensation as if sprained (*Bell., Rhus-T., Sulph.*).

Drawing pains in the limbs (*Rhus-T.*).

Stitches in the joints (*Bry., Kali-B., Nit-Ac., Sil.*).

GREAT SENSITIVENESS OF THE AFFECTED PARTS TO TOUCH (*Arn., Bell., Kali-C.*).

When handling the involved areas pain is felt as from sub-cutaneous ulceration.

INFLAMMATION ENDING IN SUPPURATION (*Calc-S., Merc., Sil.*).

Caries (*Calc-T., Fluor-Ac., Kali-B., Merc., Nit-Ac., Phos., Sil.*).

Erysipelas (*Apis, Ars., Bell., Calc-S., Ferr-P., Graph., Lach., Lyc., Merc., Puls., Rhus-T., Sil., Sulph.*).

FAINTING (IN THE EVENING FROM TRIFLING PAINS (*Lach.*).

UNHEALTHY SKIN; EVERY LITTLE WOUND SUPPURATES (*Sil., Sulph.*) (D.).

The skin is sensitive to the open air (*Sil.*); inflamed skin; injuries suppurate easily; eruptions and ulcerations are sensitive, and bleed easily (*Lach., Nit-Ac.*), and discharge a foul-smelling excretion; around the principal ulcerations there are little pimples (*Rhus-T.*) (D.).

BOILS OR ABSCESSES, WHERE THERE IS MUCH THROBBING AND STICKING IN THEM (if given low it will favour suppuration, and if given high it will sometimes abort the suppurative process (it comes always after *Bell.*) (D.).

Desire for highly seasoned food (Bl.).

Craving for strong things, as acids, etc. (D.).

Hunger and gnawing in the stomach (*Anac., Graph., Phos.*) (D.).

Craves acids, condiments or stimulants (B.).

Cannot bear anything tight about the waist (*Lach., Lyc., Nux-V.*) (D.).

Stool difficult, although soft (*Alum.*) (B.).

Diarrhœa: of children with sour smell (*Calc., Mag-C., Rheum, Sulph.*).

CLAY-COLOURED STOOL (*Aur-M-N., Berb., Calc., Card-M., Chel., Chion., Dig., Gels., Iod., Kali-B., Lach.. Lept., Merc., Nat-S., Podo., Sep.*) (A.).

Headache, as if a nail were being driven into the right side of the head (*Ign., Nit-Ac.*) (D.).

OFFENSIVE ERUPTIONS ON THE SCALP, WITH NON-EXCORIATING DISCHARGES AND GREAT TENDERNESS (D.).

Sweats profusely day and night without relief (*Merc.*); perspiration sour, offensive; easily, on every mental or physical exertion (*Bry., Calc., Psor., Sep.*) (A.).

Purulent affections about the eyes, hypo-pyon etc., worse from cold air, or cold applications (*Sil.*).

OVER-SENSITIVE, PHYSICALLY AND MENTALLY; THE SLIGHTEST CAUSE IRRITATES HIM (A.).

Quick, hasty speech and hasty drinking (*Bell.*) (A.).

Is peevish, angry at the least trifle; hycochondriacal; unreasonably anxious (A.).

Suicidal disposition (*Aur., Aur-M., Chin., Nat-S., Nit-Ac., Nux-V., Sep.*) (K.).

Hasty, violent, irritable or dissatisfied (B.).

OTALGIA, WITH SENSITIVENESS TO EXTERNAL CONTACT, OUT OF PROPORTION TO THE ACTUAL PAIN (N.).

Useful in pneumonia during the stage of resolution, when the expectoration is purulent and abscesses are threatened; also in broncho-pneumonia, when there is much mucus in the bronchial tubes, but it is difficult to raise (Bl.).

Should be remembered in chronic hepatitis and abscesses of the liver and kidneys when there is a vent for the pus, but the toxic symptoms persist (Bl.).

Asthma worse in dry, cold air and better in damp atmosphere (reverse of *Dulc., Nat-S.*) (N.).

SHARP, SPLINTER-LIKE PAINS IN THE THROAT (*Arg-N., Nit-Ac., Sil.*), OR A SENSATION AS IF THERE WERE A LUMP IN THE THROAT (*Ign., Lach., Nux-M., Phyt.*) (D.).

Quinsy, when suppuration threatens (A.).

Chronic hypertrophy of the tonsils, with hardness of hearing (*Bar-C., Calc., Lyc., Plb., Psor.*) (A.).

Urine: flow impeded, voided slowly, without force; drops vertically; is obliged to wait awhile before it passes; bladder weak, is unable to finish, seems as if some urine always remains (*Alum., Sil., Thuj.*) (A.).

HAEMORRHAGE FROM THE URETHRA AFTER URINATION (*Puls., Sars.*) (K.).

CHRONIC OTORRHOEA (*Calc., Calc-S., Merc., Nat-S., Puls., Sil., Tell.*) (B.).

Excoriation and humid soreness on the genitals, and in folds between the scrotum and the thighs (*Petr.*) (N.).

Weakness and much rattling in the chest (*Ant-T., Nat-S.*) (B.).

Whistling, choking breathing; must bend the head back (B.).

Ripened colds and old catarrhs (*Calc., Graph., Kali-S., Lyc., Puls.*) (B.).

Cough, with expectoration during the day, no expectoration at night (G.).

Suffocative attacks of breathing (*Ant-T., Ars., Samb.*) (G.).

DEEP, ROUGH, BARKING COUGH (*Spong.*), WITH HOARSENESS AND RATTLING OF MUCUS; WORSE IN COLD AIR, FROM COLD DRINKS, BEFORE MIDNIGHT OR TOWARDS MORNING (A.).

The cough of *Hepar* is never a dry one; it has a slight loose edge; the expectoration is slight, and there is little fever (D.).

WHOOPING COUGH (*Bell., Carb-V., Dros., Ipec., Kali-C., Meph., Phos., Sil.*).

WEEPING BEFORE, DURING OR AFTER COUGHING (*Arn., Bell.*) (K.).

Cough worse at night, especially after mid-night (*Dros., Kali-C.*) (K.).

CROUP, WHERE THE PATIENT IS SENSITIVE TO THE LEAST DRAUGHT OF AIR (it comes in here after *Acon.* and *Spong.*) (D.).

Cough: when any part of the body is uncovered (*Rhus-T.*).

CROUPY, CHOKING, STRANGLING COUGH (*Brom., Chlor., Iod., Spong.*) (A.).

AGGRAVATION: At night, especially during the nightly chill; from lying on the painful side (*Bell., Iod., Kali-C.*); from cold air; from uncovering; after eating or drinking cold things; and from touching the affected parts (*Arn., Lach.*).

AMELIORATION: From warmth in general (*Ars., Sil.*); from wrapping up warmly, especially the head (*Psor.,*

Sil.), and in damp, wet weather (*Caust., Nux-V.*—reverse of *Nat-S.*).

RELATIONSHIP: *Complementary to: Calend.* in injuries of soft parts, and *Spong.* in croup.

Complementary to Hep.: *Iod.* and *Sil.*

Hepar antidotes the bad effects of Mercury and other metals, Quinine, Iodine, Iodide of Potash, and Cod-liver oil.

Hydrastis Canadensis.

COMMON NAME: GOLDEN SEAL.

Adapted for debilitated persons, with viscid mucous discharges (A.).

Cachectic or malignant dyscrasia, with marked derangement of gastric and hepatic functions (A.).

Broken down by excessive use of alcohol (Carb-V., Mur-Ac., Nux-V., Puls., Sulph.) (A.).

Sensation of sinking in the epigastric region (*Dig., Hell., Hydr-Ac., Kali-B., Lept., Lyc., Merc., Murx., Nat-M., Nux-V., Sep., Staph., Tab., Verat.*) (Bl.).

Nursing sore mouth (*Bor., Merc., Nat-M., Nux-V., Puls., Rhus-T.*) (A.).

Stomatitis after mercury or potash; peppery taste; tongue as if burned or raw (N.).

Atonic dyspepsia (Carb-V., Hep., Lyc., Nux-V., Puls.) (D.).

Torpidity of the liver (Nux-V.) (D.).

TONGUE LARGE; FLABBY; SHOWS IMPRINTS OF TEETH (*Ars., Carb-V., Chel., Dulc., Ign., Iod., Kali-I., Merc., Podo., Rhus-T., Sep., Stram., Syph., Tell.*) (A.).

Catarrhal jaundice (Nux-V., Sep.) (Bl.).

Constipation: stools like sheep dung; gray, hard, knotty or large; or light-coloured (K.).

PROFUSE DISCHARGE OF THICK, YELLOW, STRINGY MUCUS FROM THE NASAL PASSAGES (*Cor-R., Kali-B.*) (A.).

The nasal discharge is more profuse when out of doors (*Ars., Carb-Ac., Dulc., Euphr., Iod., Nit-Aç., Puls., Sabad.*) (D.).

Alternate diarrhœa and constipation (*Ant-C., Chel., Nit-Ac., Nux-V., Op., Podo.*) (K.).

Hawks yellow, viscid mucus from posterior nares and fauces; ulceration, after abuse of Mercury or Chlorate of Potash; syphilitic angina (*Kali-B.*) (A.).

Constipation, especially of children and the aged (*Ant-C.*) (Bl.).

Stools often come mixed with mucus (*Graph., Nux-V., Sulph.*) (Bl.).

Constipation, after abuse of drugs (*Bry., Chin., Coloc., Nux-V.*) (K.).

After stool pain in the rectum (*Ign., Nit-Ac., Thuj.*) (N.).

LEUCORRHOEA: ROPY, THICK, VISCID, YELLOW; HANGING FROM THE OS IN LONG STRINGS (*Kali-B.*) (A.).

Pruritus vulvæ (*Ambr., Ars., Calad., Calc., Caust., Coff., Dulc., Graph., Helon., Kali-Br., Kreos., Lap-A., Merc., Nat-M.*) (A.).

Profuse albuminous leucorrhœa accompanied by sexual excitement (Bo.).

CANCER: HARD, ADHERENT; SKIN MOTTLED, PUCKERED; PAINS KNIFE-LIKE, SHARP, CUTTING; NIPPLE RETRACTED (A.).

Erosions, and superficial ulcerations of the cervix and vagina, with tenacious discharge (Ha.).

Balanitis or gonorrhœa (*Cann-S., Kali-B., Puls., Sep.*) (Bt.).

Pain the vertex every other day at 11 A.M., with excessive nausea, anguish and retching (A.).

Chronic bronchitis of old, debilitated people (*Carb-V., Kali-B., Seneg.*) (N.).

Catarrhal deafness (*Calc., Phos., Puls.*) (D.).

Muco-purulent discharge from the ears (D.).

Roaring in the ears (*Chin., Puls.*) (D.).

Small-pox: great swelling; redness and itching, with great soreness of the throat (Bt.).

Palpitation with weakness (*Kali-P., Nat-M., Phos., Sep.*) (B.).

Profuse sweating (*Calc., Con., Kali-C., Merc., Nat-M., Verat.*) (B.).

Heat alternating with chilliness (*Ars., Bry., Chin., Nux-V., Rhus-T.*) (B.).

CHRONIC CATARRH OF THE BLADDER WITH THICK, ROPY MUCUS IN THE URINE (*Kali-B.*) (R.).

Catarrhal ophthalmia, with thick, mucous discharge (*Euphr., Kali-M., Nat-S., Puls.*) (C.).

AGGRAVATION: During pregnancy; from abuse of wine; from abuse of drugs; after stool; every other day; and in the open air.

AMELIORATION: In dry weather; and from warm covering.

RELATIONSHIP: *Compare*: *Ars., Bor., Chel., Con., Graph., Hep., Kali-B., Merc-C., Nat-M., Nat-S Phyt., Puls., Sep., Sil., Stram.* and *Sulph.*

Antidote: *Sulph.*

Hydrastis antidotes: *Merc.* and *Kali Chlor.*

Hyoscyamus.

COMMON NAME: HENBANE.

Bad effects from catching cold and cold air.

Bad effects from jealousy—(a mental modality).

Internal inflammatory states with nervous symptoms.

Great sinking of strength.

Spasms and convulsions (Bell., Cic., Cupr., Gels., Kali-P., Lach., Lyc., Mosch., Nux-V., Op., Sec., Tarant., Verat.).

Epileptic attacks, ending in sleep and snoring.

St. Vitus's dance (Agar., Gels., Nux-V., Tarant.).

Vertigo, then spasm (B.).

Cold and tumbling limbs, which go to sleep.

Insensibility of the body.

INVOLUNTARY MOTIONS AND POOR BLADDER CONTROL OF MICTURITION (*Op.*).

SPASMS DURING PREGNANCY, DURING PARTURITION, WHEN TRYING TO SWALLOW FLUIDS, AND FROM WORMS (*Bell., Stram.*).

Hydrophobia (Bell., Lyss.) (G.).

Convulsions: of children, from fright or the irritation of the intestinal worms (Calc., Cina, Cupr., Mag-P.) (A.).

After meals, the child vomits; then sudden shrieks with insensibility (A.).

SPASMS WITHOUT CONSCIOUSNESS (*Arg-N., Bufo, Calc., Cic., Cocc., Cupr., Ipec., Lach., Oena., Op., Plb., Stram., Sulph., Visc.*) (A.).

Every muscle in the body twitches, from the eyes to the toes (A.).

Pupils dilated (*Bell.*) (G.).

Incipient amaurosis and a perversion of the visual sense (Gels., Phos., Puls.).

Diplopia (Bell., Gels., Stram.) (G.).

A useful remedy in mania and inflammation of the brain.

LASCIVIOUS MANIA: IMMODESTY, WILL NOT BE COVERED; KICKS OFF THE CLOTHES, EXPOSES THE PERSON; SINGS OBSCENE SONGS; LIES NAKED IN BED AND CHATTERS (A.).

Bad effects of unfortunate love; with jealousy, rage, incoherent speech, or inclination to laugh at everything (A.).

Silly, with comical acts (B.).

Plays with fingers (B.).

FEARS: BEING ALONE; POISON; BEING BITTEN; BEING SOLD; TO EAT OR DRINK; TO TAKE WHAT IS OFFERED; SUSPICIOUS OF SOME PLOT (A.).

Delirium, with restlessness; jumps out of bed, tries to escape (*Bell., Stram.*); makes irrelevant answers; thinks he is in the wrong place; talks of imaginary doings, but has no wants and make no complaints (A.).

Typhoid fever: Sensorium clouded; staring eyes; grasping at flocks or picking bed-clothes; teeth covered with sordes; tongue dry and unwieldy; involuntary stool and urine; subsultus tendinum (A.).

Talks of business (*Bry.*) (C.).

Speaks each word louder (B.).

With muttering, the lower jaw drops (*Lyc.*) (B.).

Slides down in bed (*Mur-Ac.*) (B.).

Shakes head to and fro; worse bending forward (B.).

Imbecility of the intellect; memory weak or lost (G.).

Entire loss of consciousness; sees persons who are not, and have not been present; loss of sight and hearing (N.).

Watery, painless diarrhœa (*Chin., Kali-P., Podo., Rici.*).

Much distension of the abdomen (*Carb-V., Chin., Lyc., Op., Tereb.*) (Bt.).

Nervous wakefulness (*Ambr., Coff., Gels., Nux-V.*) (B.).

STARTS OUT OF SLEEP (*Bell., Gels., Stram.*) (B.).

SPASMS OF DRY, HACKING, NIGHT COUGH; FROM A DRY SPOT IN THE LARYNX (*Con.*); WORSE FROM LYING, EATING OR TALKING (*Phos.*) (B.).

Hardness of hearing, as if stupefied, especially after apoplexy (N.).

All objects appear red, or larger than they really are, or double (Hm.).

Paralysis of the sphincter ani and vesicæ, with involuntary stool and urine (Hm.).

AGGRAVATION: In the evening; after eating and drinking; during rest; during menses; at night; from jealousy; from unhappy love; from fright; when lying down; and at the beginning of menstruation.

AMELIORATION: From sitting up; on stooping.

RELATIONSHIP: Compare *Bell., Lach., Stram.* and *Verat.*

Phos. often cures lasciviousness when *Hyos.* fails.

Antidotes: *Bell.* and *Stram.*

Hypericum.

COMMON NAME: ST. JOHN'S WORT.

It is the *Arnica* of the nerves (D.).

Consequence of spinal concussions (*Arn.*) (N.).

Injuries of the nerves in general (D.).

INJURIES FROM TREADING ON NAILS, NEEDLES, PINS, SPLINTERS, OR FROM RAT-BITES; PREVENTS LOCK-JAW (A.).

Bad effects from falls or blows upon the head, or concussion of the spine (N.).

Neuritis: the surrounding parts are inflamed; there is tingling, burning pain and numbness (Bl.).

INJURIES TO PARTS RICH IN SENTIENT NERVES, ESPECIALLY FINGERS, TOES, AND MATRICES OF NAILS (N.).

Headache and meningitis depending upon an injury to the nervous system (*Arn., Nat-S.*).

LACERATIONS, WHEN INTOLERABLE PAIN SHOWS THAT THE NERVES ARE INVOLVED; TO PREVENT OR CURE LOCK-JAW, OR CONVUL-SIONS (N.).

Tetanus (Arn., Bell., Nux-V.), after traumatic injuries (A.).

Intolerably violent, shooting or lancinating pains along the nerves (B.).

Pains, after a fall on the coccyx (A.).

Nervous depression following wounds or surgical operations (A.).

Asthma ameliorated by expectoration (K.).

Asthmatic respiration after injury of the spine (K.).

Pressure and burning in the chest (*Phos.*).

Removes bad effects of shock, fright, or mesmerism (A.).

Nightly urging to urinate, with vertigo.

Spine very sensitive to touch (*Phos.*) (A.).

Feeling of weakness and trembling of all the limbs.

Convulsions after blows on the head or concussion (A.).

After a fall, slightest motion of arms or neck extorts cries (C.).

CRUSHED, MASHED FINGER-TIPS (A.).

AGGRAVATION: From motion; from touch; from pressure; and at night.

AMELIORATION: From lying quietly.

RELATIONSHIP: Compare *Arn., Calend., Nat-S., Ruta* and *Staph.*

Ignatia.

COMMON NAME: ST. IGNATIUS BEAN.

Especially suited to women of a sensitive, easily excited nature (*Puls.*) (A.).

BAD EFFECTS FROM FRIGHT AND SORROW, OFFENCES AND UNFORTUNATE LOVE AFFAIRS.

In talking or chewing they bite themselves in the cheek or tongue (N.).

The remedy of great contradictions: the roaring in the ears relieved by music; the piles better when walking; sore-throat feels relieved when swallowing; empty feeling in the stomach not ameliorated by eating; cough aggravates the more he coughs; cough on standing still during a walk; spasmodic laughter from grief; sexual desire with impotency; headache relieved by stooping; thirst during a chill, no thirst in the fever; the colour changes in the face when at rest (A.).

Pain, as from pressing of a pointed, hard body from the inside to the outside.

Pressing asunder or constriction in the internal organs.

Pain, as if dislocation in the joints.

Tingling and sensation, as if the limbs had gone to sleep.

Change of position relieves the pains (*Kali-P., Rhus-T.*) (N.).

SPASMODIC AND HYSTERICAL COMPLAINTS (*Asaf., Bell., Cupr., Gels., Kali-P., Lach., Lyc., Mosch., Nat-C., Puls.*).

Convulsive twitches (*Agar., Bell., Cupr., Hyos., Stram., Tarant., Zinc.*).

Spasmodic yawning.

Convulsion with oppression of breathing during dentition.

Convulsive jerkings of arms and legs, or single jerks of limbs on falling asleep (N.).

Spasms in children from fright (*Acon., Hyos., Op.*) (Bt.).

Chorea: the convulsions are greatest in the mouth, producing much distortion of the face (Bt.).

Nervous headache, usually confined to one spot (R.).

Constipation, from carriage-riding (A.).

Throbbing pain in the occiput, worse from pressing at stool, smoking, or the smell of smoke (N.).

Blind piles, with pressure in the anus and rectum; painful when sitting and standing, less when walking (R.).

There is a lump in the throat and a sticking sensation, which is relieved by swallowing (D.).

Sorethroat: stitching or sticking pains only between the acts of deglutition; better swallowing solids (N.).

Cutting and stinging, as from a sharp knife.

SADNESS AND SIGHING, WITH SOBS AND TEARS, AND WILL NOT BE COMFORTED; WANTS TO BE ALONE. SILENT GRIEF (N.).

FICKLENESS (*Agar., Asaf., Bism., Cimic., Coff., Lac-C., Lach., Nat-C., Sil.*).

Amiable disposition if feeling well; every little emotion disturbs them (N.).

Introspective (D.).

Has a disposition to brood over her sorrow (D.).

INCREDIBLE CHANGE OF MOOD; JESTING AND LAUGHTER CHANGING TO SADNESS AND TEARS (*Nux-M.*) (N.).

Great sensitiveness to external impressions; patients laugh and cry alternately; face flushes on emotion; spasmodic laughing ending in screaming; globus hystericus; profuse pale urine, flatulent conditions; contortions of the muscles (D.).

Heaviness in the head as if congested, relieved by stooping; there is pain as if a nail were driven into the parietal or occipital region; clavus hystericus; the headache ends in vomiting or in a copious discharge of pale urine.

INVOLUNTARY SIGHING; MUST TAKE A LONG BREATH (*Bry., Phos.*) (N.).

Pruritus vulvæ with itching extending up into the vagnia (*Calad., Calc., Graph., Kreos., Merc., Nit-Ac., Petr., Sep., Sulph.*) (N.).

Boring pain in the front teeth, and a soreness in all the teeth; worse after drinking coffee, after smoking, after

dinner, in the evening, after lying down, and in the morning (Hr.).

Gets sleepy after every coughing spell (N.).

Dry, spasmodic cough in quick, successive shocks, as if a feather was in the throat; the more the patient coughs the more he wants to, and is only stopped by an effort of the will; the cough occurs in the evening on lying down (D.).

Pain in small, circumscribed spots (A.).

Menses: Scanty, black, of a putrid odour (*Cycl., Sep., Sulph.*) (G.).

Metrorrhagia (*Ham., Lach., Puls., Sec.. Sep.*).

Menstruation too early, and too profuse (*Sep.*).

Uterine spasms, with lancinations or labour-like pains.

Purulent, corrosive leucorrhœa (*Ars., Calc., Kreos., Merc., Nit-Ac., Sep.*) (C.).

Erection during stool (C.).

Complete loss of sexual desire (*Agn., Graph., Sep., Sulph.*) (C.)

Convulsive movements of eyes and lids (*Agar.*) (C.).

Complaints return at precisely the same hour (A.).

INTERMITTENT FEVER, WITH THIRST DUR-ING THE CHILL ONLY (*Apis, Arn., Caps., Cina, Eup-P., Ferr., Nat-M., Nux-V., Pyrog., Sep., Sil., Tub., Verat.*).

External heat with internal shuddering (*Ars., Bry., Calc., Lyc., Meny., Nux-V., Pyrog., Sep., Thuj.*).

SHAKING CHILL WITH REDNESS OF THE FACE (*Am-M., Arn., Cham., Ferr., Nux-V. Stram.*) (N.).

Chill relieved by warm room or hot stove (N.).

Hæmorrhoids: the tumors prolapse with every stool, and have to be replaced; they are sore as if excoriated; both hæmorrhage and pain are worse when the stool is loose (Dn.).

Sweats on the face while eating (N.).

Bleeding after, and during stool (*Lach., Nux-V., Sulph.*) (Dn.).

Neuralgia of the rectum (Bt.).

Constipation, associated with constant, ineffectual urging to stool (*Nux-V.*) (Bl.).

Itching about the anus, as from ascarides (*Calc., Cina, Teucr.*) (D.).

Painful contraction of the sphincter after stool (*Bell., Lach.*) (D.).

PROLAPSUS ANI (*Podo., Sulph.*).

Coarse stitches from the anus deep up into the rectum (*Nit-Ac., Sil.*) (N.).

The patient vomits simple food, but retains such things as cabbage (D.).

WEAK, EMPTY, GONE FEELING AT THE PIT OF THE STOMACH, NOT RELIEVED BY EATING (N.).

Bitter taste in the mouth (*Ars., Bry., Chin., Nat-M., Nux-V., Puls., Sep., Sulph.*) (D.).

Extreme aversion to tobacco-smoke (N.).

Regurgitation of a bitter fluid (*Eup-P., Nat-M., Puls., Sep.*) (D.).

Feeling of flabbiness in the stomach; stomach and intestines seem to hang down relaxed (N.).

Empty retching, relieved by eating (D.).

Hiccough (*Bell., Mag-P., Nux-V.*) (D.).

Distension of the abdomen after eating (*Carb-V., Lyc.*) (D.).

AGGRAVATION: In the evening; after lying down; in the morning; after awaking; after eating; after the use of tobacco and coffee; from the slightest touch; and from mental emotions.

AMELIORATION: From change of position; from lying on the painful side; from hard pressure; from profuse urination; and from warmth.

RELATIONSHIP: *Antidotes*: *Coff., Nux-V.* and *Puls.*

Similar to: *Agar., Apis, Bell., Cimic., Cycl., Ferr., Gels., Hep., Kali-B., Kali-P., Lach., Lyc., Mosch., Nat-M., Nux-V., Op., Puls., Sep.* and *Sulph.*

Complementary: *Aur., Nat-M. and Phos-Ac.*

Iodium.

COMMON NAME: IODINE.

Adapted to persons of a scrofulous diathesis, with a low, cachectic condition, profound debility and great emaciation (*Abrot., Nat-M., Sanic.*) (A.).

Bad effects of mercury (*Chin., Dulc., Hep., Lach., Nit-Ac.*) (Bt.).

EMACIATION TO A SKELETON.

Great debility; the slightest effort induces perspiration (*Calc., Chin., Kali-C., Sep.*).

Violent trembling of the limbs (*Agar., Gels., Kali-Br., Lach., Merc., Mygale, Phos., Plb., Sil., Tarant., Zinc.*)

Twitching of the muscles (*Bell., Cur., Gels., Hyos., Lach.*).

Great excitability of the whole nervous system (*Coff., Gels., Phos.*).

Violent tearing in the joints.

CHRONIC RHEUMATISM OF THE JOINTS, WITH NIGHTLY PAINS WITHOUT SWELLING.

Swelling and induration of the glands are of major importance when the remedy is indicated.

White swelling of the knee (*Apis, Bry., Kali-C., Puls., Rhus-T., Sep.*).

Struma.

Nightly pains in the bones (*Aur., Merc., Mezer., Sarsa., Sil., Syph.*).

Softening of the bones (*Calc., Calc-P., Merc., Phos., Sil.*).

Hæmorrhages from various organs (*Arn., Bell., Chin., Ferr-P., Ham., Ipec., Kali-P., Lach., Merc., Nit-Ac., Phos., Trill., Ust.*).

Pulsations (*Bell., Nat-M., Sep.*).

Warm-blooded notwithstanding emaciation; wants a cool place to move, think, or work in (N.).

Great weakness and loss of breath on going up-stairs (N.).

Inflammations of the larynx and trachea (*Brom., Chlor., Kali-M., Phos.*).

WHEEZING AND SAWING RESPIRATION (*Spong.*) (A.).

CROUP: THERE IS A HOARSE VOICE AND DIFFICULT INSPIRATION; THE CHILD GRASPS ITS THROAT; CROUP CAUSED BY LONG-CON-TINUED DAMP WEATHER (D.).

Membranous croup (*Brom., Chlor., Kali-B., Kali-M., Merc-Cyn., Phos.*) (N.)

Phthisis pulmonalis, with constant tickling and inclina-tion to cough, in the wind-pipe and under the sternum; expectoration of transparent mucus, streaked with blood; morning sweats; emaciation; wasting fever; rapid pulse; diarrhœa; and in females amenorrhœa (Hg.)

First and second stages of pneumonia, especially in the croupous form, where the hepatization tends to extend rapidly; difficulty in breathing, as if the chest would not expand; cough and blood-streaked sputa, accompanied by high fever (*Bry., Kali-M., Phos., Sulph.*) (D.).

Continual taste of salt in the mouth (*Merc., Merc-C., Nat-M., Puls.*) (G.).

Constipation, with ineffectual urging, relieved by drink-ing cold milk (A.).

HUNGER AND THIRST INCREASED (*Ars., Bism., Chel., Phos., Sulph.*).

Continual empty eructations, from morning till evening, as if every particle of food was turned into air (G.).

RAVENOUS APPETITE, WITH GREAT EMA-CIATION (*Abrot., Nat-M., Sanic.*) (D.).

Extreme hunger, but inspite of this the patient emaciates. (D.).

ALWAYS HUNGRY; EATS OR WANTS TO EAT ALL THE TIME, YET EMACIATES; AMELIO-RATED WHILE EATING (N.).

Pancreas enlarged (*Phos.*) (R.).

Pulsations all over, stomach, back, even arms, fingers and toes (*Bell.*) (N.).

The patient is subject to wasting diseases (*Calc-P., Lyc., Nat-M., Sil., Tub.*) (D.).

THERE IS WASTING OF THE MAMMAE, OVARIES, TESTICLES, ETC. (D.).

Frothy, wheyey, fatty, cheesy or lienteric stools (B.).

ENLARGEMENT OF THE THYROID GLAND OR GOITRE (*Calc-F., Spong.*) (D.).

Hypertrophy of all glands except mammary, which dwindle; while body withers glands enlarge (N.).

Tabes mesenterica, with rapid emaciation, night-sweats, slow fever, dry laryngeal cough, diarrhœa, etc. (Hg.).

ORCHITIS, WITH PAINS EXTENDING TO THE ABDOMEN (*Bell., Clem., Puls.*) (D.).

Chronic congestive headache in old people (*Gels., Lach., Nat-C., Sep., Sulph.*) (Bt.).

Hard swelling in the inguinal glands (*Bad., Carb-An., Merc-I-F.*) (R.).

Mentally anxious; anguish, wants to move, to do something, to hurry, to kill somebody, etc. (N.).

DEJECTED, OR INTOLERABLY CROSS AND RESTLESS (*Aur., Phos., Sulph.*) (B.).

Melancholy mood (*Nat-M., Puls.*) (C.).

Vertigo (*Chin., Kali-P., Lyc.*) (C.).

Urine at times turbid, dark, at others milky (R.).

Cirrhosis of the liver (*Chel., Mur-Ac., Phos., Sulph.*) (R.).

REGION OF THE LIVER SORE TO PRESSURE (*Bell., Chel., Dig., Hep., Lach., Merc., Nat-S., Phos., Sep.*) (R.).

Chronic enlargement of the spleen (*Ars., Cean., Chin., Nat-M., Sep.*) (R.).

SENSATION AS IF THE HEART WAS SQUEEZ-ED TOGETHER; AS IF GRASPED WITH AN IRON HAND (*Cact., Sulph.*) (N.).

Palpitation, worse from least exertion (*Dig.*) (A.).

Præcordial anxiety causing constant change of position (*Acon., Ars.*) (R.).

Peri-carditis attending pneumonia and rheumatism (Bl.).

Tongue loaded with thick coating (*Ant-C., Kali-M., Puls.*) (C.).

Offensive odour from the mouth (*Aur., Carb-Ac., Merc., Nit-Ac., Sulph.*) (C.).

THICK, YELLOW LEUCORRHOEA, SO CORRO-DING THAT IT EATS HOLES IN THE LINEN (N.).

Leucorrhœa, worse during the menses (G.).

Tumours in the breast (*Calc-F., Con., Carb-An., Graph., Phyt., Sil.*) (N.).

Great weakness during the menses, particularly when going upstairs (G.).

Long-lasting uterine hæmorrhages (G.).

Uterine hæmorrhage after every stool (*Ambr., Am-M., Ind., Lyc.*), *with cutting pains in the abdomen, loins and back.*

Cancerous degeneration of the cervix (*Ars., Kreos., Nit-Ac., Phos., Sep.*) (A.).

AGGRAVATION: From heat; from fasting; in warm air; in a warm room; from wrapping up the head (reverse of *Hep., Psor.* and *Sil.*); at night; during rest.

AMELIORATION: While eating; from moving; in cold air; and from bathing.

RELATIONSHIP: *Complementary to*: *Lyc.*

Compare: *Acet-Ac., Brom., Chlor., Con., Kali-B.* and *Spong.* in membranous croup.

Follows well after: *Hep.,* and *Merc.;* and is followed by *Kali-B.* in croup.

Antidotes: *Bell., Camph., Hep.,* and *Phos.*

Ipecacuanha.

COMMON NAME: IPECAC.

Adapted to cases where the gastric symptoms predominate (*Ant-C., Kali-M., Nux-V., Puls., Sep.*) (A.).

Relieves the exhaustion following bleeding from the orifices of the body (*Carb-V., Chin., Ferr., Kali-P., Sec.*).

Tetanic spasms (*Bell., Cic., Cupr., Nux-V., Op., Strych., Verat.*).

Spasmodic oppression of the chest after taking cold (*Ant-T., Phos., Stram.*).

Whooping cough (*Ant-T., Cina, Cupr., Dros., Kali-C., Meph., Puls., Verat.*).

CONVULSIVE COUGH; THE CHILD STIFFENS AND BECOMES PALE OR BLUE AND LOSES ITS BREATH; GREAT NAUSEA AND RELIEF FROM VOMITING (D.).

A sensation in the joints as if they had gone to sleep, with tingling of the same.

Tearing in the limbs when going to sleep.

Hæmorrhages (active) from all orifices, profuse, bright red (*Mill., Phos.*) (N.).

Cough with bloody expectoration (*Phos.*) (G.).

Miliary eruptions, when they come out with difficulty, or when they appear on females during the period of uterogestation.

Bad effects from the abuse of Opium, Arsenic and Quinine (*Puls.*).

Sensation as if the bones of the head were crushed or bruised; there is unilateral sick headache over one eye, with deathly nausea and very pale face: there is a drawn nauseated expression about the mouth (D.).

Incessant cough with every breath (D.).

DRY, SPASMODIC COUGH, ENDING IN CHOKING AND GAGGING (D.).

A tickling extends from the larynx to the extremities of the bronchi (D.).

Coarse rales all over the chest, with violent paroxysms of coughing and retching, pale face and great dyspnœa (D.).

TONGUE CLEAN, OR SLIGHTLY COATED (*Apis, Ars., Bell., Colch., Ferr-P., Gels., Kali-B., Lac-C., Merc., Nit-Ac., Phos., Rhus-T.*) (A.).

APPLICABLE IN ALL DISEASES WITH CONSTANT AND CONTINUAL NAUSEA (*Ant-C., Ant-T., Ars., Cadm., Dig., Graph., Kreos., Lac-C., Lyc., Mag-M., Nat-M., Nux-V., Petr., Phos., Sil., Verat.*) (A.).

Nausea accompanies most complaints (*Ant-T., Nux-V., Puls.*).

Bad effects from intemperance and cold; also from effects of pork eating.

DISTRESSING AND INTENSE NAUSEA AND INCLINATION TO VOMIT, AND AFTER VOMITING THERE IS IMMEDIATE INCLINATION TO DO SO AGAIN. CONSTANT NAUSEA WITH A CLEAN TONGUE IS THE WATCHWORD (D.).

Intense nausea and vomiting, which is followed by exhaustion and sleepiness (*Aeth., Ant-T.*) (D.).

Troubles arising from fat food, pork, pastry, candy, etc. (D.).

The stomach has a hanging down, relaxed feeling (*Carb-An., Sep., Sulph.*) (D.).

Vomiting of large quantities of tenacious, white, glairy mucus (Bt.).

DESIRE FOR DELICACIES (*Aur., Chin., Kali-C., Mag-C., Nat-C., Rhus-T., Sabad., Spong., Tub.*) (K.).

Aversion to food (*Ars., Chin., Cocc., Colch., Ferr., Lil-T., Nux-V.*) (K.).

Flatulent, cutting colic about the umbilicus (A.).

Diarrhœa of a dysenteric nature (*Acon., Bell., Colch., Coloc., Merc-C., Nux-V., Sulph.*).

Autumnal dysentery; cold nights, after hot days (*Acon., Colch., Merc.*) (A.).

STOOL: GRASSY-GREEN; OF WHITE MUCUS (*Ant-C., Colch.*); BLOODY; FERMENTED; FOAMY; SLIMY; LIKE FROTHY MOLASSES (A.).

Asiatic Cholera: First symptoms, where nausea and vomiting predominate (*Ant-C., Nux-V., Puls.*) (A.).

Often used in the secondary stage of cholera when marked nausea and persistent vomiting is present (*Ars., Bism., Colch., Cupr., Cupr-Ars., Phos., Podo., Sec., Tab., Verat.*).

Metrorrhagia (*Calc., Chin., Cinnm., Ferr., Kali-C., Lach., Nit-Ac., Phos., Sep., Sulph., Ust., Vib.*).

Hæmorrhages of bright red blood, which flows steadily (D.).

DURING HAEMORRHAGE FROM THE WOMB SHE COMMENCES TO BREATHE HEAVILY (N.).

POST-PARTUM HAEMORRHAGE; PROFUSE FLOW, BRIGHT RED AND CONSTANT NAUSEA (N.).

Threatened abortion, often with a sharp or pinching pain around the umbilicus, which runs downward to the uterus, with constant nausea and discharge of bright, red blood (G.).

Menstruation too early and too profuse (*Chin., Phos., Sep.*) (G.).

Vomiting of pregnancy (*Bry., Colch., Nux-V., Sep., Symphori., Tab.*) (A.).

Chlorosis: menses scanty; skin and mucous surfaces pale, anæmic (*Calc., Ferr., Nat-M.*) (C.).

Cutting pains across the abdomen from left to right (*Lach.;* from right to left—*Lyc.*) (A.).

Red, scanty urine (*Lyc., Puls., Sep.*) (C.).

Pains from the region of the kidneys into the thighs (*Agar., Berb., Hep., Kali-B., Nux-V.*) (K.).

Intermittent fever with slight chills and much heat, which is accompanied with much heat, gastric symptoms, and oppression of the chest in all cases.

Backache, short chill long fever; mostly heat with thirst; raging headache, nausea, cough, and sweat last; chill worse in warm room or warm covering (N.).

Better than quinine in intermittents, or after its abuse, the symptoms agreeing (N.).

One hand cold, the other hot (Hr.).

Postponing type of fever (*Alst., Bry., Chin., Cina, Gamb., Ign., Ipec.*) (K.).

Catarrhal or gastric fevers (*Acon., Ant-C., Bry., Kali-M., Nux-V., Puls.*) (B.).

PAINS IN THE EXTREMITIES DURING CHILL (*Ars., Bov., Coloc., Dulc., Eup-P.*) (K.).

EPISTAXIS WITH WHOOPING COUGH (*Arn., Bry., Cina, Cor-R., Crot-H., Dros., Led., Merc., Mur-Ac., Nux-V., Spong., Stram.*) (K.).

Sneezing with cough and expectoration (R.).

Capillary bronchitis with great accumulation of mucus in the larger tubes, violent paroxysms of coughing, retching and vomiting, also expectoration of a good deal of mucus (R.).

SPASMODIC ASTHMA, WITH WEIGHT AND ANXIETY ABOUT THE CHEST; SUDDEN WHEEZING DYSPNOEA, THREATENING SUFFOCATION; AGGRAVATED BY MOTION; THE COUGH CAUSES GAGGING AND VOMITING (D.).

Hæmoptysis: *the blood is bright red and comes in gushes, with nausea and gagging* (D.).

The chest seems full of phlegm, but does not yield to coughing (*Ant-T.*).

AGGRAVATION: From motion; in winter and dry weather; in warm moist, south winds; from the slightest motion; from stooping; and over-eating.

AMELIORATION: In the open air;

RELATIONSHIP: *Complementary*: *Ars.*, and *Cupr.* *Similar to*: *Ant-C.*, *Cocc.*, *Colch.*, *Kali-M.* and *Puls.*, in gastric troubles.

Ipec. antidotes: *Ars.*, *Chin.*, *Cupr.*, *Ferr.*, *Op.* and *Tab.*

Kali Bichromicum.

COMMON NAME: POTASSIUM BICHROMATE

Especially adapted to fat, light-haired people, and to scrofulous, catarrhal and syphilitic diseases (Bt.).

Often called for in troubles of fat, fair and chubby children (D.).

Complaints occurring in hot weather (*Ant-C.*, *Ars.*) (A.).

Cutaneous eruptions, worse in summer (*Led.*) (K.).

Liable to take cold in open air (*Bell.*, *Phos.*, *Sil.*) (A.).

Discharges from the nose, mouth, throat, stomach, vagina, or any of the mucous membranes, of a tough, stringy mucus, which sticks to the parts, and can be drawn out into strings three feet long (Bt.).

Neuralgia every day at the same hour (*Ars.*, *Chin-S.*, *Nat-M.*) (A.).

Pains in small spots; can be covered with points of finger (*Ign.*) (A.).

Pain shift rapidly from one part to another (*Kali-S.*, *Lac-C.*, *Puls.*) (A.).

Pains appear and disappear suddenly (*Bell.*, *Ign.*, *Mag-P.*) (A.).

PERIODICAL SUPRA-ORBITAL HEADACHE; AS THE HEADACHE S T A R T S THE SIGHT BECOMES LOST, BUT IT RETURNS AS THE HEADACHE INCREASES; IT IS MORE ON THE RIGHT SIDE (D.).

Headache: Blurred vision or blindness precedes the attack (Gels., Hyos., Iris, Lac-D., Nat-M., Podo., Psor., Sep.); must lie down; aversion to light and noise (A.).

Hard, painful swelling of the parotid gland (*Brom., Phyt.*) (G.).

FETID DISCHARGE FROM THE NOSE (*Aur., Calc., Graph., Hep., Kali-P., Lach., Lyc., Merc-C., Nit-Ac., Sep.*) (Bt.).

Pressive pain in the root of the nose (in the forehead and root of the nose—*Stict.*) (A.).

DISCHARGE OF PLUGS OR CLINKERS FROM THE NOSE (*Aur., Graph., Sep.*) (A.).

Lumps of hard, green mucus are hawked from the posterior nares (Hydr.) (D.).

Perfect loss of smell (Ant-C., Bell., Calc., Calc-S., Hep., Merc., Nat-M., Phos., Plb., Puls., Sep., Sil.) (Bt.).

ULCERATION OF THE S E P T U M, WITH BLOODY DISCHARGE, OR LARGE FLAKES OF HARD MUCUS (*Alum., Sep., Teucr.*) (A.).

ULCERS IN THE NOSE TEND TO PERFORATE DEEPLY (*Aur., Nit-Ac.*) (A.).

Caries of the nasal bones (Ars., Asaf., Aur., Aur-M., Aur-M-N., Calc-S., Fluor-Ac., Hekla, Hep., Hippoz., Kali-I., Merc-I-R., Phos., Phyt., Sil., Still.) (Bt.).

Violent pain from the occiput to the forehead if the nasal discharge ceases (A.).

Expired air feels hot in the nose (N.).

Eyelids red, itching, swelled, granular (B.).

Catarrhal and strumous ophthalmia (Bt.).

ULCERS OF THE CORNEA, WITH TENDENCY TO DEEP PERFORATION; LOOK AS IF PUNCHED OUT (D.).

Inflammation of the lids; agglutination in the morning (G.).

Deep-eating ulcers in the fauces, often syhphilitic (*Nit-Ac.*) (A.).

Chronic hoarseness (*Carb-V., Caust., Phos.*) (Bt.).

Cough, with expectoration of tough, stringy mucus, which sticks to the throat, mouth and lips (Bt.).

Violent, rattling cough, with gagging from viscid mucus in the throat; worse when undressing (*Hep.*) (A.).

Aggravation of the cough from the least morsel of food or drink (Bg.).

True membranous croup (Bt.).

Chronic bronchitis, with tough, stringy expectoration (Bt.).

Croup: hoarse, metallic, with expectoration of tough mucus, or fibro-elastic casts in the morning (A.).

There is great swelling of the tonsils and ulcers which secrete a purulent discharge; there are diseased follicles which exude a caseous matter; the coating of the tongue is yellow at the base; the discharge is ropy, tenacious and stringy (D.).

Oedematous, bladder-like appearance of the uvula; much swelling, but little redness (*Rhus.*) (A.).

Diphtheria: pseudo-membranous deposit, firm, pearly, fibrinous, prone to extend downwards to the larynx and trachea (*Lac-C.;* reverse of *Brom.*) (A.).

Tongue coated with a thick yellow felt (*Ant-C., Bry., Chel., Kali-S., Merc., Merc-I-F., Nat-P., Nux-M., Puls., Rhus-T., Sep., Spig., Stann., Sulph.*) (Bt.).

Mapped tongue (*Ant-C., Ars., Chæm., Lach., Lyc., Merc., Nat-M., Nit-Ac., Tarax.*) (B.).

Tongue smooth, red and cracked (N.).

Aphthous stomatitis (*Bor., Kali-M.*) (R.).

27

Gastric catarrh with vomiting (*Ant-C., Bry., Kali-M., Nux-V., Puls.*) (Bt.).

Bitter vomiting mixed with mucus, renewed by every attempt to eat or drink (D.).

Fullness in the stomach even after eating a small quantity (*Lyc., Nux-M.*), *worse from meat* (D.).

Dyspepsia from beer (D.).

ULCERATION OF THE STOMACH AND DUODENUM (*Ars., Merc-C., Nit-Ac., Phos.*) (Bt.).

Loss of appetite; weight in the pit of the stomach; flatulence, worse soon after eating (*Nux-M., Nux-V.*) (A.).

VOMITING OF ROPY MUCUS AND BLOOD; ROUND ULCER OF THE STOMACH (A.).

Sore spot in the stomach, or food lies like a load (B.).

In chronic intestinal ulceration, it vies with Mercury (Hg.).

Dull pains in the right hypochondrium, especially when limited to a small spot, with whitish stools (Hg.).

Chronic dysentery (*Aloe, Merc., Sulph.*).

Dysenteric stools with gnawing at navel and ineffectual straining (R.).

Brown, watery and frothy diarrhœa of gelatinous stools occurring in the morning (D.).

Diarrhœa alternating with rheumatism (*Cimic., Dulc.*) (K.).

Periodic dysentery coming on in the spring (R.).

Sexual desire absent in fleshy people (A.).

Jelly-like discharge from the urethra (K.).

Chancres on the penis with elevated margins and cheesy base (*Hep.*) (K.).

Prolapsus uteri, seemingly in hot weather (A.).

Menses too soon (G.).

Leucorrhœa, ropy, tough discharge, which may be drawn out in long strings (N.).

A drop remains after urinating (B.).

Deep red urine (Bt.).

Complete suppression of urine, with dull pains in the small of the back (Bt.).

Rheumatism alternating with gastric symptoms; one appearing in the fall and the other in the spring (A.).

Rheumatism and dysentery alternate (*Abrot.*) (A.).

Sciatica, relieved by flexing the leg (B.).

Pains along border of foot (B.).

Solid eruption, like measles, over the whole body (Bt.).

Large ulcers, with dark centre, and over-hanging edges (Bt.).

Dryness of the skin, with itching of the whole body (*Graph., Sulph.*) (G.).

Herpes (*Ant-T., Graph., Rhus-T., Sep.*) (G.).

Frequent micturition (*Canth., Nux-V.*) (C.).

Burning pain in the fossa navicularis and bulbus urethra (R.).

Prostatic fluid escapes at stool (*Nux-V., Sel., Sep., Sulph.*) (C.).

Pain in the coccyx while sitting (C.).

Scanty urine, with copious whitish or mucous deposit (C.).

AGGRAVATION: In heat of summer; in hot weather; in the morning; during spring; in the open air; from undressing; from beer; and suppressed catarrh.

AMELIORATION: Skin symptoms are better in cold weather (reverse of *Alum.* and *Petr.*); from heat; and motion.

RELATIONSHIP: Compare *Brom., Hep.* and *Iod.* in croupy affections.

Ant-T. follows well in catarrhal affections and skin diseases.

Complementary: *Ant-T., Ars., Phos.* and *Psor.*

Kali Bromatum.

COMMON NAME: POTASSIUM BROMIDE.

It produces blotches on the skin simulating acne, for which it is a remedy (D.).

Vertigo, as if the ground gave away (B.).

Cerebral depression (Kali-P., Phos.) (D.).

BRAIN-FAG *(Kali-P., Sil.)* (B.).

LOSS OF MEMORY *(Con., Gels., Kali-P., Lyc., Nux-V., Phos., Sil.)* (Bt.).

Forgets how to talk; absent-minded; had to be told the word before he could speak it (Anac.) (A.).

Remarkably depressed in spirits (Aur., Gels., Ign., Nat-M., Sep.) (Bt.).

Feel as if they would lose their minds (A.).

PROFOUND MELANCHOLY *(Ars., Aur., Naja, Nat-M., Puls.)* (Bt.).

Fits of uncontrollable weeping (Nat-M., Sep., Stann.) (A.).

Delirium tremens *(Ars., Hyos., Stram.)* (Bt.).

Tumbles (Bt.).

NERVOUS RESTLESS, CANNOT SIT STILL, MUST MOVE ABOUT OR KEEP OCCUPIED (A.).

STAGGERING, UNCERTAIN GAIT; FEELS AS IF THE LEGS WERE ALL OVER SIDE-WALK *(Alum., Arg-N., Nux-V.)* (A.).

Epilepsy from cerebral congestion *(Bell., Cupr., Hyos., Stram.)* (Vn.).

Loss of sensibility of the fauces, larynx, urethra and entire body (Alum., Op.) (A.).

Impotence, with diminution of sexual desire (Bt.).

Nocturnal emissions, with amorous dreams and erections *(Aur., Kali-P., Nux-V., Phos., Phos-Ac., Sulph.)* (Bt.).

Spermatorrhœa from excessive sexual desire (*Canth.*, *Phos.*) (Bl.).

Somnambulism and night terrors of children (*Sil.*, *Stram.*) (Bl.).

Spasmodic, dry, hysterical cough (Bl.).

Nervous cough during pregnancy (*Calc.*, *Caust.*, *Con.*, *Ipec.*, *Nux-M.*, *Phos.*, *Puls.*, *Sabin.*, *Sep.*, *Vib.*) (A.).

DRY, HARD, ALMOST INCESSANT COUGH, THREATENING ABORTION (*Con.*) (A.).

Induration and enlargement of the womb (*Aur.*, *Aur-M.*, *Calc.*, *Sep.*) (Bt.).

Excessive sexual desire during menses (*Agar.*, *Bell.*, *Bufo*, *Camph.*, *Canth.*, *Coff.*, *Hyos.*, *Lach.*, *Lyc.*, *Mosch.*, *Nux-V.*, *Orig.*, *Plat.*, *Puls.*, *Tarant.*, *Verat.*) (Bt.).

Menstrual ailments: before the menses—headache; during the menses—epileptic spasms, nymphomania, itching, burning and excitement in the vulva, pudenda and clitoris; after the menses—headache, insomnia and heat in the genital (Ha.).

Scanty menstruation (*Graph.*, *Puls.*, *Sep.*) (Bt.).

Pruritus of the vulva (*Calad.*, *Kreos.*, *Merc.*, *Nit-Ac.*, *Sep.*, *Sulph.*).

Vaginismus (*Bell.*, *Cact.*, *Canth.*, *Con.*, *Ferr-P.*, *Gels.*, *Ham.*, *Ign.*, *Lyc.*, *Mag-P.*, *Merc.*, *Nat-M.*, *Nux-V.*, *Plat.*, *Puls.*, *Sil.*) (Bt.).

Morning sickness (*Cocc.*, *Nux-V.*, *Puls.*, *Sep.*) (Bt.).

Spasms: From fright, anger or emotional causes; during parturition, teething, whooping cough, or Bright's disease (A.).

Stammering (*Bell.*, *Bufo*, *Cann-I.*, *Caust.*, *Cupr.*, *Dulc.*, *Euphr.*, *Glon.*, *Hyos.*, *Iod.*, *Lac-C.*, *Lach.*, *Mag-C.*, *Mag-P.*, *Merc.*, *Nat-C.*, *Nux-V.*, *Phos.*, *Plat.*, *Sec.*, *Sel.*, *Spig.*, *Stram.*, *Sulph.*, *Verat.*) (A)

Slow, difficult speech (*Bov.*) (A.).

Diabetes: Urine loaded with sugar, copious pale and watery urine (C.).

Sick and giddy, with repeated retching and vomiting (*Ipec.*, *Nux-V.*, *Tab.*, *Verat.*) (C.).

Grinding teeth in sleep (*Ant-C., Ars., Bell., Bry., Calc., Cann-I., Caust., Cina, Coff., Colch., Con., Crot-H., Hell., Hyos., Ign.*) (A.).

The child screams, moans or cries in sleep (A.).

Sees horrible dreams, cannot be comforted by friends (A.).

Restlessness and sleeplessness due to worry and grief, loss of property or reputation, or from business embarrassments (*Ambr., Gels., Sep.*) (A.).

Cholera infantum: Green, watery stool, with rapid collapse (*Acon., Verat.*) (B.).

In-coordination of muscles (*Gels.*) (A.).

Nervous weakness or paralysis of motion and numbness (A.).

HANDS AND FINGERS IN CONSTANT MOTION (A.).

FIDGETY HANDS (fidgety feet—*Zinc.*) (A.).

Twitching of fingers (*Agar., Cupr., Merc., Osm., Phos., Stann., Sulph-Ac.*) (A.).

AGGRAVATION: From mental exertions; from emotion; from sexual excesses; at night; during pregnancy; and before, during and after menses.

AMELIORATION: When occupied.

RELATIONSHIP: *Compare*: *Ambr., Bell., Camph., Cupr., Gels., Hyos., Ign., Kali-P., Lach., Lyc., Merc., Nux-V., Op., Plb., Sil., Tarant.* and *Zinc.*

One of the antidotes for lead-poisoning.

Kali Carbonicum.

COMMON NAME: POTASSIUM CARBONATE.

Adapted to weak, anæmic and easily exhausted patients, who are always tired and suffer from backache (D.).

Swelling and induration of the glands (after contusions) (*Con.*).

Sensation of hollowness in the whole body (*Cocc.*).

Great liability to catch cold after having been heated.

Aversion to open air and air draughts.

Stinging pain in the muscles and in internal parts (*Apis, Nit-Ac., Sil.*).

Tearing pain in the limbs, with swelling and aggravation during rest.

After exertion, like exercise in walking, attacks of faintness and trembling come on.

Very great weakness, drops down in chair (N.).

Painful sensitiveness of the limbs on pressure.

Twitching of the muscles (*Bell., Cupr., Hyos., Mygale, Tarant.*).

In the open air she appears to be better than in the room; only the fever is higher in the open air.

Parotitis (*Apis, Bell., Brom., Merc., Puls., Rhus-T., Sil.*).

When he shuts his eyes painful sensation from light penetrating into the brain.

DRYNESS OF THE SKIN (*Apis, Ars., Bell., Bry., Cham., Chin., Colch., Dulc., Eup-P., Kali-Ars., Led., Lyc., Nux-M., Olnd., Op., Petr., Phos., Plb., Sec., Seneg., Stram., Sulph., Teucr.*).

Itching of the body during menstruation (*Graph., Phos.*) (D.).

Great dryness of the hair (*Alum., Calc., Fluor-Ac., Med., Phos., Plb., Psor., Sulph., Thuj.*) (N.).

SAC-LIKE SWELLING BETWEEN THE EYE-BROWS AND EYE-LIDS (N.).

Wakes in the morning at about 1 or 3 o'clock and cannot sleep again, from wakefulness (N.).

Pain in the back at 3 A.M., driving out of bed (N.).

Backache extending into gluteal muscles and thighs or down legs (N.).

Constipation (*Ant-C., Bry., Coloc., Merc., Nat-M., Nux-V., Op., Plb., Sep., Sulph.*).

Stool large and difficult, with stitching pains an hour or two before (A.).

Amenorrhœa with backache (*Sep.*) (D.).

Menses too early and too profuse and too long-lasting (*Chin., Ferr., Puls., Sab., Sec., Ust.*) (D.).

FEELS BADLY WEAK BEFORE MENSTRUATION (*Cimic., Cocc., Ferr., Mag-C., Nat-M., Nux-M.*) (A.).

BACKACHE, BEFORE AND DURING MENSES (*Am-C., Bar-C., Berb., Calc., Caust., Hydr., Kreos., Lach., Lyc., Mag-C., Mag-M., Nux-V., Puls., Sang., Zinc.*) (A.).
"Will bring on the menses, when Nat-M., though apparently indicated fails" (Hn.).

DELAYED FIRST MENSES (*Calc-P., Caust., Ferr., Graph., Lyc., Nat-M., Puls., Senec., Sep., Sulph., Tub., Zinc.*). (B)

Yellow leucorrhœa, with much burning and itching (*Kreos., Sep.*) (G.).

In labour the pains begin in the back, and instead of coming around in front like labour-pains pass off down the buttocks or gluteal muscles (N.).

LABOUR-PAINS INSUFFICIENT: VIOLENT BACKACHE; WANTS THE BACK PRESSED (*Caul., Caust., Nux-V.*) (A.).

Complaints after parturition (*Chin., Ferr., Nat-M., Sep., Sulph.*) (G.).

Complaints in the male from coition, from involuntary seminal emissions (G.).

Weakness in the knee after coition (*Agar., Calc., Con., Lyc., Petr., Sep., Sil.*) (K.).

DIM VISION, AFTER COITION (*Chin., Kali-P., Nat-P., Phos., Sep., Sil.*) (K.).

Foamy urine, with thick, tough, red sediment (B.).

OEDEMATOUS SWELLING OF ONE FOOT ONLY (K.).

Stitches in the liver; worse in the cold air. (*Bry., Chel., Phos.*) (Mr.).

Heat and burning pain in the hepatic region (*Sulph.*) (C.).

Great aversion to being alone (Ars., Bism., Lyc., Stram.; desires to be alone—Ign., Nux-V., Sep.) (A.).

Peevish (Bry., Nux-V., Sulph.) (B.).

Easily startled (Bor., Gels., Puls.) (B.).

CANNOT BEAR TO BE TOUCHED; STARTS WHEN TOUCHED LIGHTLY, ESPECIALLY ON THE FEET (*Arn.*) (A.).

Talks of pigeons flying in the room, which he tries to catch with his hand (Bt.).

Very easily frightened (Nit-Ac.) (C.).

Anxiety with fear about her disease (C.).

Vertigo, when rapidly turning the head or body (Con.) (C.).

Headache, in the mornings, on waking (*Lach., Nat-M., Nux-V.*) (C.).

Roaring, wheezing, cracking noises in the ears (*Bor., Chin., Graph.*) (C.).

Nose-bleed, when washing the face in the morning (Am-C., Ant-S., Arn., Calc-S., Dros., Kali-B., Tarant.) (A.).

Periodic epistaxis (Carb-V., Puls.) (K.).

Offensive odour from the mouth every morning, like old cheese (C.).

Foul, slimy taste in the mouth (*Anac., Arn., Ars., Bry., Caps., Carb-V., Dros., Graph., Hep., Kali-B., Merc.*) (C.).

Toothache: only when eating; throbbing; worse when touched by anything warm or cold (A.).

Face bloated (Apis, Ars., Ferr., Rhus-T., Sep., Sulph.) (C.).

Water-brash, after eating (*Am-M., Bry., Calc., Chin., Ferr., Merc., Nat-M., Nux-V., Phos., Sep., Sil., Sulph.*) (K.).

Pit of the stomach sensitive to touch (*Nux-V.*) (C.).

A constant feeling, as if the stomach were full of water (C.).

Dyspepsia of the aged (*Ant-C., Carb-V., Lyc., Sulph.*) (D.).

Before eating there is a faint feeling, sour eructations and heart-burn, and a nervous feeling; during meals the patient is sleepy, and after meals there is great flatulence; the belching is putrid, but it relieves (D.).

STOMACH FEELS AS IF IT WOULD BURST; EVERY THING EATEN SEEMS TO BE CONVERTED INTO GRASS (N.).

EXCESSIVE FLATULENCY (*Arg-N., Carb-V., Chin., Lyc.*) (A.).

Intense thirst: morning, noon and night (G.).

Disgust of food in general (*Chin., Lyc., Sep., Sil.*) (G.).

Sensation of a lump in the stomach (*Bry., Nux-V., Puls.*) (R.).

Distension of the abdomen after eating even a little (*Lyc.*) (R.).

Pain in the back when swallowing (A.).

Food easily goes into the wind-pipe (A.).

Stricture of the œsophagus (*Nat-M.*) (R.).

Swallowing difficult; food descends œsophagus very slowly (*Ign., Phos.*) (R.).

Sticking in the pharynx, as from a fish-bone (*Bell., Hep., Nit-Ac., Sil.*) (R.).

Dry cough, night-sweats, hectic fever; sometimes expectorates bloody pus (Bt.).

Yellow, green or crusty discharge from the nose (*Kali-S., Puls., Sep.*) (B.).

Respiration short, worse from least motion or walking (*Ars., Dig., Phos.*) (B.).

Pleurisy (*Bell., Bry., Carb-An., Kali-B., Phos., Sil., Sulph.*) (B.).

Dry, paroxysmal cough (*Bell., Dros., Sil., Spong.*) (A.).

While in the act of coughing, loosens viscid mucus or pus, which must be swallowed (A.).

Hard, white or smoky masses fly from the throat when coughing (Bad., Chel.) (A.).

Pain in the lower right chest through to the back (N.).

" Persons suffering from ulceration of the lungs can scarcely get well without this anti-psoric " (Hn.).

ASTHMA, RELIEVED WHEN SITTING UP OR BENDING FORWARD, OR BY ROCKING (*Ars.*); WORSE FROM 2 TO 4 A.M. (N.).

Pneumonia, after measles (K.).

Heart weak, irregular, intermits (Ferr., Nat-M., Phos.) (N.).

Tendency to fatty degeneration of the heart (Phos.) (A.).

Sensation as if the heart is suspended by a thread (*Lach.*) (A.).

Pneumonia in infants (*Acon., Ant-T., Bry., Ferr-P., Ipec., Lob., Lyc., Merc., Nux-V., Op., Phos., Sulph.*) (K.).

SPASMODIC COUGH, WITH GAGGING OR VOMITING OF INGESTA (*Ipec.*) (A.).

AGGRAVATION : In the morning; after exertion; in the open air; during rest; at 3 A.M.; after sexual intercourse; after eating; during menstruation; from suppressed menses; and lying on the painful side.

AMELIORATION : From eructation; while sitting in a bent position; on getting warm; from warmth in general; and in the open air.

RELATIONSHIP : *Complementary to : Carb-V., Nit-Ac.* and *Phos.*

Compare : *Bry., Cact., Calc-Hyp., Carb-V., Chin., Dig., Kali-P., Lach., Lyc., Nat-M., Nit-Ac., Nux-V., Phos., Sep., Stann., Sulph.* and *Vib.*

Follows well after : *Kali-S.. Phos.* and *Stann.* in loose, rattling cough.

Antidotes : *Spirits of Nitre and Dulc.*

Kalmia Latifolia.

COMMON NAME: MOUNTAIN LAUREL.

Adapted to acute neuralgia, rheumatism and gouty complaints, especially when the heart is involved as a sequel of rheumatism and gout (A.).

Maddening supra-orbital pain (*Spig.*) (B.).

Severe stitching pain in the right eye and orbit (left eye —*Spig.*); *stiffness in muscles, pain worse when turning the eyes* (*Spig.*); *begins at sunrise, aggravates at noon and leaves at sunset* (*Nat-M.*) (A.).

Brachialgia (B.).

Pulse, very slow, weak and tremulous (*Gels., Mur-Ac.*) (B.).

Scarcely perceptible pulse (*Carb-V.*) (A.).

Useful in heart diseases that have developed from rheumatism, or alternate with it.

Aching, bruised, stiff feeling (*Arn., Bry., Eup-P.*) (B.).

RHEUMATISM: PAINS INTENSE, CHANGE PLACES SUDDENLY; GOING FROM JOINT TO JOINT; JOINT HOT, RED, SWOLLEN; WORSE FROM LEAST MOVEMENT (*Kali-S.*) (A.).

Changing pains, shoot outward along nerves (B.).

Pains sticking, darting, pressing, shooting in a downward direction (*Cact.; in an upward direction—Led.*) (A.).

PAINS ARE ATTENDED OR SUCCEEDED BY NUMBNESS OF THE AFFECTED PART (*Acon., Cham., Plat.*) (A.).

Cardiac hypertrophy and valvular insufficiency (C.).

Difficult and oppressed breathing (*Apis, Cact., Cupr., Lyc., Phos.*) (C.).

Sharp pains about the heart, shooting in the abdomen, which take away breath, and a very slow pulse, with *numbness and tingling in the left arm* (.D.).

Angina pectoris (*Amyl-N., Cact.*) (C.).

The face is pale and the extremities are cold (*Acon.,* *Carb-V., Verat.*) (Bl.).

Fluttering of the heart (*Spig.*) (C.).

Vertigo when stooping, or looking down (*Spig.*) (A.).

Tearing pains in the head and neck (*Cimic.*) (C.).

Rheumatic pains in the limbs from the hips to the feet (N.).

Prosopalgia (or facial neuralgia), mostly on the right side (left side—*Spig.*) (C.).

Tearing pains down the legs (D.).

Rheumatism shifting from joint to joint, from external applications (D.).

Bright's disease, with heart symptoms (C.).

AGGRAVATION: When turning the eyes; at noon; from least movement; soon after going to bed; and during early part of the night.

AMELIORATION: After sun-set; from sitting; or when standing upright.

RELATIONSHIP: *Complementary*: *Benz-Ac.* and *Spig.*

Similar to: *Acon., Bell., Ferr., Led., Rhod., Rhus-T.* and *Spig.* in rheumatic affections and gout.

Antidotes: *Acon.* and *Bell.*

Kreosotum.

COMMON NAME: KREOSOTE.

Acrid, fœtid, decomposed, mucous secretions; sometimes ulcerating, bleeding, malignant (N.).

Difficulty of hearing, before and during the menses, with buzzing and humming in the head (G.).

Intense itching of the margins of the eye-lids, greatly aggravated by rubbing or touching them (Bt.).

HAEMORRHAGIC DIATHESIS; SMALL WOUND BLEEDS PROFUSELY (*Lach., Phos.*) (N.).

Oedema of the feet (*Apis, Ars., Chel., Graph., Lyc., Med., Merc-C., Phos., Samb.*) (Bt.).

Fetid sweat of the feet (*Bar-C., Calc., Graph., Kali-C., Lyc., Nit-Ac., Puls., Sil.*) (Bt.).

Herpes: Humid, scaly, pustulous on ears, eyelids, cheeks, mouth, elbows, fingers and malleoli (*Sep.*).

Eruptions on the extensor surfaces (eruptions on the flexor surfaces—*Nat-M.*) (D.).

Large, greasy, pox-shaped pustules all over the body.

Itching, so violent toward evening as to drive one almost wild (itching, without eruption—*Dol.*) (A.).

Cholera infantum: profuse vomiting; cadaverous smelling stools (*Calc-P., Kali-P., Podo., Sulph.*) (N.).

Children old-looking and wrinkled (*Arg-N., Lyc., Op.*) (A.).

PUTRID, ACRID, AND CORROSIVE LEUCOR-RHOEA (*Ars., Carb-Ac., Merc-C., Nit-Ac., Sulph.*), STAINING THE LINEN YELLOW (N.).

The parts with which the leucorrhœal discharge comes in contact itch and burn, while scratching does not relieve but inflames the parts (N.).

Leucorrhœa worse between the periods (*Bor., Bov.*) (A.).

Cancer of the uterus, with profuse discharge of dark, coagulated blood, or of a pungent bloody ichor, preceded by a pain in the back (G.).

Voluptuous itching, deep in the vagina (Hr.).

Leucorrhœa, with great debility, particularly of the lower extremities (G.).

Post-climacteric diseases of women (*Cimic., Graph., Lach., Sang., Sulph.*) (A.).

She always feels chilly at the menstrual period (*Puls.*) (G.).

MENSES FLOW ON LYING DOWN, CEASE ON SITTING OR WALKING ABOUT (A.).

BURNING AND SWELLING OF THE EXTERNAL AND INTERNAL LABIA (G.).

Lochia: dark, brown, lumpy, offensive, acrid; almost ceases, then freshens up again (*Con., Sulph.*) (A.).

AWEFUL BURNING, AS OF RED-HOT COAL IN THE PELVIS, WITH DISCHARGE OF CLOTS OF BLOOD HAVING A FOUL SMELL (G.).

Leucorrhœa gushing like bloody water (Calc., Cocc., Graph., Lyc., Sep., Sil., Thuj.).

In cancer, the whole mammœ is hard, bluish-red, and covered with little, scurfy protuberances (G.).

BLEEDING FROM THE FEMALE GENITALIA AFTER COITUS (*Arg-N., Arn., Ars., Hydr., Sep., Tarant.*). (K.).

BURNING IN THE VAGINA DURING COITION (*Kali-B., Lyc., Nat-M., Sulph.*) (K.).

Dragging from back to genitals, as if to come out (*Sep.*) (B.).

Scraping and roughness of the throat, with hoarseness (*Mezer., Nux-V.*) (C.).

Shortness of breath (*Acon., Ars., Dig., Phos., Seneg.*) (C.).

Chronic bronchitis with offensive expectoration (*Puls., Seneg., Sil.*) (Bl.).

Tormenting cough, with little expectoration (*Con., Dros., Hyos.*) (B.).

Neglected phthisis (*Kali-C.*) (B.).

AGGRAVATION: In the open air; during and after menstruation; during cold weather; when growing cold; during dentition period; from washing or bathing with cold water; from rest, especially when lying; while eating; and during pregnancy.

VOMITING OF SWEETISH WATER (*Cupr., Iris, Kali-B., Plb., Psor., Tub.*) (A.).

Vomiting of pregnancy (*Bry., Ign., Puls., Nat-M., Sep.*) (A.).

COLICKY PAINS DURING, BUT ESPECIALLY AFTER MENSES (A.).

Cold drinks relieve menstrual pains (A.).

Severe headache before and during menses (*Am-C., Bell., Glon., Graph., Lyc., Nat-M., Sep.*) (A.).

GUMS PAINFUL, DARK RED OR BLUE, TEETH DECAY AS SOON AS THEY COME (*Merc., Staph.*) (N.).

Gums scorbutic (*Merc-C., Nat-M., Nit-Ac., Sulph.*) (A.).

Soft, spongy and bleeding gums (*Carb-V., Merc., Nat-M.*) (A.).

Sad and irritable (*Aur., Ign., Nat-M., Stann.*) (G.).

Cross, wilful and obstinate (*Bry., Cham., Nux-V., Sulph.*) (B.).

Desire for death (*Aur., Lac-C., Nat-M.*) (B.).

Copious, pale urine (*Acet-Ac., Gels., Merc., Nat-S., Phos-Ac., Sars., Sulph.*) (A.).

INCONTINENCE OF URINE (*Sep., Sulph., Thuj., Uran., Verb., Viol-T.*) (A.).

Smarting and burning during and after micturition (*Sulph.*) (A.).

Can only urinate when lying (only when sitting bent back—*Zinc.*) (N.).

SUDDEN URGING TO URINATE OR DURING FIRST SLEEP, WHICH IS VERY PROFOUND (N.).

Menses too early, too profuse, and last too long; inclined to be intermittent; she thinks she is almost well, when the discharge returns afresh (G.).

Stitches in the vagina (G.).

AMELIORATION. From warmth; from hot food; and motion.

RELATIONSHIP: *Antidotes*: *Carb-V.* and *Nux-V.*
Similar to: *Arum-T., Ars., Bism., Calc., Carb-Ac., Graph., Lach., Lyc., Merc-C., Nat-M., Nit-Ac., Nux-V., Petr., Rhus-T., Sep., Sil., Sulph.* and *Thuj.*

Kreosote is followed well by *Ars., Phos.* and *Sulph.* in cancer and diseases of a malignant tendency.

Lac Caninum.

COMMON NAME: DOG'S MILK.

Inflammatory affections travel crosswise, from side to side, back and forth (rheumatism, sore-throat, etc.).

Symptoms erratic, pains constantly flying from one part to another (Kali-B., Puls.); changing from side to side every few hours or days.

SHINING, GLAZED APPEARANCE OF DIPH-THERITIC DEPOSITS, CHANCRES AND ULCERS· (N.).

Diphtheria: the membrane forms on one side and goes to the other; or is constantly changing sides; the membrane is mother-of-pearl like (D.).

Throat sensitive to touch externally (*Lach.*) (A.).

Sorethroat: aggravated by empty swallowing (Ign.); constant inclination to swallow; swallowing painful, almost impossible (Bell., Merc.); pains extend to the ears (Hep., Kali-B.); begins on the left side (Lach.) (A.).

Tonsillitis: symptoms change from side to side (Bl.).

Great prostration (*Ars., Lach.*) (Bl.).

Breasts inflamed, painful, aggravated by least jar; must hold them when stepping up or down stairs (Bell.) (N.):

Breasts and throat get sore at every menstrual period (N.).

MASTITIS: BREASTS VERY SORE AND TENDER; CANNOT BEAR A JAR OF THE BED (N.).

Loss of milk while nursing without any known cause (*Asaf.*) (A.).

Serviceable in almost all cases when it is required to dry up milk (*Asaf.*; to bring back or increase it—*Lac-D.*) (A.).

Galactorrhœa (*Asaf., Bry., Puls.*) (B.).

Breasts swollen, painful, sensitive before and during menses (*Con.*) (A.).

Menses: Green, gushing or ammoniacal (B.).

Menses too early and too profuse (*Chin., Ferr., Sab.*) (A.).

Discharge of bright red, viscid and stringy blood during the catamenia (dark, black and stringy blood—*Croc.*) (A.).

Hoarseness during menses (*Calc., Graph., Spong.*) (B.).

Sexual organs easily excited, from touch, pressure on sitting, or friction by walking (*Cinn., Coff., Murx., Plat.*) (A.).

Discharge of flatus from the vagina (*Brom., Lyc., Nux-M., Sang.*) (A.).

Delusions of snakes in and around her (*Arg-N., Bell., Calc., Hyos., Lach., Op.*) (K.).

Attacks of rage, cursing and swearing at the slightest provocation (*Anac., Bell., Hyos., Lil-T., Nit-Ac., Stram.*) (A.).

Intense ugliness (*Nit-Ac.*) (A.).

Full of imaginations (B.).

Fears to be alone (*Kali-C., Phos.*); *of dying* (*Ars., Puls.*); *of becoming insane* (*Lil-T.*); of falling down-stairs (*Bor.*) (A.).

Despondent, hopeless; thinks her disease incurable; has not a friend living; nothing worth living for; could weep at any moment (*Act-R., Aur., Calc., Lach.*) (A.).

VERY FORGETFUL, ABSENT-MINDED; MAKES PURCHASES AND WALKS AWAY WITHOUT THEM (*Agn., Anac., Caust., Nat-M.*) (A.).

In writing, uses too many words, or not the right ones; omits final letter or letters in a word; cannot concentrate the mind to read or study; very nervous (*Bov., Graph., Lach., Nat-C., Sep.*) (A.).

Cross, irritable; child cries and screams all the time, especially at night (*Jal., Nux-V., Psor.*) (A.).

CORYZA: ONE NOSTRIL STUFFED UP, THE OTHER FREE AND DISCHARGING; THESE CONDITIONS ALTERNATE: DISCHARGE—ACRID; NOSE AND LIPS RAW (*Arum-T., Cepa*) (A.).

Sorethroat and cough are apt to begin and end with menstruation (A.).

Pains (*in the throat*) *shoot to the ear* (*Kali-B., Kali-C., Merc., Phyt.*) (A.).

Sinking at the epigastrium (*Carb-A., Sep., Sulph.*) (A.).

Faintness in the stomach (A.).

Very hungry, cannot eat enough to satisfy (*Chel., Ind., Tub.*) ; as hungry *after eating as before* (*Calc., Casc., Cina, Lyc., Stront.*) (A.).

Sensation as if breath would leave her when lying down; must get up and walk (*Am-C., Grind., Lach.*) (A.).

Palpitation violent when lying on the left side, better from turning on the right (*Tab.*) (A.).

When walking, seems to be walking on the air; when lying, does not seem to touch the bed (*Asàr.*) (A.).

Spine aches from the base of the brain to the coccyx (A.).

Spine very sensitive to touch or pressure (*Chin-S., Phos., Zinc.*) (A.).

Backache: Intense, unbearable, across super-sacral region, extending to the right natis and right sciatic nerve; aggravation by rest and on first moving (*Rhus-T.*) (A.).

AGGRAVATION: From touch; from jar; during menses; from empty swallowing; from pressure; during rest; and at night.

AMELIORATION: In the open air; from turning on the right side; and from walking.

RELATIONSHIP: *Similar to: Apis, Ars., Bell., Con., Kali-B., Lach., Lyas., Murx., Nit-Ac., Puls., Sep.* and *Sulph.*

Lac Defloratum.

COMMON NAME: SKIMMED MILK.
Great prostration (*Ars., Camph., Kali-P.*) (A.).
Sick headache relieved by a profuse flow of urine (Gels.) (N.).
Pain begins in the forehead and extends to the occiput, in the morning on rising (Bry.) (A.).

DIM VISION, BEFORE HEADACHE (*Gels., Hyos., Iris, Kali-B., Nat-M., Podo., Psor., Sep.;* during headache— *Ars., Bell., Caust., Cycl., Gels., Iris, Nat-M., Petr., Phos., Psor., Sil., Stram., Sulph.;* after headache—*Sil.*) (K.).

INTENSE THROBBING IN THE HEAD, WITH NAUSEA AND VOMITING (*Bell., Bry., Verat-V.*) (A.).
Hemicrania (Alum., Arg-N., Coff., Ign., Kali-C., Kali-I., Kali-P., Phos-Ac., Plat., Puls., Sang., Sars., Spig., Sulph-Ac., Verb., Zinc.) (Bl.).
Headache increased by noise, light and motion (*Bell., Bry., Nat-M.*) (A.).
Sick headache, with icy coldness all through the body, even near the fire, and profuse emission of urine (N.).
Pale, sickly look (*Ferr., Graph., Sep.*) (B.).
Headache during menses (Kreos., Sep.).
Headache relieved by pressure or by bandaging the head lightly (Arg-N., Puls.) (A.).
Photophobia (*Acon., Bell., Calc., Con., Merc., Nat-M., Phos., Sep., Sulph., Thuj.*) (B.).

AVERSE TO MILK (*Aeth., Ant-T., Arn., Bry., Calc., Calc-S., Carb-V., Cina, Ferr-P., Guai., Ign., Lec., Mag-C., Nat-C., Nat-S., Nux-V., Phos., Puls., Sep., Sil., Sulph.*) (B.).

NAUSEA (*Ars., Bry., Chin., Dig., Eup-P.*) (B.).

SOUR VOMITING (*Calc., Caust., Chin., Iris, Lyc., Mag-C., Nat-P., Nux-V., Phos., Psor., Puls., Rob., Sulph.. Sulph-Ac., Tab., Verat.*) (B.).

Vomiting, first of undigested food, intensely acid, then of bitter water (*Iris*) (A.).

PROFUSE AND COLOURLESS URINE (*Apis, Gels., Phos-Ac.*) (N.).

Globus hystericus: Sensation of a large ball rising from the stomach to the throat, causing a sense of suffocation (*Asaf., Ign., Nux-M.*) (A.).

Vomiting of pregnancy (*Bry., Lac-Ac., Nux-V., Petr., Psor., Sep., Symphori.*) (A.).

Scanty flow of milk (*Bry., Lac-C., Puls.*) (B.).

Menses: Delayed or suppressed by putting hands in cold water (*Con.*) (A.).

Amenorrhœa (*Cimic., Cycl., Ferr., Puls., Sep., Sulph.*) (B.).

Drinking a glass of milk will promptly suppress the (menstrual) flow until the next period (*Phos.*) (A.).

Feels completely exhausted, whether she does anything or not; great fatigue when walking (A.).

Despondency (*Aur., Gels., Kali-P.*) (B.).

Does not care to live (*Ars., Aur., Hep:, Naja, Nit-Ac., Nux-V.*) (A.).

Has no fear of death, but is sure he is going to die (*Ars.*) (A.).

Vertigo, worse from lying on the left side (B.).

CONSTIPATION, WITH INEFFECTUAL URG-ING (*Anac., Carb-V., Ign., Nux-V., Sulph.*) (A.).

DRY, LARGE AND PAINFUL STOOLS (*Bry.,
Nat-M., Sel., Sulph.*) (B.).

GREAT STRAINING (DURING AN EVACUA-
TION), LACERATING THE ANUS (*Nat-M., Sulph.*)
(A.).

PAINFUL MOTION, EXTORTING CRIES (*Sulph.*)
(A.).

ALWAYS CHILLY (*Nux-V., Psor., Sil.*) (B.).

Sensation as if cold air was blowing on her, even while
covered up; as if sheets were damp (A.).

Skin is super-sensitive to cold (*Sil.*) (B.).

Dropsy from organic heart disease, chronic liver complaint, and far advanced albuminuria, or following intermittent fever (*Ars., Kali-C., Lyc., Phos., Sep.*) (A.).

*Great restlessness, extreme and protracted suffering from
loss of sleep* (*Cocc., Nit-Ac.*) (A.).

AGGRAVATION: From least draught of air; in the
morning; from rising; from noise; from light; from motion;
during menses; during pregnancy; and from putting hands
in cold water.

AMELIORATION: From a profuse flow of urine;
from rest; from pressure of a bandage; and from warm
covering.

RELATIONSHIP: *Similar to*: *Acet-Ac., Bry., Cycl.,
Gels., Kali-B., Nat-M., Psor., Puls., Sep., Sil.,* and*Sulph.*

Lachesis.

COMMON NAME: SURUKUKU SNAKE
POISON.

Better adapted to thin and emaciated than to fleshy persons; to those who have been changed, both mentally and
physically, by their illness (A.).

Generally called for women who have not recovered from the change of life, "have never felt well since that time" (A.).

Dimness of vision (Cycl., Gels., Kali-P., Phos., Sep.) (N.).

Conjunctiva yellow or orange-coloured (*Chel., Iod., Merc., Sep.*) (A.).

Black flickering before the eyes (N.).

Photophobia, always worse in the morning, after sleeping (N.).

LEFT SIDE PRINCIPALLY AFFECTED; DISEASES BEGIN ON THE LEFT SIDE AND GO TO THE RIGHT SIDE—LEFT OVARY, TESTICLE, CHEST, ETC. (A.).

Pains in the ear with sore-throat (*Bell., Kali-B., Merc., Nit-Ac., Phyt., Sil.*) (N.).

Roaring and singing in the ears, relieved by putting the finger in the ear and shaking it (D.).

Hardness of hearing, with want of wax (N.).

Ears full of pasty, offensive wax (D.).

Dryness of the ears (Calc., Carb-V., Graph., Nit-Ac., Nux-V., Onos., Petr., Phos., Puls., Sulph.) (N.).

Tearing extending from the zygoma into the ears; raises the hand to the back of ear with each scream (hydrocephalus) (N.).

Bluish colour of the affected part (N.).

Great hyper-sensitiveness of the body (D.).

SMALL WOUNDS BLEED MUCH (*Phos.*); BLOOD DARK AND UNCOAGULABLE (N.).

Great physical and mental exhaustion—sinks down from weakness. Worse A.M. and after sleep (N.).

Paroxysms of sneezing in hay fever, especially if worse after sleeping (N.).

Watery discharge from the nose, worse on the left side (D.).

Cannot put the tongue out but with difficulty; trying it the tongue trembles or catches behind the lower teeth (N.).

Dry tongue, cracked at the tip and brown on the dorsum (D.).

Sensation of a lump in the left side of the throat, which seems to go down when swallowing, but returns again (D.).

Empty swallowing is painful and fluids escape from the nose (D.).

Liquids are more painful than solids when swallowing (A.).

THROAT COMPLAINTS BEGIN IN THE LEFT AND GO TO THE RIGHT SIDE (*reverse of Lyc.*) (N.).

Throat sensitive externally (*Apis, Bell., Hep.*) (D.).

TONSILLITIS OR DIPHTHERIA, WORSE ON THE LEFT SIDE; CHOKING WHEN SWALLOWING, OR PAINS FROM THE THROAT INTO THE EAR; NECK VERY SENSITIVE TO TOUCH; AGGRAVATION AFTER SLEEP (N.).

Diphtheria aggravated by hot drinks (by cold drinks—*Lyc.*) (N.).

Intolerance of bands about the neck or waist (A.).

GREAT SENSITIVENESS TO TOUCH: THROAT, STOMACH, ABDOMEN (A.).

Cannot bear bed-clothes or night dress to touch the throat or abdomen, not because sore or tender, as in Apis or Bell., but clothes cause an uneasiness, make her nervous (A.).

Desire for oysters (D.).

Horribly offensive diarrhœa, preceded by sopor; the offensiveness of the stools indicates it in low forms of diseases (D.).

Constipation from inactivity of the rectum (*Bry., Ign., Op.*); stool lies in the rectum, without urging (A.).

Sensation of constriction of the sphincter (*Caust., Nit-Ac.*) (A.).

A tormenting, constant urging in the rectum, but not for a stool (N.).

Pain in the rectum from coughing (*Kali-C.*) (K.).

Stools extremely offensive; hard or soft (N.).

BEATING IN THE ANUS, AS WITH LITTLE HAMMERS (*Aloe, Nat-M., Sulph.*) (N.).

Hæmorrhage from the bowels, as in typhoid; when kept in a vessel, black particles like charred straw rest in the bottom (N.).

With every single cough a stitch in the hæmorrhoidal tumour (N.).

Piles: With scanty menses or at climaxis; strangulated; with stitches shooting upward (*Ign., Nit-Ac.*) (A.).

Bad effects of poison wounds (*Ars.*) (A.).

Diarrhœa in warm weather, aggravated by acid fruits; worse at night and after sleep (Hr.).

Sensation as if a ball were rolling in the abdomen (*Aur-S., Lyc., Sabad., Sep.*).

Sensation as of a ball rolling in the bladder (A.).

URINE ALMOST BLACK, FOAMY, FREQUENT AND DARK (N.).

Pressure in the bladder, with frequent urging (*Bell., Canth., Gels.*) (C.).

Sticking, cutting pains, or soreness in the fore part of the urethra (C.).

Mouth sore, parched, dry, aphthous (*Bry., Nux-V., Sulph.*) (C.).

Feeling as if the teeth were too long when biting them together.

Toothache: from warm and cold drinks (C.).

Odontalgia with swollen, dark, purplish and bleeding gums (R.).

Great mental activity; ideas crowd rapidly (*Coff.*) (C.).

Ailments from long-lasting grief, sorrow, fright, vexation, jealousy or disappointed love (*Aur., Ign., Nat-M Phos-Ac.*) (A.).

THINKS HERSELF UNDER SUPER-HUMAN CONTROL (*Anac.*) (N.).

GREAT LOQUACITY (*Agar., Hyos., Stram.*); WANTS TO TALK ALL THE TIME; JUMPS FROM ONE IDEA TO ANOTHER; ONE WORD OFTEN LEADS INTO ANOTHER STORY (A.).

Great sadness, particularly on waking in the morning (N.).

Mental excitability (*Bell., Hyos., Stram., Verat.*) (A.).

ECSTASY, WITH ALMOST PROPHETIC PERCEPTIONS (*Coff.*), OR WITH A VIVID IMAGINATION (*Stram.*) (A.).

Jealousy (*Apis, Nux-V.*) (D.).

Low, muttering delirium (*Hyos.*) (R.).

Fear of being poisoned (*Hyos.*); *refuses the medicine* (D.).

Has been used with success in cases of religious melancholia when the patient was continually moaning the fact that he was lost (R.).

Very unhappy and distressed after sleeping (Bt.).

Fright from seeing snakes (Bt.).

Thinks she is dead (*in typhoid*), *and that preparations are made for the funeral, or that she is nearly dead, and wishes some one would help her off* (Be.).

Amativeness (*Croc., Phos., Plat.*) (G.).

No desire at all to mix with the world (G.).

Restless and uneasy; does not wish to attend to business, but wants to be off somewhere all the time (G.).

FACIAL ERYSIPELAS, MORE ON THE LEFT SIDE; AT FIRST BRIGHT RED. THEN DARK BLUISH OR PURPLISH (D.).

Great infiltration of cellular tissues and great weakness (D.).

INFLAMED PARTS VERY TENDER TO TOUCH AND OF BLUISH OR DARK COLOUR (N.).

BURNING ON THE VERTEX (*Sulph.*) (N.).

Headache over the left eye accompanying a cold, but as soon as the discharge is established headache is better (D.).

PRESSING OR BURSTING PAIN IN THE TEMPLES. WORSE FROM MOTION, PRESSURE, STOOPING, LYING, AND AFTER SLEEP. DREADS TO GO TO SLEEP, BECAUSE SHE WAKENS WITH SUCH A HEADACHE (A.).

Rush of blood to the head: after alcohol; from mental emotions; during suppressed or irregular menses or at climaxis (A.).

Left-sided apoplexy (A.).

Heart feels too large for the cavity; can bear no pressure on the throat or chest (N.).

Constriction about the heart (*Cact.*) (D.).

EPILEPSY: COMES ON DURING SLEEP (*Bufo*); FROM LOSS OF VITAL FLUIDS; ONANISM OR JEALOUSY (A.).

FAINTNESS FROM PAIN IN THE HEART (*Aur.*), OR DURING PALPITATION (*Cact., Cimic., Cocc., Iod., Nux-M., Petr., Verat.*) (K.).

Must take deep breaths (*Bry., Ign., Phos.*) (R.).

Cough during sleep; patient seems to sleep into the cough, or worse also after a nap (N.).

Spasm of the glottis: suddenly something runs from the neck to the larynx, and interrupts breathing completely; it wakens at night (N.).

WANTS TO BE FANNED (*Ant-T., Apis, Carb-V., Chin., Ferr., Med., Sulph.*), BUT SLOWLY AND AT A DISTANCE (N.).

The least thing coming near the mouth or nose interferes with breathing (A.).

AS SOON AS HE FALLS ASLEEP THE BREATHING STOPS (*Am-C., Grind., Lac-C., Op.*) (A.).

Deglutition painful, with regurgitation through the nose (G.).

Pressure upon the larynx causes cough (G.).

Hot flushes, metrorrhagia and other troubles during the climacteric (N.).

Pain in the left ovary relieved by a discharge from the uterus; can bear nothing heavy on this region (D.).

CATAMENIA AT THE REGULAR TIME, BUT TOO SHORT AND FEEBLE (N.).

Menses scanty and feeble, black and offensive, with pain in the hips and bearing down in the left ovary; better when the flow is established (D.)

Uterus does not bear contact, or has to be relieved of all pressure by frequently lifting the clothes, they cause an uneasiness in the abdomen; no tenderness (N.).

Left ovary swollen, with tensive pressing, stitching pains; inability to lie on the right side, on account of a sensation as if something were rolling over to that side (G.).

Pains in the uterine region, increased at times more and more until relieved by a flow of blood from the vagina; after a few hours or days the same again, etc. (N.).

Is of great service in the fainting tendency of nervous women (Ba.).

Gnawing in the stomach; relieved after eating, but returns when the stomach gets empty (Anac.) (C.).

Typhlitis: Swelling in the cæcal region. Must lie on the back, with limbs drawn up (Bell.) (C.).

Peritonitis (Bell., Lyc., Merc., Rhus-T.) (C.).

Burning of the palms and soles, especially at night (K.).

Seems to sleep into troubles, such as cramp, cough, etc. (N.).

Extremes of heat and cold cause great debility (A.).

Fever annually returning; paroxysm **every spring** *(Carb-V., Sulph.)*; after suppression by quinine the previous autumn (A.).

CHILD MUST BE HELD TO RELIEVE HEAD AND CHEST AND PREVENT SHAKING; FEELS BETTER IF HELD OR PRESSED DOWN (*Gels.*) (N.).

Heat at night, especially after sleep, from orgasm of blood (N.).

Muttering delirium, with dropping of the lower jaw (*Lyc.*) and illusions (D.).

Typhoid pneumonia: Indicated late in the disease, when pus forms in the lungs (*Kali-C.*), and the patient is bathed in a profuse sweat and sputa is mixed with blood and pus (D.).

Much pain of an aching kind in the shin-bones only (N.).

Boils, carbuncles, ulcers with intense pain (*Tarant.*) (A.).

Red, bluish, painful swelling on the limbs; very sensitive; impending gangrene (N.).

MALIGNANT PUSTULES, WITH DARK BLUISH OR PURPLE APPEARANCE (A.).

Perspiration cold, or stains yellow or bloody (*Lyc.*) (A.).

Sticking, drawing pains in the spine extending into the hips and legs, especially the ischium (R.).

Sticking, tearing in the arms and legs (R.).

Post-diphtheritic paralysis (R.).

Thirsty, but fears to drink (*Lyss.*) (R.).

AGGRAVATION: At climacteric; from touch; from constriction or pressure; from the heat of the sun; after sleeping; from suppressed or delayed discharges; during spring, or summer; from acids; from alcohol; from empty deglutition; from extremes of temperature; from hot drink; and from hot room.

AMELIORATION: From the onset of a discharge; during menses; in the open air; and from cold application.

RELATIONSHIP: *Incompatible*: *Acet-Ac.*, and *Carb-Ac.*

Complementary: *Hep.*, *Lyc.* and *Nit-Ac.*

In intermittent fever *Nat-M.* follows *Lach.* well when the type changes.

Latrodectus Mactans.

COMMON NAME: SPIDER.

The præcordial region seems to be centre of the attack (Br.).

Præcordial anxiety (*Acon., Cact., Lach., Naja, Spig., Verat.*) (B.).

GASPS, FEARS TO LOSE BREATH AND DIE (*Ars., Dig., Lach.*) (B.).

Screams with pain (Br.).

ANGINA PECTORIS (*Ars., Spig., Verat.*) (Bl.).

PAIN IN THE REGION OF THE HEART, EXTENDING TO THE LEFT ARM (*Acon., Kalm., Rhus-T.*) (K.).

Constriction of chest muscles, with radiation to the shoulders and back (Br.).

Cardiac pain: violent, sharp to shoulder or both arms, with numbness (B.).

Skin as cold as marble (*Camph., Carb-V., Laur., Verat.*) (Br.).

Quick, feeble, thready pulse (*Acon., Camph., Phos., Verat.*) (B.).

Sinking at the epigastrium (*Carb-An., Dig., Sep.*) (B.).

Paræsthesia of the lower limbs (Br.).

Weakness of the legs followed by cramps in the abdominal muscles (Br.).

AGGRAVATION: From least motion: even of hands; from exertion; and from talking.

AMELIORATION: From sitting quietly.

RELATIONSHIP: *Similar to: Acon., Ars., Cact., Dig., Lach., Laur., Naja, Phos.* and *Verat.*

Laurocerasus.

COMMON NAME: CHERRY LAUREL.

This remedy contains Hydrocyanic Acid; consequently many of the symptoms are similar to those produced by that Acid (Bl.).

Stinging and tearing in the limbs.

Want of reaction, and vital powers are low.

Lack of power, as regards the action of the sphincters.

Want of vital heat (*Sil.*).

Want of energy, of vital power; want of reaction, especially in chest and heart affections (N.).

TETANIC SPASMS (*Bell., Cupr., Hyos., Nux-V., Op., Stram., Verat.*).

Convulsions, with foam before the closed mouth.

Painlessness accompanies the symptoms.

Acute suppuration of the lungs.

SUFFOCATIVE SPELLS ABOUT THE HEART, WORSE FROM SITTING, BETTER FROM LYING DOWN (N.).

Mitral regurgitation (*Lach., Naja, Phos., Rhus-T.*) (Br.).

Clutching at heart and palpitation (Br.).

A slow, weak pulse (*Mur-Ac.*).

Short, titillating cough (N.).

Cardiac cough (*Dig., Lach., Phos.*) (N.).

Low-spiritedness (*Kali-P., Puls., Sep.*).

Cough, with copious expectoration of mucus, interspersed here and there with bright red points of blood (*Stann.*) (N.).

Sensation as if the heart would turn over; gasps for breath; better on lying down (N.).

Heart trouble, with continuous cough as soon as he lies down.

DRINK ROLLS AUDIBLY DOWN THROUGH THE OESOPHAGUS AND INTESTINES (N.).

Internal chilliness and external heat (*Ars.*) (G.).

The patient puts his hand to the cardiac region, as is observed after even a short run (Bl.).

Heart action irregular (N.).

Catamenia too early and too profuse (Ferr., Sab., Sec.).

Catamenia with thin blood (Alum., Cycl., Ferr., Graph., Nat-M.).

LONG-LASTING FAINTS, WITH A PALE, BLUE FACE AND COLD SURFACE (Bl.).

Cyanosis neonatorum: *face blue; gasping* (N.).

Spells of deep sleep, with snoring and stertorous breathing (*Op.*) (Br.).

Cold, clammy feet and legs (Br.).

Persistent hiccough (*Mag-P.*) (B.).

Cold, livid skin (*Camph., Sec.*) (B.).

Eyes, open and staring; distorted (*Hyos., Lyc., Op., Stram.*) (C.).

Stupefaction with vertigo (*Gels.*) (C.).

Loss of speech (*Caust., Dulc., Gels., Naja*) (C.).

Perspiration from least exertion (*Bry., Calc., Chin.. Verat.*) (C.).

Diarrhœa: Green mucous stools (C.).

Cholera, with suffocative spells about the heart (*Arg-N., Hydr-Ac.*), and rapid sinking of the forces (*Ars., Camph., Sec.*) (C.).

AGGRAVATION: In · the evening; before eating; from sitting up; and from least exertion.

AMELIORATION: At night; in the open air; and from lying down.

RELATIONSHIP: *Antidotes*: *Coff.* and *Op.*

Compare: *Ambr., Am-C., Cact., Camph., Dig., Hydr-Ac., Kali-P., Lach., Naja, Nat-M., Phos., Sec.,* and *Verat.*

Ledum Palustre.

COMMON NAME: MARSH TEA.

Adapted to rheumatic or gouty diathesis, and constitutions abused by alcohol (*Colch.*) (A.).

Painful knots on the joints.

Hot swelling of the painful joints (*Bell.*).

Easy spraining of ankles and feet (*Carb-A.*) (A.).

RHEUMATIC TEARING FROM THE HEAT OF THE BED, MOSTLY IN THE EVENING UNTIL MID-NIGHT.

The heat of the bed is insupportable, on account of the heat in the limbs.

In the evening heat in the hands and feet.

Emaciation of the affected parts (*Graph.*, *Plb.*).

Dropsical swelling of single parts, or in internal organs, or of the whole skin.

GOUT (*Calc-F.*, *Colch.*, *Kalm.*).

Boils, especially on the extremities.

Hives (*Apis*, *Ars.*, *Rhus-T.*, *Sep.*).

RHEUMATISM BEGINS BELOW AND TRAVELS UPWARD (descends—*Kalm.*) (N.).

Acute and chronic arthritis (B*ry.*) (A.).

Swelling of the feet up to the knees (A.).

Perspiration in the palms of the hand (*Calc.*, *Sil.*).

Affects the left shoulder and right hip-joint (*Agar.*, *Ant-T.*, *Stram.*) (A.).

BALL OF GREAT TOE SWOLLEN AND PAINFUL (*Colch.*) (A.).

Bad effects from the abuse of spirituous liquors (*Bry.*, *Nux-V.*, *Sulph.*).

Ecchymosis of the lids or conjunctivæ, especially after contusion (*Arn.*, *Ham.*, *Nux-V.*) (N.).

Hæmorrhage into the anterior chamber after iridectomy (A.).

Swelling of the ankle, with unbearable pain when walking, as from a sprain or false step (A.).

ALWAYS FEEL COLD AND CHILLY (*Sil.*) (A.).

Lack of animal or vital heat (*Sep., Sil.*) (A.).

Cracking of the joints, on moving them (G.).

Itching worse by scratching (G.).

The wounded parts are cold to the touch (A.).

Parts cold to the touch, but not cold subjectively to the patient (A.).

Punctured wounds (*Hyper.*) (N.).

STINGS OF INSECTS, ESPECIALLY MOSQUI-TOES (N.).

Rat-bites (*Ars., Lach., Sulph.*) (A.).

May be used to prevent or remove black and blue spots after blows (N.).

Long-remaining discloration after injuries; " black or blue " spots turn green (N.).

Red pimples or tubercles on the forehead and cheeks, as in brandy drinkers, stinging when touched (A.).

Stiffness in the back, as after sitting a long time (*Rhus-T.*) (D.).

Drawing pain in the joints (D.).

Bruised feeling in various parts of the body (D.).

Intense itching of feet and ankles, worse from scratching and warmth of bed (*Puls., Rhus-T.*) (A.).

Lumbago (*Calc., Calc-F., Kali-P., Nat-M., Rhus-T., Sep., Sulph.*) (B.).

Tetanus with twitching of muscles near wound (Br.).

Soles painful, can hardly step on them (Br.).

Sleeplessness, with restlessness and tossing about (*Rhus-T.*) (C.).

Night-sweats, with inclination to uncover (*Sulph.*) (C.).

Raging, pulsating headache (*Bell., Glon.*) (C.).

Hæmoptysis, alternating with rheumatism (B.).

Hollow, racking cough, with purulent expectoration, or of bright-red and foaming blood (C.).

AGGRAVATION: From motion; at night; from warmth of bed and bed-covering (*Merc.*); while walking; and from alcohol.

AMELIORATION: From holding feet in ice-water (*Sec.*); from getting out of bed; while reposing; and in cool air.

RELATIONSHIP: *Compare*: *Arn., Bellis., Con., Crot-T., Ham., Ruta* and *Sulph-Ac.* in traumatism.
Antidote: *Camph.*
It antidotes *Rhus poisoning.*

Lilium Tigrinum.

COMMON NAME: TIGER LILY.

Faint in warm room (*Acon., Ipec., Kreos., Lach., Lyc., Nat-M., Nux-V., Puls., Sep., Spig., Tab.*) (Br.).

Sensation of constriction in the heart with uterine troubles (N.).

Cold feeling about the heart (*Nat-M., Petr.*) (Br.).

Feeling as if the heart contained too much blood, which might be relieved by throwing it up (N.).

Palpitation (*Kali-P., Nat-M., Puls.*) (A.).

Rapid heart-beat, 150 to 170 per minute (A.).

Faint, hurried, anxious sensation about the apex (A.).

Continual pressure upon the bladder; wants to urinate all the time (N.).

Urine scanty, milky and hot (Br.).

Irregular pulse (*Dig., Ign., Nat-M., Phos., Verat.*) (A.).

Frequent desire for stool and urine with uterine displacements; tenesmus (N.).

Severe pain in the rectum and anus (*Aesc., Aloe, Ign., Lach., Nit-Ac.*) (Py.).

Constant pressure on the bladder (G.).

Great depression of spirits, with constant inclination to weep (*Ign., Puls., Stann.*) (Bt.).

Confused ideas (*Glon.*) (A.).

Constant hurried feeling, as if of imperative duties, and utter inability to perform them (N.).

Tormented about her salvation (*Aur., Puls., Verat.*) (N.).

Consolation aggravates (*Nat-M.*) (Br.).

Anxious; fears some organic and incurable disease (Br.)
Melancholia (*Aur., Gels., Ign., Nat-M.*) (Bl.).

Listless, yet does not want to sit still; restless, yet does not want to walk; hurried manner, desire to do something, yet no ambition (N.).

Indifferent about anything being done for her (N.).

Disposed to curse, strike, think obscene things (*Hyos., Stram.*) (Br.).

Desires finery (B.).

Prolapsus uteri, with bearing down sensation, accompanied with palpitation of the heart (*Nat-M., Sep.*) (Bt.).

BEARING DOWN IN THE LOWER PART OF THE ABDOMEN; WORSE WHEN STANDING, WITH PRESSURE UPON THE PERINAEUM, RELIEVED BY PRESSING WITH THE HAND AGAINST THE VULVA (Py.).

Soreness in the pelvic region (*Apis, Bell., Lach.*) (D.).

Menses flow only when moving about, cease when she ceases to walk (N.).

Weak and atonic condition of the ovaries, uterus and pelvic tissues, resulting in anteversion, retroversion, and sub-involution (*Helon., Sep.*) (A.).

Slow recovery after labour (*Carb-V., Chin., Ferr., Sep.*)

Wild, crazy feeling on the vertex (A.).

Sensation of a lump in the stomach (Br.).

Aversion to food (*Ars., Bry., Cycl., Ferr., Nux-V., Puls., Sep.*) (N.).

Abdomen feels as if it must be supported, as if it must be held up with both hands (G.).

Affects principally the left side of the body (*Lach., Thuj.;* the right side (*Apis, Lyc.*) (A.).

Morning diarrhœa in cases with prolapsus of uterus (G.).

Frequent small stools, with tenesmus (B.).

Menses early, scanty, dark and offensive (*Sep.*) (A.).

Must keep busy, to repress sexual desire (A.).

Voluptuous itching in the vagina (C.).

Air hunger (*Carb-V.*); takes long breaths (B.).

Sharp pains in the ovarian region (*Bell.*) (C.).

Sensation as if the heart was grasped in a vise (*Cact.*); *as if blood had all gone to the heart; feels full to bursting* (A.).

Sharp pain in the left chest (*Lach.*) (A.).

Pains in small spots (*Ign.*); *constantly shifting* (*Bell., Kali-B., Kali-S.*) (A.).

Pains in the ovaries, extending down into the inside of the thighs (G.).

Leucorrhœa: Thin, acrid; excoriating; staining the linen brown; after the menses (G.).

Blurred vision, with heat in the eyes and lids (C.).

Hollow, empty sensation in the stomach and bowels (C.).

Pulsations over the whole body (*Ferr., Nat-M., Sep., Sulph-Ac.*) (A.).

Dull pain in the sacrum (*Aesc.*) (C.).

Cannot walk on uneven ground (A.).

Inability to walk erect (*Bell.*) (A.).

Burning palms and soles (*Lach.*) (Br.).

Extremities cold and covered with cold sweat (*Carb-V., Sec., Verat.*) (A.).

AGGRAVATION: In the evening; at night; from standing; in a warm room; from consolation; after menses; and when moving about.

AMELIORATION: During the day; from sitting down; from pressure with the hand; from fresh air; and from keeping busy.

RELATIONSHIP: *Compare*: *Act-R., Agar., Bell., Cact., Dig., Helon., Kali-P., Lach., Murx., Nat-M., Pallad., Plat., Puls., Sep., Tarant.*, and *Verat.*

ANTIDOTES: *Helon.* and *Nux-V.*

Lobelia Inflata.

COMMON NAME: INDIAN TOBACCO.

Extreme sensitiveness of the sacrum; can't bear least touch; sits leaning forward to avoid contact of chair or cushion (N.).

Sick headache with vertigo (Bt.).

Dull headache, with violent nausea, vomiting and great prostration (Bt.).

Face bathed in cold sweat (*Ars., Bry., Cact., Calc., Calc-P., Camph., Carb-S., Carb-V., Chin., Cina, Cocc., Cupr., Dig., Dros., Glon., Ipec., Kali-B., Lach., Lyc., Merc., Merc-C., Spong., Verat.*) (Br.).

Shortness of breath after eating (*Nux-V.*) (Br.).

A deep pain about the heart (*Spig.*) (N.).

Sense as if the heart would stand still (*Dig.*) (N.).

Cannot bear smell or taste of tobacco (Br.).

Nausea and vomiting, with great relaxation of muscular system and profuse accumulation of saliva (N.).

DEATHLY NAUSEA, WITH VERTIGO (B.).

VOMITING WITH COLD SWEAT ON THE FACE (*Verat.*) (B.).

Violent nausea and vomiting, with great loss of strength (Bt.).

After vomiting, breaks out all over with sweat (Smi.).

Heartburn with profuse flow of saliva (Br.).

WEAK, SINKING FEELING AT THE STOMACH (*Carb-An., Dig., Sep.*) (B.).

Chronic vomiting with good appetite, with nausea, profuse sweat and marked prostration (A.).

Faintness, weakness and an indescribable feeling at the epigastrium, from excessive use of tea or tobacco (A.).

Loss of appetite, with acrid, burning taste in the mouth (*Ars.*) (C.).

Burning in the stomach (*Ars., Carb-V.*) (A.).

Deep red urine, with red sediment (*Lyc.*) (B.).

Sense of pressure or weight in the chest (Br.).

Hawking up copious quantities of mucus (*Lyc., Puls.*) (Bt.).

Spasmodic cough, with sneezing (*All-C., Bell., Bry., Cina, Con., Eup-P., Hep., Iod., Kali-C., Merc., Nat-M., Sil., Squil., Sulph.*) (B.).

SPASMODIC ASTHMA; WORSE FROM EXERTION (*Ars., Dig., Phos.*) (Bt.).

RATTLE IN THE CHEST, BUT DON'T EXPECTORATE (*Am-C., Ant-T., Carb-V., Nat-S.*) (B.).

Dyspnœa, with a sense of a lump in the pit of the stomach rising into the mouth (Bt.).

EMPHYSEMA (*Am-C., Ant-Ars., Ant-T., Ars., Bell., Brom., Camph., Carb-V., Chlor., Cupr., Dig., Hep., Ipec., Lach., Merc., Nat-M., Phel., Phos., Seneg., Sep., Stann., Sulph.*) (Bt.).

Pertussis, with dyspnœa threatening suffocation (*Ipec.*).

Morning sickness (*Bry., Colch., Ipec., Puls., Sep.*) (Br.).

AGGRAVATION: From the slightest motion; in the afternoon; from cold; from touch; from going up or down-stairs (*Ipec.*).

AMELIORATION: From warmth; from walking rapidly (chest pain).

RELATIONSHIP: *Antidote*: *Ipec.*
Compare: *Ant-T., Ars., Cocc., Colch., Cupr., Dig., Ipec., Phos., Sep.* and *Verat.*

Lycopodium Clavatum.

COMMON NAME: CLUB MOSS.

It is especially adapted to ailments gradually developing (D.).

Often useful for persons who are intellectually keen, but physically weak (A.).

Functional power weakening with failure of the digestive power (D.).

Great emaciation (*Abrot., Iod., Nat-M., Sil.*).

Involuntary spasmodic contraction and stretching of the limbs.

Drawing and tearing in the limbs, especially while at rest and at night.

Numbness of the limbs (*Acon., Kalm., Rhus-T.*).

Contraction of the limbs (*Am-M., Cupr., Sec.*).

Limbs go to sleep (*Puls.*).

There is inclination to lie about and real aversion to movement.

RIGHT-SIDED AFFECTIONS (THROAT, CHEST, ABDOMEN, LIVER AND OVARIES) (A.).

Twitchings through the body (*Ign.*).

Varices (*Calc-T., Ham., Nat-M., Sep.*).

Chronic gout, with chalky deposits in the joints (Br.).

COMPLAINTS FROM RIGHT TO LEFT (reverse of *Lach.*) (D.).

Offensiveness of the discharges (*Bapt., Merc., Nit-Ac., Petr., Sil., Sulph.*) (D.).

Inflammation of the bones with nightly pains (*Asaf., Calc-F., Calc-S., Fluor-Ac., Merc., Mezer., Nit-Ac., Phyt., Sil.*).

Softening of the bones (*Calc., Merc., Sil.*).

Caries (*Asaf., Calc., Kali-B., Merc., Nit-Ac., Phos., Sil.*).

Deep-seated, progressive, chronic diseases (*Calc., Merc., Sil., Sulph.*) (A.).

DROPSY (*Acet-Ac., Chel., Dig., Kali-C.*).

Child screams before passing urine (*Bor., Sars.*) (A.).

Soreness in children (*Cham.*).

Children weak, emaciated; with well-developed head, but puny and sickly bodies (A.).

LOOKS OLDER THAN HE IS (*Arg-N.*) (N.).

BABY CRIES ALL DAY, SLEEPS ALL NIGHT (reverse of *Jal., Psor.*) (A.).

Snuffles: Child starts from sleep rubbing its nose (A.).

Nose stopped at night, due to dry catarrh; must breathe through the mouth (*Am-C., Nux-V., Samb.*) (A.).

Enlarged tonsils; studded with small ulcers (D.).

Tonsils and tongue are both swollen (*Apis, Merc., Rhus-T.*) (D.).

Diphtheritic deposits on the right side of the throat (D.).

Diphtheria: Fauces brownish-red; deposit spreads from the right tonsil to the left, or descends from the nose (A.).

SORETHROAT: WORSE AFTER SLEEP AND FROM COLD DRINKS (worse from warm drinks— *Lach.*) (A.).

Aching pain in the lumbar region, ameliorated after urinating (K.).

RENAL COLIC (*Berb., Canth., Ocim.*) (F.).

SANDY SEDIMENT OF URINE (*Am-C., Berb., Nit-Ac., Sep.*).

Urinary disturbances are marked (*Canth., Merc., Sep., Tereb.*) (D.).

Stitches in the neck of the bladder and anus at the same time (N.).

HEAVY, RED SEDIMENT IN THE URINE (*Arn., Ars., Arund., Dig., Lob., Merc-C., Ocim., Ox-Ac., Pareir., Phos., Plan., Sel., Senec., Sep., Tarant.*) (D.).

Terrific pain in the back previous to every urination, with relief as soon as the urine begins to flow (G.).

Lithic acid diathesis (N.).

IMPOTENCE, OR SEXUAL DESIRE TOO STRONG (*Agar., Calad., Con., Phos.*).

Premature emission (*Sulph.*) (A.).

Impotence, with cold, relaxed sexual organs, and diminished sexual powers (*Agn.*) (D.).

Aversion to coition (*Graph.*) (K.).

Incomplete erection during coition (*Camph., Graph., Phos-Ac., Sulph.*) (K.).

Falls asleep during an embrace (A.).

Profuse leucorrhœa, with cutting pains across the right side to the left (G.).

Catamenia too profuse (*Calc., Erig., Ferr., Graph., Sec.*).

Dryness of the vagina (*Ars., Ferr., Graph., Nat-M., Sep.*). (A.).

Burning in the vagina during and after coition (*Kreos.*) (A.).

Discharge of blood from the genitals during every stool (*Ambr., Am-M., Ind.*) (A.).

Nipples bleed much and are very sore (G.).

Fœtus appears to be turning somersault (*Thuj.*) (A.).

Discharge of wind from the vagina (*Brom.*) (G.).

Snoring breathing (*Brom., Camph., Cupr., Hep., Ign., Lac-C., Lach., Nux-V., Op., Stram.*) (D.).

Nose stuffed up; cannot breathe through it night or day (*Nux-V., Stict.*) (D.).

Discharge of yellowish-green matter from the nose (*Arg-N., Kali-B., Kali-S., Merc., Nat-S.*) (D.).

FAN-LIKE MOTION OF THE ALAE-NASI (*Ant-T.*) (D.).

Very often of great service in pneumonia with great dyspnœa, flaying of the alæ nasi, and the presence of the mucous rattle (*Phos.*).

Cough deep, hollow; even raising mucus in large quantities affords little relief (A.).

CHRONIC DRY COUGH IN PINING BOYS (K.).

MALTREATED OR NEGLECTED PNEUMONIA (*Kali-C.*); THE BASE OF THE RIGHT LUNG IS INVOLVED ESPECIALLY (A.).

In intermittents, flatulence, sour eructations, sour taste, sour sweat and sour vomiting (N.).

Chill on the left side of the body (*Caust., Carb-V.*) (N.).

Perspiration immediately after the chill (N.).

Thirst after sweating stage (N.). (

Sour vomiting between chill and heat; must uncover (N.).

Old, broken-down cases of malaria (N.).

AFRAID TO BE LEFT ALONE (*Arg-N., Ars., Bism., Crot-C., Hyos., Kali-C., Lil-T., Phos.*) (D.).

Avaricious, greedy, miserly, malicious, and pusillanimous (A.).

Ailments from fright, anger, mortification, or vexation with reserved displeasure (*Staph.*) (A.).

IMPERIOUS AND DOMINEERING (*Plat.*) (D.).

Depression of mind and sensorium; stupid; lower jaw drops (*Hyos.*) (N.).

Sad and melancholic (*Ign.*, *Nat-M.*, *Sep.*) (D.).

Weeps all day, cannot calm herself (*Nat-M.*, *Puls.*, *Stann.*) (A.).

Makes mistakes in speech (*Arg-N.*, *Arn.*, *Bar-C.*, *Both.*, *Cann-I.*, *Chin-Ars.*, *Kali-Br.*, *Kali-P.*, *Lach.*, *Med.*, *Nat-M.*, *Nux-V.*, *Onos.*, *Phos-Ac.*, *Sulph.*, *Verat.*) (D.).

VERY SENSITIVE, EVEN CRIES WHEN THANKED (A.).

Averse to undertaking new things (Br.).

Irritable; peevish and cross on waking; ugly, kick and scream; easily angered; cannot endure opposition (*Aur.*, *Cham.*, *Nux-V.*)·; *or contradiction; seeks disputes; is beside himself* (A.).

Plica polonica (Hg.).

Dry porrigo of children (G.).

Greyish yellow colour of the face (Bt.).

Shakes head without apparent cause (Br.).

Boils, which bleed a great deal all the time (G.).

PALPITATION DURING DIGESTION (*Sep.*) (K.).

CONVULSIONS IN THE RIGHT SIDE OF THE BODY (*Bell.*, *Caust.*, *Nux-V.*; left side of the body—*Calc-P.*, *Cupr.*, *Elaps*, *Graph.*, *Ipec.*, *Nat-M.*, *Plb.*, *Sulph.*) (K.).

Ulcers and vesicles on and under the tongue (N.).

Chronic eczema, associated with urinary, gastric and hepatic disorders (Br.).

GREAT DEBILITY—LOWER JAW HANGING DOWN, EYES HALF OPEN AND SLOW BREATH-ING THROUGH THE MOUTH.

Twitching and jerking during sleep (*Bell.*, *Hyos.*, *Stram.*).

While at rest he feels the debility most, but is disinclined to move.

Debility in the morning when awakening (*Lach.*).

Twitchings through the body.

Ebullition in the evening, with trembling and restlessness.

A sensation as if the circulation had ceased.

Weakness and relaxation (*Gels.*) (D.).

Bad effects of tobacco-smoking and chewing (*Ars.*) (A.).

Early senility (*Arg-N.*) (B.).

Hemiopia (*Aur., Bov., Calc., Cocc., Dig., Gels., Glon., Lith., Nat-M., Sep.*) (B.).

TONGUE OSCILLATING FROM SIDE TO SIDE LIKE A PENDULUM (*Cupr., Lach.*) (N.).

Oversensitiveness of the organs of sense (*Cham., Coff., Lach., Nux-V.*).

Wrinkled forehead; frowning (B.).

Purulent, ichorous otorrhœa, with impaired hearing, after scarlatina (N.).

Evening light blinds him very much; can see nothing on the table (N.).

Sees only left half of an object distinctly (right half of objects invisible—*Lith.*) (N.).

Throbbing headache after every paroxysm of coughing (N.).

Swelling, inflammation and suppuration of the glands (*Calc., Hep., Iod., Merc., Sil.*).

Shuddering as if from a shock in both temples and chest (when coughing) (N.).

Upper part of the body emaciated, lower part semi-dropsical (reverse of *Am--M.*) (A.).

ONE FOOT HOT AND THE OTHER COLD (N.).

Burning as of hot coals between the scapulæ (*Berb., Kali-B., Med., Nux-V., Phos., Sulph., Thuj.*) (D.).

Night-sweats; perspiration cold, clammy, sour, fetid, or smelling like onions.

Right-sided hernia (A.).

Constipation; almost impossible to evacuate the stools (G.).

Bleeding piles (*Aloe, Nux-V., Sulph.*) (D.).

Constipation: Since puberty; since last confinement; when away from home (A.).

Constipation with inffectual urging and a sensation as if something remained behind due to constriction of the rectum and anus (*Sep.*) (D.).

There is sour taste, sour belching and sometims sour vomiting (*Arg-N., Carb-V., Nat-P.*) (D.).

Function of the liver seriously disturbed (*Berb., Chel., Dig., Hep., Iod., Kali-M., Lach., Merc., Nat-S., Phos., Sep., Sulph.*) (D.).

Predisposed to lung and hepatic affections (*Calc., Phos., Sulph.*) (A.).

BITTER TASTE IN THE MOUTH AT NIGHT (*Ant-T., Lach., Rhus-T.*) (K.).

Constant sensation of satiety (A.).

Desire for sweets (*Arg-N., Calc., Merc.*) (D.).

FERMENTATION IN THE ABDOMEN, WITH LOUD GRUMBLING, CROAKING, ESPECIALLY IN THE LOWER ABDOMEN (upper abdomen—*Carb-V.,* entire abdomen—*Chin.*) (A.).

SOUR VOMITING, DURING CHILL OR FEVER (*Rob.*) (K.).

Goes to meals with a vigorous appetite, but a few mouthfuls fills him up full (D.).

Waking at night feeling hungry (*Cina, Psor.*) (A.).

Canine hunger; the more he eats, the more he craves; head aches if he does not eat (*Chel., Phos.*) (A.).

Excessive accumulation of flatulence; fulness, not relieved by belching (*Chin.*) (A.).

Very sleepy after eating (*Agar., Anac., Bov., Carb-V., Chin., Kali-C., Nat-M., Nux-V., Op., Phos., Sil., Sulph.*) (D.).

Great accumulation of flatus in the intestines, which presses up and causes difficulty in breathing (*Arg-N.*) (D.).

ERUCTATIONS AMELIORATE G A S T R I C TROUBLES (*Ant-T., Arg-N., Carb-S., Carb-V., Graph., Ign., Kali-B., Kali-C., Sang.*) (K.).

Slow digestion (*Chin., Hep.*) (C.).

Heart-burn; water-brash (*Nat-P.*) (C.).

Pit of the stomach swollen and sensitive, and intolerant to tight clothing (D.).

AGGRAVATION: In the afternoon; at night; from 4 to 8 P.M.; from cold; in a warm room; after eating; from wrapping up the head; while lying down; and while urinating.

AMELIORATION: By motion; in the heat of the bed; in the cool, open air; from warm food and drinks; from loosening the garments; from uncovering the head; and from eructation.

RELATIONSHIP: *Complementary: Iod., Kali-C., Lach.*

Follows well after: Calc., Carb-V., Chel., Graph., Iod., Lach., Nux-V., and *Sulph.*

Antidotes: Camph., Caust., and *Puls.*

It antidotes: Chin.

Lyssin.

COMMON NAME: THE SALIVA OF A RABID DOG.

May be used as a prophylactic in hydrophobia (Hr.).

Complaints resulting from abnormal sexual desire (*Canth., Phos., Plat.;* from abstinence—*Con.*) (A.).

There is a desire to urinate on seeing running water (*Canth., Sulph.*) (Bl.).

There is a pressing, boring pain in the forehead (Bl.).

Headache: From bites of dogs, whether rabid or not; chronic, from mental emotion or exertion; aggravated by noise of running water or bright light (A.).

Urine scanty, cloudy, contains sugar (A.).

Chronic headaches (*Arg-N., Nat-M., Puls., Sep., Sil., Sulph., Syph.*) (D.).

CANNOT BEAR HEAT OF THE SUN (*Acon., Bell., Gels., Glon., Lach., Nat-C., Nat-M., Sep.*) (A.).

Dysphagia (*Bell., Hyos., Ign., Lach., Lyc., Merc., Nit-Ac., Stram.*) (Bl.).

Spasms of the œsophagus from attempting to swallow water (Bl.).

Gagging when swallowing water (A.).

Lasciviousness (*Bell., Canth., Hyos.*) (Br.).

LYSSOPHOBIA (*Bell., Stram.*) (A.).

PATIENT CANNOT HEAR WATER RUN (D.).

Fear of becoming mad (*Calc., Cann-I., Manc., Puls., Sep., Stram.*) (A.).

Difficult and incoherent speech (*Bell., Hyos., Stram.*) (Hr.).

Rapid speech (*Bell., Lach., Stram.*) (B.).

IMPATIENCE AND VIOLENT TEMPER (*Bell., Bufo, Nux-V., Stram.*) (B.).

Roams about (B.).

Hypersensitiveness of all senses (*Bell., Cham., Coff., Lach., Stram.*) (Br.).

Voice altered in tone (*Arum-T.*) (Br.).

Aching in the bones (*Eup-P.*) (Br.).

Bluish discoloration of wounds (*Lach.*) (A.).

Atrophy of the testicles (*Aur., Bar-C., Caps., Carb-An., Gels., Iod., Kali-I., Plb.*) (Br.).

Priapism (*Canth., Pic-Ac.*), *with frequent emissions* (Br.).

No emission during coition (*Graph.*) (Br.).

Froths at mouth (*Cupr.*) (Br.).

The saliva is tough and ropy (*Kali-B.*), *and causes a constant spitting* (Bl.).

Wants water, but cannot drink it (Bt.).

Sorethroat, with constant desire to swallow (*Bell., Ign., Lac-C., Lach., Merc.*) (A.).

Barking cough (*Acon., Bell., Coc-C., Dros., Dulc., Hep., Kali-B., Merc., Nit-Ac., Phos., Rumex, Spong., Stram.*) (B.).

DIARRHOEA, AGGRAVATED FROM HEARING RUNNING WATER (K.).

Profuse watery stools, from six to twenty a day, with pain in the bowels; worse in the morning (*Aloe, Podo., Sulph.*) (Ha.).

Sexual excitement (*Bell., Canth., Phos., Plat., Stram.*) (B.).

Sensitive womb (*Apis, Bell., Canth., Lach.*) (B.).

Sensitiveness of the vagina, rendering coition painful (*Plat.*) (A.).

Conscious of womb (Br.).

Prolapsus uteri (*Bell., Murx., Sep.*) (A.).

Convulsions in pregnancy (D.).

CONVULSIONS ON HEARING WATER POURED OUT (D.).

CONVULSIONS AS THE RESULT OF REFLECTED LIGHT, OR FROM WATER, OR A MIRROR (Bl.).

SPASMS ARE EXCITED AT EVERY ATTEMPT TO DRINK WATER, OR AT THE SOUND OF WATER (Bt.).

Convulsions from even thinking of fluids of any kind, or from the slightest touch or current of air (A.).

Breathing held for a time (*Cupr.*) (Br.).

AGGRAVATION: From the sight or sound of running water or pouring water; from mental emotion; from mortifying news; from the heat of the sun; from draughts; from glistening objects; from bright, dazzling light; from carriage-riding, and from stooping.

AMELIORATION: From bending backward; from gentle rubbing.

RELATIONSHIP: *Compare*: *Apis*, *Bell.*, *Canth.*, *Hyos.*, *Ign.*, *Kali-B.*, *Lach.*, *Merc.*, *Nit-Ac.*, and *Stram.*

Magnesia Carbonica.

COMMON NAME: CARBONATE OF MAGNESIA.

Useful for persons, especially children, of irritable disposition and nervous temperament (*Cham.*, *Nux-V.*, *Staph.*) (A.).

Painless twitching, here and there.

In the evening, after sitting, restlessness in the limbs, which compels one to walk about.

Swelling of the glands (*Bell.*, *Calc.*, *Graph.*, *Hep.*, *Iod.*, *Kali-I.*, *Lyc.*, *Merc.*).

Great sensation of fatigue whilst sitting.

The knees are painful when walking (*Bry.*) (G.).

Oedema of the feet up to the calves (G.).

Sudden falling down with consciousness (*Cupr.*, *Nux-V.*, *Sulph.*).

Sad and disconsolate (G.).

Insupportable pains during repose; she must get up and walk about (G.).

Craves open air (*Apis*, *Puls.*) (B.).

Sudden deafness (B.).

Paroxysmal cough (*Bell.*, *Dros.*) (B.).

Toothache of a bothersome nature often calls for exhibition of the remedy (*Cham.*, *Coff.*, *Merc.*, *Puls.*).

TOOTHACHE AT NIGHT, COMPELLING ONE TO RISE AND WALK ABOUT; PAIN INSUPPORTABLE WHILE AT REST; WORSE IN COLD (C.).

Toothache of pregnancy (*Acon.*, *Bell.*, *Calc.*, *Cham.*, *Hyos.*, *Lyss.*, *Merc.*, *Nux-M.*, *Nux-V.*, *Puls.*, *Rat.*, *Rhus-T.* *Sep.*, *Staph. Tab.*) (D.).

Labour-like pain, cutting colic, backache, weakness and chilliness during menses (A.).

It should be remembered in acid dyspepsia, with heart-burn (Bl.).

The tongue is coated dirty yellow (G.).

Doubling up colic, relieved after stool (Nux-V.) (N.).

Starchy foods disagree, as does milk (Bl.).

The child is improperly nourished; its mouth is full of ulcers (Bor.) (D.).

Sour smell of the whole body (Rheum).

Pale, sickly children, with colic and green stools (D.).

White, tallow-like masses are found floating in the stool (A.).

Diarrhœa occurs regularly every three weeks (A.).

THE STOOLS ARE SOUR AND GREEN AS GRASS *(Merc.)* (D.).

THE STOOLS ARE GREEN AND FROTHY—LIKE THE SCUM OF A FROG-POND (A.).

Diarrhœa, preceded by cutting, doubling up colic (Nux-V.) (A.).

When milk is taken into the stomach it causes pain and is vomited undigested (in puny, sickly children) (D.).

Many stools day and night (G.).

Sour vomiting (Lyc., Nat-P.) (G.).

Griping, cutting, rumbling in the whole abdomen, followed by thin, green stools (N.).

Disposition to furuncles and headache (G.).

Inordinate craving for meat in children of tuberculous parentage (A.).

Unrefreshing sleep; more tired on rising than when retiring *(Bry., Con., Hep., Op., Sulph.)* (A.).

Dreams anxious; for dead persons; of fire; and of thieves (G.).

Heart-burn: Sour, belching, eructations, taste and *vomiting; of pregnancy* (A.).

Ailments from cutting wisdom teeth (*Bell., Merc., Sil.*) (Br.).

Sticking pain in • the throat; hawking up fetid, pea-coloured particles (Br.).

Desire for fruits, acids and vegetables (Br.).

Pains in the top of the shoulder-joints, generally left side, which prevent raising the arm (G.).

Whole body feels tired and painful, especially legs and feet (Br.).

Face dirty, dark yellow (Bt.).

Nightly tearing, digging and boring in the cheek bones; insupportable during rest, and driving from one place to another (C.).

Pressive headache; rush of blood to the head (*Bell., Glon., Nat-M.*) (C.).

Tetter on the scalp, itching during wet, rainy weather (C.).

Chilly in the evening; fever at night; sour, greasy perspiration (Br.).

Tickling cough, with salty, bloody expectoration (Br.).

Constrictive pain in the chest with dyspnœa (*Cact., Naja, Phos.*) (Br.).

Catamenia retarded (*Cycl., Graph., Nat-M., Puls., Sep.*).

Before the catamenia there is toothache (*Am-C., Ant-C., Bar-C., Nat-M., Phos., Puls., Sulph., Thuj.*).

MENSES BLACK AND FLOW AT NIGHT ONLY (D.).

Has a sorethroat during every menstruation (G.)

Menses dark, acrid and thick; washed out with great difficulty (G.).

Menses flow only in the absence of pain and at night (G.).

Too frequent and too profuse menstruation (Dn.).

Menses too late, and too scanty (G.).

Mucous leucorrhœa (*Hydr.*) (G.).

Menses flow when lying, cease when walking (N.)

AGGRAVATION: In the evening; at night; while standing; during rest; before and during menses; every third week; from milk; from warmth of bed; from change of temperature; and during pregnancy.

AMELIORATION: After stool; in warm air; and from walking in the open air.

RELATIONSHIP: *Antidotes*: *Ars., Cham., Merc., Nux-V.* and *Puls.*

Complementary to: *Cham.*

Magnesia Muriatica.

COMMON NAME: CHLORIDE OF MAGNESIA.

It is useful in women and children; in hysteria, scrofula and liver affections (D.).

Great tendency of the head to sweat (*Calc., Sanic., Sil.*) (A.).

Aptness to take cold (*Calc-P., Hep., Kali-C., Psor., Sil., Sulph., Tub.*) (G.).

Much weakness of the limbs (*Gels., Kali-P., Pic-Ac., Zinc.*) (G.).

Swelling of the glands (*Brom., Carb-An., Iod., Merc., Sil.*).

Blood boils (*Arn., Hep., Lach.*).

Great sensitiveness to noise (*Ign., Nux-V., Ther.*) (A.).

Enlargement of the liver; pains worse from touch or from lying on the right side (D.).

Hyperæmia of the liver with constipation (*Bry., Chel., Sep., Sulph.*) (Bl.).

Pressing pain in the liver, when walking and touching it (A.).

Jaundice (*Chin., Iod., Merc., Plb., Sep.*) (B.).

Violent hiccough during and after dinner (R.).

The tongue is large and yellow and takes the imprints of the teeth (*Chel., Merc., Plb.*) (D.).

Poor appetite (*Chin.. Lyc., Puls., Sep.*) (G.).

Bad taste in the mouth (*Carb-V., Nux-V., Puls.*) (G.)

Continual rising of white froth into the mouth (A.).

Throbbing in the pit of stomach (R.).

Palpitation of the heart when the patient is quiet, better when moving about (N.).

Acidity after dinner (*Nux-V.*) (C.).

Dreams of robbers in the house; on awaking will not believe to the contrary until a search is made (G.).

Painful, smarting hæmorrhoids (Br.).

Headache: Every six weeks, in the forehead and around the eyes; as if it would burst; worse from motion and in the open air; better from lying down, strong pressure (*Puls.*), and wrapping up warmly (*Sil., Stront.*) (A.).

CONSTIPATION: STOOLS KNOTTY OR LUMPY, LIKE SHEEP DUNG (*Op., Plb., Verat.*); CRUMBLING AT THE VERGE OF THE ANUS (N.).

Slow dentition (*Calc., Sil.*), with large, distended abdomen (G.).

CHILDREN ARE UNABLE TO DIGEST MILK: IT CAUSES PAIN IN THE STOMACH AND PASSES UNDIGESTED (*Mag-C.*) (A.).

Useful particularly for puny and rachitic children, who crave sweets (*Arg-N.. Calc.. Lyc., Merc., Sulph.*) (A.).

Constipation of infants during dentition (*Sil.*) (A.).

Micturition in drops (*Clem., Hep.*) (R.).

Urine pale yellow; can only be passed by bearing down with the abdominal muscles; weakness of the bladder (*Alum., Op.*) (N.).

Sensation as if a ball were ascending from abdomen into œsophagus, ameliorated by eructations (R.).

Dysuria due to partial paralysis of the muscles of the bladder (R.).

Eructations, tasting like rotten eggs, like onions (breath smells of onions—*Sinap.*) (A.).

Toothache: Unbearable when food touches the teeth (A.).

Much excited at the menstrual crisis (G.).

Uterine spasms extending to the thighs (G.).

Metrorrhagia, worse at night in bed, causing hysteria (Act-R., Caul.) (A.).

Menstrual flow black and clotted (Cham.) (A.).

Profuse, dark, lumpy menses; like pitch; with cramps, backache and pains in the thighs (B.).

Leucorrhœa, after every stool (G.).

Leucorrhœa, two weeks after menses, for three or four days *(Bar-C., Bov., Con.)* (A.).

Hysterical complaints and spasmodic turns; many spasms day and night; with great sleeplessness; fainting fits (G.).

Bruised or burning feeling in the hips and back (B.).

Coryza: Nose stopped; cannot lie down; must breathe through the mouth *(Lyc., Nux-V.)* (Br.).

Loss of smell and taste, following catarrh (Nat-M.) (Br.).

Gums swollen; bleed easily (Carb-V., Merc., Nit-Ac.) (Br.).

Fretful, morose, peevish (Cina, Nux-V., Sulph.) (C.).

Chilliness every evening; disappears after going to bed (C.).

Sleep unrefreshing; tired in the morning *(Nux-V.)* (C.).

AGGRAVATION: While sitting; from lying on the right side; immediately after eating; from sea-bathing; at night; from noise; from milk; and from salt foods.

AMELIORATION: By motion; from exercise; in the open air; and from hard pressure.

RELATIONSHIP: *Antidotes: Camph.* and *Cham.*
Similar to: Am-M., Bry., Calc., Caust., Cham., Chel., Chin., Cycl., Ferr., Graph., Hep., Iod., Kali-C., Lach., Lyc., Merc., Nat-M., Puls., Sep., Sulph. and *Zinc.*

Magnesia Phosphorica.

COMMON NAME: PHOSPHATE OF MAGNESIA.

General action: It corresponds to darting, spasmodic pains along the course of the nerves; spasms in different parts of the body; colic, cramps, etc. (D.).

The patient is languid, tired and exhausted (D.).

Pains lightning-like, coming and going (Bell.) (N.).

Darting, spasmodic pains, which are relieved by pressure and warmth—are its main characteristics (D.).

Affections of the right side of the body: Head, ear, face, chest, ovary and sciatic nerve (Bell., Bry., Chel., Kali-C., Lyc., Podo.) (A.).

Spasmodic twitching of the eyelids or facial muscles (*Ign.*) (D.).

Great dread: of cold air, of uncovering; of touching the affected part; of cold bathing or washing; and of moving (A.).

SPASMODIC HICCOUGH DAY AND NIGHT, WITH RETCHING (N.).

Hiccough and spasms in teething children (*Bell., Cupr., Ign.*) (D.).

Colic, accompanied by belching of gas (*Coloc., Nux-V., Puls.*) (D.).

Severe cramping pains, especially in the stomach, abdomen and pelvis, amelioration by hot applications (N.).

FLATULENT COLIC, FORCING THE PATIENT TO BEND DOUBLE, RELIEVED FROM HEAT AND RUBBING (N.).

Spasmodic cough, coming on in paroxysms, without expectoration (D.).

Asthmatic oppression of the chest (*Ant-T., Ars., Blatta, Carb-V., Dig., Ferr., Graph., Hep., Ipec., Kali-C.*) (Br.).

Whooping cough, worse at night and accompanied with difficulty in lying down (Dros.) (D.).

Inter-costal neuralgia (Ran-B.) (Br.).

Constricting pains around heart (Br.).

Angina pectoris (Lach., Naja) (Br.).

Dull headache; as if the brain were too heavy (*Bry., Nux-V.*) (R.).

Cramps of the extremities, during pregnancy (A.).

Complaints from standing in cold water, or working in cold clay (*Calc.*) (A.).

Chorea, with contortions of the limbs (D.).

Piano or violin player's cramps (D.).

WRITER'S CRAMPS (*Bry.*) (D.).

SCIATICA (*Coloc., Phyt.*) (Br.).

Menses: Early; flow dark, stringy; pains worse before, better when the flow begins; pains drifting, like lightning, shooting, worse on the right side, ameliorated by heat and bending double (A.).

Spasmodic retention of urine (*Bell.*) (D.).

Headache of school girls (*Calc-P., Nat-M.*) (A.).

Headache, from mental emotion, exertion or hard study; relieved by pressure and external heat (A.).

Headache from 10 to 11 A.M., or 4 to 5 P.M. (A.).

Headache, begins in the occiput and extends over the head, with red or flushed face (A.).

Vaginismus (*Canth., Plat.*) (A.).

SPASMODIC DYSMENORRHOEA (*Act-R., Bell., Cupr., Gels., Lach., Puls., Sec.*) (D.).

Sudden paroxysms of pain; shooting like lightning; suddenly changing place; extorting cries; causing restlessness, prostration, etc. (B.).

Sobbing, crying, lamenting all the time about pain in the affected parts (R.).

Spasmodic convulsions, with stiffness of the limbs, clenched fingers and thumbs drawn in (D.).

SPASMS DURING DENTITION, WITHOUT FEVER (with fever, hot head and skin—*Bell.*) (A.).

Photophobia, with increased lachrymation (*Euphr., Merc., Nat-M.*) (R.).

Intermittent darting pains in and above the orbit (*Spig.*) (R.).

Double vision (*Bell., Gels., Stram.*) (R.).

Toothache aggravated after going to bed, aggravated by eating and drinking cold things, and ameliorated by heat (R.).

Severe neuralgic pains in the ears; worse by going into cold air and washing the face and neck with cold water (C.).

AGGRAVATION: From cold air; from cold water; from touch; from cold bathing; from motion; from uncovering; and at night.

AMELIORATION: From pressure; from heat; from warmth; from hot bathing; and from friction.

RELATIONSHIP: *Compare*: *Acon., Bell., Caul., Coloc., Ign., Lac-C., Lyc., Puls. and Rhus-T.*

Cham. is its vegetable analogue.

Manganum.

COMMON NAME: MANGANESE.

This is a close analogue of Iron, and will be found adapted to similar diseases (Bt.).

Violent tearing and drawing in the extremities.

Violent, nightly, digging pains in the joints.

After catching cold a red, shining swelling of the joints

Rheumatism in the joints, with stinging and digging worse at night, often one-sided, or oblique, in association with which there is a glistening red swelling of the joints.

The whole body feels sore to contact (*Arn., Bapt., Lach.*).

Insupportable nightly digging in the bones and periosteum (*Aur., Merc., Mezer., Nit-Ac., Syph.*).

Inflammation of the bones and periosteum (*Calc-F., Fluor-Ac., Merc., Nit-Ac., Phyt., Sil.*).

Rhagades in the joints.

Burning heat and dryness of the eyes; lids pain on moving them, and become dry in bright light (N.).

Skin does not heal readily (*Calc-S., Graph., Hep., Sil., Sulph.*).

Chronic suppurations of the skin, especially about the joints (*Petr.*) (Bt.).

Paralysis of the nerves of motion (*Con., Gels., Nux-V. Plb.*) (Bt.).

Diagonal pains (B.).

Headache, worse from straining at stool (*Bry., Con., Glon., Ind., Lyc., Nux-V.*) (B.).

Toothaches, with suddenly shifting painfulness to other parts of the body.

Many ailments change with the weather.

Difficult, dry, and knotty evacuations (*Mag-M., Plb., Sep.*) (C.).

Loud cracking noise in the ears, when blowing the nose or swallowing (*Graph.*) (C.).

Congestion of blood to the head (*Bell., Ferr., Glon.*) (C.).

SPASMODIC COUGH. BETTER ON LYING DOWN (N.).

Hoarse voice (*Arg-N., Carb-V., Phos., Rhus-T.*) (G.).

Raw, dry, larynx (*Caust.*) (B.).

Expectorating a lump of mucus (*Calc., Kali-C., Phos., Sil.*) (B.).

Cough worse from reading or laughing (*Phos.*) (B.).

Hemming all the time (Br.).

Tuberculosis of larynx (*Calc., Carb-V., Kali-B., Phos., Sulph.*) (Br.).

Every cold rouses up a bronchitis (*Hep., Kali-C., Lyc., Nat-S., Sil.*) (Br.).

Hæmoptysis (*Caust., Kali-P., Lach., Nit-Ac., Phos., Rhus-T., Sep.*) (Br.).

Greenish or yellow expectoration (K.).

Menses too early and too scanty (*Cycl., Ferr., Puls.*) (C.).

AGGRAVATION: At night; on stooping; from talking; from touch; in cold, damp weather; in feather bed; from motion; from straining at stool; from reading; and from laughing.

AMELIORATION: From lying down; and in open air.

RELATIONSHIP: *Antidotes*: *Camph., Coff.* and *Merc.*

Remedies following: *Puls., Rhus-T.* and *Sulph.*

Medorrhinum.

COMMON NAME: THE GONORRHOEAL VIRUS.

For the constitutional effects of mal-treated and suppressed gonorrhœa, when the best selected remedy fails to relieve or permanently improve (A.).

BURNING OF HANDS AND FEET (*Lach., Phos., Sep., Sulph.*); WANTS THEM UNCOVERED AND FANNED (N.).

Great heat and soreness, with enlargement of lymphatic glands all over the body (A.).

Is of service in the chronic pelvic diseases of women that date from a gonorrhœal infection (Bl.).

Useful in obstinate rheumatism, when this obstinacy is due to a latent sycotic taint (D.).

Trembling all over (*subjective*); *intense nervousness and profound exhaustion* (A.).

Headache of exhaustion, or from hard work (D.).

Head feels heavy and is drawn backwards (*Cocc.*) (A.).

Intense burning pain in the brain (A.).

Headache from jarring of cars (A.).

Sensation of tightness and contraction in the head (A.).

Desire for ale, ice, acids, oranges and green fruits (A.).

Morning nausea (*Bry., Nux-V., Sep.*) (B.).

Vomiting of pregnancy (Cycl., Ign., Ipec., Kali-M., Nux-V., Petr., Puls.) (B.).

Craves stimulants (*Nux-V.*) (B.).

Ravenous hunger, immediately after eating (Chel., Cina, Iod., Lyc., Psor.) (A.).

Cravings for liquor, salt, sweets, etc. (Br.).

Often restores a gonorrhœal discharge (Puls., Thuj.) (Br.).

Constant thirst; even in dreams she is drinking (A.).

Sore all over, as if bruised (*Arn., Bapt., Eup-P., Pyrog.*) (A.).

Children are pale and rachitic, dull and weak (Bl.).

Children are dwarfed and stunted in growth (*Bar-C.*) (A.).

Sleeps in knee-chest position (Br.).

Lower limbs ache all night, preventing sleep (A.).

Sweat easy; towards morning (B.).

Burning heat, with sweat; wants to uncover, but is chilled thereby (B.).

Is cold and bathed with cold perspiration (Carb-V., Verat.) (A.).

Skin cold, yet throws off the covers (*Camph., Sec.*) (A.).

State of collapse; wants to be fanned all the time; craves fresh air (Carb-V.) (N.).

Is in a great hurry; when doing anything is in such a hurry that it fatigues her (Arg-N.) (N.).

Weakness of memory; cannot remember names, words or initial letters; has to ask name of the most intimate friend; even forgets his own name (A.).

Loses the thread of conversation (Br.).

Cannot spell correctly; wonders how a well-known name is spelled (A.).

CANNOT SPEAK WITHOUT WEEPING (*Kali-C., Puls., Sep.*) (Br.).

Great difficulty in stating her symptoms; question has to be repeated as she loses herself (A.).

TIME PASSES TOO SLOWLY (*Arg-N.*) (Br.).

Irritated at trifles (*Bry., Cham., Ign., Nux-V., Sulph.*) (A.).

Hopeless of recovery (*Ars., Calc., Ign., Nux-V., Psor., Sep.*) (Br.).

Cross during the day, exhilarated at night (A.).

Fear of going insane (*Calc.*) (Br.).

Anxious, nervous, extremely sensitive; starts at the least sound (*Bor., Kali-C.*) (A.).

Melancholy, with suicidal thoughts (*Aur., Hep., Nit-Ac., Nux-V.*) (Br.).

Anticipates death (*Ars.*) (A.).

Many symptoms are worse when thinking of them (A.).

Throat sore and swollen; deglutition of either liquids or solids impossible (*Merc.*) (A.).

Throat constantly filled with thick, gray or bloody mucus from the posterior nares (*Hydr.*) (A.).

Oozing of fetid moisture from the anus (*Pæon.*) (Br.).

Can pass stool only by leaning very far back (C.).

Sharp, needle-like pains in the rectum (A.).

Intense itching of the anus (*Calc., Sulph., Teucr.*) (Br.).

Constriction and inertia of the bowels with ball-like stools (*Lach.*) (A.).

Diarrhœa from jarring of cars (A.).

Painful tenesmus when urinating (*Bell., Canth., Merc.*) (C.).

Severe pain in the renal region (backache), relieved by profuse urination (*Lyc.*) (A.).

Renal colic (*Berb., Canth., Lyc., Nux-V., Ocim., Puls.*) (Br.).

Urine flows very slowly (*Clem., Con., Hep., Thuj.*) (C.).

NOCTURNAL ENURESIS (*Calc., Kreos., Sep.*) (A.).

Nocturnal emissions, followed by great weakness (*Phos-Ac.*) (Br.).

GLEET; WHOLE URETHRA FEELS SORE (*Hep.*) (C.).

Enlarged and painful prostate with frequent urging and painful urination (*Staph.*) (Br.).

Impotence (*Agn., Calad.*) (C.).

Intense menstrual colic, with drawing up of the knees and terrible bearing down (labour-like) pains; must press feet against support, as in labour (A.).

Menses offensive, profuse, dark and clotted; stains difficult to wash out (Br.).

Sycotic warts on the female genitals (*Nit-Ac., Staph., Thuj.*) (C.).

Metrorrhagia at the climacteric; profuse for weeks; in gushes, on moving; with malignant disease of the uterus (A.).

Sterility (*Agn.*) (Br.).

BREASTS AND NIPPLES SORE AND SENSITIVE TO TOUCH (A.).

Leucorrhœa thin, acrid, excoriating and emitting a fishy odour (C.).

Dyspnœa and sense of constriction; can inhale with ease, but no power to exhale (*Samb.*) (A.).

Incipient tuberculosis (C.).

ASTHMA, ONLY RELIEVED BY LYING ON THE FACE AND PROTRUDING THE TONGUE (A.).

Incessant, dry night cough (*Con.*) (C.).

Cough, better from lying on the stomach (Br.).

Sputa viscid, difficult to raise (*Kali-B., Kali-C., Spong.*) (A.).

Larynx feel sore (*Caust., Phos.*) (C.).

AGGRAVATION: When thinking of ailment; from heat; from day-light to sunset; during thunder-storm; from covering; and from least movement.

AMELIORATION: At the sea-shore; from lying on the stomach; and in damp weather.

RELATIONSHIP: *Compare*: *Ars., Bry., Calc., Carb-V., Ferr., Kali-B., Kali-C., Kali-P., Kali-S., Lach., Lyc., Merc., Nit-Ac., Puls., Sep., Sulph.* and *Thuj.*

Melilotus Alba.

COMMON NAME: SWEET CLOVER.

" The provers all had fearful headaches and hæmorrhages except myself " (Bw.).

Engorgement of blood-vessels in any part or organ (*Acon., Bell., Ferr-P.*) (A.).

GREAT CONGESTION TO THE HEAD, WITH PAIN AND SENSE OF FULLNESS (N.).

VIOLENT CONGESTIVE HEADACHE (*Acon., Bell., Glon., Sang.*) (A.).

INTENSE REDNESS (GLOWING REDNESS) OF THE FACE IN ASSOCIATION WITH HEADACHE (*Bell.*) (N.).

Headache, with throbbing of the carotids (*Bell., Glon., Verat-V.*) ; *this is often relieved by a profuse epistaxis* (N.).

Swaying sensation in the brain (C.).

Infantile spasms (*Bell.*) (A.).

Religious melancholy, with an intensely red face (A.).

Congestions, relieved by hæmorrhages (*Bell.*, *Lach.*) (A.).

It seems as if the brain would burst through the forehead (D.).

Constipation: The passage is difficult and painful; the anus feels constricted and throbs (Bl.).

Undulating sensation in the brain (Br.).

Sick headache relieved by epistaxis or menstural flow (*Lach.*) (Br.).

Dull, congestive headache relieved by profuse, watery urine (*Gels.*) (C.).

Dysmenorrhœa (*Bell.*, *Mag-P.*, *Puls.*, *Sep.*) (Br.).

Feels as if smothering, especially from rapid walking (*Ferr-P.*) (Br.).

AGGRAVATION: From approach of a storm; in rainy, changeable weather; during climacteric; and from rapid walking.

AMELIORATION: From bleeding; from vinegar; after profuse urine; from walking; from change of position; and in the open air.

RELATIONSHIP: *Similar to*: *Amyl-N.*, *Bell.*, *Cact.*, *Ferr.*, *Ferr-P.*, *Glon.*, *Lach.*, *Nat-M.*, *Op.*, *Sang.* and *Sulph.*

Menyanthes.

COMMON NAME: BUCK BEAN.

This remedy is indicated in malarial disorders, when the coldness predominates (Bl.).

Great debility, often accompanied by chilliness.

THE HANDS AND FEET ARE ICY COLD DURING CHILL (*Aur.*, *Phos.*, *Verat.*) (K.).

Intermittent fever, with coldness in the abdomen.

Heat in the face, with cold hands and feet.

Heat without thirst (*Apis, Gels., Puls.*)

Shivering, with yawning (B.).

Rheumatic pains in the extremities (*Bry., Ipec., Rhus-T.*).

Pinching and stinging in the limbs and joints.

Coldness of the tip of the nose during chill (*Apis, Ant-C., Cedr., Tarax.*) (K.).

Tension in the root of the nose (A.).

Sensation of pressure on the vertex, relieved by hard pressure with the hand (Bl.).

Complaints from abuse of Cinchona and Quinine (*Ipec., Nat-M., Puls., Sep., Sulph.*) (A.).

Visible, but painless twitching of the muscles.

Pinching and stinging in the limbs and joints.

Anxiety about the heart, as if some evil was impending (A.).

Inclination to shed tears (*Puls., Sep.*).

Feeling as of a heavy weight pressing upon the head at every step (*Glon., Lach.*); *worse on ascending* (*Calc.*) (A.).

As soon as the patient lies down, legs jerk and twitch (Br.).

Tension in the arms, hands, and fingers (A.).

Sensation of coldness extending up the œsophagus; with great nausea (C.).

Desire for meat (*Ferr-M., Iod., Kreos., Lil-T., Mag-C., Merc., Nat-M., Sanic., Sulph., Tub.*) (Br.).

FULLNESS IN THE ABDOMEN, MUCH INCREASED BY SMOKING TOBACCO (C.).

Frequent desire to urinate with scanty discharge (*Bell., Canth., Nux-V.*) (C.).

Misty vision (*Calc., Cycl., Gels., Kali-C., Phos., Puls.*) (B.).

Vivid dreams (B.).

Hoarseness (*Arg-N., Calc., Carb-V., Phos., Rhus-T.*) (C.).

Dyspnœa (*Ars., Chin., Dig.*) (C.).

AGGRAVATION: By rest; towards evening; from lying down; and from ascending.

AMELIORATION: By motion; from pressure on the affected part; and from stooping.

RELATIONSHIP: *Compare*: *Apis, Arn., Aur., Bell., Calc., Caps., Carb-An., Carb-V., Gels., Kali-Ars., Mag-M., Paris, Puls., Sang., Sep., Stram. and Verat.*

Follows well: *Caps., Lach., Lyc., Puls., Rhus-T.* and *Verat.*

Mercurius Biniodide.

COMMON NAME: RED IODIDE OF MERCURY.

It is useful in chronic syphilitic lesions in scrofulous subjects (Bl.).

Early stages of cold, especially in children (*Acon., Bry., Rhus-T.*) (Br.).

Phlegm in the nose and throat (Br.).

Tubercular pharyngitis (*Arg-N., Bar-C., Calc., Hep., Iod., Kali-B., Lach., Lyc., Merc., Nat-M., Phos., Sil., Sulph., Tub.*) (A.).

Disposition to hawk, with sensation of a lump in the throat (Br.).

Laryngeal troubles with aphonia (*Am-Caust., Arg-N., Caust., Phos., Sil.*) (Br.).

DIPHTHERITIC AND GLANDULAR AFFECTIONS OF THE LEFT SIDE; FAUCES DARK-RED; SOLIDS OR LIQUIDS PAINFUL WHEN SWALLOWING; EXUDATION SLIGHT, EASILY DETACHED; CASES ATTENDING EPIDEMIC SCARLET FEVER; ULCERS ON FAUCES OR TONSILS (A.).

Profuse saliva in the mouth (*Kali-B., Merc., Nit-Ac.*) (Br.).

HARD CHANCRES (*Merc-P-I.*).

Glands enlarged (*Bad., Carb-An., Hep., Sil.*) (A.).

CHRONIC SUPPURATING BUBOES (*Merc., Sil.*) (Br.).

Profuse, acrid, green leucorrhœa (B.).

Greenish, tough lumps from the pharynx or posterior nares (*Kali-I.*) (A.).

Wandering pains (*Bell., Ign., Kali-S., Lac-C., Puls.*) (B.).

Copious sweat at night (*Calc., Hep., Nit-Ac., Sil.*) (C.).

Turbinated bones swollen (*Aur., Calc., Hep., Nit-Ac., Sil.*) (C.).

AGGRAVATION: From swallowing; and at night.

AMELIORATION: From warm application.

RELATIONSHIP: *Compare*: *Apis, Bell., Carb-An., Kali-B., Kali-I., Lach., Lyc., Merc., Merc-P-I., Mezer., Nit-Ac., Phos., Rhus-T., Sil.* and *Sulph.*

Mercurius Corrosivus.

COMMON NAME: CORROSIVE SUBLIMATE.

Its action is very similar to that of *Mercurius Sol.*, only much intensified (R.).

Syphilitic diseases of men (*Fluor-Ac., Kali-B., Kali-I., Nit-Ac.*) (A.).

Tearing in the periosteum, as from intermittent fever, with sensation of heat about the head.

Salivation of salty taste—a very valuable indication for the *Sublimatus.*

Swelling of the upper lip (*Apis, Bar-C., Bell., Calc., Hep., Nat-M., Nit-Ac., Staph., Sulph.*).

Useful in painful and acute swelling of the mammary glands and the nipples (*Bell., Graph., Phyt.*).

Cystitis (*Apis, Bell., Canth.*) (B.).

Brick-dust-like sediment in the urine (*Lyc., Sars.*) (A.).

Bright's disease (especially during pregnancy) (*Apis, Canth., Phos., Sep.*) (A.).

Urine hot, burning, scanty or suppressed (A.).

ALBUMINOUS URINE (*Apis*) (A.).

Dysentery and summer complaints of intestinal canal, occurring from May to November (A.).

Chilliness from the least motion, with cutting in the abdomen and tenesmus.

DYSENTERY IS MORE FAVOURABLY EFFECT-ED BY THE SUBLIMATUS THAN BY ANY OTHER HOMOEOPATHIC PREPARATION AS YET USED.

BLOODY, FREQUENT MOTIONS OF DYSEN-TERY AT ONCE BENEFITTED—THAT STATE OF DIARRHOEAL DISEASE TERMED " THE BLOODY FLUX " IN THE LATE AMERICAN CIVIL WAR; ALSO GREEN MOTIONS CONSISTING OF MUCUS, LIKE SCRAPINGS OF THE INTESTINES WITH CONTINUED CUTTING IN THE ABDOMEN, TENESMUS AND CLOTTED BLOOD.

TENESMUS OF THE RECTUM, NOT RELIEVED BY STOOL (*ameliorated by stool—Coloc., Nux-V., Sulph.*) (A.).

A NEVER-GET-DONE FEELING IN THE RECTUM (DURING AN EVACUATION) (B.).

Chilly after stool (*Canth., Dios., Petr.*) (B.).

INCESSANT AND PERSISTENT TENESMUS (A.).

Passes pure blood, or bloody water (*Phos.*) (B.).

Stool: Hot (*Aloe, Cham., Sulph.*); *scanty* (*Aloe, Nux-V. Sulph.*); *bloody* (*Canth., Kali-P., Lach., Nit-Ac.*); *slimy* (*Aloe, Nux-V.*); *and offensive* (*Bapt., Carb-Ac., Lach.*) (A.).

Great burning at the anus (*Sulph.*) (D.).

Colicky pain before, during and after stool (N.).

Nightly toothache (B.).

Gums are apt to be purple, swollen and spongy (*Plb.*) (Bl.).

The uvula is swollen, and there is intense burning, worse from pressure (D.).

Constriction of the throat; swallowing causes spasm (*Bell.*) (D.).

Gluey nasal discharge; swelled nose (*Graph., Kali-B.*) (B.).

Patchy tongue (B.).

Intense inflammation of the vulva (C.).

Paraphimosis (*Coloc., Lach., Merc., Nit-Ac., Rhus-T.*) (K.)

Syphilis in all its various manifestations (*Aur., Fluor-Ac., Kali-B., Kali-I., Lach., Merc., Nit-Ac.*).

ULCERS, WITH CORRODING AND ACRID PUS (*Nit-Ac.*) (A.).

PHAGEDENIC CHANCRES (*Ars., Aur-M-N., Caust., Kali-P., Lach., Nit-Ac., Sulph.*) (K.).

GANGRENOUS OR SPREADING ULCERS (*Ars.*) (K.).

Spasms of the rectum, during coition (B.).

Gonorrhœa: Second stage; greenish discharge; worse at night; great burning and tenesmus (A.).

The urethral orifice is red and swollen (*Canth., Sulph.*) (Bl.).

Gonorrhœal ophthalmia (*Arg-N., Kali-S., Puls.*)

Swelling of the testicles after suppressed gonorrhœal disease (*Puls.*).

Urethra bleeds after urinating (*Hep.*) (B.).

Tenesmus of the bladder, with intense burning in the urethra; urine in drops, with great pain (*Canth., Tereb., Thuj.*) (A.).

Great tenesmus of the rectum and bladder at the same time (N.).

BLOODY URINE (*Ars., Both., Canth., Coc-C., Crot-H., Ham., Mill., Phos., Puls., Sec., Squil., Tereb., Uva, Vesp.*) (A.).

Excessive photophobia and lachrymation (*Euphr.*); the discharges are acrid, excoriating the lids and cheeks; pains very severe, especially at night (*Aur., Hep., Nit-Ac.*) (N.).

Tearing in the bones around the eye (D.).

ULCERATION OF THE CORNEA, WITH TENDENCY TO PERFORATION (*Sil.*) (D.).

Albuminuric retinitis (*Phos.*) (Br.).

IS ALMOST A SPECIFIC FOR SYPHILITIC IRITIS.

Keratitis (*Fluor-Ac., Kali-B., Nit-Ac., Sil.*) (B.).

Insatiable thirst (*Ars., Nat-M., Phos., Sulph.*) (B.).

Vomits slime and blood (*Kali-B., Kreos., Lach., Phos.*) (B.).

Gastritis (*Ars., Bism., Phos.*) (B.).

Sweats from every motion (*Bry., Calc., Chin.*) (B.).

Foul perspiration at night (*Hep., Nit-Ac., Psor., Sil.*) (B.).

Throat instensely inflamed, swollen, burning, with swollen gums, which bleed easily (N.).

Ozæna, with perforation of the septum nasi (*Aur., Fluor-Ac., Kali-B., Nit-Ac.*) (Br.).

Surface cold and covered with profuse perspiration, especially on the forehead (*Camph., Verat.*) (C.).

AGGRAVATION: In the evening; at night; in the open air; from motion; from fat food; from acids; from cold; during autumn; during hot days and cool nights; after urination, stool or swallowing; and from pressure.

AMELIORATION: While at rest; and from warm application.

RELATIONSHIP: *Antidotes*: *Hep., Nit-Ac.* and *Sil.*

Similar to: *Ars., Aur., Bism., Canth., Kali-B., Kreos., Lach., Merc., Nit-Ac., Phos., Sil., Tereb.* and *Thuj.*

Mercurius Cyanatus.

COMMON NAME: CYANIDE OF MERCURY.

It seems to spread its action all over the buccal cavity (N.).

Is of great value in that much dreaded disease—diphtheria (N.).

MALIGNANT DIPHTHERIA, WITH INTENSE REDNESS OF FAUCES AND GREAT DIFFICULTY OF SWALLOWING (A.).

Diphtheria of the larynx and nose (Br.).

Pseudo-membranous formation extends all over fauces and down the throat (A.).

Putrid, gangrenous diphtheria, with phagedenic ulceration (*Lach., Nit-Ac.*) (A.).

Membranous croup (*Brom., Kali-B., Phos.*) (A.).

GREAT WEAKNESS; EXTREME PROSTRATION (this is attributed by Dr. T. F. Allen to the *cyanogen element* in it) (A.).

Cannot stand up from weakness (*Ars., Gels., Kali-P., Phos.*) (A.).

Chronic sorethroat of public speakers (N.).

Hoarseness (*Arg-N., Brom., Carb-V., Phos.*) (N.).

Fetid breath (*Ars., Bapt., Nit-Ac.*) (D.).

Epistaxis (*Kali-P., Lach., Nit-Ac.*) in association with diphtheria (D.).

Is useful in syphilitic ulceration, when perforation is threatened. The soft parts of the palate and fauces are necrosed (*Aur.*) (Bl.).

Urine albuminous, scant, in some cases completely suppressed (*Apis, Canth., Stram.*) (R.).

Coldness and cyanosis (*Carb-V., Hydr-Ac., Verat.*) (B.).

Weak heart (*Ars., Dig., Gels., Kali-P., Lach., Mur-Ac., Naja*) (B.).

Rapid respiration and heart action (*Ant-T., Carb-V., Lach., Phos.*) (Br.).

Hiccough (*Bell., Carb-V., Mag-P.*) (Br.).

Twitching and jerking of muscles (*Hyos., Ign., Stram.*) (Br.).

AGGRAVATION: From swallowing; and from speaking.

AMELIORATION: From warmth.

RELATIONSHIP: *Similar to*: *Ars., Bapt., Carb-V., Kali-P., Lach., Mur-Ac.,* and *Phos.*

Mercurius Dulcis.

COMMON NAME: CALOMEL.

Catarrhal affections of mucous membranes, especially of the eye and ear (A.).

Otitis media (*Calc-S., Kali-M., Puls.*) (Br.).

Eustachian catarrh, with deafness and tinnitus aurium (D.).

Catarrhal deafness and otorrhœa in psoric children (*Kali-M., Sil.*) (A.).

Deafness of old age (*Caust., Kali-M., Phos.*) (A.).

Salivation with sore-mouth and offensive breath (*Bor., Kali-P., Lach., Nit-Ac., Podo.*) (Bl.).

Cirrhosis of the liver, especially in the hypertrophic form (Br.).

DIARRHOEA: OF CHILDREN; STOOLS GRASS-GREEN (*Ipec.*); LIKE CHOPPED EGGS (*Cham.*);

PROFUSE (*Podo.*); CAUSING SORENESS OF ANUS (*Sulph.*) (A.).

Is also of use in dysentery when the stool is small in quantity and consists of mucus and blood, covered with bile (Bl.).

Acute affections of prostate after mal-treated stricture (*Acon., Arn., Canth., Ferr-P., Staph.*) (A.).

Ulceration of throat, with dysphagia (*Lach., Nit-Ac., Sil.*) (Br.).

Blows lumps from nose (*Sep.*) (B.).

Slimy, pussy expectoration (B.).

Tonsil inflamed, relieved by cold drinks (B.).

Copper-coloured eruptions (*Kali-I., Mezer., Syph.*) (Br.).

Mucous membrane of mouth pale, sometimes covered with aphthous patches (R.).

Liver enlarged and tender (*Chel.*) (R.).

Swollen glands (*Iod., Lyc., Phyt.*) (Br.).

Scrofulous ophthalmia (*Calc.*) (C.).

Ulceration of the cornea (*Kali-B., Nat-M., Sil.*) (C.).

AGGRAVATION: From acids; at night; and in cold weather.

AMELIORATION: From cold drinks; and after stool.

RELATIONSHIP: *Similar to:* *Calc-S., Cham., Chel., Ipec., Kali-M., Lach., Lyc., Merc., Nit-Ac., Podo., Puls., Sil.,* and *Sulph.*

Antidotes: *Hep.* and *Podo.*

Mercurius Protoiodide.

COMMON NAME: YELLOW IODIDE OF MERCURY.

The Iodide of Mercury acts especially upon the glands and mucous membranes of the throat, after the manner of other *Mercuries,* though partaking somewhat the action of the *Iodine* (C.).

Right side of the throat and neck most affected (*Lyc.*) (A.).

Cervical and parotid glands are enormously swollen (*Phyt.*) (A.).

Swelling of the parotids and tonsils during scarlatina (Co.).

Deep bone-pains, especially at night (*Mezer., Nit-Ac., Phyt.*) (Bt.).

SYPHILITIC IRITIS (*Aur., Flour-Ac., Merc-C., Nit-Ac., Sil.*).

Cornea looks scratched or chipped (B.).

Pyorrhœa (*Calc-F., Hep., Kali-P., Merc., Nit-Ac., Sil., Sulph.*) (B.).

Superficial ulceration of the cornea and other especially scrofulous affections of the eyes (N.).

Faint or dizzy on rising (*Puls.*) (B.).

BASE OF THE TONGUE COVERED WITH A THICK, DIRTY YELLOW COAT (*Chel., Kali-B., Nat-P.*) (N.).

Mammary tumours, with warm perspiration and gastric disturbances (Bl.).

Flat warts (*Acet-Ac.*) (B.).

PAINLESS, HARD CHANCRES, WITH SWELL-ING OF THE INGUINAL GLANDS (*Merc-B-I.*) (D.).

Great swelling of the inguinal glands, with no disposition to suppurate (*Carb-An., Kali-M., Merc., Sil.*) (A.).

Yellow leucorrhœa (*Ars., Calc., Hydr., Kreos., Sep., Sulph.*) (B.).

DIPHTHERITIC DEPOSITS BEGINNING ON THE RIGHT SIDE, WITH GREAT SWELLING OF THE GLANDS, AND ACCUMULATION OF THICK, TENACIOUS MUCUS IN THE THROAT; THE TONGUE IS COATED YELLOW AT THE BASE, THE TIP AND SIDES BEING RED (D.).

Diphtheritic and throat affections aggravated by warm drinks, and empty swallowing (*Lach.*) (A.).

Great soreness and stiffness of the neck (*Bell., Phyt., Rhus-T.*) (Bt.).

Polypus of the nose (*Calc.*) (Hm.).

Palpitation, with dyspnœa, aggravated by lying on the back (*Ars., Lyc.*) (B.).

Follicular tonsillitis (*Kali-C.*) (R.).

Suppuration of the middle ear (*Calc-S., Hep., Merc., Puls., Sil., Tell.*) (R.).

Dull frontal headache, with pain in the root of the nose (*Kali-B., Nat-Ars., Stict.*) (C.).

Troublesome itching over the whole body; worse at night, especially while in bed (C.).

Sensation of a lump in the throat (*Ign., Lach., Phyt.*) (Br.).

Sometimes useful in chronic nasal catarrh, the posterior nares being most affected (*Hydr.*) (C.).

AGGRAVATION: At night; from warm drinks; from swallowing; in a warm room; during rest; and from lying on the back.

AMELIORATION: In the open air; when exercising actively; from cold drinks; and during the day.

RELATIONSHIP: *Similar to*: *Bad., Bell., Carb-An., Iod., Kali-B., Lach., Lyc., Merc., Merc-B-I., Nit-Ac., Phyt., Sil., Sulph.* and *Syph.*

Mercurius Solubilis.

COMMON NAME: BLACK OXIDE; HAHNE-MANN'S SOLUBLE MERCURY.

Nervous affections after suppressed discharges, especially in psoric patients (*Asaf.*) (A.).

Trembling of all the limbs, especially of hands and feet (N.).

Stinging pain in the limbs (*Apis*).

Rheumatism of the joints, with swelling and sensation of coldness.

NIGHTLY TEARING PAINS WITH PERSPIRATION (*Hep., Nit-Ac., Sil.*).

Rheumatic, shining red swellings (*Bell.*).

All parts go to sleep while sleeping.

Cold perspiration on the forehead (*Verat.*).

PERSPIRATIONS, WHICH DO NOT RELIEVE (*Bell.*).

Weakness and debility from exertion (*Ars., Bry., Calc., Con., Crot-H., Lach., Nat-C., Phos-Ac., Pic-Ac., Rhus-T., Sil., Sep., Spong., Stann.*).

GLANDULAR AND SCROFULOUS AFFECTIONS OF CHILDREN (*Calc., Sil.*) (A.).

SALIVATION VERY MARKED (*Chin., Dulc., Kali-B., Kali-I., Nit-Ac., Rhus-T., Sep., Sil.*).

Teeth sore and loose, and feel too long (*Ant-T., Caust., Cham., Lach., Mag-C., Mezer.*) (Bt.).

The gums bleed, and are inclined to ulcerate about the teeth (G.).

Odontalgia, worse at night, with periosteal inflammations, and ulceration (*Hep., Sil.*) (Bt.).

Teeth all feel on edge (Bt.).

Very fetid breath (*Bapt., Carb-Ac., Kali-P., Nit-Ac., Sil.*).

Saltish, metallic taste in the mouth (Bt.).

MOIST TONGUE WITH GREAT THIRST (G.).

Red tongue, with much burning and great thirst.

Flabby tongue, showing imprints of teeth (D.).

Bleeding of the nose (*Am-C., Bry., Carb-V., Kali-P., Lach., Nit-Ac., Phos., Rhus-T., Sep., Sulph.*).

Acrid nasal secretion, having odour of old cheese (A.).

Nostrils red, raw and ulcerated (*Ars., Kali-B., Nit-Ac., Sulph.*) (A.).

Epistaxis: When coughing; at night during sleep; hangs in a dark clotted string from the nose, like an icicle (A.).

No remedy prevents suppuration as certainly as *Mercury,* especially in the glandular system (Bt.).

Ulceration of the tonsils (Hn.).

Grayish ulcers on the inner surface of the lips, cheeks, gums, tongue and palate (Hn.).

Otorrhœa: Bloody, offensive discharge, with stabbing, tearing pain; worse in the right side, at night and lying on the affected side (A.).

Furuncles and boils in the external meatus (*Pic-Ac.*) (A.).

Congestion of blood to the chest, head and abdomen, with pulsation in the arteries (*Bell., Ferr-P.*).

Icteric complaints very beneficially affected (*Dig., Kali-M., Lyc., Mag-M., Nat-P., Nat-S., Podo., Sep., Sulph.*).

Ascarides creep out of the anus, and can be seen on the perineum and buttocks, even at night in bed (G.).

Lumbricoids escape easily and freely (G.).

Weakness and weariness of the limbs, which feel sore and bruised (*Bapt., Kali-P., Rhus-T.*) (A.).

Cold, clammy sweat on the thighs and legs at night (G.).

Yellow, or mucous and bloody, or dark green stools, with tenesmus (G.).

Passes frequently almost pure blood (*Sulph.*) (Bt.).

Very sensitive about the pit of the stomach and abdomen (G.).

A very valuable remedy for the cure of dysentery (*Kali-M., Nux-V., Sulph.*).

Much colic, relieved by a bloody stool, with tenesmus (*Nux-V.*) (G.).

Polypi and fungous excrescences in the external meatus (*Teucr., Thuj.*) (A.).

VIOLENT TENESMUS AND CONTINUED URGING AFTER STOOL; A "NEVER-GET-DONE" FEELING (N.).

DRY ITCH, WHICH BLEEDS AFTER SCRATCHING (*Ars., Sulph.*).

Intolerable biting, itching over the body, as from insect-bites; worse in the evening and from warmth of bed; becomes pleasant on scratching (A.).

Of great service in the treatment of all forms of syphilitic disorders (all stages and varying conditions of luetic disease).

PRIMARY CHANCRE, OR REGULAR INDURATED HUNTERIAN CHANCRE WITH A LARDACEOUS BASE, OR WITH A CHEESY BOTTOM AND INVERTED RED EDGES (A.).

Primary sore, with phimosis or paraphimosis (Sulph.) (A.).

Impotency, from syphilis (K.).

Bleeding and painful ulcer, with yellowish and fœtid discharge (Hep., Nit-Ac.) (A.).

DEEP, ROUND, PENETRATING CHANCRE, EATING THROUGH THE FRAENUM AND PREPUCE (*Kali-B.*) (A.).

Gonorrhœa with phimosis or chancroids; green discharge, worse at night; urging to urinate; intolerable burning in the forepart of the urethra when passing last few drops; prepuce hot, swollen, œdematous and sensitive to touch; of a torpid character, with threatening or suppurating bubo.

Testicles swollen, hard and shining (C.).

The boy often handles his genital organ (K.).

Bloody emissions (B.).

Itching, burning, smarting, corroding leucorrhœa, with sensation of rawness in the vagina; discharges of clots of pus and mucus as large as hazel-nuts; worse at night (G.).

Prolapsus of the vagina, with sensation of great rawness (Bt.).

Vulva much swollen, with a raw, sore feeling; worse at night (Bt.).

Pain in the mammæ, as if they would ulcerate, at every menstrual period (Bt.).

Intolerance of eyes to fire-light, with dimness of vision (D.).

Muco-purulent discharges from the eyes, which cause soreness of the lids and ulceration (*Calc., Euphr., Hep., Sil.*) (D.).

Momentary loss of sight (*Cycl., Phos., Puls., Sep.*) (G.).

Hypo-pyon (*Hep., Sil.*) (Br.).

Parenchymatous keratitis of syphilitic origin (Br.).

Affects lower lobe of the right lung (left lobe—Phos.); stitches through to the back (Chel., Kali-C.) (N.).

Cough with yellow, muco-purulent expectoration (*Puls.*) (Br.).

Paroxysms of two coughs (Phos., Puls., Sulph., Thuj.) in quick succession (K.).

Shortness of breath, on ascending or walking (*Am-C., Ars., Calc.*) (C.).

Short, dry, fatiguing cough, principally in bed, in the evening or at night, caused by tickling in the upper part of the chest (C.).

Sweat stains the linen yellow (Carls.) (C.).

Itching of the skin, aggravated during perspiration (*Mang., Rhod.*) (K.).

Inflammatory states going on even to suppuration of the parts (Hep., Sil.).

Especially useful in bilious fevers, with prominent hepatic symptoms (Bt.).

Urine scanty and red, with a strong smell (*Berb., Lyc.*) (Bt.).

Urine highly albuminous (*Apis, Canth., Phos.*) (Bt.).

Suppression of urine, or it is passed with great difficulty, with tenesmus of the bladder (Bt.).

Creeping chilliness in the beginning of a cold, or threatened suppuration (N.).

Heat and shuddering at the sametime, or heat and shuddering alternately (G.).

AGGRAVATION: At night; in damp, cold weather; from warmth of bed; from lying on the affected side; while sweating; from cold; during stool; from artificial light; while urinating; and when blowing the nose.

AMELIORATION: In the morning; whilst lying down; and from scratching.

RELATIONSHIP: *Antidotes*: *Aur., Carb-V., Chin., Dulc., Hep., Kali-B., Kali-I., Lach., Lyc., Nit-Ac., Podo., Sil., Sulph.* and *Thuj.*

It sometimes completes the action of *Bell. Podo.* is its vegetable analogue.

Mercurius Sulphuricus.

COMMON NAME: SULPHATE OF MERCURY.

It is as important, as *Arsenicum*, in hydrothorax. When it acts well it produces a profuse, watery diarrhœa with great relief to the patient).

Hydrothorax, occurring from heart or liver diseases (*Dig., Phos.*) (A.).

DYSPNOEA: HAS TO SIT, CANNOT LIE DOWN (*Ars., Lyc., Sulph.*) (A.).

Short and rapid respirations (Bl.).

Extremities become swollen (*Apis, Ars., Dig., Lach., Lyc., Phos., Sep., Sulph.*) (A.).

Burning in the chest (*Calc., Phos., Sulph.*) (A.).

Diarrhœa: Stool loose, watery, causing severe burning and soreness (*Aloe, Ars., Sulph.*) (A.).

Morning diarrhœa; the passage is forcible and consists of yellow matter (*Aloe*) (Bl.).

Scanty, clear, scalding urine (*Apis, Sulph.*) (Br.).

Sore tip of tongue (*Rhus-T.*) (Br.).

Cardiac pain and weakness (*Ars., Kali-C., Naja*) (Br.).

AGGRAVATION: In the morning; at night; and from lying down.

AMELIORATION: From sitting up.

RELATIONSHIP: *Compare*: *Acet-Ac., Apis, Ars., Blatta, Canth., Dig., Kali-C., Kali-P., Lach., Lyc., Nux-V., Phos., Sep., Sulph.* and *Tereb.*

Mezerium.

COMMON NAMES: DAPHNE MEZERIUM; SPURGE OLIVE.

Bad effects of Mercury and Alcohol (*Podo., Sulph.*) (A.).

Headache: Violent after slight vexation; painful on the slightest touch, right-sided (A.).

Heaviness in the limbs (*Plb.*).

Paralytic tension in the limbs and twitching of the muscles.

Burning in internal parts and quivering in external parts.

Neuralgic burning pains after zona (*Ars.*) (A.).

Sensitiveness to cold air (*Hep., Sil.*).

External chilliness associated with internal burning.

PERIOSTITIS AND SWELLING OF THE BONES, ESPECIALLY ON THE TIBIA, WITH MOST VIOLENT NIGHTLY PAINS (G.).

Desquamation of the skin (G.).

Eczema and itching eruptions after vaccination (*Sil., Thuj.*) (A.).

The head is covered with a thick, leather-like crust, under which thick and white pus collects here and there; hair is glued and matted together; pus after a time is ichorous, becomes offensive and breeds vermin (A.).

Eczema with intolerable itching; worse in bed and from touch; with copious and serous exudation (A.).

Child scratches his face continually, which is covered with blood; eruptions moist; itching worse at night (A.).

Inflammatory redness of the face (*Bell., Stram.*) (A.).

Pruritus of the aged; there is itching after getting warm in bed (Bl.).

Boring, pressing pains, coming like lightning, which leave the parts numbed (G.).

Collection of water in the mouth (*Merc.*) (G.).

Roots of the teeth decay (*Am-C., Thuj.*) (A.).

Dull pain in the teeth when biting on them and when touched with the tongue, aggravated at night and ameliorated with mouth open and drawing in air (A.).

Violent nightly toothache (*Merc., Rhus-T.*) (Bt.).

Toothache in carious teeth (*Calc-T., Kreos., Merc., Staph.*); *teeth feel elongated* (*Alum., Am-C., Bry., Calc., Caust., Glon., Hep., Kali-I., Lach., Lyc., Merc.*) (A.).

Deep, hard, painful ulcers (B.).

Linen or charpie sticks to the ulcers; they bleed when it is torn away (A.).

Shining, fiery red areola around the ulcers (A.).

Vesicles appear around the ulcers; they itch violently or burn like fire (*Hep.*) (A.).

Vesicular eruptions on the nose, with excoriations and formation of thick scabs (N.).

Sensation as if the ears were too open and air were pouring into them (N.).

Herpes zoster, with intercostal neuralgia, worse at night and in warmth of bed (N.).

Gonorrhœa, with hæmaturia (*Canth., Hep., Nit-Ac., Thuj.*) (Br.).

Biting, burning in the fore part of the urethra at the close of urination (*Sulph.*) (Br.).

Enlargement of the testicles (*Puls., Rhod., Sil.*) (Br.).

Sleeplessness from itching (*Anac., Bar-C., Gels., Merc., Psor., Puls., Raph., Zinc.*) (K.).

CILIARY NEURALGIA (*Ars., Spig.*) (D.).

Neuralgia of cheek-bones with numbness (*Cham.*) (D.).

Pressing and tearing pains in and about the eyes (R.).

Sharp, constricting pains transversely across the abdomen, especially about the heart (R.).

Burning in the pit of the stomach (*Ars., Phos., Sulph.*) (C.).

Loud flatulence (*Aloe, Arg-N., Caust., Nat-S.*) (C.).

Constipation (*Caust., Nux-V.*) (C.).

AGGRAVATION: In the evening; at night; from cold air; from cold washing; from touch; from motion; from warmth of bed; and from suppressions.

AMELIORATION: From wrapping up; from eating; in the open air; and from radiated heat.

RELATIONSHIP: *Compare*: *Ars., Caust., Guai., Kreos., Lyc., Merc., Phos., Phyt., Rhus-T., Sil., Staph., Sulph.,* and *Thuj.*

Antidote: *Merc.*

Millefolium.

COMMON NAME: YARROW.

It stands at the head of the long list of our remedies for hæmorrhages (Bt.).

Ailments from over-lifting, over-exertion, or a fall (*Arn., Rhus-T., Sulph-Ac.*) (A.).

Vertigo when moving slowly, but not when taking violent exercise (A.).

Hæmorrhage, from the nose, lungs, kidneys, bowels and sexual organs of women (Bt.).

Hæmorrhages of mechanical origin (*Arn.*) (A.).

PAINLESS HAEMORRHAGE (*Ham.*) (A.).

HAEMORRHAGE WITHOUT FEVER (with fever —*Ferr-P.*) (A.).

HAEMORRHAGE OF BRIGHT RED, FLUID BLOOD (*Acon., Ipec., Sab.*) (A.).

Hæmoptysis, and other hæmorrhages in consequence of violent exertions (*Rhus-T.*) (Bt.).

HAEMORRHAGE AFTER LABOUR, ABORTION OR MISCARRIAGE (*Chin., Ferr-P., Sec.*) (A.).

Spasms after suppressed secretions, menses, etc. (B.).

Lochia suppressed, or too copious (*Sec.*) (C.).

Menses suppressed, with colicky pain in the abdomen (*Puls.*) (A.).

MENSES TOO EARLY AND TOO PROFUSE AND PROTRACTED (*Calc., Phos., Sec.*) (A.).

Leucorrhœa: *Of children* (*Calc., Caul., Puls.*); *from uterine atony* (*Alet., Helon., Puls., Sep.*) (A.).

Cough with raising of blood, in suppressed menses or hæmorrhoids (A.).

Cough with oppression and palpitation (*Ferr., Phos.*) (A.).

Excessive accumulation of mucus in the bronchi (*Hep., Nat-S.*) (C.).

Wounds bleed profusely, especially from a fall (C.).

Bleeding hæmorrhoids (*Carb-V., Nux-V., Sulph.*) (B.).

Hæmaturia (*Canth., Sars.*) (Bl.).

Hæmorrhage without anxiety (with anxiety—*Acon.*) (D.).

Painful varices in the female genitalia during pregnancy (*Ham., Puls., Sep.*) (Br.).

Piercing pain from the eyes to the root of the nose (Br.).

The head seems full of blood (*Acon., Bell., Ferr-P., Glon., Lach., Sep., Sulph.*) (Br.).

Bad effects from fall from a height (*Arn.*) (Br.).

AGGRAVATION: After violent exertion; at 4 P.M.; from suppression of habitual discharge; from slow motion; in the evening; and during night.

AMELIORATION: When taking violent exercise; from re-establishment of the discharges; and during the day.

RELATIONSHIP: *Follows well after*: *Acon.* and *Arn.* in hæmorrhages.

Compare: *Acon.*, *Arn.*, *Bell.*, *Calc.*, *Carb-V.*, *Erig.*, *Ferr-P.*, *Ham.*, *Ipec.*, *Kali-P.*, *Led.*, *Merc.*, *Nit-Ac.*, *Phos.*, *Rhus-T.*, *Sab.*, *Sec.*, *Senec.*, *Sep.*, *Sulph.*, *Sulph-Ac.*, *Tril.*, and *Ust.*

Moschus.

COMMON NAME: MUSK.

Through the cerebro-spinal system it especially affects the sexual organs and nerves of motion (Bt.).

The open air appears to him sensitively cold.

The symptoms, especially those pertaining to the respiration, are aggravated by becoming cold.

Tightness of the chest; is obliged to take a deeper breath (*Ign.*, *Phos.*) (Br.).

Trembling and quaking through the whole body.

Debility, which is more felt during rest than during motion.

FAINTING, FOLLOWED BY HEADACHE.

SPASM OF THE CHEST (*Cupr.*, *Phos.*).

Nervous, suffocative constrictions of the chest (N.).

Spasm of the glottis (*Brom.*) (Br.).

Tingling with heaviness in the limbs (*Acon.*, *Rhus-T.*, *Zinc.*).

The parts on which he lies pain as if dislocated and broken.

Much nervous trembling and frequent fainting (*Agar.*, *Ign.*, *Phos.*) (Br.).

Catalepsy (*Agar.*, *Art-V.*, *Cann-I.*) (Br.).

Hypochondriacal and hysterical complaints originating from the genital systems (*Ign.*, *Staph.*).

Palpitation of the heart from nervous excitement (*Acon.*, *Ars.*, *Kali-P.*, *Phos.*) (Bt.).

HYPOCHONDRIACAL ANXIETY, WITH PALPITATION OF THE HEART (*Kali-P.*, *Nat-C.*).

PALPITATION (HYSTERIC) W I T H DYSPNOEA, PROSTRATION, FAINTING, EXCLAIMING, " I SHALL DIE! I SHALL DIE!" ETC., GREATLY EXCITED (N.).

HYSTERIC SPASMS, WITH FAINTING: CRYING ONE MOMENT, AND THE NEXT MOMENT BURSTS OUT IN INCONTROLLABLE LAUGHTER (G.).

LAUGHS IMMODERATELY, OR CRIES OR SCOLDS UNTIL HER LIPS TURN BLUE, EYES STARE AND SHE FALLS DOWN FAINTING OR UNCONSCIOUS (N.).

Globus hystericus (*Asaf.*, *Ign.*, *Nux-M.*) (Br.).

The sight of food makes her sick (*Colch.*, *Kali-C.*, *Lyc.*, *Phos-Ac.*, *Sil.*, *Sulph.*) (G.).

Eructations, with hot saliva in the mouth (G.).

Eructations tasting of garlic (*Aesc.*, *Asaf.*, *Mag-M.*, *Sulph.*, *Sulph-Ac.*) (Bt.).

Great flatulence (*Lyc.*, *Nux-M.*) (Br.).

Vomiting of the food, then subsequent vomiting and more vomiting (G.).

Spasmodic hiccough (*Mag-P.*) (Bt.).

Diabetes: Profuse urination, great thirst, emaciation, perfect loss of sexual desire, and sugar in the urine (*Kali-P.*, *Lyc.*, *Merc.*, *Nat-M.*, *Sulph.*) (Y.).

Vertigo on least motion (*Am-C., Bry., Calc-P., Con., Gels., Glon., Graph., Kalm.*) (Br.).

SEXUAL DESIRE EXCITED (*Canth., Nux-V., Phos., Plat., Stram.*).

VIOLENT SEXUAL DESIRE, WITH INTOLERABLE TITILLATION IN THE GENITAL ORGANS (*Plat.*) (G.).

MENSES TOO EARLY, TOO PROFUSE, WITH INTOLERABLE TITILLATION IN THE GENITAL ORGANS (G.).

Drawing and pushing in the direction of the female genitals (*Bell., Murx., Nat-M., Sep.*) (Br.).

NAUSEA AND VOMITING AFTER COITION (Br.).

Involuntary, seminal emissions (*Con., Gels., Kali-P., Phos-Ac.*) (Br.).

VIOLENT SEXUAL DESIRE, OR IMPOTENCE (*Nux-V., Phos., Pic-Ac.*) (Br.).

Premature senility (*Arg-N., Lyc.*) (Br.).

Impending paralysis of the lungs (*Ant-T., Lyc.*) (Br.).

Cough ceases, mucus cannot be expectorated (*Ant-T.*) (Br.).

Asthma, with intense anxiety, fear, and smothering sensation (*Ars.*) (Br.).

Sleepy by day; sleepless at night (*Nux-V.*) (B.).

FREQUENTLY RECURRING, EASY FAINTING (*Ign., Nux-M., Puls.*) (R.).

FAINTS COMPLETELY AWAY FROM THE LEAST EXCITEMENT (R.).

Faints when eating (Br.).

Aversion to food (*Calc., Kali-M., Puls.*) (Br.).

Desire for black coffee and stimulants (Br.).

Burning heat, with restlessness (*Ars., Phos., Sulph.*) (B.).

Rigor or chilliness, or shuddering, as though the patient were very cold (G.).

External chilliness with internal heat (*Ars., Lyc., Nux-V., Sulph.*) (G.).

AGGRAVATION: From cold; from cold open air; from excitement; from suppressions; and while eating.

AMELIORATION: In the fresh, open air; from rubbing; on getting warm; and from warmth in general.

RELATIONSHIP: *Compare*: *Ant-T., Asaf., Brom., Bry., Canth., Carb-V., Castor., Con., Dig., Ferr-P., Ign., Kali-C., Kali-P., Lach., Lyc., Murx., Nux-M., Op., Phos., Phos-Ac., Pic-Ac., Plat., Sep., Sulph., Sumbul, Valer., Verat.* and *Zinc.*

Compatible: *Ambr.*

Antidotes: *Camph., Coff.*

Murex Purpurea.

COMMON NAME: MOLLUSK.

Especially adapted to nervous, lively, and affectionate women (Br.).

Useful for the sufferings during climacteric (*Amyl-N., Glon., Graph., Lach., Sep., Sulph.*) (A.).

Very weak and tired (*Kali-P., Nux-M., Sep.*) (B.).

Aching in the sacrum (*Rhus-T.*) (Bl.).

Lumbar pain impels walking, which ameliorates (*Rhus-T.*) (B.).

The secretions are profuse, such as the menses and urination (D.).

NYMPHOMANIA (*Hyos., Plat., Stram.*) (B.).

Fearful and anxious (*Ars., Kali-P.*) (B.).

Great depression of spirits (*Aur., Ign., Kali-P., Nat-M., Puls., Sep.*) (A.).

Violent excitement in the female sexual organs (*Mosch., Plat.*) (A.).

EXCESSIVE DESIRE FOR AN EMBRACE (*Canth., Phos., Plat., Stram.*) (A.).

LEAST CONTACT OF PARTS, CAUSES VIOLENT SEXUAL EXCITEMENT (*Plat.*) (A.).

Leucorrhœa alternating with mental symptoms (B.).

Leucorrhœa, worse from mental depression; happier when the leucorrhœa is worse (A.).

SORE PAIN IN THE UTERUS (A.).

A distinct sensation of a womb (*Helon., Lyss.*) (A.).

Menses: irregular; too early and too profuse; protracted; consisting of large clots (A.).

BEARING DOWN SENSATION, AS IF THE INTERNAL ORGANS WOULD BE PUSHED OUT; MUST SIT DOWN AND CROSS THE LIMBS TO RELIEVE THE PRESSURE (but no sexual desire— *Sep.*) (A.).

Sensation as if something were pressing on a sore part in the pelvis (D.).

Sinking, all-gone sensation in the stomach (*Carb-An., Sep., Sulph.*) (A.).

Violent hunger, even after eating (*Arg-M., Bov., Chin-S., Cina, Iod., Kali-P., Lyc., Phos., Staph., Sulph.*) (B.).

Benign tumours in breast (*Carb-An., Con., Sil.*) (Br.).

Dysmenorrhœa (*Cqul., Coloc., Cupr., Mag-P., Nux-V., Plat., Sep., Xanth.*) (Br.).

Chronic endo-metritis (*Apis, Bry., Calc., Graph., Hydr., Kali-C., Lyc., Merc., Nat-M., Puls., Sep., Sulph., Thuj.*) (Br.).

Pain in the breast during menstrual period (*Puls.*) (Br.).

Urging in the bladder (*Bell., Canth., Nux-V., Sep., Tereb.*) (Br.).

Urine smells like valerian (B.).

Frequent urination at night (*Merc., Phos-A., Sulph.*) (Br.).

AGGRAVATION: In the sun; from touch; during climacteric; during menses; after eating; and at night.

AMELIORATION: From sitting and crossing the limbs; and from walking.

RELATIONSHIP: *Compare*: *Lil-T.* and *Plat.* in nymphomania and *Sep.* in bearing down sensation (with lack of sexual erethism).

Muriatic Acid.

COMMON NAME: HYDROCHLORIC ACID.

Mouth and anus are chiefly affected; the tongue and sphincter ani are paralysed (A.).

Often called for asthenic type of diseases (*Ars., Bapt., Hyos., Lyc., Phos-Ac., Sec., Verat.*) (A.).

Great sensivity to moist air (*Nux-M.*).

All the joints feel as if bruised (*Arn.*).

Drawing and tearing in the extremities during rest and relieved by motion (*Kali-P., Rhus-T.*).

The periosteum pains in intermittent fever (*Rhus-T.*).

Eczema solaris (*Petr.*) (A.).

Cures muscular weakness following excessive use of opium and tobacco (A.).

Offensive discharges (*Ars., Bapt., Lach.*) (D.).

Bed-sores (*Arn., Ars., Bapt., Lach.*) (D.).

Vertigo (*Ars., Bry., Calc., Kali-P., Lyc.*) (A.).

Palpitation of the heart felt in the face (A.).

The heart is feeble, irregular and intermits every third beat (D.).

GREAT DEBILITY—AS SOON AS HE SITS DOWN, HIS EYES CLOSE.

SLIDING DOWN IN BED, BECAUSE OF BODILY INERTIA.

LOWER JAW HANGS DOWN (*Hyos., Lyc.*) (A.).
INTENSE PROSTRATION (*Ars., Kali-P., Phos.*) (A.).

TYPHOID OR TYPHUS: DEEP STUPID SLEEP; UNCONSCIOUS WHILE AWAKE; LOUD MOANING OR MUTTERING; TONGUE COATED AT THE EDGES, SHRUNKEN, DRY, LEATHER-LIKE, PARALYZED; INVOLUNTARY FOETID STOOLS WHILE PASSING URINE; SLIDING DOWN IN BED; PULSE INTERMITS EVERY THIRD BEAT (A.).

Intense burning heat, with aversion to coverings (R.).

Putrid ulcers (*Ars., Carb-Ac., Nit-Ac.*) (G.).

A sensation of emptiness in the stomach and abdomen (*Sep., Sulph.*).

Cannot bear the thought or sight of meat (*Nit-Ac.*) (A.).

The hæmorrhoids are aggravated by cold water, and ameliorated by warmth (reverse of *Aloe*) (R.).

Ascites (*Acet-Ac., Ars., Chel., Iod., Lyc.*) (B.).

Severe pain at the conclusion of urination (*Berb., Puls., Sars., Thuj.*) (N.).

CANNOT URINATE WITHOUT HAVING THE BOWELS MOVED AT THE SAME TIME (A.).

Bladder weak, must wait a time for the passage of urine; has to press, so that the anus protrudes (A.).

URINE PASSES SLOWLY (*Alum., Arg-N., Arn., Berb., Calc-P., Camph., Caust., Clem., Dig., Gels., Hell., Hep., Merc., Merc-C., Op., Prun., Sars., Sulph., Thuj.*) (A.).

Want of good sphincteric control (*Aloe, Apis, Phos., Squil., Sulph.*), *and trembling, due to loss of power, of the tongue* (*Gels., Lach.*).

WHILE URINATING INVOLUNTARY DIS-CHARGE OF STOOL (*Aloe, Bell., Carb-Ac., Carb-S., Hyos., Ind., Nat-S., Phos., Squil., Sulph., Verat.*).

Diarrhœa (*Aloe, Ars., Bapt., Chin., Ferr., Nux-V., Sulph.*).

Involuntary stool on passing wind (*Aloe*) (A.).

Increased urinary secretion, with prolapsus ani.

Anus sore during menses (A.).

HAEMORRHOIDS: SWOLLEN, BLUE, SENSITIVE AND PAINFUL TO TOUCH; TOO SORE TO BEAR LEAST TOUCH; EVEN THE SHEET IS UNCOMFORTABLE (*Lach.*) (A.).

Prolapsus ani while urinating (*Valer.*) (A.).

Irritable, peevish, disposed to anger and chagrin (*Nux-V.*) (A.).

Restlessness (*Ars., Rhus-T.*).

Moaning and fretfulness (*Bell., Hyos.*) (A.).

UNCONSCIOUSNESS (*Bapt., Lyc., Op., Stram.*) (A.).

SAD AND TACITURN (B.).

Vertigo in the open air and unsteadiness while walking (C.).

Hardness of hearing (*Calc., Chin., Ferr., Graph., Nit-Ac., Phos., Puls., Sep.*) (C.).

Nose-bleed (*Acon., Bry., Ferr., Merc., Phos., Sep.*) (C.).

Weakness of the thighs, causing a tottering gait (*Nux-V., Plb.*) (C.).

Coldness of the extremities (*Camph., Carb-V., Phos., Verat.*) (C.).

Impotence (*Agn., Calad., Graph., Phos., Sel., Sulph.*).

CIRRHOSIS OF THE LIVER (*Chel., Iod., Lyc., Merc., Podo., Sulph.*) (C.).

Carbuncles, with low states of the system (*Ars., Carb-V., Hep., Lach., Sil.*) (C.).

Dysentery, with typhoid symptoms (*Bapt., Phos., Rhus-T.*) (C.).

Catamenia too early and too profuse (*Calc-C., Sep.*).

Cannot bear the least touch, not even of the sheet on the female genitals (*Murx., Plat.*).

Ulcers in the female genitals, with putrid discharge (*Kreos.*) (C.).

Frequent waking at night (*Bell., Stram., Sulph.*) (C.).

Anxious dreams (*Ars., Nat-M., Phos.*) (C.).

Malignant affections of the mouth: Diphtheria, scarlatina, cancer (A.).

The buccal cavity is studded with ulcers, deep, perforating, having a black or dark base; offensive, foul breath (*Bapt., Carb-Ac., Kali-P., Merc-C., Nit-Ac.*) (A.).

The dry tongue rattles in the mouth (D.).

Tongue dry, leathery and shrunken, one-third its natural size (typhoid) (N.).

Tongue heavy as lead; hinders talking (N.).

Attempting to swallow produces violent spasms and choking (C.).

Deep respiration (*Arg-N., Aur., Brom., Bry., Caps., Cupr., Dig., Glon., Hep., Hydr-Ac., Ign., Ipec., Lach., Nat-S., Op., Phos., Sel., Sil., Sulph., Zinc.*) (C.).

Sighing and groaning respiration (C.).

AGGRAVATION: During menses; while urinating; from least touch; during wet weather; from walking; from sitting; from cold drinks; and bathing.

AMELIORATION: From warmth; from motion; lying on the left side.

RELATIONSHIP: *Follows well after:* Bry., Merc. and *Rhus-T.*

Remedies following: Calc-C., Kali-C., Nux-V., Puls., Sep., Sil. and Sulph.

Antidotes: Bry. and Camph.

It antidotes: Op.

THE END OF PART I.

LIPPE'S KEY NOTES
&
RED LINE SYMPTOMS

PART II.

NAJA TRIPUDIANS
to
ZINCUM METALLICUM.

PART II

Naja Tripudians.

COMMON NAME: COBRA POISON.

Often called for restoring a heart damaged by acute inflammation or for relief of sufferings or chronic hypertrophy and valvular lesions (A.).

Body cold and collapsed (*Camph., Carb-V.*) (C.).

Pain in the left ovary during cough (D.).

Excited, tremendous action of the heart (B.).

Cardiac asthma (*Ars., Lach., Phos.*) (B.).

Endo-carditis (*Apis, Lach., Nat-M.*) (B.).

Simple hypertrophy of the heart (*Arn., Rhus-T.*) (A.).

Valvular diseases of the heart, with a dry, teasing cough (*Dig., Lach., Phos.*) (D.).

Threatened paralysis of the heart, post-diphtheretic (*Lach.*) (A.).

UNABLE TO SPEAK FROM PALPITATION (K.).

PALPITATION OF THE HEART FROM EXERTION, OR TALKING, OR WALKING (K.).

SEVERE STITCHING PAIN IN THE REGION OF THE HEART (*Apis, Bry., Caust., Kalm., Lach., Mag-M., Petr., Psor., Spig., Spong., Staph., Sulph.*) (A.).

Nervous palpitation, especially after public speaking (A.).

Pulse irregular in force, but regular in rhythm (A.).

Inability to speak with choking (A.).

Weak and thready pulse (*Carb-V.*) (C.).

Suffocative choking; grasps the throat (B.).

Puffing breathing (*Am-C., Ant-T., Ars., Camph., Chin., Glon., Laur., Lyc., Nux-V., Op., Puls., Stram.*) (B.).

Suicidal insanity (*Ars., Nit-Ac.*) (A.).

Broods constantly over imaginary troubles (*Aur.*) (A.).

Aversion to talking (*Ign., Sep.*) (Br.).

Anxiety and fear of death (*Acon., Ars., Kali-C.*) (Br.).

Irritating, dry, sympathetic cough in the acute stage of rheumatic carditis, or chronic organic lesions (*Spong.*) (A.).

Violent pain in the heart, shooting to the left scapula or shoulder (B.).

Cardiac cough, with sweat in the palms (N.).

Dyspnœa and prostration from weak heart (*Ars., Kali-P., Phos.*) (N.).

Suffocative spells after sleeping (*Lach.*) (Br.).

Pale, haggard countenance (C.).

Rheumatic pains in the limbs (*Bry., Cimic., Kali-M., Rhus-T.*) (C.).

AGGRAVATION: By carriage riding; from lying on the left side; from exertion; from talking; from walking; after sleep; from alcohol; after menses; from pressure of clothes and from cold, draught of air.

AMELIORATION: From sneezing; from riding in open air; and from lying on the right side.

RELATIONSHIP: *Compare. Ars., Bry., Cact., Crot-H., Dig., Kali-P., Lach., Mygal., Nat-M., Phos., Puls., Rhus-T., Spig. and Verat.*

Antidotes: Alcohol and *Salt.*

Naphthalinum.

COMMON NAME: A CHEMICAL COMPOUND FROM COAL TAR; NAPHTHALIN.

The secretions are highly acrid (*All-C., Ars., Nat-M., Sulph.*) (Bl.).

Hay-fever (*All-C., Ars., Sabad., Squil.*) (Br.).

Constant sneezing (All-C., Anac., Ars., Dulc., Gamb., Indg., Iris, Merc., Nat-C., Squil. (Bl.).

WHOOPING COUGH: LONG AND CONTINUED PAROXYSMS OF COUGHING; UNABLE TO GET A RESPIRATION (*Ipec.*) (Br.).

During the paroxysms the face becomes purple, the perspiration starts and there is expectorated a quantity of thick, tenacious mucus (Bl.).

Spasmodic asthma (Ars., Cupr., Ipec., Lob., Nux-V., Phos., Samb.) (Br.).

Soreness in the chest and stomach (*Nux-V., Rhus-T.*) (Bl.).

Emphysema (*Carb-V.*) (Br.).

Great dyspnœa, with a sighing respiration (Bl.).

Gonorrhœa, with a violent desire to urinate; the meatus urinarius is reddened and tumefied (Bl.).

Cutting pain down the penis (*Canth.*) (Br.).

Oedema of the prepuce (*Merc., Rhus-T., Sulph.*) (Bl.).

Black urine (*Ars., Lach.*) (Br.).

Terribly offensive odour of the decomposing (ammoniacal) urine (Br.).

AGGRAVATION: During night, while urinating.

AMELIORATION: In the open air; and from loosening clothing.

RELATIONSHIP: *Similar to*: *All-C., Ars. Bry., Cocc-C., Cupr., Dros., Ipec., Kali-C., Lach., Nux-V., Op., Phos., Rhus-T., Samb., Sulph. and Thuj.*

Natrum Carbonicum.

COMMON NAME: CARBONATE OF SODA.

Debility and headache from the sun (*Lach.*, *Nat-M.*) (D.).

Vertigo from drinking wine, or from mental exertion, from sun, or working under gas-light (N.).

Involuntary twitching of the muscles and limbs (*Bell.*, *Ign.*, *Mag-P.*).

Instability of the whole body (*Nux-V.*).

Great weakness in the limbs, especially in the morning (*Alum.*, *Dulc.*, *Nit-Ac.*, *Ox-Ac.*, *Pall.*, *Phos.*, *Sulph.*).

Easy dislocation and spraining of ankle (*Led.*); so weak that it gives way; foot bends under (*Carb-An.*, *Nat-M.*) (A.).

Cramp-like tearing in the arms and legs.

After a short walk the patient is very weak (*Alum.*, *Calc.*, *Con.*, *Ferr.*, *Mur-Ac.*, *Nit-Ac.*, *Phos.*, *Pic-Ac.*).

DRY SKIN OR VIOLENT PERSPIRATION AFTER THE LEAST EXERTION (*Agar.*, *Ars-I.*, *Calc.*, *Chin.*, *Ferr.*, *Graph.*, *Iod.*, *Kali-C.*, *Kali-P.*, *Lyc.*, *Nat-S.*, *Nit-Ac.*, *Phos.*, *Psor.*, *Rhus-T.*, *Sep.*, *Sulph.*).

Aversion to the open air (*Am-C.*, *Bapt.*, *Calc.*, *Calc-P.*, *Cham.*, *Ign.*, *Kali-C.*, *Nux-V.*, *Petr.*, *Rumx.*, *Sil.*, *Sulph.*).

In the morning great restlessness in the body when not mentally occupied.

With the pain anxiety, trembling and cold sweat (*Acon.*).

HYPOCHONDRIACAL HUMOUR (*Nux-V.*).

AFFECTIONS OF THE MIND WITH MIS-ANTHROPY (*Aur.*, *Bar-C.*, *Con.*, *Ign.*, *Lach.*, *Lyc.*, *Nat-M.*, *Phos.*, *Plat.*, *Puls.*).

Depressed and irritable, especially after a meal (*Bry.*, *Nux-V.*, *Puls.*).

This hypochondriasis decreases as the food gets out of the stomach into the bowels (D.).

GETS VERY NERVOUS DURING THUNDER-STORMS AND HIDES IN THE CELLAR (D.).

Imbecility (Bar-C., Bar-M., Op.) (A.).

Exhaustion from least effort, mental or physical; ready to drop after a walk (A.).

Mental symptoms worse from music (A.).

Inability to think or perform any mental labour, causes headache; feels stupefied if he tries to exert himself; comprehension slow, difficult .(A.).

Intolerable melancholy and apprehension; is wholly occupied with sad thoughts *(Ign., Sep.)* (A.).

Face pale, with blue rings around the eyes *(Cina, Staph.)* (A.).

CHRONIC EFFECTS OF SUN-STROKE *(Nat-M.)* (A.).

Forgetfulness *(Agn., Calc., Kali-P., Lyc., Nat-M., Sep.)* (C.).

Makes mistakes in writing *(Cann-I., Nux-V.)* (C.).

HEADACHE: *from the slightest mental exertion (Calc-P., Nat-M.)* ; *from the sun or working under gaslight (Glon., Lach.)* (A.).

Head feels too large (Glon., Nux-V.) ; *as if it would burst (Arg-N., Bry.)* (A.).

Headache with tension in the nape or occiput before menses (A.).

Catarrh extends to the posterior nares and throat; profuse discharge during the day, stopped at night *(Nux-V.)* (A.).

MUCH NASAL MUCUS PASSES THROUGH THE MOUTH; HAWKS AND HAWKS (N.).

THICK, YELLOW, GREEN, OFFENSIVE, MUSTY OR HARD DISCHARGE FROM THE NOSE; OFTEN CEASING AFTER A MEAL (A.).

Dry cough when he comes from the open air into a warm room (or going from warm room to open air—*Acon., Con.*).

Cough with salty, purulent, greenish sputa, and rawness in the chest (*Nat-S.*) (C.).

Short breath, with difficult respiration (*Ars., Carb-V., Phos., Samb.*) (C.).

Violent palpitation of the heart, especially on going up-stairs or at night, and when lying on the left side (*Nat-M., Phos.*) (C.).

Falls asleep late at night (*Nux-V.*) (C.).

Palpitation, worse from every strange noise (*Agar., Nat-M., Nat-P., Nat-S.*) (K.).

Drowsy during the day (*Nux-V.*) (Br.).

Sleepy after meals (*Nux-V.*) (B.).

Amorous dreams (*Nux-V., Phos., Sulph.*) (Br.).

Nocturnal pollutions (*Nux-V., Sulph.*) (G.).

Incomplete coition; erections weak; emissions speedy (*Calc., Nux-V., Sulph.*) (C.).

VERY WEAK DIGESTION (*Carb-V., Hep., Nux-V., Puls.*).

SOUR ERUCTATIONS (*Ars., Calc., Mag-P., Nat-P,. Nux-V., Puls., Sulph.*) (D.).

A weak hungry feeling about 11 A.M. (*Sep., Sulph.*) (D.).

GREAT FLATULENCY (*Aloe, Carb-V., Chin., Kali-B., Lyc., Nux-M., Podo., Puls., Sulph.*).

The patient is worse from vegetable and starchy foods (*Nat-S.*). (D.).

Dyspepsia from eating soda biscuits (D.).

Aversion to milk (*Calc., Lac-D., Nat-S., Nux-V., Sil.*) (A.).

DIARRHOEA FROM TAKING MILK (*Calc., Kali-C., Mag-M., Sep., Sulph.*) (A.).

Stools escapes with great haste, noise and rushing (G.).
Stools like orange pulp (Aloe, Chin.) (B.).

TOOTHACHE AFTER TAKING SWEETS *(Am-C., Phos., Sep.)* (K.).

Discharge of mucus from the vagina after an embrace, causing sterility (A.).

Leucorrhœa: thick, yellow *(Calc., Hydr., Kali-B., Puls.)*; putrid, ceasing after urination (C.).

Menses late, scanty, like meat-washing (Br.).

Bearing down, as if everything would come out (Agar., Lil-T., Murx., Sep.); *heaviness, worse from sitting and better from moving* (A.).

Induration of the cervix *(Aur., Carb-An., Con., Kreos., Mag-M., Plat., Sep., Sil.)* (Br.).

Violent pain in the small of back after walking (C.).

Itching over the whole body as from fleas (C.).

AGGRAVATION: During a thunder-storm; whilst sitting; in the sun; from excessive heat of summer; from music; from mental exertion; and in the forenoon.

AMELIORATION: During motion; from pressing; from rubbing; and after eating.

RELATIONSHIP: *Follows well after: Sep.* in bearing down.

Remedies following: Calc-C., Nux-V., Puls., Sep. and *Sulph.*

Antidotes: Ars., Camph. and *Nitr-Sp-D.*

It antidotes: Chin.

Natrum Muriaticum.

COMMON NAMES: COMMON SALT; CHLORIDE OF SODIUM.

Often of great benefit in the treatment of malarial disease and intermitting fevers.

Hard chill about 11 A.M., with great thirst which continues through all stages; the heat is characterized by the most violent headache (Ra.).

Continued chilliness and want of animal heat very marked (Nux-V., Sil.).

Intermittent fever made inveterate by the use of quinine (*Apis, Ars., Ign., Ipec., Nux-V., Puls., Sep., Sulph.*) (N.).

Pulse intermitting (Dig., Ign.).

Twitching in the muscles and limbs (*Bell., Cupr., Kali-P., Mag-P., Stram.*).

Shortening of the muscles (Am-M., Caust., Sil.).

Painful contraction of the hamstrings (Hr.).

Great coldness of the body, with disposition to put on more clothing.

INTERMITTENT FEVER WITH SPLITTING HEADACHE (*Nux-V.*).

The most weakness is felt in the morning in bed (Ambr., Carb-V., Con., Puls.).

Continuous heat in the after-noon, with violent headache and unconsciousness.

Intermittent fever from living in damp regions (D.).

Great weakness and debility of mind and body after exertion.

Every movement accelerates the circulation (*Bry., Dig.*).

GREAT EMACIATION (*Abrot., Calc-P., Op., Sars., Sanic., Sil.*).

Great emaciation while living well; especially seen in the neck (N.)

CHILL AT 10 TO 11 A.M. (*Agar., Ars., Carb-V., Lob., Nux-V., Sulph.*) (N.).

Continuous chilliness from morning till noon.

Any fever with violent headache, heat in the face and great thirst, if it is regularly aggravated at 10 to 11 A.M. (N.).

There is vomiting with the chill (Eup-P.) (D.).

Complete relief during sweat (Ars.) (N.).

Sallow complexion or very pale countenance (Bt.).

After great bodily exertion an itching nettle-rash appears (N.).

Hang-nails: skin around the nails dry and cracked (N.).

Congestion of blood to the head, chest and stomach, with coldness of the legs (Bell., Stram.).

SPLITTING HEADACHE *(Bry., Glon.).*

Hammering in the frontal region on the head (D.).

Headache, accompanied by constipation *(Bry.)* (D.).

Headache as if bursting; beating or sticking through to the neck and chest, with heat in the head, red face, nausea and vomiting before, during or after the catamenia, or during the fever stage, decreasing gradually after the sweat (N.).

School girls' headache (Calc-P.) (N.).

Useful (in eye diseases) after all kinds of cauterizations with Arg-Nit. (N.).

Unsteadiness of vision; objects become confused, on looking at them; letters and stitches run together (N.).

Drawing, stiff sensation in the muscles of the eyes on moving them (N.).

Of value in bringing up power of vision after debilitating illness (Chin.).

Excessively sore, red, disgusting eyelids (Ra.).

Asthenopia (Calc-P., Phos., Ruta, Sep.) (D.).

CILIARY NEURALGIA, WHICH COMES AND GOES WITH THE SUN *(Spig.)* (D.).

Blepharitis (Bor., Euphr., Graph., Sulph.) (D.).

Lachrymation and scalding tears (D.).

Bad effects from anger (Bry., Ign., Nux-V., Staph.) and illness induced from much talking.

HYSTERICAL CONDITIONS *(Ign., Nux-M., Puls., Sep., Valer.).*

CONSOLATION AGGRAVATES (*Calc-P., Cham., Ign., Sep., Sil., Thuj.;* consolation ameliorates—*Puls.*) (N.).

SAD AND WEEPING (*Aur., Ign., Sep., Stann.*) (N.). Hypochondriacal mood (*Nat-C.*) (D.).

Hopeless about the future (*Bry., Calc-O., Chin-S., Cic., Dig., Ferr., Gels., Iod., Lach., Mur-Ac., Nux-V., Phos., Puls.*) (D.).

Cold sores or herpes (so-called fever blisters) on the lips, or on the wings of the nose (D.).

Clear, watery discharge from coryza accompanied with loss of smell and taste (D.).

Vertigo, as if falling on closing the eyes (B.).

Brain-fag (*Calc-P., Kali-P.*) (D.).

Pain in the stomach, ameliorated by bandaging the abdomen (*Cupr.*) (K.).

Gastric complaints often beneficially affected by use of this remedy.

VIOLENT THIRST (*Ars., Bry., Phos., Sulph., Verat.*) (D.).

Bad effects from acids and bread.

Pressing in the stomach, with nausea and sudden sinking of strength.

Has always heart-burn after eating (*Lyc.*) (G.).

GREAT AVERSION TO BREAD, OF WHICH SHE WAS ONCE VERY FOND (N.).

Bad effects of using too much salt (*Phos.*) (N.).

Craves salt and salty things (N.).

Great dryness of the mucous membranes from the lips to the anus; lips dry and cracked, especially in the middle; anus dry, cracked, fissured (N.).

Difficult expulsion of stool fissuring the anus, with flow of blood, leaving a sensation of much soreness in the anus (N.).

CONSTIPATION (*Bry., Ign., Lyc., Nux-V., Sep.*).

Sensation of constriction of the anus (*Bell., Lach.*) (N.).

Herpes about the anus (N.).

The stools are dry, crumbling, hard, and difficult to expel (*Mag-M.*) (D.).

Alternate constipation and diarrhœa (*Nux-V.*) (Bl.).

The nightly pains cause shortness of breath and a kind of one-sided loss of power.

Diarrhœa, accompanied with great weakness of the abdominal muscles (D.).

The stools are sometimes involuntary (*Aloe, Nat-S., Podo., Sulph.*) (D.).

Chronic bronchial catarrh with profuse secretion of mucus (D.).

HEART PALPITATES, FLUTTERS, INTERMITS, PULSATES VIOLENTLY, SHAKING THE WHOLE BODY; WORSE FROM LYING ON THE LEFT SIDE (N.).

Cold feeling in the heart when exerting the mind, or from mental over-exertion (N.).

White-coated tongue (*Ant-C., Bry., Kali-M.*) (Ra.).

Mapped tongue, with red, insular patches (N.).

Excoriating diarrhœa like water, only in the day-time (*Petr.*) (Hr.).

Scorbutic, putrid inflammation of the gums (*Kreos., Merc., Nit-Ac., Phos., Sulph.*) (Ra.).

Difficulty of talking, as if the organs of speech were weak (*Bar-C.*) (Ra.).

Dryness of the vagina, which is painful during an embrace (*Graph., Lyc., Sep.*) (G.).

Very sad and gloomy during the menses, with much palpitation of the heart, and morning headache (G.).

SCANTY AND DELAYING MENSTRUATION—IS A PROMINENT INDICATION FOR THE USE OF THIS SALT (Bt.).

WATERY LEUCORRHOEA (*Graph., Nit-Ac., Puls.*) (D.).

Especially useful in uterine troubles, accompanied by backache, which is relieved by laying on the back, or on something hard (D.).

Every morning pressing and pushing towards the genitals; has to sit to prevent prolapse (*Sep.*) (N.).

Cutting in the urethra after micturition (*Berb., Calc-P., Canth., Con., Dig., Lyc., Petros., Rhus-T., Sulph.*) (N.).

Catarrh of the bladder, with burning on urinating (*Hydr., Kali-B., Lyc.*) (D.).

Pain in the urethra just after urinating (*Sars.*).

Has to wait a long time for the urine to pass if others are present (Br.).

SEMINAL EMISSION, EVEN AFTER COITUS (Br.).

Gleet: Clear mucus; chronic after abuse of *Argent-Nit.* (or *Nitrate of Silver*) (N.).

Averse to coition, or painful coition (B.).

Hair falling off the pubes (N.).

PAIN IN THE BACK AS IF BROKEN, RELIEVED BY LYING ON SOMETHING (N.).

Chlorosis: Chronic cases; cachectic individuals, with dead, dirty skin; frequent palpitation and fluttering of the heart; oppression and anxiety in the chest (G.).

Herpetic eruptions of little, watery blisters (*Rhus-T.*) (D.).

Affections of the scalp accompanied by falling off of the hairs (D.).

Eruptions on the flexor surfaces; (eruptions on the extensor surfaces—*Kreos.*) (D.).

Warts on the palms of hands (N.).

Itching eruptions, dry or moist; worse at the roots of the hairs (*Rhus-T.*) (N.).

Tormenting sleeplessness after gnawing grief (*Ign., Kali-Br.*) (N.).

Frequent dreams of robbers in the house, and on waking will not believe the contrary until a search is made (N.).

AGGRAVATION: In the morning; at night; from 10 to 11 A.M.; on lying down, especially on the left side; from the heat in general; from the heat of the sun; after abuse of quinine; during hot weather; at sea-shore; from mental exertion; and from noises.

AMELIORATION: By sweat; in the open air; from cold bathing; from lying on the right side; from pressure; from tight clothing; and while fasting.

RELATIONSHIP: *Complementary to*: *Apis, Ign.,* and *Sep.*

ANTIDOTES: *Ars., Phos.* and *Nit-Spir-Dulc.*

Nat-Mur. antidotes: *Apis, Arg-N.* and *Quin.*

Compare: *Alum., Apis, Ars., Bry., Calc., Carb-V., Chin., Dig., Euphr., Ferr., Graph., Hydr., Ign., Ipec., Kali-P., Lach., Lyc., Merc., Mur-Ac., Nit-Ac., Nux-V., Op., Petr., Phos., Plb., Puls., Rhus-T., Sep., Sil., Sulph., Thuj., Urt., Verat.* and *Zinc.*

Natrum Sulphuricum.

COMMON NAMES: GAUBER'S SALT; SULPHATE OF SODA.

It corresponds to the hydrogenoid constitution and sycotic dyscrasia (D.).

Feels every change from dry to wet weather, and cannot eat even plants that grow near water (Bl.).

Chilly, can't get warm, even in bed (B.).

Meningitis (*Apis, Bell., Cupr., Glon.*) (B.).

Crushing or gnawing in the occiput (B.).

Chronic effects of blows, falls, etc. (*Arn.*) (N.).

Ill-effects of falls and injuries to the head, and mental troubles arising therefrom (D.).

Slow digestion (*Carb-V., Chin., Hep., Lyc., Nux-V., Puls., Sep.*) (B.).

A dirty, brownish coating on the tongue (*Bry., Nat-P.*) (D.).

Bitter taste in the mouth (*Bry., Chin., Nat-M., Nux-V., Puls., Sep., Sulph.*) (D.).

Toothache relieved by cold water, or cool air (*Coff., uls.*) (N.).

Diarrhœa, acute or chronic, with much flatulence (*Aloe, ilc-P., Podo.*) (N.).

Rumbling in the abdomen, especially in the right ileo-cæcal region (N.).

Diarrhœa: Dark, bilious or greenish stools, accompanied with an irritable liver and flatulent colic (D.).

THIN YELLOW FLUID, GUSHING STOOLS IN THE MORNING AFTER RISING AND MOVING ABOUT (N.).

Lead colic (*Alum., Bry., Coloc., Dios., Graph., Mag-A., Nux-V., Op., Sep., Sulph., Verat.*) (N.).

Pain in the abdomen ameliorated by lying on the side (K.).

Flatus becomes incarcerated here and there in the abdomen (R.).

Aching and cutting in the region of the liver (D.).

THE LIVER IS ENGORGED AND THE SYMPTOMS ARE WORSE FROM LYING ON THE LEFT SIDE (*Arn., Bry., Card-M., Mag-M., Ptel.*) (D.).

There is jaundice, bilious colic, and vomiting of bile and bitter mucus (D.).

Painful sensitiveness of the hepatic region to touch, during a walk or to a sudden jar (R.).

Stitches, throbbing, tension and lancinations in the hepatic region (*Chel., Merc., Podo.*) (R.).

Rheumatism, worse in damp, cold weather (*Dulc., Rhus-T.*) (Br.).

Oedema of the feet (*Apis, Bry., Kali-C., Lyc., Sep.*) (Br.).

Is a useful remedy in bilious intermittent fevers, accompanied by liver affections, jaundice and bilious diarrhœa (D.).

Thirst at start of fever only (B.).

Heat with aversion to uncover (*Ars., Nux-V., Rhus-T.*) (B.).

Pain in the small of the back with scanty urine (R.).

Nose-bleed during menses (*Ambr., Bry., Puls., Sep., Sulph.*) (Br.).

YELLOWISH-GREEN LEUCORRHOEA FOL-
LOWING GONORRHOEA (*Puls.*) (Br.).

Menses too late and too scanty (*Graph., Sep.*) (C.).

Herpetic vulvitis (*Graph., Kreos., Rhus-T., Sulph.*) (Br.).

Nasal catarrh with thick, yellow discharge (*Calc., Hydr., Kali-S.*) (Br.).

Constant desire to take deep, long breath (*Bry., Ign., Phos.*) (Br.).

Useful in asthma, worse upon change to damp weather. Moist asthma, with a great deal of rattling on the chest. The shortness of breath is especially worse in damp weather (D.).

PAIN IN THE LOWER CHEST ON COUGHING,
SPRINGS UP IN BED AND GRASPS THE CHEST
WITH HANDS. LOOSE COUGH (*dry cough—Bry.*) (N.).

The sputum is copious and of a greenish colour (*Puls., Stann.*) (Bl.).

Humid asthma, especially in children (*Ant.-T., Brom., Hep., Kali-S.*) (Bl.).

Granular conjunctivitis with much redness of the lids (*Sulph.*) (R.).

Pain in the eyes in the evening when reading by candle light (*Merc.*) (R.).

Agglutination of the lids in the morning with photophobia (*Calc., Graph.*) (R.).

Delayed resolution in pneumonia (*Hep., Kali-C., Lyc., Sulph.*) (Br.).

Every fresh cold brings on attack of asthma (*Hep.*) (Br.).

Diabetes (*Acet-Ac., Kali-P., Lyc., Sulph.*) (Br.).

Urine copious, and passed more frequently than normal; so that she had to get up several times in the night (R.).

It is one of the principal remedies in sycosis, especially where there are condylomata (D.).

GONORRHOEA: YELLOWISH GREEN DISCHARGE; THICK CONSISTENCY; LITTLE PAIN; ESPECIALLY IN HYDROGENOID CONSTITUTION (N.).

Sexual desire excited in the evening (C.).

Burning in the urethra during micturition (*Canth., Merc., Sulph.*) (R.).

Urine with brick-dust sediment (*Berb., Lyc., Sars.*) (R.).

Enlarged prostate causing retention of urine (*Con., Dig., Hep., Kali-C., Lyc., Pareir., Staph., Thuj.*) (R.).

Tendency to warts (*Nit-Ac., Thuj.*) (Br.).

Chronic gout (*Benz-Ac., Calc., Lyc.*) (Br.).

Music makes her sad (*Acon., Cham., Dig., Graph., Kreos., Lyc., Nat-C., Nat-P., Nux-V., Phos., Sabin., Sep., Tarent.; Thuj.*; sad music ameliorate—*Mang.*) (Br.).

Very irritable, ill-humoured (*Bry., Nux-V., Sulph.*) (C.).

Tearful (*Cham., Ign., Med., Puls., Sep.*) (C.).

Melancholy, with periodical attacks of mania (Br.).

Suicidal tendency; must exercise restraint (*Ars., Aur., Naj.*) (Br.).

WANTS TO COMMIT SUICIDE BY SHOOTING (*Anac., Ant-C., Aur., Carb-V., Hep., Med., Nux-V.*), OR BY HANGING (*Ars., Bell., Ter.*) (Br.).

Dislike to speak, or to be spoken to (*Ars., Aur., Cocc., Ferr., Hyos., Kali-C., Mag-M., Nat-C., Nit-Ac., Nux-V., Sep.*) (Br.).

Inability to think (*Con., Nux-V., Pic-Ac.*) (Br.).

AGGRAVATION: In cold, wet weather; from living in damp cellars; lying on the back; from lying on the left side; from motion; and in the morning.

AMELIORATION: From pressure; from changing position; and in dry, hot weather.

RELATIONSHIP: Compare: *Ars., Bry., Calc-P., Dulc., Euphr., Ferr., Graph., Hep., Ipec., Kali-C., Lyc., Med., Merc., Nat-M., Nit-Ac., Nux-V., Puls., Rhus-T., Sil., Staph., Sulph.* and *Thuj.*

Complementary: *Ars.,* and *Thuj.*

Nitric Acid.

COMMON NAME: NITRIC ACID.

Affects principally the mucous outlets of the body where the skin and mucous membrane join, viz., the mouth, nose, rectum, anus, urethra, and vagina (*Mur-Ac.*) (A.).

Generally indicated for persons suffering with chronic diseases, who take cold easily and are easily disposed to diarrhœa (A.).

Ailments from the change of weather (*Calc-P., Dulc., Nat-S., Phos., Rhod., Rhus-T.*).

Tearing in the limbs after catching cold (*Bell., Phyt., Rhus-T.*).

CRACKING IN THE JOINTS (ON MOTION), (*Ang., Ant-C., Brom., Calc., Camph., Caps., Cham., Cocc., Ferr., Kali-B., Kali-C., Kali-S., Led., Lyc., Merc., Nat-C., Nat-M., Nat-S., Nux-V., Petr., Phos., Rhus-T., Sabad., Sep., Sulph., Thuj.*).

Great debility and trembling, especially in the morning (*Arg-M., Ars., Calc., Cimic., Con., Graph., Lyc., Mag-C., Nat-M., Nux-V., Petr., Phos., Sil., Sulph.*).

Soreness of the shin and cranial bones, worse from damp weather (D.).

Inflammation, swelling and suppuration of the glands (*Ars-I., Brom., Calc-S., Hep., Iod., Kali-I., Lach., Lyc., Merc., Phos., Rhus-T., Sil.*).

Chilblains (*Agar., Calc., Petr.*).

NIGHTLY PAINS, ESPECIALLY TO THE TOUCH AS FROM SPLINTERS.

SYPHILITIC BONE-PAINS, ESPECIALLY AFTER ABUSE OF MERCURY (*Aur., Mezer., Phyt.*) (N.).

The pains are felt during sleep (*Lach.*).
Pains suddenly appearing and disappearing (*Bell.*) (A.).
Bad effects from catching cold (*Hep., Psor., Tub.*).
Painfulness and inflammation of the bones (*Asaf., Aur., Calc., Fluor-Ac., Merc., Mezer., Phos., Sil.*).
Softening of the bones (*Phos.*).
Caries (*Aur., Calc-F., Flour-Ac.*).

SENSATION OF A BAND AROUND THE HEAD (*Am-Br., Arg-N., Bell., Carb-Ac., Carb-V., Chel., Cocc., Cycl., Gels., Hep., Iod., Merc., Spig., Sulph., Tereb.*). (A.).

HEADACHE FROM PRESSURE OF HAT (*Calc-P., Carb-V., Crot-T., Glon., Lach., Sil., Valer.*) (A.).

Very sensitive to rattle of wagons over paved streets (*Therid.*) (A.).

Cracking in the ears, on masticating (A.).

HARDNESS OF HEARING RELIEVED BY RID-ING IN A CARRIAGE OR A TRAIN (*Graph.*) (A.).

This remedy is very often of curative value in angry, deep-seated ulcers of a perforating character (*Fluor-Ac., Kali-B., Sil.*).

EASILY BLEEDING ULCERS, WITH SPLINTER-LIKE PAINS, ESPECIALLY ON CONTACT (A.).

SYPHILITIC ULCERS (*Aur., Calc-S., Merc.*).

SYCOTIC EXCRESCENCES ON THE GLANS, SOMETIMES BLEEDING WHEN TOUCHED (N.).

ULCERS WITH ZIG-ZAG, IRREGULAR EDGES; THEIR BASES LOOK LIKE RAW FLESH AND CONSIST OF EXUBERANT GRANULATIONS (A.).

Discharges from the ulcers are thin, offensive, acrid; of a brown or dirty yellowish-green colour; rarely laudable pus.

Milk does not agree (*Calc., Carb-V., Nat-C., Sep., Sil., Sulph.*).

DESIRE FOR F^ :H, CHALK AND LIME (*Alum., Calc., Cic., Ferr., Nat-M., Nux-V.*).

Bleeding after miscarraige, or post-partum hæmorrhage (*Chin., Sab., Sec.*) (A.).

Discharge of profuse, bright red or dark blood (*Sab.*) (A.).

HAEMORRHAGE FROM THE BOWELS IN TYPHOID OR TYPHUS (*Alum., Crot-H.*) (A.).

. Great straining but little passes, as if fæces remained and cannot be expelled (*Alum.*) (A.).

PAIN IN THE RECTUM, WHICH LASTS FOR HOURS AFTER A STOOL (*Ign., Thuj.*) (N.).

Lancinating pain in the rectum, even after soft stools (*Alumn., Nat-M., Rat.*) (A.).

FISSURE OF THE RECTUM (*Graph., Nat-M., Sil., Sulph.*) (N.).

Ulceration about the anus (*Sulph.*) (D.).

Diarrhœa: .The stools are offensive, green and putrid, and are accompanied by a great deal of straining and soreness about the anus (D.).

Much discharge of blood after stool (*Sulph.*) (G.).

Fistula lachrymalis (*Fluor-Ac., Puls., Sil.*).

Syphilitic iritis (*Merc-C.*) (Bl.).

Ophthalmia (*Euphr., Merc., Sil.*) (D.).

Corneal ulcers (*Calc., Sil.*) (Bl.).

Anguish from the loss of his dearest friend (*Nat-M., Phos-Ac.*) (A.).

IRRITABLE, HEADSTRONG; HATEFUL AND VINDICTIVE; INVETERATE, ILL-WILLED, UN-MOVED BY APOLOGIES (A.).

Indifference (*Aur., Ign., Sep.*) (A.).

Suicidal disposition (*Aur., Aur-M., Hep., Nat-S., Nux-V., Sep., Thuj.*) (K.).

Restlessness (*Ars., Phos., Rhus-T.*) (D.).

Tired of life (*Ars., Aur., Nux-V.*), (A.).

Constantly thinking about his past troubles (*Ambr., Benz-Ac., Chin., Nat-M., Sep., Sulph.*) (A.).

Great anxiety about his disease (*Ars., Calc., Nux-V., Phos., Puls., Sep.*) (A.).

Hateful, profane (*Anac., Nux-V.*) (B.).

MORBID FEAR OF CHOLERA (*Ars.*) (A.).

Depressed and anxious in the evening (A.).

Sadness before menses (*Caust., Nat-M., Puls.*) (A.).

Ulcers in the mouth and throat (*Ars., Calc., Fluor-Ac., Hep., Kali-B., Lach., Merc., Nat-M., Rhus-T., Sil., Sulph.*).

Ulcerated spots on the inner surface of the cheeks, with pricking pains as from splinters (N.).

CORNERS OF THE MOUTH ULCERATED (N.).

FOUL ODOUR FROM THE MOUTH, (*Ars., Aur., Bapt., Carb-Ac., Kali-P., Lach., Merc., Sulph.*) (N.).

PTYALISM (*Dulc., Kali-B., Lach., Merc., Nat-M., Puls., Rhus-T., Sil.*) (D.).

Sour taste in the mouth (*Calc., Lyc., Nux-V., Puls., Sulph.*) (C.).

Tongue coated yellow, white or green (C.).

Ulcers in the throat, irregular in outline (D.).

Pricking pains in the throat, worse when swallowing (*Kali-B.*) (N.).

Tearing and cutting in the abdomen (*Aloe, Ars., Cham., Coloc., Nux-V.*).

Soreness and ulceration of the external genitals of the females (Bl.).

Menses are too early and too profuse, and often irregular (*Puls., Sep.*) (Bl.).

ITCHING OF THE VAGINA, ESPECIALLY AFTER COITION (*Agar.*), OR FROM LEUCOR-RHOEA (*Calc., Kreos., Sep.*) (K.).

Leucorrhœa: Brown, flesh-coloured, watery, or stringy (Br.).

Metrorrhagia after parturition (*Sec.*) (Br.).

Stitches through the vagina (Br.).

Excrescences on the cervix uteri (C.).

Profuse, offensive night sweats (*Chin., Hep., Merc., Sil.*) (C.).

Epileptic attacks after midnight, beginning like a mouse moving up and down in the left side, then loss of consciousness (C.).

Secondary syphilis (*Aur., Kali-B., Lach., Merc., Thuj.*) (D.).

Yellowish-brown or copper coloured spots over the body (*Aur., Cinnb., Kali-I., Merc., Mezer., Sep.*) (D.).

Dry, tickling cough, worse at night, and often starting from a particular spot in the larynx (*Con., Spong.*) (D.).

Phthisis: Difficult, green, purulent expectoration; night sweats; soreness of the chest, hectic fever; hæmorrhages; dyspnœa and hoarseness, worse in the morning (D.).

Rattling breathing (*Ant-T., Hep., Nat-S.*) (D.).

Yellow, sickly face (*Sep.*) (B.).

Moist, fissured or mapped tongue (*Kali-B., Tarax.*) (B.).

GUMS FLABBY, SORE AND BLEEDING (B.).

Cough, coryza, and pain in the back (*Bry., Nat-S., Rhus-T.*).

Stitches as from a splinter in the nose, on touch (N.).

OZAENA, WITH GREEN CASTS FROM THE NOSE EVERY MORNING (*Kali-B.*) (A.).

Offensive, excoriating discharge from the nose, accompanied by nose-bleed (D.).

Hard plugs in the nose, which, when detached, leave a raw surface (D.).

Sycotic or syphilitic warts or condylomata; large, jagged, pedunculated; bleeding readily on washing; moist, oozing; with sticking pain (A.).

URINE: SCANTY, DARK-BROWN, STRONG SMELLING, "LIKE HORSE'S URINE"; COLD WHEN IT PASSES; TURBID, "LOOKS LIKE REMAINS OF A CIDER BARREL" (A.).

AGGRAVATION: In the evening; at night; from milk; during sleep; on change of temperature or weather; after midnight; from contact; during sweat; on waking; and while walking.

AMELIORATION: From riding in a carriage; from warm covering; and from hot application.

RELATIONSHIP: *Complementary*: *Ars.* and *Calad.*

Inimical to: *Hep., Lach.*

Follows well after: *Calc., Hep., Kali-C., Merc., Nat-C., Puls.,* or *Thuj.*

Similar to: *Ars., Aur., Bapt., Calc., Dulc., Ferr., Graph., Hep., Iod., Kali-B., Kali-I., Lach., Lyc., Merc., Nat-M., Op., Phos., Rhus-T., Sil., Thuj.* and *Verat.*

Nitrum.

COMMON NAME: NITRATE OF POTASH.

In the morning sensation of debility with sensation of heat in the face and hot forehead.

Greater debility when sitting than when moderately exercising.

Tearing and stinging in the limbs and joints.

Tingling in the ears (*Am-C., Bell., Calc., Carb-V., Chin-S., Colch., Graph., Ign., Kali-C., Laur., Mur-Ac., Nux-V., Sep., Sulph., Verat.*) (N.).

Deafness from paralysis of auditory nerve (*Phos.*) (N.).

Inflammation of internal organs (*Ferr-P.*).

Bad effects from veal.

Useful in bronchitis (*Bry., Kali-C., Lyc., Nat-S., Phos., Puls., Seneg.*).

Cough aggravates.

ONE OF THE VERY BEST REMEDIES, GENERALLY IN CASES OF ASTHMA (*Ars., Kali-B., Lyc., Nat-S., Sulph.*).

VERY VALUABLE IN CARDIO-ASTHMA (*Ars., Aur., Cact., Dig., Lach., Nat-M., Spig., Sulph.*).

ABUNDANT PALE URINE (*Acet-Ac., Ars., Gels., Helon., Lyc., Merc., Nat-M., Phos-Ac., Sep., Sulph., Uran.*).

Frequent and profuse urine (Phos-Ac., Sulph.) (G.).

Of very great value in sudden dropsical swellings over the whole body (Apis, Ars., Kali-C., Phos.).

Catamenia too early and too profuse with black blood. (Cycl., Kali-N.).

AGGRAVATION: In the after-noon; towards morning; from taking veal; and from coughing.

AMELIORATION: From moderate exercise; and from sitting.

RELATIONSHIP: *Remedies following*: Bell., Calc.,
Puls., Rhus-T., Sep. and Sulph.

ANTIDOTE: *Dulc.*

Nux Moschata.

COMMON NAME: NUTMEG.

Especially suitable for women and children (*Ign.*).

Great sensitivity of the body and pain of the parts on
which one lies (*Bell.*).

*Wandering and pressing pains, which always . only
occupy a small spot (Ign., Kali-B.), last only a short time
(Bell.), but soon returns (Mag-P.).*

*Drawing in the limbs, especially after catching cold,
worse while at rest (Rhus-T.).*

PAIN IN THE LIMBS, CAUSED BY WET, COLD
WEATHER (*Dulc., Rhod., Rhus-T.*).

Great restlessness in the muscular system (*Rhus-T.*).

Weakness of old age (*Gels., Lyc., Sil.*) (A.).

Vertigo, as if intoxicated (*Cocc., Gels.*) (C.).

Headache from eating a little too much. (*Coff., Puls.*)
(N.).

Painless pulsation in the head, with fear to go to sleep,
(N.).

Dryness of the eyes; too dry to close the lids (A.).

Fatigue, must lie down after the least exertion (A.).

UNCONQUERABLE SLEEP (*Op.*) (A.).

Drowsy, with other complaints, particularly with pain
(N.).

Lies in stupid slumber (Apis, Gels., Hyos., Op.) (N.).

*Cold, from sudden cooling off, after having perspired,
with pain in the neck and in all the bones.*

Oversensitive: to light; of hearing; of smell; and to
touch (*Bell., Coff., Nux-V.*) (A.).

Emaciation of scrofulous individuals (*Iod., Nat-M., Phos., Tub.*).

Irresolute and thoughtless (*Puls.*) (N.).

Stupor and insensibility (Apis, Arn., Bapt., Hell., Hyos., Kali-P., Lach., Lyc., Nat-M., Nux-V., Op., Phos-Ac., Stram.) (A.).

SLOW THINKING (*Gels., Lyc., Sil.*) (N.).

WEAKNESS OR LOSS OF MEMORY (*Anac., Con., Kali-P., Lac-C., Lyc., Nux-V., Phos., Sil.*) (A.).

Absence of mind; cannot think (Agn., Gels., Nux-V.) (A.).

Great indifference to everything (*Sep.*) (A.).

Vanishing of thoughts while reading, talking, or writing; uses wrong words; does not recognise well-known streets (*Cann-I., Glon., Lach.*) (A.).

CHANGEABLE HUMOUR; ONE MOMENT LAUGHING, THE NEXT MOMENT CRYING (*Apis, Croc., Ign.*) (A.).

Sudden change from grave to gay, and from lively to serene (*Plat.*) (A.).

During menses great pressure in the back from within outward, abdominal bearing down and drawing in the limbs (N.).

At every menstrual nisus, mouth, throat and tongue become intolerably dry, especially when sleeping (N.).

Physometra (Brom., Chin., Lac-C., Lyc., Mag-C., Nat-C., Nux-V., Phos-Ac.) (K.).

Menorrhagia, blood thick, dark, with such as have had catamenia very irregularly (N.).

Leucorrhœa in place of menses (Coc.) (A.).

Inclination to faintness and great debility, especially in the small of the back and in the knees, with sleepiness (*Kali-C.*).

DISPOSITION TO FAINT FROM THE PAINS.

EVEN WHEN SLIGHT (*Asaf., Cham., Cocc:, Hep., Nux-V., Valer., Verat.*) (N.).

Dreamy, clairvoyant state (B.).

HYSTERICAL ATTACKS (*Ambr., Arg-N., Calc-P., Ferr., Gels., Ign., Kali-Br., Lach., Mosch., Nat-C., Op., Puls., Sep.*).

Fainting and palpitation of heart followed by sleep (N.).

Nausea and vomiting during pregnancy, or from wearing pessaries (A.).

Constipation: Stool difficult, although soft (*Alum.*) (B.).

Of use in the spasms in children (*Acon., Aeth., Bell., Cina, Cupr., Ign., Mag-P., Stram.*).

Pains in the teeth from inhaling cold air, or taking warm drinks (Hr.).

Dyspepsia of old people (*Ant-C., Carb-V., Lyc.*) (A.).

Craving for highly seasoned food (*Hep.*) (Br.).

Saliva seemed like cotton (A.).

Tongue so dry, that it adheres to the roof of the mouth (A.).

Painfulness and distress in the stomach while eating, or immediately after (*Kali-B.*) (A.).

Greatly troubled with dryness in the mouth and throat while sleeping; always awake with a very dry tongue, but without thirst (N.).

THIRSTLESSNESS, WITH DRYNESS IN THE MOUTH AND THROAT (*Puls.*).

WHILE EATING SOON SATISFIED (*Lyc.*) (N.).

ABDOMEN ENORMOUSLY DISTENDED AFTER EVERY MEAL (*Arg-N., Carb-V., Lyc.*) (N.).

Diarrhœa: in children; in summer (*Ant-C., Podo.*) (N.)

Flatulent colic (*Coloc., Nux-V., Pul.*) (B.).

White fœtid stools (*Podo.*) (A.).

Stools contain undigested particles or are like chopped eggs (*Cham.*) (N.).

Diarrhœa: from cold drinks; from boiled milk; during dentition; and during pregnancy (A.).

Rheumatism of the left shoulder (*Rhus-T.*) (A.).

Pain in the back while riding in a carriage (N.).

Rheumatic affections from getting feet wet, or from exposure to draught of air while heated (*Acon., Bry.*) (A.).

Intermittent fever, with sleepiness during the heat (*Apis, Gels., Op.*).

Cold, dry skin.

Dry, nervous, hysterical cough (*Ign.*) (Bt.).

Cough caused by getting warm in bed, being overheated, bathing, standing in water, or living in cold damp places (*Nat-S.*) (A.).

Cough loose after eating, dry after drinking (A.).

Sudden hoarseness from walking against the wind (*Hep., Phos.*) (N.).

Cough during pregnancy (*Sep.*) (A.).

AGGRAVATION: From cold, wet weather; from lying on the painful side; during menstruation; from carriage driving; from emotions; during pregnancy; from cold food; from cold water; from cold washing; from spirituous liquors; and after eating or drinking.

AMELIORATION: From external heat; in dry, warm weather; in a warm room; and from wrapping up warmly.

RELATIONSHIP: *Nux-M.,* antidotes mercurial inhalation, lead colic, oil of turpentine, spirituous liquors, and escpecially the effects of bad beer.

Complementary: *Calc.* and *Lyc.*

ANTIDOTES: *Camph., Gels., Nux-V.* and *Valer.*

Nux Vomica.

COMMON NAME: POISON NUT.

Is the greatest of polychrests, because the bulk of its symptoms correspond in similarity with those of the commonest and most frequent diseases (Br.).

One of the best remedies with which to commence treatment of cases that have been drugged by mixtures, bitters, vegetable pills, nostrums or quack remedies, especially aromatic or " hot medicines," but only if symptoms correspond (A.).

NUX is pre-eminently · the remedy for many of the conditions incident to modern life. The typical *Nux* patient is rather thin, spare, quick, active, nervous and irritable. He does a good deal of mental work; has mental strains and leads a sedentary life, found in prolonged office-work, over-study, and close application to business, with its cares and anxieties. This indoor life and mental strain seeks stimulants, coffee, wine, possibly in excess; or again, he hopes to quiet his excitement, by indulging in the sedative effects of tobacco if not really a victim to the seductive drugs, like opium, etc. These things are associated with other indulgences: at table, he takes preferably rich and stimulating food; and wine and women play their part to make him forget the close application of the day. Late hours are a consequence; a thick head, dyspepsia, and irritable temper are the next day's inheritance. Now he takes some cathartic, liver pills, or mineral water, and soon gets into the habit of taking these things, which still further complicate matters. *Since these frailties are more yielded to by men than women Nux is pre-eminently a male remedy* (Br.).

These conditions (just mentioned) produce an irritable nervous system, *hyper-sensitive and over-impressionable*, which *Nux* will do much to soothe and calm (Br.).

Especially adapted to digestive disturbances, portal congestion, and hypochondriacal states depending thereon (Br.).

NAUSEA AND VOMITING EVERY MORNING WITH DEPRESSION OF SPIRITS (A.).

NAUSEA AND VOMITING AFTER EATING (*Ars., Bry., Cocc., Puls.*) (A.).

CONSTANT NAUSEA (*Ipec.*) (A.).

The patient feels, "If I could only vomit, I would be so much better." (A.).

Pressure in the stomach an hour or two after eating (A.).

Pressure as from a stone in the stomach (*Bry., Puls.*) (A.).

Feeling of tightness in the abdomen after a meal; must loosen clothing (A.).

Sleepy after dinner (A.).

Flatulent distension after eating or drinking (Hr.).

Cannot use the mind for two or three hours after a meal (A.).

PYROSIS (*Ars., Bar-C., Bry., Calc., Carb-V., Lyc., Mezer., Par., Petr., Puls., Sabad., Sang., Sil., Staph., Sulph., Verat.*) (A.).

PAIN IN THE STOMACH (GASTRALGIA) TWO OR THREE HOURS AFTER EATING (*Anac., Con., Mag-M., Nat-P., Phos., Puls.*) (K.).

SOUR OR BITTER ERUCTATIONS (*Bry., Chin., Puls., Sep., Sulph.*) (A.).

RISING OF WATER AND BITTER FLUID FROM THE STOMACH (Ra.).

Vertigo from excessive use of coffee or liquor (Bt.).

Vertigo with momentary loss of consciousness (*Cann-I., Kali-P., Sep.*) (Br.).

Vertigo, with tendency to fall sideways (*Calc., Cocc., Con., Puls., Sil.*) (K.).

Mouth and fauces full of fetid ulcers (*Bor., Kali-M., Merc., Nit-Ac.*) (G.).

Mouth dry and sore, with bloody saliva (G.).

Sour taste in the mouth (*Calc., Lyc., Sulph.*) (G.).

Offensive odour from the mouth (*Aur., Bapt., Carb-Ac., Kali-P., Lach.*) (K.).

Tongue coated thick white (*Ant-C., Kali-M., Puls.*) (C.).

Gums scorbutic (*Ars., Nat-M.,*) (C.).

Throat raw, sore, rough, as if scraped (*Caust., Merc.*) (C.).

Stitches in the ear when swallowing. Hepatic troubles arising from drastic purgatives and allopathic dosing (*Podo., Sulph.*).

Jaundice (*Chin., Merc., Nat-S.*) (B.).

ENLARGEMENT OF THE LIVER FROM ALCO-HOLIC EXCESSES (*Aur., Chin., Sulph.*) (D.).

Sticking pains and soreness in the liver (*Hep., Lach., Merc., Sulph.*) (D.).

Gall-stone colic (*Berb., Chel., Chin., Podo., Sep.*) (B.).

Colic with pressure upwards towards the thorax (*Arg-N.*) (Ra.).

Flatulent colic with desire to stool (*Aloe, Coloc., Puls.*) (D.).

Sensation as if the intestines were squeezed between stones (*Coloc.*) (D.).

CONSTIPATION, DUE TO IRREGULARITY OF THE PERISTALTIC ACTIONS (D.).

CONSTANT INEFFECTUAL URGING TO STOOL (*Sulph.*) (D.).

Frequent, small, slimy, or bloody stools, with pain low down in the back and urging or tenesmus, relieved immediately after the stool (N.).

Incomplete and unsatisfactory motions (*Alum., Mag-M., Sep.*) (D.).

Sensation as if a part of stool remained behind (*Ign.*) (D.).

Itching hæmorrhoids, which keep the patient awake (*Sulph.*) (D.).

BLEEDING PILES, WITH INEFFECTUAL URGING TO STOOL (*Lyc.*) (D.).

Alternate constipation and diarrhœa (*Aloe, Podo., Sulph., Verat.*) (A.).

DYSENTERY (*Aloe, Merc., Sulph.*) (K.).

Strangulated hernia (*Coloc., Lyc.*) (A.).

Painful, ineffectual efforts to pass urine, with scanty discharge and burning (**Canth., Merc., Tereb.**) (D.).

Strangury (*Bell., Canth., Clem., Con., Equiset., Merc-C., Puls., Sep.*) (D.).

Dribbling of urine in old people from enlarged prostate (*Con., Hep., Lyc., Sep.*) (D.).

PAINFUL URGING FOR URINE WITH URGING TO STOOL (*Alum., Canth., Dig., Kreos., Nat-M., Prun., Staph.*) (K.).

Renal colic (*Berb., Canth., Lyc., Mag-P., Ocim., Puls., Sep.,*) ; pain extending to the genitals (Br.).

Urine passes in drops, with burning and tearing in the urethra and neck of the bladder (**Canth., Puls.**) (N.).

Cannot keep awake in the evening; falls asleep long before bed-time, and awakes at 3 or 4 A.M. (Bl.).

Falls into a dreamy sleep at day-break, from which he is hard to arouse, and then complains a great deal and feels tired and weak (Bl.).

Tendency to faint (*Ign., Nux-M.*), from odours, after eating, in the morning, and after every labour-pain (A.)

WEAKNESS AND PARALYSIS (*Con., Kali-P., Plb., Sil.*) (R.).

LEFT-SIDED PARALYSIS (*Lach., Rhus-T.*) (K.).

Paralysis after apoplexy (*Bar-C., Phos.*) (K.).

Paralysis with coldness of the paralyzed part (*Caust., Dulc., Plb.*) (K.).

Convulsions with consciousness (*Cina, Stram.*) (K.).

SPASMS, WITH TETANIC RIGIDITY OF NEARLY ALL MUSCLES, WITH INTERRUPTIONS OF A FEW MINUTES, DURING WHICH MUSCLES ARE RELAXED (R.).

Convulsions brought on by the slightest touch, or draught of air (R.).

Opisthotonos, with inability to move, but wants to be held (R.).

Jaws snap shut, stiff (B.).

Trismus or lock-jaw (*Bell., Cic., Hyper., Op., Strych.*) (K.).

Tired, worn out feeling in the morning on waking (D.).

Cannot tolerate noise, music, talking, strong odours, or bright light (*Bell., Colch., Stram.*) (C.).

VIOLENT (SUICIDAL) IMPULSES (*Ars., Merc., Nit-Ac.*) (B.).

ANGRY AND IMPATIENT; CAN'T STAND PAIN (B.).

Ailments after continual mental labour (N.).

Oversensitiveness (*Ign., Staph.*) (N.).

Finds fault and scolds (*Lyc., Sulph.*) (C.).

Gives surly answer (*Cham.*) (G.).

Easily offended (*Ign., Puls., Staph.*) (N.).

Ill-humoured (*Bell., Ign., Puls.*) (C.).

Disinclination to do or say anything (G.).

SPITEFUL, MALICIOUS DISPOSITION (*Nit-Ac.*) (N.).

QUARRELSOME, EVEN TO VIOLENCE (*Anac., Aur., Bry., Sulph.*) (C.).

Disinclination to do or say anything (*Bry., Ign., Sep.*) (G.).

Even the least ailment affects her greatly (*Acon., Cham., Ign.*) (Br.).

Cannot bear to be opposed (Aur., Bry., Cham., Hep., Nit-Ac.) (D.).

IRRITABLE AND IRASCIBLE *(Sulph.)*(D.).

Great disinclination to mental work (D.).

Catarrh, from sitting in cold places, or stone steps (A.).

Catarrh, worse in a warm room, and better in the cold air (A.).

Headache: Worse in the morning, from mental exertion, exercising in the open air, after eating, or from wine or coffee; better in the warm room and from sitting quietly, or lying down (N.).

Sick headache, commences in the morning, increases through the day, growing milder in the evening; with dimness of vision and sour or bitter vomiting *(Kali-B.)* (G.).

SENSATION AS IF HIS HEAD WERE IMMENSELY LARGER THAN HIS BODY; AS LARGE AS A CHURCH *(Arg-N.)* (G.).

Nose running through the day, at night stopped up (N.).

Snuffles of infants *(Am-C., Lyc., Samb.)* (A.).

Dry coryza; worse at night; nose completely filled up *(Puls., Sticta)* (Bt.).

Dry, hard cough, with great soreness of the abdomen *(Bry., Puls.)* (G.).

Dry, racking cough (Bry., Con., Sticta) (Bt.).

Photophobia, much worse in the morning (C.).

Cough brings on bursting headache *(Bry.)* (Br.)

Spasmodic asthma; muscles of the chest become rigid; great anxiety and suffocation (Ars., Cupr., Lobel.).

Dyspnœa, while coughing, after eating, on lying down and from walking; and relieved by eructations *(Aur., Carb-V.)* (K.).

Palpitation after eating, or on lying down after dinner (C.).

Pressure towards the genital organs early in the morning, in bed, or during a walk, with a sensation of contraction of the abdomen (G.).

3

EVERY PAIN DURING LABOUR PRODUCES A DESIRE TO DEFAECATE, OR TO URINATE, PARTICULARLY THE FORMER (G.).

Much pain in the lumbar region (*Aesc.*, *Calc.*, *Rhus-T.*) (Hm.).

Painless injection of the whites of the eye (ecchymoses) (N.).

Blood-shot eyes (*Bell.*, *Stram.*) (B.).

MUCH PAIN IN THE SMALL OF THE BACK, WHICH IS MADE WORSE BY TURNING IN BED (G.).

BACKACHE, MUST SIT UP TO TURN OVER IN BED (N.).

Easily excited sexual desire (*Phos.*) (Br.).

NOCTURNAL EMISSIONS (*Chin.*, *Phos.*, *Sulph.*) (Hm.).

Troublesome erections (*Canth.*, *Phos.*, *Pic-Ac.*, *Plat.*) (K.).

Erections wanting (impotency) (*Agn.*, *Bar-C.*, *Calad.*, *Calc.*, *Calc-S.*, *Chin.*, *Con.*, *Lyc.*, *Med.*, *Phos.*, *Sel.*, *Sep.*, *Sulph.*) (K.).

Spermatorrhœa (*Con.*, *Phos-Ac.*) (Br.).

Gonorrhœa with thin or greenish-yellow discharge (*Merc.*, *Nat-S.*, *Puls.*) (K.).

Soft sore or chancroid (*Merc.*) (F.).

Smegma increased (*Canth.*, *Caust.*, *Sang.*, *Sulph.*, *Sumb.*) (K.).

Bad effects of sexual excesses (*Phos-Ac.*) (Br.).

Menstruation very irregular (*Puls.*) (Bt.).

Menses too early and too profuse, with weak, faint spells (Bt.).

Catamenia before the time, and rather too copious, or keeping on too long, with complaints at the onset and remaining after it is over (N.).

Fetid leucorrhœa, tinging the linen yellow (*Ars., Kali-P., Nit-Ac., Sep.*), with pain in the uterus, as if bruised (G.).

Morning sickness during pregnancy (*Puls., Sep.*) (T.).

Threatened abortion (*Caul., Sep.*) (G.).

Pain in the extremities during fever (*Bry., Eup-P., Rhus-T.*) (K.).

Repugnance to cold or to cold air (*Hep., Psor., Sil.*) (A.).

Chill at 10 or 11 A.M. (*Nat-M., Sulph.*) (K.).

Chilly, on least movement, from being uncovered (*Rhus-T.*) (A.).

MUST BE COVERED IN EVERY STAGE OF FEVER VIZ., CHILL, HEAT OR SWEAT (A.).

Great chilliness and coldness, with blue nails, decreased neither by warmth of stove, nor by covering; mostly in A.M. (N.).

ANTICIPATING TYPE OF FEVER (*Ars., Bry., Chin., Chin-Ars., Chin-S., Eup-P., Gamb., Ign., Nat-M., Sep.*) (K.).

Great heat, whole body burning hot (*Acon., Ars., Bell., Sulph.*), *yet must be covered, as the least uncovering or motion makes him chilly* (N.).

The face becomes red and hot during fever (*Bell., Stram.*) (A.).

Sweat after midnight and in the morning (C.).

Sour perspiration, only on one side of the body (Br.).

AGGRAVATION: In the morning; soon after awaking; after mental exertion; after eating; at 3 A.M.; from touch; at 10 or 11 A.M.; from noise; in cold weather; from anger; from lying down; from uncovering; from liquors; after debauchery; from coffee; from over-eating; and use of purgatives.

AMELIORATION: In the evening; while at rest; in damp, wet weather (*Caust.*); in a warm room; on covering; after stool; after discharging wind; from warmth; from hot drinks; from free discharges; and from loosening the garments.

RELATIONSHIP: *Complementary: Kali-C., Merc., Phos., Sep. and Sulph.* (in nearly all diseases).

N.B. *Nux-V.,* acts best when given at night, during repose of mind and body; *Sulph.* in the morning.

Inimical to: Zinc. (must not be used before or after).

Follows well after: Aloe, Ars., Ipec., Phos., Sep. and *Sulph.*

Is followed well by: Bry., Puls. and Sulph.

Similar to: Anac., Bell., Bry., Canth., Caust., Cocc., Hydr., Ign., Lyc., Merc., Sep., Sulph., Thuj. and Zinc.

ANTIDOTES: *Cocc., Coff.* and *Ign.*

Oleander.

COMMON NAME: ROSE LAUREL.

Dull pressing in the limbs (*Nux-V.*).

Great pressing, as from spasms, in many places.

Want of sensation in the whole body (Op.).

Tension through the whole body.

Want of animal heat in the limbs.

Faintish debility (*Kali-P.*).

Memory weak; slow perception (*Sil.*) (Br.).

Headache relieved by looking sideways (worse from looking sideways —*Acon., Dig., Sil.*) (D.).

When standing, trembling of the limbs; when writing, trembling of the hands.

Great sensitiveness of the skin to rubbing; it becomes red and sore.

An eruption on the back of the scalp and ears, oozing a sticky fluid and breeding vermin (*Graph., Mezer., Petr.*) (D.).

Itching, relieved on first scratching, but it soon becomes sore (*Sulph.*) (D.).

Eruptions at the margin of the hair (*Rhus-T.*) (Bl.).

Chapping of the skin (G.).

Useful in paralytic conditions (hemiplegia, paraplegia, etc.) (Bl.)

Painless stiffness and paralysis of the limbs.

Painless paralysis with swelling, burning and stiffness of the fingers (Bl.).

Diarrhœa of a watery, painless and undigested character.

CHRONIC DIARRHOEA; PASSES STOOL WITH THE LEAST EMISSION OF FLATUS (*Aloe, Nat-S.*) (N.).

Thin, undigested stools, the patient passing undigested food that was eaten a day or two before (*Podo.*) (D.).

Morning diarrhœa (*Aloe, Bry., Calc-P., Dios., Nux-V., Podo., Sulph., Thuj.*).

Burning pain in the anus (*Aloe*) (Br.).

Sensation of emptiness in the abdomen (*Sep.*) *and chest* (*Phos.*).

Ravenous appetite with diarrhœa (*Aloe, Asaf., Calc., Fluor-Ac., Iod., Lyc., Petr., Stram., Sulph., Verat., Zinc.,* preceding diarrhœa—*Psor.*) (K.).

Much thirst, especially for cold water (*Phos.*) (C.).

Empty belching (*Ars., Bism., Carb-V., Dios., Iod., Kali-B., Lyc., Puls., Sulph.*) (Br.).

Borborygmus, with profuse fœtid flatus (*Aloe, Carb-V., Lyc., Nat-S.*) (Br.).

Vertigo when looking down, or when looking fixedly at an object (Br.).

Heat from mental exertion (B.).

Double vision (*Bell., Gels., Stram.*) (Br.).

Momentary loss of sight (*Cycl., Kali-B., Phos., Sep.*) (G.).

AGGRAVATION: From rubbing; in the morning; from undressing; after eating; looking fixedly; on rising in bed: looking downwards; and when passing flatus.

AMELIORATION: From scratching; from looking sidewise; and while lying.

RELATIONSHIP: *Antidotes*: *Camph.* and *Sulph.*

Compare: *Aloe, Asaf., Carb-V., Con., Dios., Graph., Kali-P., Kali-S., Lathy., Lyc., Merc., Nat-S., Nux-V., Op., Petr., Phos., Podo., Rhus-T., Sep., Staph., Sulph.*

Opium.

COMMON NAME: POPPY.

Want of sensation of the whole body (*Anac., Cocc., Graph., Kali-C., Lyc., Olnd., Phos-Ac., Phos., Plb., Sec., Sep., Stram.*).

Increased sensitiveness and activity of the muscles subject to the will, and diminutions of it in the muscles not subject to the will.

PAINLESSNESS WITH ALMOST ALL AILMENTS.

Trembling of the whole body, with external coldness and startings of the limbs (*Nux-V.*).

TREMBLING OF THE LIMBS AFTER FRIGHT.

CONVULSIONS AFTER FRIGHT (*Ign.*) (N.).

WANT OF SENSITIVENESS TO EXTERNAL IMPRESSIONS (reverse of *Bell., Coff., Nux-V.*) AND MEDICINES, WITH A WANT OF REACTION OF THE VITAL POWER (*Laur., Psor., Sulph.*).

Renewal and aggravation of the symptoms from getting heated.

State of stupor (*Arn., Bapt., Hyos., Kali-P., Lach., Lyc., Nux-V., Phos-Ac., Stram.*).

Profound coma; the patient cannot be aroused from the stupor (Bt.).

COMPLETE LOSS OF CONSCIOUSNESS, WITH SLOW, STERTOROUS BREATHING (*Arn.*) (N.).

Drunkenness with stupor, as if from smoke (N.).

Delirium tremens (*Hyos., Stram.*) (A.).

COMPLAINS OF NOTHING; WANTS NOTHING (A.).

Screaming before or during a spasm (*Apis, Bell., Cupr., Hell., Stram.*) (A.).

Thinks she is not at home (*Bry.*) (A.).

Delirious, talking, eyes wide open, face red and puffed up (N.).

Picking of bed-clothes during sleep (while awake—*Bell., Hyos.*) (A.).

Full and slow pulse (*Gels.*).

Twitching of the head, arms and hands; now and then jerks, as if the flexors were over-active; body cold; inclination to stupid sopor; motion of the body and uncovering the head ameliorates (N.).

Pupils greatly contracted, or widely dilated and insensible to light (Bt.).

FACE BLOATED, DARK-RED, AND HOT; FEATURES DISTORTED (*Bapt., Gels., Stram.*) (N.).

The lower lip and jaw hangs down (*Hyos., Lyc.*) (N.).

Spasms of children, from approach of strangers, from nursing after fright of mother and from crying; eyes half-open and up-turned (A.).

Cessation of the labour-pains, with snoring, stupor and twitchings.

Ailments from charcoal vapors, or from inhaling gas (A.).

PUERPERAL CONVULSIONS (*Apis, Bell., Cupr., Lyc.*), WITH DROWSINESS OR COMA BETWEEN THE PAROXYSMS (Br.).

Very often indicated in states of diarrhœa, especially where the patient is suffering greatly with abdominal cramp and sharp, shooting and twisting pains in the whole belly area (*Coloc., Dios., Mag-P., Nux-V., Verat.*).

Involuntary stools (*Sulph.*) (A.).

Sleepy but cannot sleep (*Bell.*); her bed feels so hot that she can hardly lie on it (*Sulph.*) (N.).

Unrefreshing, soporous sleep, with eyes half-open (*Lyc.*) (N.).

Sleeplessness, with acuteness of hearing; clocks striking and cocks crowing at a great distance keeps her awake (N.).

Paralysis of the lungs (*Ant-T., Lach., Lyc.*).

SNORING DURING INSPIRATION AND EXPIRATION (*Arn.*) (N.).

Loss of breath on falling asleep (*Grind., Lach.*) (A.).

HEAVY, STUPID SLEEP, WITH STERTOROUS BREATHING, RED FACE, EYES HALF-CLOSED, BLOOD-SHOT, AND SKIN COVERED WITH HOT SWEAT (A.).

LEAD-POISONING VERY FAVORABLY AFFECTED BY ITS USE (*Alum., Coloc., Nux-V., Sep., Verat.*).

CONSTIPATION (*Bry., Mag-M., Plb., Sep., Sil., Thuj.*).

Hard tympany (*Carb-V., Lyc., Tereb.*) (B.).

Acute and serious effects from colicky pains in the abdomen.

Lead colic (*Alum., Coloc., Verat.*) (Bt.).

PASSES NOTHING BUT HARD, BLACK BALLS FROM THE BOWELS (*Plb.*) (N.).

FAECAL VOMITING (*Ars., Bell., Bry., Colch., Cupr., Nux-V., Plb., Sulph., Thuj.*).

INTESTINAL OBSTRUCTION (*Plb.*).

Peristaltic motion reversed or paralyzed; bowels seemed closed (*Plb.*) (A.).

Constipation, from inaction or paresis of the rectum (A.).

Fæces protrude and recede (*Sil., Thuj.*) (A.).

Sexual desire increased (*Canth . Nux-V., Phos., Plat., Sulph.*).

Frequent erections and pollutions (*Canth., Nux-V., Phos., Sulph.*) (C.).

Impotency (*Agn., Calad., Con., Lyc.*) (K.).

Erections during sleep (*Aster., Fluor-Ac., Merc-C., Nat-C., Nux-V., Rhod.*), *with impotence when awake* (K.).

Suppressed menses from fright (*Acon.*) (Br.).

Threatened abortion and suppression of lochia from fright, with stupor (Br.).

APOPLEXY, WITH STERTOROUS BREATHING (*Arn.*) (G.).

Sudden retrocession of acute eruptions (*Ant-T., Apis, Bry., Cupr., Zinc.*) (Bt.).

Dry, tickling cough, relieved by a drink of water (*Caust.*) (D.).

Dry, spasmodic, nightly cough, preventing sleep (*Con., Hyos., Puls.*) (Bt.).

Spasmodic, dry, titillating cough, especially tormenting at night, with scanty expectoration (Bhr.).

Body burning even when bathed in sweat (N.).

Colic, with great pressure downwards upon the rectum and bladder, without any passing off of fæces, gas or urine (Ra.).

Child makes no water, with full bladder, and has no stool; from nursing after the nurse had a furious fit of passion (N.).

DISTENSION OF THE BLADDER, BUT NO POWER TO EXPEL THE URINE AND A CATHETER HAS TO BE USED (*Caust.*) (N.).

RETENTION OF URINE, AFTER CONFINEMENT (*Arn., Ars., Bell., Canth., Caust., Equiset., Hyos., Ign., Lyc., Nux-V., Puls., Rhus-T., Sec., Sep., Stann., Staph., Stram.*) (A.).

THE CHILD WITH A WRINKLED SKIN, LOOKS LIKE A DRIED UP OLD MAN (*Arg-N.*) (A.).

Marasmus of children (*Abrot., Nat-M., Sanic.*) (A.).

AGGRAVATION: During and after sleep (*Apis, Lach.*) ; while perspiring: from warmth; from stimulants; from spirituous liquors; from fear; from furious fit of passion; and at night.

AMELIORATION: From cold; from constant walking; and from open air.

RELATIONSHIP: *Antidotes for poisonous doses*: Strong coffee, *Ipec., Nux-V., Kali-Per.*, and constant motion.

When symptoms correspond, the potencies may antidote bad effects of *Opium*-drugging.

Compare: *Ant-T., Apis, Arn., Bell., Bry., Canth., Dig., Ferr-P., Gels., Hyos., Kali-P., Lach., Nux-M., Nux-V., Sang., Stram., Verat-V.* and *Zinc*.

COMPLEMENTARIES: *Alum., Bar-C., Bry., Phos.,* and *Plb*.

Paris Quadrifolia.

COMMON NAME: ONE-BERRY.

Stinging pain in the body and limbs.

Heaviness through the whole body (*Bry., Gels.*).

One-sided coldness of the body with heat of the other side.

Continued internal coldness with trembling (*Ars., Nux-V., Rhus-T.*).

SENSATION AS IF A WEIGHT WERE LYING ON THE NECK (*Agar., Calc-P., Chel., Nux-V., Petr., Phos., Plb., Rhus-T., Sep., Tab., Verat.*).

Disease of the bronchi (*Calc., Euphr., Hep.*)

BRONCHITIS (*Bry., Kali-B., Kali-S., Lyc., Phos.*).

GREENISH EXPECTORATION (*Carb-V.*, *Lyc.*, *Phos.*, *Puls.*, *Sulph.*) (N.).

Stitches in the chest (*Bry.*, *Kali-C.*, *Nit-Ac.*) (C.).

Periodical (*Nux-V.*), *painless hoarseness* (*Ant-C.*, *Calc.*, *Carb-V.*, *Calc-Sil.*, *Caust.*, *Dig.*, *Phos.*) (Br.).

Constant hawking, on account of viscid, green mucus in the larynx and trachea (*Arg-N.*, *Kali-C.*, *Lyc.*, *Nat-C.*, *Phos.*, *Sep.*) (Br.).

Cough with expectoration in the morning, without expectoration in the evening (*Calc.*, *Hep.*, *Squil.*) (G.).

Oppression, with desire to draw a long breath (*Bry.*, *Ign.*, *Phos.*) (C.).

Stuffed condition and fullness at the root of the nose (*Kali-B.*, *Stict.*) (Br.).

Imaginary foul smells (*Bell.*, *Graph.*, *Phos.*, *Sulph.*) (Br.).

Bread and milk smell putrid (K.).

Great sensitiveness to offensive odours (*Sulph.*) (G.).

Collection of water in the mouth (*Arum-T.*, *Merc.*, *Puls.*, *Rhus-T.*) (G.).

Sensation as of a ball in the throat (*Asaf.*, *Ign.*, *Lach.*, *Nat-M.*, *Psor.*) (B.).

Palpitation during motion and in the evening (*Agar.*, *Arg-N.*, *Brom.*, *Cact.*, *Carb-S.*, *Carb-V.*, *Dig.*, *Ferr.*, *Graph.*, *Kalm.*, *Nat-M.*, *Phos.*, *Sil.*) (C.).

Hard mouth swellings (*Kali-Chl.*, *Merc.*, *Nit-Ac.*).

SENSATION AS IF THE EYES WERE BEING DRAWN BACK INTO THE HEAD (*Crot-T.*, *Graph.*, *Hep.*, *Lach.*, *Mezer.*, *Puls.*, *Rhod.*, *Sep.*, *Sil.*, *Sulph.*, *Zinc.*) (D.).

Foolish talk and silly actions (*Apis*) (C.).

Talkative mania. (*Bell.*, *Hyos.*, *Lach.*, *Stram.*, *Verat.*).

Garrulous, prattling, vivacious (*Cann-I.*, *Stram.*) (Br.).

Soreness of the top of the head; cannot brush hair (Br.).

The head seems enormously large (Agar., Arg-N., Arn., Bapt., Bell., Bov., Caps., Cimic., Dulc., Gels., Glon., Lac-D., Nux-M., Nux-V., Ran-B.) (D.).

Headache of spinal origin; the pains come up over the head from the occiput (*Cocc., Nat-M., Sil.*) (D.).

When moving, a sensation as if the joints were broken, swelled, or dislocated.

URINE WITH GREASY CUTICLE ON THE SURFACE (*All-C., Alumn., Calc., Dulc., Graph., Hep., Lyc., Med., Petr., Phos., Psor., Sars., Sep., Sulph., Sumb., Thuj., Verat., Zinc.*) (G.).

Dark red urine with red sediment (*Lyc.*) (C.).

Frequent micturition, with burning (*Canth., Merc., Sulph., Thuj.*) (C.).

Sticking in the forepart of the urethra (C.).

Hic-cough after eating (Ars., Bry., Carb-V., Cycl., Graph., Hyos., Ign., Lyc., Mag-M., Nat-C., Nux-V., Phos., Sep., Sil., Staph., Teucr., Verat.) (C.).

Weak, slow, digestion (*Carb-V., Hep., Nux-V., Puls., Sep.*) (C.).

Heaviness in the stomach, as from a stone (*Ars., Bry., Nux-V., Puls.*) : better from eructations (*Aloe, Chel., Fago*) (C.).

AGGRAVATION: From thinking; from eye-strain; from touch; in the evening; in the morning; from motion; and after eating.

AMELIORATION: From pressure; and from eructation.

RELATIONSHIP: *Compare: Arg-N., Bapt., Bry., Calc., Cocc., Hyos., Lach., Lyc., Nux-V., Petr., Phos., Plb., Rhus-T., Sep., Sil., Stict., Stram., Sulph., Thuj.* and *Verat.*

Incompatible: Ferr-P.

Antidote: Coff.

Passiflora Incarnata.

COMMON NAME: PASSION FLOWER.

Given in large doses PASSIFLORA causes spasms and paralysis (C.).

Muscular twitching and nervous excitement of children (*Bell., Ign., Mag-P.*) (Bl.).

Acute mania (*Acon., Bell., Hyos.*) (Br.).

TETANUS (*Bell., Cupr., Hyos., Hyper., Ign., Nux-V., Strych.*) (C.).

TRISMUS (*Bell., Cic., Hyper., Nux-V., Op., Strych., Verat.*) (C.).

Opisthotonos (*Bell., Cupr., Nux-V.*) (Bl.).

Puerperal convulsions (*Apis, Bell., Canth., Cupr., Ign., Kali-P., Lach., Lyc., Puls., Stram.*) (C.).

Delirium tremens (*Agar., Ars., Bell.,Hyos., Ign., Lach., Nux-V., Plb., Stram.*) (Br.).

Spinal meningitis (*Apis, Hell., Zinc.*) (Bl.).

Hysteria (*Apis, Bell., Calc-P., Ign., Lach., Nat-M., Puls., Sep.*) (C.).

Violent headache (*Bell., Glon.*), as if the top of the head would come off (Br.).

Eyes felt as if pushed out (*Bell., Com., Ferr-I., Guai., Nat-M., Stram.*) (Br.)).

Insomnia resulting from nervousness, mental worry or excitement, or from exhaustion (*Gels., Kali-P., Nux-V.*) (C.).

Insomnia of the infants (*Acon., Bell., Cham.*) *and the aged* (*Bar-C.*) (Br.).

Flatulence and sour eructations (*Carb-V., Lyc., Nux-V.*) (Br.).

Painful diarrhœa (*Acon., Coloc., Dios.*) (Br.).

Asthma (*Ars., Blatta, Carb-V., Ferr-P.*) (C.).

Whooping cough (*Brom., Cocc-C., Dros., Kali-C., Naphth., Sulph.*) (Br.).

Nocturnal cough (*Con., Hyos., Puls.*) (Br.).

Neuralgia (*Bell., Mag-P., Sil.*) (Br.).

Worm fever (*Bell., Cina, Hyos., Merc., Nat-M.*) (C.).

AGGRAVATION: From mental worries; from exhaustion; from mental excitement; at night; after a meal; and from nervousness.

AMELIORATION: From remaining quiet.

RELATIONSHIP: *Similar to*: ACON., *Bell., Cham., Dros., Ferr-P., Gels., Hyper., Ign., Kali-C., Lach., Merc., Nux-V., Op., Puls., Sil., Sulph., Verat.*, and *Zinc.*

Petroleum.

COMMON NAMES: ROCK OIL; COAL OIL.

It acts prominently on the skin, producing eczema, fissures and pustules, and upon the glandular and digestive systems (D.).

Particularly indicated in diseases of the ears, mucous membranes, skin, and joints (Ml.).

Symptoms appear and disappear rapidly (*Bell., Mag-P.*; reverse of *Plat., Stann.*) (A.).

Ailments from riding in a carriage, railroad car, or in a ship (*Cocc.*) (A.).

Salt-rheum on hands; red, raw, burning, or moist, or covered with thick crusts (N.).

Ailments which are worse before and during a thunderstorm (*Nat-C., Phos., Psor.*) (A.).

Heat and burning of soles of feet and palms of hands (*Lach., Med., Sep., Sulph.*) (A.).

THE SKIN SYMPTOMS ARE WORSE IN WINTER, BETTER IN SUMMER (*Alum.*); AND IF SUPPRESSED, CAUSES DIARRHOEA (A.).

Salt-rheum on lower legs from knee to ankles; purplish oozing, or covered with scales or scabs, which are easily detached; itching and burning like fire (N.).

Headache: *In the occiput, which is as heavy as lead; pressing, pulsating pain; as if everything in the head were alive; numb, bruised;* as if *made of wood* (A.).

Vertigo in the occiput, like sea-sickness (*Cocc.*) (A.).

· *Vertigo, when rising from a recumbent posture* (*Bry., Chin., Nux-V., Puls., Sep.*) (Py.).

Vertigo on closing the eyes (*Arn., Chel., Lach., Sep., Ther.*) (K.).

Ozæna, with scabs and muco-purulent discharge (*Aur., Hep.*) (Br.).

The nostrils are cracked and ulcerated (*Alum., Graph., Nat-M.*) (Bl.).

Post-nasal catarrh (*Hydr., Kali-B., Nat-S.*) (Bl.).

Easily offended at trifles (*Ign., Med., Puls., Staph.*) (A.).

Irritable, quarrelsome disposition (*Bry., Nat-M., Nux-V., Sulph.*) (A.).

Feeling as if intoxicated (*Bapt., Gels., Nux-V.*) (A.).

Vexed at everything (*Bry., Cham., Nux-V., Sulph.*) (A.).

SENSE OF DUALITY (*Anac., Bapt.*) (B.).

IMAGINES THAT ANOTHER PERSON LIES IN THE SAME BED (*Bapt.*) (Be.).

DELUSION THAT THERE ARE TWO BABIES IN THE BED (A.).

THINKS HE IS DOUBLE, (*Anac., Bapt., Cann-I., Glon., Lach., Mosch., Nux-M., Stram.*) (Br.)., OR SOME ONE ELSE LYING ALONG-SIDE (Br.).

Imagines that one leg is double (A.).

Irresolute (*Puls.*) (B.).

Feels that death is near, and must hurry to settle affairs. (*Ars.*) (Br.).

CHRONIC FOETID DISCHARGE FROM THE EAR (*Calc-S., Graph., Hep., Merc., Sil., Tell.*) (Ml.).

Chronic Eustachian catarrh (*Puls.*) (Br.).

IMPAIRED HEARING (*Calc., Phos., Puls.*) (Ra.).
A large quantity of thick or thin wax in the ear, which is dry or hard, and of a brown colour (Ra.).
Humid soreness behind the ear (*Graph.*) (N.).

CHRONIC MOIST ECZEMA; PARTS SEEM EXCORIATED (*Ars., Graph., Nat-M., Rhus-T.*) (N.).

CRACKING OF THE JOINTS (*Led., Lyc., Merc., Nat-C., Nat-M., Nat-S., Nit-Ac., Nux-V., Phos., Plb., Rhus-T., Sep., Sulph., Thuj.*) (G.).
Inflexibility of the joints (*Ars., Bell., Caust., Led., Lyc., Rhus-T., Sep., Sil., Sulph.*) (G.).
Chronic sprains (*Rhus-T.*) (G.).

COLD FEELING IN THE HEART (*Arn., Carb-An,. Graph., Helo., Kali-B., Kali-Chl., Kali-N., Lil-T., Nat-M., Pyrog.*) (G.).
Fainting, with ebullitions, heat and palpitation (Br.).
FETID SWEAT FROM THE AXILLAE (*Merc.*) (G.).
Brown or yellow spots on the skin (G.).
Painful sensitiveness of the skin of the whole body (*Hep., Lach.*) ; *all clothing* is painful (A.).

SLIGHT INJURY SUPPURATES (*Hep., Merc., Sil., Sulph.*) (A.).
Skin of hands rough, cracked; tips of fingers rough, cracked, fissured, every winter (A.).
Vesicular eruptions, turning into pustules, which are covered with scabs (D.).
Tenderness of the feet, which are bathed in foul-smelling sweat (*Graph., Sanic., Sil.*) (A.).
Painful, itching chilblains and chapped hands, worse in cold weather (A.).
Many furuncles on the neck and arms, with ulceration of the ears (Ml.).

Bitter or sour taste in the mouth (*Chin., Nux-V., Sep.*) (G.).

DISGUST FOR MEAT (*Calc., Chin., Graph.*) (G.).

Deep, fistulous ulcers (*Sil.*) (G.).

RAVENOUS APPETITE OR CANINE HUNGER WITH DIARRHOEA (*Aloe, Calc., Fluor-Ac., Iod., Lyc., Olnd., Stram., Sulph., Verat.*) (K.).

Aversion to fat food (*Chin., Merc., Ptel., Puls.*) (G.).

Empty, hungry feeling and nausea, which lasts all day (D.).

Particularly applicable in all gastric troubles of pregnant females (*Puls., Sep.*) (G.).

Sensation of repletion after a little food (*Lyc., Nux-M.*) (Mr.).

GASTRALGIA, WHENEVER THE STOMACH BECOMES EMPTY (*Bar-C., Calc., Cocc., Graph., Ign., Lach., Nit-Ac., Psor., Sep.*) (Dr. Brs.).

Gastralgia with pressing, drawing pains; ameliorated by keeping on eating something constantly (*Anac., Brom., Chel., Cina, Dios., Graph., Hep., Ign.*) (G.).

SEA-SICKNESS (*Carb-Ac., Cocc., Colch., Con., Glon., Hyos., Kali-B., Kreos., Lac-Ac., Nat-M., Nux-V., Sep., Staph., Tab., Ther.*) (K.).

Nausea when riding (*Calc-P., Cocc., Mag-C., Nux-M., Sep.*) (G.).

COLD FEELING IN THE ABDOMEN (*Ambr., Calc., Camph., Crot-T., Grat., Kali-S., Meny., Nat-M., Phos., Sec., Verat.*) (G.).

Nausea, worse from motion or riding, and accompanied by vertigo (D.).

Diarrhœa, preceded by colic (*Aloe, Nux-V.*) (N.).

Diarrhœa: After cabbage, sour-crout; during pregnancy; and during stormy weather (A.).

Chronic diarrhœa (*Aloe, Podo., Sulph.*) (Br.).

4

DIARRHOEA, ALWAYS IN THE DAY TIME (A.).

Stools yellow, watery, gushing (*Aloe, Chin., Crot-T., Sulph.*) (A.).

Slimy stools with pain in the bowels (*Coloc., Dios., Merc., Nux-V., Sulph.*) (Bt.).

Burning and stinging in the anus and rectum (*Aloe, Sulph.*) (G.).

Raw hæmorrhoids; scurf on the anus (G.).

Great desire to urinate, with itching of the meatus (*Cann-I., Caust., Cocc-C., Hydr., Kali-C., Merc-C., Nat-M., Sulph.*) (Ra.).

Chronic gonorrhœa (*Calc-S., Kali-S., Med., Nat-M., Nat-S., Petrosel., Sep., Thuj.*) (K.).

Itching in the urethra (*Petrosel.*) (Br.).

HERPES OF THE GENITAL ORGANS EXTENDING TO THE PERINEUM, AND THIGHS; ITCHING, REDNESS; SKIN CRACKED, ROUGH, BLEEDING; DRY OR MOIST (A.).

Sweat and moisture of the external genitals, both sexes (*Lyc., Merc., Sulph., Thuj.*) (A.).

Menses cause an itching in the genitals (*Calc., Caust., Kreos., Lyc., Merc., Nat-M., Sep., Sil., Zinc.*) (G.).

Profuse leucorrhœa every day, with lascivious dreams every night (G.).

Labia majoræ perspire and itch much (G.).

INFLAMED TARSI (*Alum., Graph., Sep., Sulph.*) (B.).

Cough at night only (*Ambr., Caust.*) or worse then (*Con., Hyos., Nux-V., Puls.*) (B.).

Cough produces headache (*Bry., Sep.*) (Br.).

MARGINAL BLEPHARITIS (*Alum., Arg-N., Bor., Graph., Sep., Sulph.*) (Br.).

FISTULA LACHRYMALIS (*Calc., Fluor-Ac., Puls., Sil.*) (K.).

AGGRAVATION: From carriage-riding; before and during a thunder-storm; in winter; during the day time; in a ship; on rising; when fasting; during pregnancy; from touch; and from taking sauer-kraut or cabbage.

AMELIORATION: At night; in summer; after eating; in warm air; and from lying with the head high.

RELATIONSHIP: One of our best antidotes for lead-poisoning.

Remedies following: *Bry., Calc-C., Lyc., Nux-V., Puls., Sep., Sil., Sulph.*

Antidotes: *Cocc.* and *Nux-V.*

Complementary: *Sep.*

Petroselinum.

COMMON NAME: PARSLEY.

Acts decidedly upon the urethral mucous membrane, producing a considerable degree of irritation and inflammation (C.).

The urinary symptoms give the keynotes for this remedy (Br.).

Piles with much itching (*Aloe, Ign., Nux-V., Sulph.*) (Br.).

Thirsty and hungry, yet as soon as they begin to eat or drink they lose all desire (reverse of *Calc.*) (A.).

Intermittent fever complicating with traumatic or chronic urethritis or stricture; with abdominal affections and perverted or defective assimilation (A.).

Priapismus, with curvature of the penis (*Cann-S., Canth., Nux-V., Sulph.*) (C.).

Profuse emission toward morning (*Carb-V., Nux-V., Psor.*) (C.).

SUDDEN DESIRE TO URINATE (*Cann-S., Canth., Merc.*) (A.).

CHILD JUMPS UP AND DOWN WITH PAIN IF CANNOT BE GRATIFIED AT ONCE (A.).

Pain at the root of the penis, or neck of the bladder (A.).

Burning, tingling from the perineum throughout the whole urethra (A.).

INTENSE ITCHING IN THE URETHRA (*Berb., Cann-S., Chim., Ferr., Graph., Kali-Chl., Led., Lyc., Merc., Merc-C., Mezer., Nat-M., Nit-Ac., Nux-V., Petr., Sep., Sulph., Sulph-I., Thuj.*) (N.).

ITCHING IN THE URETHRA WITH GONORRHOEA (*Merc-C., Nat-M., Petr.*; following gonorrhœa—*Nit-Ac.*; with gleet—*Nat-M., Nit-Ac., Nux-V., Petr.*) (K.).

VOLUPTUOUS ITCHING IN THE FOSSA NAVICULARIS (*Thuj.*) (K.).

Gonorrhœa: Sudden irresistible desire to urinate; intense biting, itching, deep in the urethra; must rub it with some rough article for relieving the pain (A.).

Gleet (or chronic gonorrhœa) (*Agn., Brom., Calc-P., Ferr., Hydr., Kali-S., Med., Nat-M., Nat-S., Petr., Sep., Sil., Sulph., Thuj.*) (A.).

Must hasten to urinate, or urine will escape (*Arn., Canth., Clem., Kreos., Nux-V., Puls., Sep., Sulph.*) (K.).

Milky discharge from the urethra (*Cann-S., Caps., Cop., Ferr., Iod., Kali-C., Kali-Chl., Lach., Merc., Nat-M., Nux-V., Sep.*) (Br.).

Burning in the navicular fossa while urinating (*Clem., Kali-B., Nat-M., Thuj.*) (C.).

Orifice of the urethra agglutinated with mucus (*Sep.*) (C.).

AGGRAVATION: Before and during urination; during acute or chronic gonorrhœa; and towards morning.

AMELIORATION: From rubbing the urethra with some rough article.

RELATIONSHIP: *Compare*: *Alum., Berb., Cann-S., Canth., Graph., Hep., Kali-B., Kali-S., Lyc., Merc., Nat-M., Nat-S., Petr., Puls., Rhus-T., Sep., Sulph., Thuj.* and *Zinc.*

Phosphoric Acid.

COMMON NAME: GLACIAL PHOSPHORIC ACID.

It produces nervous prostration and debility; an atonic condition of the gastro-intestinal tract and bone affections (D.).

Best suited to persons of originally strong constitutions, who have become debilitated by loss of vital fluids, sexual excesses (*Chin.*), violent acute diseases (*Calc-P., Psor., Sel.*), chagrin, or a long succession of moral emotions, as grief, care, disappointed affection (A.).

Also useful in diseases of children and young people who grow too rapidly (*Calc.* for those who grow too fat) (A.).

Pale, sickly complexion (Ferr., Puls., Sep.) (A.).

Eyes sunken and surrounded by blue margins (*Cina, Staph.*) (A.).

Eyes like glass, without lustre (*Lyc.*).

Chronic effects of grief; hair turns gray; hopeless, haggard look (N.).

GROWS TOO FAST AND TOO TALL (N.).

Palpitation in young persons growing too fast, after onanism (Phos.) (N.).

Great physical and mental weakness from ovarian diseases or sexual excesses (N.).

Great debility with perspiration during the day (not so marked as *Acon.*, however).

Nervous debility arising from continued grief or over-exertion of mind (D.).

Debility from loss of fluids, without pain, or only with burning (Phos.).

Pain in the back and limbs as if beaten (A.).

Soreness in the limbs, as from rowing, especially in the morning.

FORMICATION (*Agar., Alum., Bar-C., Carb-S., Cocc., Ferr., Lyc., Nat-M., Nux-V., Phos., Rhod., Rhus-T., Sec., Sulph., Tarent.*).

Burning of the lower half of the body: the limbs feeling cold.

The pains are only severe during rest, relieved by motion (*Rhus-T.*), *and the nightly pains from pressure* (*Rhus-T.*).

Pains, as from a knife, scraping the periosteum.

Inflammation of the bones, with burning at night.

Swelling of the bones (*Calc-P., Merc., Sil.*).

Offensive caries of the osseous structures (*Asaf., Aur., Calc-F.*).

Bruised feeling in the muscles (*Arn., Bry., Cimic.*) and burning in the spine (*Phos.*) (D.).

Patient trembles, legs weak; stumbles easily or makes missteps (*Nat-M.*) (A.).

Neurosis in stump after amputations (*Cepa, Hyper.*) (A.).

CLAMMY, STICKY TONGUE (*Puls.*) (Ra.).

Ulceration of the soft palate (*Aur., Cinnb., Kali-B., Lach., Lyc., Merc., Merc-C., Nat-M., Nit-Ac., Phos., Sanic., Sil.*).

Mercurial syphilitic ulceration of the lips, guns and soft palate, with swelling of the bones (Hm.).

Bread tastes bitter (*Asaf., Calc-P., Chin., Chin-S., Dig., Ferr., Merc., Nux-V., Phos., Puls.*) (G.).

Gluey matter on the tongue, in choleraic diseases (Puls.) (G.).

At night he bites his tongue involuntarily.

Useful in typhus or *typhoid fever* (*Bapt., Hyos., Kali-P., Lach., Nux-V., Op., Rhus-T.*).

Meteoristic distension of the abdomen, with rumbling and gurgling (*Carb-V., Lyc., Nat-S., Nux-M., Puls.*) (N.).

Cerebral typhoid or typhus; complete apathy and stupor; takes no notice, "lies like a log" (*Carb-V.*), utterly regardless of surrounding (A.).

Aversion to acids (*Abies-C., Bell., Cocc., Ferr., Ferr-M., Ign., Nux-V., Sabad., Sulph.*) (K.).

Desire for pungent things (*Ars., Ast-R., Cist., Fluor-Ac., Hep., Lac-C., Nat-P., Sang.*) (K.).

Intestinal hæmorrhage; blood dark (*Ham.*) (A.).

Diarrhœa after fright (*Acon., Arg-N., Gels., Ign., Kali-P., Op., Phos., Puls., Verat.*) (K.).

Diarrhœa from taking acids (*Aloe, Ant-C., Brom., Coloc., Lach., Nux-V., Sulph.*) (A.).

Involuntary stools with passage of flatus (*Aloe, Nat-S., Sulph.*) (A.).

Soft stools (*Alum., Aur-M., Bapt., Calc., Hep., Merc., Nit-Ac., Phos., Plat., Sulph., Sulph-Ac.*).

PAINLESS, WATERY DIARRHOEA (*Chin., Podo., Puls., Ricin.*) (N.).

White or gray watery diarrhœa (*Calc., Iod., Podo.*) (N.).

Undigested, painless stools (*Arg-N., Chin., Ferr., Podo., Sulph.*) (Bt.).

The diarrhœa, although of long continuance, does not seem to debilitate much; the mother wonders that the child remains so strong with it all (G.).

DIARRHOEA WITH RUMBLING (*Podo.*), METEORISM; BUT NOT SO MUCH WEAKNESS AS WOULD BE EXPECTED (N.).

Urine loaded with phosphates and showing a greasy pellicle (D.).

GLYCOSURIA AND POLYURIA (*Nat-M., Sulph.*) (D.).

Very profuse, watery or milky urine (N.).

MUST OFTEN RISE AT NIGHT IN ORDER TO PASS LARGE QUANTITIES OF COLOURLESS URINE (*Merc., Sulph.*) (N.).

Urine like milk mixed with jelly-like pieces and pain in the kidneys (N.).

White jelly-like flocculi in the urine (N.).
He lies down stupid (*Arn., Bapt., Hell., Hyos., Lyc.*).

BAD EFFECTS FROM SORROW (*Gels., Ign., Nat-M., Puls., Sep.*).
Disinclination to talk, with moroseness and low-spiritedness (*Ign., Nat-M., Sep.*).

APATHETIC, LISTLESS (*Apis, Carb-V., Chin., Crot-C., Hell., Lil-T., Mezer., Nat-C., Nat-M., Nat-P., Onos., Op., Phos., Plat., Puls., Sep., Staph.*) (N.).

WANTS NOTHING AND CARES FOR NOTHING (G.).
Indifferent to the affairs of life (*Sep.*) (N.).
Indifferent to those things that used to interest her the most (G.).

HOME-SICKNESS (*Aur., Caps., Carb-An., Caust., Ign., Kali-P., Mag-M., Merc., Nat-M., Nit-Ac., Petr., Puls., Sil., Sulph., Verat.*) (K.).

UNCONSCIOUS OF ALL SURROUNDINGS, BUT CAN BE AROUSED TO FULL CONSCIOUSNESS (*Arn., Bapt.*) (N.).
Slow grasp (*Nat-M., Sil.*) (B.).
Can't collect his ideas, hunts for words (*Nux-M.*) (B.).
Hysteric affections of young women, with excessive sensibility and irritability (*Apis, Ign., Nux-M., Puls.*) (G.).
Hypochondriasis from sexual abuse (Bt.).

LOSS OF MEMORY (*Calc., Kali-P., Lyc.*) (Bt.).
Disposed to weep (*Ign., Nat-M., Puls., Sep.*) (A.).

ABASHED, SAD, DESPAIR OF CURE (A.).
Mild, yielding disposition (*Puls.*) (A.).

MUTTERING OR UNINTELLIGIBLE DELIRIUM (*Hyos.*) (A.).
Headache, usually from behind forward, made worse by least motion and noise, especially music (A.).

Dreadful pain on the top of the head, as though the brain were crushed (after long-continued grief) (G.).

Cerebral weakness from brain-fag (*Kali-P.*) (Bt.).

Headache of school-girls from eye-strain, or overuse of eyes (*Calc-P., Nat-M.*) (N.).

OCCIPITAL HEADACHE AND PAINS IN THE NAPE OF THE NECK, FROM EXHAUSTED NERVE POWER, OR EXCESSIVE GRIEF (N.).

SEVERAL EMISSIONS IN ONE NIGHT (*Nux-V.*) (A.).

ONANISM (*Chin., Dios., Nux-V., Staph.*); WHEN THE PATIENT IS DISTRESSED BY THE CULPABILITY OF HIS INDULGENCE (N.).

SEMINAL EMISSIONS WHEN PRESSING AT STOOL (*Nat-M., Sel., Sulph.,*) (C.).

DEBILITY, RELAXATION OR IMPOTENCE FROM SEXUAL EXCESSES (*Agn., Calad.*) (D.).

THE SEMEN IS DISCHARGED SHORTLY AFTER AN ERECTION, OR WITHOUT ERECTION (*Graph., Lyc., Nux-V., Sulph.*).

FREQUENT, PROFUSE AND DEBILITATING EMISSIONS (*Nat-P., Nux-V., Phos., Sulph., Zinc.*) (A.).

SEMINAL EMISSIONS AFTER COITUS (*Calc., Graph., Nat-M.*) (A.).

Dragging pains in the testicles (*Cann-S., Gels., Iod., Kali-C., Lach., Med., Sumb.*), especially after seminal emissions (K.).

Exhaustion after coition (*Calc.*), also after pollutions (*Chin.*) (C.).

Spermatorrhœa (*Arg.-N., Gels., Kali-P., Nat-M., Phos., Sep.*) (D.).

Too early and too long menstruation (*Calc., Ferr., Sec.*) (G.).

Profuse leucorrhœa, with itching, some days after the menses (*Alum., Ars., Calc., Caust., Hydr., Kali-P., Kreos., Merc., Nat-M., Nit-Ac., Puls., Sab., Sulph.*) (G.).

Metritis with great debility and slow fever (*Calc., Chin., Kali-P., Lach.*) (G.).

Scanty milk (*Agn., Bry., Caust., Dulc., Puls., Urt-U.*) (G.).

Vertigo in the morning, towards evening, when standing and walking (*Chin., Kali-P., Nux-V., Phos.*) (C.).

Roaring in the ears, with difficult hearing (*Puls.*) (C.).

Pulse irregular, intermittent (*Dig., Mur-Ac., Nat-M.*) (C.).

Hair turns grey early (*Lyc.*), or falls off (*Nat-M., Sep.*) (C.).

FREQUENT URINATION DURING CHILL OR FEVER (*Merc.*) (K.).

FAINTNESS AFTER EATING (*Bar-C., Bufo, Caust., Mag-M., Nux-V., Plan., Sang.*), AFTER EMISSION (*Asaf.*), OR ON EXCITEMENT (*Coff., Ign., Lach., Nux-M., Op., Sumb., Verat.*) (K.).

Chest weak from talking or coughing (*Stann.*) (N.).

Cough with purulent and offensive expectoration (*Calc., Merc., Sep.*) *and pains in the chest,* (*Bry., Kali-C., Phos.*) (N.).

Cough with salty expectoration (*Kali-I., Nat-M., Puls.*) (N.).

Cough on slightest exposure (*Hep., Kali-C., Rumx, Sil.*) (D.).

Cough from tickling in the chest about the ensiform cartilage, worse in the evening on lying down (*Puls.*) (D.).

Weakness of the chest causes dyspnœa; the patient can hardly talk (D.).

NIGHT-SWEATS TOWARDS MORNING (*Kali-C., Merc., Nit-Ac.*) (A.).

Sleepy by day, but wakeful at night (*Nux-V., Staph.*) (B.).

AGGRAVATION: From bad news; from depressing emotions; from masturbation; from sexual excesses; from draft or wind; from snowy air; from mental affections; from over-study; from loss of vital fluids; from talking; from noise; from music; and from acids.

AMELIORATION: After short sleep; from warmth; from pressure; and by motion.

RELATIONSHIP: *Compare: Arn., Bapt., Chin., Ferr., Graph., Hep., Ign., Kali-P., Lach., Lyc., Mur-Ac., Nat-M., Nit-Sp-D., Nux-V., Op., Phos., Pic-Ac., Puls., Rhus-T., Sep., Sil., Sulph., Thuj., Verat.* and *Zinc.*

Phos-Ac. acts well before or after *Chin.,* in colliquative sweats, diarrhœa, debility, etc., and after *Nux-V.* in fainting after a meal and seminal emissions.

Antidotes: Camph., Coff.

Phosphorus.

COMMON NAME: PHOSPHORUS.

Adapted to tall, slender persons of sanguine temperament, fair skin, delicate eye-lashes, fine blond or red hair, quick perceptions, and very sensitive nature (A.).

Useful for young people, who grow too rapidly, are inclined to stoop (to walk stooped—*Sulph.*) (A.).

Fistulous ulcers, with callous edges, secreting a thin, foul pus and of a blue appearance (*Carb-V.*) (Bt.).

Flushes all over, beginning in hands (N.).

BURNING HEAT RUNNING UP THE BACK AND BETWEEN SHOULDERS (N.).

Glandular swellings, especially after contusions (*Con.*).

Great debility of the nervous system (Ars., Con., Gels., Kali-P., Phos-Ac., Pic-Ac.).

EMACIATION (*Abrot., Bar-C., Calc-P., Nat-M., Sanic., Sil., Tub.*).

Burning in the body and limbs (*Ars., Camph., Carb-V., Kali-P., Lach., Sec., Sulph.*).

Morning weakness in the limbs in bed (*Canth., Nat-M.*).

Sensitiveness to cold weather and open air.

Easy-catching cold and from it tearing and stinging in the limbs.

TREMBLING OF THE LIMBS FROM SLIGHT EXERTIONS (*Merc., Nat-M., Rhus-T., Sec.*).

Weakness of the joints, especially the knees (*Calc., Con., Kali-C., Lyc., Merc., Nat-M., Plb., Psor., Sep., Sulph.*).

Cold legs and feet (*Calc., Carb-V., Sep.*) (Bt.).

Necrosis of the (left) lower jaw (A.).

Rachitis (*Calc., Merc., Phos-Ac., Sil.*).

SWELLING AND CARIOUS AFFECTIONS OF THE BONES (*Asaf., Aur., Aur-M., Calc-F., Calc-P., Calc-S., Fluor-Ac., Merc., Sil.*).

HAEMORRHAGES FROM VARIOUS ORGANS (*Bell., Crot-H., Lach., Merc., Nit-Ac., Sec.*).

SMALL WOUNDS BLEED MUCH (*Lach., Nit-Ac.*).

Sneezing and coryza from putting hands in water (*Lac-D.*) (A.).

Frequent blowing of blood in small quantity from the nose (*Arn., Carb-S., Lach., Phos-Ac., Sulph.*) (N.).

Polypus of the nose; easily bleeding (*Calc., Calc-P., Thuj.*) (N.).

Caries of the nasal bones (*Aur., Kali-B.*) (D.).

DIFFICULT HEARING, ESPECIALLY OF THE HUMAN VOICE (N.).

Oedema of the face, especially of the lids and around the eyes (*Apis, Ars., Kali-C.*) (N.).

Re-echoing of sounds in the ears (D.).

TOOTHACHE OF WASHER-WOMEN, OR FROM WASHING CLOTHES (N.).

Face semi-transparent, like polished ivory (*Nat-M.*) (Hm.).

Small bald spot over the ear (Dg.).

Hair falls out in bunches (*Nat-M.*) (A.).

Violent ebullitions and congestions (*Acon., Bell., Ferr-P., Sang., Sulph., Verat-V.*).

Great sensitiveness of the senses and giddiness (*Bell., Coff., Nux-V.*).

Great depression at twilight (G.).

Amativeness (*Canth., Nux-V.*) (G.).

Anxious and fearful before and during a thunder-storm (*Gels., Nat-C., Nat-M., Sep.*) (N.).

FEAR OF BEING ALONE (*Arg-N., Ars., Bism., Camph., Crot-C., Gels., Hyos., Kali-C., Lyc.*) (N.).

NYMPHOMANIA (*Canth., Hyos., Stram., Verat.*) (G.).

Fearfulness, as if something were creeping out at every corner (*Hyos., Stram.*) (G.).

Apathetic; unwilling to talk (*Phos-Ac.*) ; *answers slowly; moves sluggishly* (*Gels.*) (A.).

Clairvoyance (*Anac., Cann-I., Crot-C., Hyos., Lach., Lyss., Nux-M., Op., Pyrus., Sil., Stram., Tarent.*) (Bt.).

Laughing against the will (*Cann-I., Ign., Nat-M., Sep., Tarent.*) (Bt.).

DESIRES TO BE MAGNETIZED (*Calc., Lach., Nat-C., Sil.*) (A.).

Restless, fidgety; moves continually; cannot sit or stand still for a moment (A.).

Dread of mental exertion (*Kali-P., Lyc., Sil.*) (D.).

Weary of life (*Aur., Nux-V., Sep.*) (A.).

FULL OF GLOOMY FOREBODINGS (*Ars., Lach.*) (A.).

Stools are soft (*Alum., Hep., Merc., Nit-Ac., Sulph., Sulph-Ac., Thuj.*).

Stools watery, with lumps of white mucus, or like little grains of tallow or sago (N.).

DISCHARGE OF MUCUS FROM THE WIDE OPEN ANUS, WITH TENESMUS (N.).

Chronic painless diarrhœa of undigested food (*Ferr., Podo.*) with much thirst for water during night (N.).

Diarrhœa, during cholera time (*Camph.*) (A.).

Diarrhœa, as soon as anything enters the rectum (A.).

Morning diarrhœa of old people (*Ant-C., Gamb., Nat-S.*) (A.).

Involuntary stool on coughing or sneezing (*Bell., Merc., Rumx., Squil., Sulph.*) (K.).

PROFUSE, EXHAUSTING DIARRHOEA POURING AWAY AS IF FROM A HYDRANT (*Podo., Sulph.*) (Ra.).

Green and bloody passages; the anus remaining open (*Apis*) (Ho.).

Constipation: *The fæces being slender, long, narrow, dry, tough, and hard like a dog's; voided with difficulty* (N.).

PAINLESS DIARRHOEA, WITH EXHAUSTION AND PROSTRATION (D.).

Acute yellow atrophy of the liver, or acute hepatitis, with tendency to formation of abscesses (D.).

Stitches in the liver (*Bry., Chel., Merc.*) (Bt.).

FATTY DEGENERATION OF THE LIVER, WITH MALIGNANT JAUNDICE (*Crot-H., Lach., Merc.*) (Bt.).

ENLARGED, CIRRHOSED LIVER (*Mur-Ac.*) (D.).

Fistulous openings and abscesses of the breast (*Sil.*) (Bt.).

CATAMENIA TOO EARLY, TOO PROFUSE AND OF TOO LONG DURATION (*Cycl., Ferr., Nat-M., Nux-V., Sabin.*).

Acrid, corrosive, smarting leucorrhœa, drawing blisters (N.).

Metrorrhagia, in cancer (*Lach., Nit-Ac., Sec.*) (A.).

Vicarious hæmorrhage from the nose, stomach, anus, urethra, etc., in association with amenorrhœa (A.).

Is unable to drink water during pregnancy; sight of it causes vomiting; must close her eyes while bathing (*Lyss.*) (A.).

The patient is hungry, especially at night; wakes up hungry and longs for cold thing (D.).

Tongue parched, dry, cracked, and covered black, or glazed (Hi. & Ht.).

Thirst and dryness of the mouth (*Ars., Bry., Nat-M., Sulph.*) (Bt.).

Perforating ulcer of the stomach, with vomiting of coffee-ground-like matters (*Con.*) (D.).

The victuals, which have been scarcely swallowed, come up again in the mouth.

Hiccough in typhoid (*Ars., Carb-V., Cic., Crot-H., Mag-P.*) (K.).

Belching large quantities of wind after eating (*Arg-N., Carb-V., Lyc.*) (Bt.).

WANTS COLD FOOD AND DRINK, ICECREAM; IS RELIEVED BY THEM (N.).

Longs for juicy, refreshing things (A.).

Desire for fish (*Nat-M., Nat-P.*), *cold milk, and highly seasoned food* (*Chin., Hep., Sulph.*) (K.).

AS SOON AS WATER BECOMES WARM IN THE STOMACH IT IS THROWN UP (*Chlf., Pyrog.*) (N.).

Nausea from placing hands in warm water (A.).

Sensation of weakness and emptiness in the abdomen (*Ign., Sep.*) (Bt.).

Sharp, cutting pains in the bowels, sometimes with sour vomiting (G.).

Objects have a cloudiness about them by candle-light (D.).

Hemicrania (*Nat-M., Sang., Spig.*) (Hr.).

Hemi-plegia from apoplexy, with formication in the paralyzed limbs (Hm.).

Typhus with paralysis impending (Bt.).

GLAUCOMA (*Bry., Spig., Sulph.*) (B.).

Green halo about objects (D.).

Deprivation of sight, with dilatation of the pupils, and darting pains in the eyeballs (Hr.).

LETTERS APPEAR RED (D.).

SHORT-SIGHTEDNESS (*Nat-M.,*) (G.).

ATTACKS OF SUDDEN BLINDNESS; OBJECTS APPEAR VEILED (*Merc.*) (Bt.).

DEGENERATION OR GREY ATROPHY OF THE OPTIC NERVE (D.).

Cataract (*Calc., Nat-M., Sep., Sil.*) (K.).

Retinitis albuminurica (*Ars., Nat-M.*) (B.).

Dim vision after coition (*Chin., Kali-C., Kali-P., Nat-P., Sep., Sil*), or during headache (*Cycl., Iris, Sulph.*) (K.).

Green mucus in the nostrils (*Merc., Puls.*) (Bt.).

Strong effect on the respiratory organs and the capillary vessels, with inflammation of the lung on the left side.

ACUTE PAIN IN THE LOWER PART OF THE LEFT LUNG, GREATLY AGGRAVATED BY LYING ON THE LEFT SIDE (Bt.).

Cough in the evening, when reading, laughing, or loudly talking, or from lying on the left side (N.).

Trembling of the whole body while coughing (Hr.).

CANNOT TALK ON ACCOUNT OF PAIN IN THE LARYNX (N.).

HOARSENESS, WITH LOSS OF VOICE, WORSE IN THE EVENING (*Brom., Carb-V., Caust., Graph., Kali-B., Mang., Rumx., Sulph.*) (Bt.).

Cough worse when coming from the warm room into the cold air (Hr.).

Capillary bronchitis; severe, hard, dry, exhausting cough (Bry., Squil.) (Bt.).

Pain in the chest with coughing, better by external pressure (*Bry.*) (N.).

Tightness across the chest, with a dry tight cough (*Bry.*) (Bt.).

Heaviness of the chest, as if a weight were lying on it (Bry.) ((A.).

PNEUMONIA WITH SANGUINEOUS INFILTRATION OF THE PARENCHYMA, AND RED HEPATIZATION.

RUSTY SPUTUM OR BRICK-DUST EXPECTORATION; OR EXPECTORATION OF MUCUS, PUS AND BLOOD (Bt.).

OPPRESSION OF THE CHEST (*Bry., Ferr-P., Lach.*) (D.).

Very sleepy during menstruation (*Eupi., Kali-C., Nux-M., Sulph., Uran.*) (Bt.).

Very sleepy after meals, especially after dinner (*Agar., Calc., Nux-V.*) (G.).

HAEMOPTYSIS, WITH OCCASIONAL ATTACKS OF PROFUSE HAEMORRHAGE (*Ferr-P., Ipec., Lach., Nit-Ac., Sulph-Ac.*) (Bt.).

It should be borne in mind in incipient as well as the more advanced cases of phthisis (Bl.).

Gums inflamed, bleed easily, and are separated from the teeth (*Merc., Nit-Ac.*) (R.).

PERSISTENT BLEEDING AFTER EXTRACTION OF TEETH (*Merc.*) (R.).

RAVENOUS HUNGER DURING FEVER. (*Chin., Cina, Cur., Eup-Pur., Hell.*) (K.).

Fungous hæmatodes and exerescences (B.).

Perspiration has the odour of sulphur (A.).

Acute and chronic nephritis (*Apis, Canth., Lyc., Merc-C., Nit-Ac., Sep.*) (K.).

THICK, TURBID AND SCANTY URINE (*Apis, Canth., Kali-C., Puls., Sep.*) (Bt.).

Albumen and exudation cells in the urine (*Apis, Canth., Merc-C., Tereb.*) (Hm.).

LASCIVIOUS; STRIPS HIMSELF; SEXUAL MANIA; IRRESISTIBLE DESIRE FOR COITION (*Canth., Stram.*) (N.).

Nocturnal emissions with or without lascivious dreams (*Anac., Camph., Dios., Gels., Graph., Nat-P., Pic-Ac., Sep., Stann., Zinc.*) (K.).

IMPOTENCE FROM SEXUAL ABUSE (*Agn., Calad., Chin., Lyc., Nat-M., Phos-Ac., Sulph., Zinc.*) (Hm.).

THE PATIENT HAS DESIRES AND FANCIES, BUT NO POWER (*Con.*) (D.).

Discharge of prostatic juice, during hard stools (*Agn., Alum., Cann-I., Carb-V., Con., Gels., Hep., Nat-C., Nit-Ac., Phos-Ac., Psor., Sep., Sil., Staph., Sulph., Zinc.*) (Bt.).

Sexual abuse producing dorsal consumption, trembling, imbecility, mania, epileptic fits and impaired digestion (Bt.).

Moisture in the meatus urinarius (*Nat-M.*), *causing a yellow stain* (K.).

AGGRAVATION: From change of weather; during a thunder-storm; in the morning; in the evening; while in bed; after eating; after drinking; before midnight; when lying on the back; and when lying on the left side.

Cold air relieves the head and face symptoms, but aggravates those of the chest, throat and neck.

AMELIORATION: After eating; from drinking cold water; from cold food; from lying on the right side; from being rubbed or mesmerized; and after sleep.

RELATIONSHIP: *Complementary*: *Ars.*, with which it is isomorphic; *All-C.*, its vegetable analogue.

Incompatible: with *Caust.;* must not be used before or after.

Phos. removes the bad effects of *Iod.* (*Hep.*), and excessive use of table salt.

Follows well after: *Calc.* or *Chin.*

Antidotes: *Coff.*, *Nux-V.*

Physostigma.

COMMON NAME: CALABAR BEAN.

Contraction of the pupil (*Acon.*, *Bell.*, *Chin-S.*, *Daph.*, *Euphr.*, *Gels.*, *Hyos.*, *Merc.*, *Nat-M.*, *Op.*, *Plb.*, *Puls.*) (D.).

Night blindness (*Chin.*, *Hyos.*, *Lyc.*, *Merc.*, *Nit-Ac.*, *Nux-V.*, *Puls.*, *Ran-B.*, *Stram.*, *Verat.*, *Zinc.*) (Bl.).

Twitching of the ocular muscles (*Agar.*) (Bl.)

MYOPIA (*Arg-N.*, *Calc.*, *Gels.*, *Phos.*, *Puls.*) (K.).

Spinal irritation (*Kali-P.*, *Phos.*, *Zinc.*) (D.).

Impaired locomotion (*Con.*, *Gels.*) (A.).

TETANUS (*Arn.*, *Bell.*, *Cupr.*, *Nux-V.*, *Op.*, *Phyt.*, *Strych.*, *Verat.*) (D.).

Slightest draught of air renews the spasm (*Ars.*, *Lyss.*, *Nux-V.*, *Strych.*).

Violent trembling all over (*Gels.*) (C.).

Trismus or lock-jaw (*Cic.*, *Cup.*, *Ign.*, *Nux-V.*, *Strych.*) (D.).

Great prostration of the muscular system and tenderness of the spine (*Phos.*) (Bl.).

Progressive muscular atrophy (*Iod.*, *Nat-M.*, *Op.*, *Plb.*) (Bl.).

Unsteadiness from knee downward, when walking, especially with the eyes shut (*Con.*) (C.).

Locomotor ataxia (*Alum.*, *Con.*, *Gels.*, *Nux-V.*, *Phos.*, *Sil.*) (Br.).

Numbness in the paralyzed parts (*Cocc., Op., Rhus-T.*) (*Br.*).

Staggering gait (*Alum., Gels.*) (*C.*).

Laboured, sighing respiration (*Laur., Op., Phos.*) (*C.*).

Tremors or trembling from mental or physical disturbances (*A.*).

Uncommon mental activity (*Cann-I., Coff., Pip-M., Phos.*) (*A.*).

Cannot stop thinking (*Coff.*) (*A.*).

Cannot concentrate the mind (*Gels., Nux-V.*, (*C.*).

Nothing right; too many things in the room; continually counting them (*C.*).

Dim vision from blur or film (*Chin., Euphr., Nat-M.*); objects appear mixed (*A.*).

Pain after using the eyes (*Calc-P., Nat-M., Ruta*) (*A.*).

FLOATING BLACK SPOTS BEFORE THE EYES (*Chin., Cocc., Nat-M., Phos., Sep., Sil., Sulph.*) (*K.*).

Nystagmus (*Agar., Bell.*) (*A.*).

Photophobia (*Bell., Con., Euphr., Merc., Nat-M., Phos., Sulph.*) (*Br.*).

FLASHES OF LIGHT (*Bell., Calc., Cedr., Croc., Glon., Merc., Nat-C., Phos., Puls., Sil., Stram., Sulph., Valer.*) (*Br.*).

Profuse lachrymation (*Euphr., Merc., Nat-M., Rhus-T.*) (*Br.*).

Heart's action irregular and tumultuous (*Dig., Lach., Mur-Ac., Nat-M.*) (*C.*).

Pain over the orbits; cannot bear to raise the eyelids (*Br.*).

Pain from forehead down nose (*B.*).

Sensation as of a band around the head (*Arg-N., Bell., Cann-S., Carb-Ac., Cocc., Gels., Iod., Merc., Nat-M., Nit-Ac., Op., Sang., Spig., Sulph., Sulph-Ac., Tereb.*) (*B.*).

Feeling as if a ball were coming up in the throat (*Asaf., Ign., Lyc., Nux-M.*) (*C.*).

Gastralgia; great pain immediately after eating (*Calc-P., Mag-P., Nux-V.*) (Br.).

Torpid bowels (*Alum., Bry., Lyc., Sil., Sulph.*) (B.).

Painful evacuations (*Aloe, Nux-V., Sulph.*) (C.).

Piles: Hard, protruding, painful and very sensitive (*Lach.*) (C.).

Heart seems to flutter in the throat (B.).

Perspires very easily (*Calc., Chin., Merc., Rhus-T., Sil.*) (C.).

Dull, heavy, stupid feeling in the head (*Bapt., Bry., Gels., Kali-P.*) (C.).

Omits bath on account of horror for cold water (*Ant-C., Psor., Sulph.*) (C.).

Jerking limbs (*Bell., Cupr., Hyos.*) (B.).

AGGRAVATION: From straining the eyes; after injury; from the draught of air; from walking; during night; after eating; and from mental activity.

AMELIORATION: From lying with the head low; from warmth; and in a warm room;

RELATIONSHIP: *Compare*: *Agar., Bell., Calc-P., Chin., Con., Daph., Euphr., Ferr., Gels., Hyper., Ign., Kali-P., Lyc., Merc., Nat-M., Op., Puls., Ruta, Sep., Strych., Sulph., Verat., Zinc.*

Phytolacca.

COMMON NAME: POKE ROOT.
Patient of a rheumatic diathesis, suffering from the bad effects of syphilis (*Merc., Nit-Ac., Syph.*) (Bt.).

RHEUMATISM OF FIBROUS AND PERIOSTEAL TISSUES (*Rhus-T.*) (A.).

CHRONIC RHEUMATISM, WORSE IN DAMP WEATHER (*Dulc., Nat-S., Rhus-T.*) (Bt.).

Rheumatism after gonorrhœa, syphilis or abuse of mercury (*Hep., Kali-P., Lyc., Nat-S., Sil.*) (A.).

Aching heels, ameliorated by elevating the feet (B.).

Hips and thighs pain on change of weather (*Rhus-T.*) (B.).

SCIATIC PAINS RUN FROM THE HIP DOWN-WARD AND MOSTLY ON THE OUTWARD SIDE OF THIGHS; WORSE AT NIGHT (N.).

A SORE, ACHING, BRUISED FEELING ALL OVER THE BODY, CAUSING THE PATIENT TO GROAN, AND WHILE, LIKE RHUS TOXICODEN-DRON, HE FEELS AS IF HE MUST MOVE, THE ACT OF MOVING GREATLY AGGRAVATES ALL HIS PAINS AND SORENESS (N.).

Pain flying like electric shocks; shooting, lancinating; rapidly shifting (*Bell., Lac-C., Mag-P., Puls.*); worse from motion and at night (A.).

Rheumatic pains in the arms, especially about the attachment of the deltoid muscles (*Ferr., Rhus-T.*) (N.).

Entire indifference to life (*Ars., Aur.*) (A.).

Is sure she will die (*Ars.*) (A.).

Chronic induration of the glands (*Carb-An., Iod., Merc., Rhus-T., Sil.*) (Bt.).

Great pain at the root of the tongue when swallowing (A.).

Diphtheritic inflammation and ulceration of the throat (*Merc-B-I., Merc-P-I., Rhus-T.*) (Bt.).

TONSILS RED, SWOLLEN, WITH WHITE SPOTS, WHICH SOMETIMES COALESCE AND FORM PATCHES; PAINS RUN UP INTO THE EARS (*Kali-B., Merc., Nit-Ac.*) (N.).

Sensation as if there was a lump in the throat that causes constant efforts to swallow (*Bell., Lach.*) (Bt.).

Induration and ulceration of the tonsils (*Merc., Sil.*) (Bt.).

THROAT OF A DARK RED COLOUR (*Lach.*) (A.).

Tonsils, uvula and back part of the throat covered with ash-coloured membrane (*Ars.*, *Merc-B-I.*, *Merc-P.I.*) (A.).

With every attempt to swallow shooting pains through both ears (N.).

Uvula large, dropsical, almost translucent (*Kali-B.*, *Rhus-T.*) (A.).

Tongue fiery red at tip (*Fluor-Ac.*) (B.).

CANNOT DRINK HOT FLUIDS (*Lach.*).

Breath very fetid (*Ars.*, *Bapt.*, *Carb-Ac.*, *Kali-P.*, *Lach.*, *Mur-Ac.*, *Nit-Ac.*, *Sil.*, *Sulph.*) (Bt.).

Great roughness and rawness of the throat (*Caust.*, *Nux-V.*) (Bt.).

FEELING AS IF A BALL OF RED-HOT IRON HAD LODGED IN THE THROAT (Bt.).

Great exhaustion and profound prostration (*Ars.*, *Bapt.*, *Gels.*, *Kali-P.*, *Lach.*, *Mur-Ac.*, *Phos.*) (A.).

Induration of the parotid glands (*Brom.*, *Iod.*) (Bt.).

Painful menstruation in barren females (*Cham.*, *Nux-V.*, *Puls.*) (Bt.).

Galactorrhœa (*Bell.*, *Bry.*, *Calc.*, *Puls.*) (Br.).

BREASTS VERY HARD, SWOLLEN, HOT AND PAINFUL (*Bell.*, *Merc.*, *Sil.*) (N.).

MAMMARY ABSCESS (*Bell.*, *Bry.*, *Merc.*, *Phos.*, *Sil.*); HASTENS SUPPURATIONS (*Hep.*, *Lach.*, *Merc.*, *Sil.*) (A.).

FISTULOUS, GAPING, ANGRY ULCERS IN THE MAMMAE (*Sil.*); PUS SANIOUS, ICHOROUS, FOETID AND UNHEALTHY (A.).

Pain from the breast radiates all over the back when the child nurses (*Crot-T.*) (N.).

Tumefied breast neither heals, nor suppurates (*Merc.*); *is of a purple hue and " hard as old cheese "* (*Bry.*, *Lac-C.*, *Phel.*) (A.).

Mammæ full of hard, painful nodosities (*Carb-An., Sil.*) (A.).

Cancer of the mammæ (*Ars., Bufo, Carb-An., Con., Graph., Merc., Nit-Ac., Phos., Sep., Sil., Sulph., Thuj.*) (Bt.).

Nipples, sensitive, sore and fissured (*Graph.*) (A.).

Chalk-like sediment in the urine (N.).

Albuminous urine (*Apis, Canth., Merc., Phos., Sep.*) (Bt.).

Dark-red urine, leaving a deep red stain in the vessel (*Berb., Colch., Lyc.*) (Bt.).

Vertigo; when rising from bed feels faint (*Bry., Con.*) (A.).

Vertigo, with dimness of vision (*Cycl., Kali-P., Sep.*) (C.).

Intense headache (*Bell., Ferr-P., Glon., Sang., Spig.*) (A.).

Headache, commencing in frontal region and extending backward (C.).

Chronic endocarditis from rheumatism (*Lach., Naja, Phos.*) (C.).

Shock of pain in the cardiac region alternating with pain in the right arm. (Br.).

Chlorosis (*Alum., Cycl., Ferr., Graph., Kali-I., Nat-M., Puls.*) (A.).

Emaciation with loss of fat (A.).

IRRESISTIBLE INCLINATION TO BITE THE TEETH OR GUMS TOGETHER (DURING DENTITION) (N.).

Salivation, with metallic taste in the mouth (*Ars., Calc., Cup-Ars., Kali-B., Merc., Nat-C., Rhus-T., Sep.*) (Bt.).

Mucous and bloody stools, or like scrapings from the intestines (*Canth., Merc-C.*) (C.).

Painful induration of the testicles (*Bell., Puls.*); shooting along perineum to penis (Br.).

Stitches in various parts, always from without inward and near the surface (C.).

Carotid and sub-maxillary glands indurated after diphtheria, scarlet fever (A.).

AGGRAVATION: From exposure to damp, cold weather; from motion; at night; when swallowing; from hot drinks; from nursing the child; and when rising from bed:

AMELIORATION: From cold drinks; from lying on the abdomen; from rest; from warmth; and in dry weather.

RELATIONSHIP: *Phyt.* occupies a position between *Bry.* and *Rhus-T.;* cures when these fail, though apparently well-indicated.

Complementary: *Sil.*

Picric Acid.

COMMON NAME: PICRIC ACID.

It corresponds in general to symptoms of neurasthenia or brain fag. It also has a marked action on the sexual organs (D.).

Is often restorative of a wasted and worn-out system (A.).

Depression and weariness from slight fatigue (*Kali-P., Phos.*) (D.).

MENTAL INACTIVITY (*Agn., Calc., Gels., Phos-Ac., Sil.*) (C.).

Lack of will power (*Gels., Puls.*) (C.).

Indifference to everything (*Phos-Ac., Sep.*) (C.).

Great weakness of the spine and back (*Cocc., Nat-M., Sil.*) (A.).

Burning along the spine (*Kali-P., Phos., Zinc.*) (A.).

Softening of the spinal cord (*Phos.*) (A.).

Dementia with prostration (Br.).

BRAIN-FAG (*Con., Kali-P., Phos-Ac., Zinc.*) (D.).

SLIGHTEST EXERTION BRINGS ON SPEEDY EXHAUSTION (*Ars., Camph., Kali-P., Phos., Verat.*) (D.).

NEURASTHENIA (*Ars., Calc-P., Kali-P., Lyc., Mosch., Nux-V., Op., Phos., Sep., Sil.*) (A.).

Desire to lie down and rest (*Gels., Nux-V., Sep.*) (D.).

Headache of students, teachers and over-worked business-men (*Nux-V.*); aggravated or brought on by the slightest motion or mental exertion (*Nat-M.*) (A.).

Pain in the occipito-cervical region (*Bry., Cocc.. Nat-M., Petr., Sil.*) (A.).

Tired, heavy feeling all over the body, especially of the limbs, worse on exertion (*Nux-V., Phos-Ac.*) (A.).

PRIAPISM ASSOCIATED WITH SPINAL DIS-EASE; TERRIBLE ERECTIONS (*Canth., Phos.*) (N.).

THE PENIS IS SO DISTENDED THAT IT FEELS AS THOUGH IT WOULD BURST (*Canth., Fluor-Ac., Phos.*) (Bl.).

EXCESSIVE ERECTION DURING LASCIVIOUS THOUGHTS (*Cop.*) (K.).

ERECTIONS WORSE AT NIGHT (*Aur., Canth., Fluor-Ac., Nit-Ac., Phos., Plat., Sil., Thuj.*) (K.).

Profuse seminal emissions (*Agar., Carb-V., Kali-C., Merc-I-F., Nat-M., Petr., Phos-Ac., Sep., Staph., Sulph., Zinc.*) (A.).

Satyriasis; erections violent and long-lasting (*Canth., Phos.*) (A.).

Weariness, progressing from a slight feeling of fatigue on motion to complete paralysis (*Caust., Nux-V., Phos., Zinc.*) (A.).

Numbness or formication (*Kali-P., Phos.*) (B.).

Small painful boils in any part of the body (*Arn., Hep., Merc., Sulph.*), but not especially in the external auditory canal (*Calc-Pic., Merc., Sulph.*) (A.).

Oily or greasy stool (*Iod.*, *Thuj.*) (K.).

Diarrhœa worse in the evening (*Aloe*, *Bov.*, *Calc.*, *Cycl.*, *Gels.*, *Kali-C.*, *Kali-P.*, *Lach.*, *Merc.*, *Nat-S.*, *Phos-Ac.*, *Phos.*, *Sang.*, *Sars.*, *Sulph.*, *Verat.*) (K.).

Ammoniacal, dribbling urine (*Merc.*, *Petr.*, *Phos.*) (B.).

AGGRAVATION: From least mental exertion; from motion; from study; in wet weather; from sexual excitement; and from loss of semen.

AMELIORATION: From cold air; from cold water; from bandaging; and from repose.

RELATIONSHIP: *Compare*: *Arg-N.*, *Bar-C.*, *Calc-Pic.*, *Canth.*, *Gels.*, *Graph.*, *Hep.*, *Kali-P.*, *Merc.*, *Nat-M.*, *Petr.*, *Phos-Ac.*, *Phos.*, *Rhus-T.*, *Sep.*, *Sil.*, *Sulph.*, *Thuj.*, and *Zinc*.

Plantago Major.

COMMON NAME: PLANTAIN.

Has considerable reputation in the treatment of earache, toothache, and enuresis (Br.).

Pains centre in ears and teeth, or alternate between them (B.).

Pyorrhœa alveolaris (*Fluor-Ac.*, *Hep.*, *Merc.*, *Nit-Ac.*, *Phos.*, *Sil.*) (Br.).

Teeth feel too long (*Ant-T.*, *Caust.*, *Cham.*, *Hep.*, *Lach.*, *Mag-C.*, *Mezer.*, *Nux-V.*, *Rhus-T.*, *Sep.*, *Sil.*, *Staph.*, *Sulph.*) (Br.).

TOOTHACHE: WORSE IN THE COLD AIR, FROM COLD DRINKS, FROM TOUCH, AND WARM THINGS (K.).

Pain in the sound teeth (*Acon.*, *Am-C.*, *Ars.*, *Bell.*, *Bry.*, *Carb-V.*, *Cham.*, *Coff.*, *Hyos.*, *Mag-C.*, *Nux-V.*, *Rhus-T.*, *Sulph.*, *Zinc.*) (K.).

Toothache, better while eating (*Am-C.*, *Cham.*, *Chin.*, *Coff.*, *Ipec.*, *Selen.*, *Sil.*, *Spig.*) (Br.).

Toothache extending to the ears (*Bell., Cham., Kreos.,* *Mang., Merc., Rhod., Sep., Staph., Sulph., Thuj.*) (K.).

Neuralgic earache, with sticking pains in the ears (Bl.).

Salivation (*Merc., Nat-M., Rhus-T.*) (Br.).

SALIVA FLOWS WITH THE PAINS (B.).

Dirty taste in the mouth (B.).

Periodical prosopalgia (*Ars.*), worse 7 A.M. to 2 P.M., accompanied with flow of tears, photophobia (Br.).

Brown, frothy stools (Br.).

Eye-ball very tender to touch (Br.).

Polyuria (*Kali-P., Lyc., Merc., Sil.*) (B.).

The urine is profuse and colourless (*Gels., Merc., Phos-Ac., Sulph.*) (Bl.).

Nocturnal enuresis (*Calc., Kreos., Sep., Sulph.*) (Bl.).

AGGRAVATION: In the cold air; from touch; from warm things; from cold drinks; from 7 A.M. to 2 P.M.; and at night.

AMELIORATION: While eating.

RELATIONSHIP: *Similar to*: *Ars., Bell., Chin., Ferr-P., Gels., Hep., Kali-P., Lyc., Merc., Nat-M., Puls., Rhus-T., Sep. and Sulph.*

Platinum Metallicum.

COMMON NAME: PLATINUM.

Is pre-eminently a woman's remedy (*Ign., Puls.*) (Br.).

Hysteria, with much depression of spirits (*Ign., Mosch., Nat-M., Puls., Sep.*)(Bt.).

Hysterical spasms, with full consciousness (*Cina, Mag-C., Nat-M., Nux-V., Phos., Sep., Stram., Sulph.*).

Lead poisonings (*Alum., Hep., Op.*).

Catalepsy (*Graph., Ign., Op., Phos-Ac.*) (K.).

Dull, stinging pains, which press inwardly, as from a plug (*Anac.*).

Tension in the limbs, as if they were tightly bandaged (Arund., Chin.).

Debility and tired feeling of the limbs, especially while at rest.

Numbness and sensation of stiffness of many parts mostly accompanied by sensations of coldness.

Pains like constrictions in character.

Pains, as from contusions.

THE PAINS BEGIN SLOWLY, INCREASE GRADUALLY, AND DISAPPEAR JUST AS SLOWLY (*Kalm., Nat-M., Phos., Spig., Stann., Sulph-Ac.*).

Feeling of numbness, with trembling and palpitation of the heart (Bt.).

Bad effects from fright, insults or anger (*Ign., Op., Stram.*).

Alternating symptoms of mind and body.

Anxiety with fear of the approaching death (Acon., Apis, Ars.).

Low-spiritedness, with shedding of tears (Ign., Kali-P., Med., Nat-M., Puls., Stann.).

GRANDIOSE IDEAS; HE THINKS HIMSELF VERY GREAT.

PROFOUND CONCEIT; HE THINKS LITTLE OF ANYTHING OUTSIDE OF HIMSELF.

PRIDE WITH OVER-ESTIMATION OF ONE'S OWN SELF.

Proud, haughty and egotistical; everything seems inferior to her in mind and body; she looks down upon everything with contempt (D.).

Much anguish; she feels as if she would lose her senses and die soon (G.).

Past events trouble her (*Ign., Staph.*) (G.).

CHANGING MOODS; GAY AND SAD ALTER-NATELY (*Croc., Ign., Nux-M., Puls.*) (N.).

Sensation of growing larger in every direction (A.).

Trifling things produce profound vexation (*Ign., Staph., Sulph.*) (A.).

Satiety of life (*Aur.*), with taciturnity and fear of death (*Acon., Ars., Nux-V.*) (A.).

Weary of everything (*Phos-Ac., Sep.*) (Br.).

Irresistible impulse to kill (*Ars., Bell., Hep., Hyos., Nux-V., Phos., Sec., Stram., Thea.*) (Br.).

Eyes feel cold (*Calc., Euphr., Kali-C.*) (Br.).

Objects appear smaller than they are.

Cramp-like pain in the orbits (Br.).

Indurations of the uterus (*Aur.*) (Bt.).

Menses in excess; blood dark and thick, with chilliness and sensitiveness of the vulva (G.).

Premature or excessive development of sexual instinct (N.).

EXCESSIVE SEXUAL DESIRE, PARTICULARLY IN VIRGIN FEMALES (*Phos.*) (G.).

Voluptuous tingling in the vulva, and abdomen, with depression of spirits, anxiety, and palpitation of the heart (G.).

Mons veneris cold and excessively sensitive to the touch; cannot bear the napkin usually applied (G.).

Amenorrhœa, with painful pressure, as if the menses would appear, with pain in the small of the back (G.).

Albuminous leucorrhœa, only in the day-time, with great sensitiveness of the vagina (G.).

Gradually increasing, then slowly lessening headache (B.).

Painful, cramp-like numbness in the left malar bone (R.).

Ravenous hunger (*Anac., Lyc., Phos.*) (Br.).

COSTIVE STATE (*Alum., Bry., Ign., Nat-M.*).

Constipation due to inertia of the bowels (*Alum., Bry., Op., Plb.*) (D.).

There are frequent and unsuccessful attempts to stool (*Carb-V., Ign., Nux-V., Sep., Sulph., Thuj.*) (D.).

THE STOOLS ARE LIKE PUTTY, AND ADHERE TO THE ANUS (*Alum.*) (D.).

CONSTIPATION OF EMIGRANTS AND TRAVELLERS (*Ign.*) (D.).

Stools as if burnt (*Bry.*) (Br.).

Catamenia too early and too profuse (*Calc., Ferr., Sep.*).

Metrorrhagia (*Chin., Mille., Sab., Sec.*).

NYMPHOMANIA (*Canth., Phos., Stram.*).

Early and profuse menses of dark, clotted blood, accompanied by bearing down pains (D.).

Ovaritis with sterility (Br.).

The ovaries are sensitive and have burning pains in them (*Apis*) (D.).

GENITALS EXCESSIVELY SENSITIVE; CANNOT BEAR TO BE TOUCHED; WILL ALMOST GO INTO A SPASM FROM AN EXAMINATION, AND ALMOST FAINT DURING INTERCOURSE (N.).

Vaginismus (*Bell., Cact., Ferr-P., Ign., Lyc., Nat-M., Nux-V., Plb., Puls., Sil.*) (K.).

Puerperal mania, with suppressed lochia (R.).

Pruritus vulvæ (*Ambr., Am-C., Calad., Calc., Kreos., Merc., Nat-M., Nit-Ac., Petr., Rhus-T., Sep., Sil., Sulph., Tarent.*) (A.).

Spasms and screaming at every menstrual period (G.).

Globus hystericus (*Asaf., Ign., Sep.*) (R.).

Cramp in the calves (*Arg-N., Calc., Cham., Coloc., Cupr., Graph., Hep., Lyc., Plb., Sec., Sil., Sulph.*) (B.).

TETANIC RIGIDITY (*Cic., Cupr., Hyper., Nux-V., Petr., Sep.*) (K.).

Bruised backache, aggravated by pressure or bending backward (B.).

Epistaxis, with dark coagulated blood (G.).

Pale, easily fatigued (*Stann.*) (A.).

Chlorosis (*Alum., Calc-P., Ferr., Graph., Puls.*) (G.).

Erections in sleep with amorous dreams (*Phos.*) (R.).

Onanism (*Nux-V., Phos-Ac., Staph.*) (B.).

CONVULSIONS AFTER ONANISM (*Bufo, Calc., Dig., Kali-Br., Lach., Nux-V., Plb., Sep., Sil., Stram., Sulph.*) (K.).

Inclination to draw a long breath, prevented by a sensation of weakness in the chest (*Stann.*) (C.).

Sensation of numbness in the head or temples, zygomata and mastoid, as if the head were constricted or too tightly bound (N.).

Sensation of coldness, crawling and numbness in the right side of the face (N.).

Sleeps with legs far apart (*Cham.*) (Br.).

AGGRAVATION: In the evening; whilst at rest; in the open air; during the lying-in period; from anger; during menses; after rising; from standing; and during coition.

AMELIORATION: In the room; from walking; and from motion.

RELATIONSHIP: *Compare*: *Ars., Aur., Bry., Bufo, Calc., Croc., Ferr-P., Graph., Ign., Kali-P., Lach., Lyc., Merc., Mosch., Nat-M., Nux-V., Op., Petr., Puls., Rhus-T., Sep., Stann., Sulph., Thuj., Valer.*

Antidotes: PULS., and *Sp-Nitr-D.*

Plumbum Metallicum.

COMMON NAME: LEAD.

Especially adapted to diseases, where they arise from disease of the spinal cord (Bt.).

The patient's complexion is waxy, pallid and greasy, or shiny looking (D.).

Excessive and rapid emaciation (*Ars.*) (N.).

Locomotor Ataxia (*Alum., Kali-P., Zinc.*) (Bl.).

GENERAL OR PARTIAL PARALYSIS (*Caust., Nux-V.*) (N.).

PARALYSIS OF THE EXTENSOR MUSCLES OF THE WRIST; WRIST-DROP; THE PARALYSIS IS ACCOMPANIED BY ATROPHY OF THE AFFECTED PARTS (D.).

Stinging and tearing in the limbs.

Twitching of the limbs, with paralysis of the same (*Merc., Zinc.*).

Infantile paralysis (*Bar-C., Calc.*) (Bl.).

The pains in the limbs are aggravated at night and relieved by rubbing.

Badly smelling sweat of the feet (*Bar-C., Graph., Nit-Ac., Sil.*) (G.).

A sensation of tingling on the bones themselves.

Burning in many parts (*Canth., Phos., Sec., Sulph.*).

Sensation of constriction in the internal organs (*Bell., Cact., Lach.*).

Sciatica, with drawing, pressing pains (*Coloc., Dios., Mag-P., Rhus-T.*) (Hr.).

Convulsions followed by paralysis (*Cupr., Nux-V., Zinc.*).

Retracted testes (*Clem., Nux-V., Op., Rhod.*) (B.).

Complete impotence (*Agn., Graph., Lyc.*), with excessive emaciation, and great debility (Hm.).

Threatening abortion (*Apis, Sep.*) (A.).

Undeveloped uterus (R.).

Hypersensitiveness of the vulva and vagina (*Plat.*) (R.).

Loss of sexual desire (*Arg-N., Camph., Sep.*) (C.).

Menorrhagia, with a sensation of a string pulling from the abdomen to the back (G.).

Milk scanty (*Bry., Calc.*) (C.).

Sweetish taste in the mouth; everything tastes sweet (D.)

There is a blue line along the border of the gums (D.).

Fluids can be swallowed without difficulty; solids come back into the mouth again (G.).

Loss of appetite (*Bry., Kali-M., Nux-V.*) (C.).

Violent thirst (*Ars., Bry., Merc., Phos-Ac., Sulph.* (C.).

Colic during the costive state—a highly prominent indication for its use.

Colicky pains proceeding from the spinal cord (Bhr.).

Constipation during pregnancy (*Plat.*) · (A.).

Obstinate constipation from constriction of the intestinal muscular fibres.

THE STOOL IS PASSED IN LITTLE, ROUND BALLS, WHICH ARE BLACK AND HARD (D.).

The stools are passed with great difficulty (*Alum., Nat-M., Op., Sep., Sulph.*) (D.).

FAECAL VOMITING (*Nux-V., Op., Sulph.*).
Incessant vomiting of food (*Ipec., Puls.*) (C.).

HORRIBLE GRIPING PAIN IN THE ABDOMEN; THE PAINS RADIATE IN ALL DIRECTIONS (D.).

LEAD COLIC (*Alum., Bell., Coloc., Nux-V., Op.*); THE WALLS OF THE ABDOMEN BECOME RETRACTED (D.).

INTUSSUSCEPTION WITH COLIC AND FAECAL VOMITING (A.).

Spasm or contraction of the sphincter ani (Bell.). (D.).

Sensation of a string pulling the anus up into the rectum (D.).

Gastralgia; the pains are very sudden and severe, better from hard pressure and eructations (*Coloc., Nux-V., Puls.*) (R.).

Typhlitis with a large, hard swelling developed in the ileo-cæcal region, very sensitive to contact or to the least motion (Bell., Bry., Lach.) (N.).

Chronic spinal meningitis (Hn.).

Useful in granular kidney (*Aur., Kali-C., Lyc., Merc-C., Nit-Ac., Phos., Rhus-T.*).

Complete paralysis of the urinary organs (*Op.*) (Bt.).

Much troubled with the urine, in not being able to pass it, apparently from want of sensation to do so; the will to do so cannot effect it, as if from paralysis (G.).

Albuminous urine (*Apis, Merc-C., Phos.*) (R.).

Chronic interstitial nephritis (*Lyc., Sep.*) (R.).

Hectic fever, with dry, hacking cough, and great exhaustion (Hm.).

Pale, dry skin with liver spots (*Sep.*) (G.).

Jaundice: the whites of eyes, skin, stool and urine—all are very yellow (*Chel., Iod., Nat-S., Sep.*) (N.).

Intellectual torpor (*Op., Phos-Ac.*) (A.).

Slow of perception (*Nux-M., Op.*) (R.).

Memory lost, so that when talking he was unable to find the right word (*Anac., Lac-C., Lyc., Phos-Ac.*) (R.).

Fears assasins (*Absin., Cimic., Op., Phos., Stram.*) (B.).

DELIRIUM (*Bell., Canth., Hyos., Stram., Verat.*), ALTERNATING WITH COLIC (A.).

Timid and anxious (*Phos., Puls.*) (B.).

COMA (*Hyos., Op., Sulph.*) (R.).

Taciturn (*Bry., Ign., Phos-Ac.*) (B.).

Tongue trembling (*Camph., Gels., Lach., Lyc., Merc., Phos-Ac.*); cannot be put out (*Apis, Brom., Carb-Ac., Dulc., Hyos., Lyc., Merc-C.*) (R.).

Assumes strangest attitudes and positions in bed (A.).

Imperfect articulation (*Bar-C., Caust., Gels.*), sometimes only confused sounds (R.).

Paralysis of the upper eyelid (*Caust., Gels.*) (C.).

Diplopia (*Bell., Hyos., Stram.*) (C.).

Femoral, inguinal or umbilical hernia ((*Lyc., Nux-V.*) (A.).

Strangulated hernia (*Nux-V.*) (A.).

Dilatation of veins on the back of hands, arms and calves (C.).

Pulse rapid, jerky, weak (*Acon., Aur., Bar-C.*) (C.).

AGGRAVATION: From exertion; from excitement; at night; and from motion; from drinking.

AMELIORATION: From hard pressure; and from rubbing.

RELATIONSHIP: The bad effects of lead or *Plumb.* are antidoted by *Alum., Hep., Nux-V., Op., Petr., Plat., Sulph-Ac.* and *Zinc.*

Complementary: *Rhus-T.*

Podophyllum Peltatum.

COMMON NAMES: MAY APPLE: MANDRAKE.

Acts especially upon the liver and digestive tracts, its special affinity being for the mucous membranes, more especially of the duodenum and rectum, and for glandular structures, producing irritation, excessive secretions, inflammation and even ulceration or suppuration (C.).

Adapted to persons of bilious temperament (*Bry., Nat-S., Sulph.*), who suffer from gastro-intestinal derangements (A.).

"BILIOUS ATTACKS"—ESPECIALLY AFTER ABUSE OF MERCURY (*Nux-V.*) (A.).

Affects the right side of the throat, right ovary and right hypochondrium (*Lyc.*) (A.).

The liver is swollen and sensitive (*Chin., Merc., Nat-S.*) (D.).

Chronic congestion and torpidity of the liver; chronic hepatitis (*Chel., Dig., Merc., Nat-S., Nux-V., Sep., Sulph.*) (C.).

Gall-stone colic with jaundice (*Chin., Mag-M., Merc., Nat-S., Sep.*) (C.).

CONSTANTLY RUBBING AND SHAKING THE REGION OF THE LIVER WITH HIS HAND (A.).

Biliousness, with nausea and giddiness; bitter taste and risings; tendency to bilious vomiting and purging, with dark urine (Hg.).

Bad taste in the mouth (*Nux-V., Puls.*) (D.).

Vomits bilious matter mixed with blood (*Bry., Nat-S., Sep.*) (Bt.).

Vomiting, with very severe spasms of the stomach (*Ant-T., Cupr., Ipec., Sec., Verat.*) (Bt.).

Food turns sour, with belching of hot flatus, which is very sour (Ra.).

Colicky pain in the abdomen ameliorated by flexing the limbs (*Bell., Bry., Chel. Coloc.*) (K.).

Indented tongue (*Ars., Carb-V., Chel., Dulc., Glon., Hydr., Ign., Iod., Kali-I., Merc., Plb., Rhus-T., Sep., Stram., Syph., Tell., Vib.*) (K.).

Tongue seems too broad (*Kali-B., Nat-M., Par., Plb., Puls., Vib., Ziz.*) (K.).

Desire for something sour (*Ant-T., Ars., Hep., Puls., Sep.*) (C.).

Thirst for large quantities of cold water (*Ars., Bry., Ferr-P., Nat-M., Phos., Sulph., Verat.*)

Cramp-like pain in the abdomen with actual retraction of the abdominal muscles (N.).

Sudden shocks of jerking pains (A.).

RUMBLING AND GURGLING IN THE ABDOMEN BEFORE STOOL (*Aloe, Coloc., Merc., Olnd.*) (K.).

Flatulence during dentition, with green, sour stools in the morning (G.).

Diarrhœa of children during teething, after eating and drinking, or being bathed or washed. (A.).

SEEMS TO DRAIN ONE DRY, BUT SOON IS FULL AGAIN (A.).

Diarrhœa of long-standing (*Aloe, Merc., Nat-S., Sulph.*)
(A.).

DIARRHOEA EARLY IN THE MORNING CONTINUES THROUGH FORENOON, FOLLOWED BY NATURAL STOOL IN THE EVENING (*Aloe*) (A.).

Stools watery and green, or they may be natural, but
exhaustive (Bt.).

Changeable stools (*Am-M., Berb., Cham., Colch., Dulc.,
Puls., Sanic., Sulph.*) (K.).

Diarrhœa accompanied by sensation of weakness or
sinking in the abdomen or rectum (*Aloe, Sulph.*) (A.)

Black stools only in the morning (*Sulph.*) (Ha.).

Stool: Green, watery, fetid, profuse, gushing out (*Gamb.,
Jatr., Phos.*); *chalk-like* (*Calc.*); *jelly-like* (*Aloe, Kali-B.*);
undigested (*Aloe, Chin., Ferr.*); *or, with yellow meal-like
sediment* (A.).

PROFUSE, WATERY STOOLS, POURING OUT LIKE WATER FROM A HYDRANT (D.).

Diarrhœic stools are preceded by retching and vomiting,
and followed by a sensation of great weakness in the abdomen, and especially in the rectum (D.).

PROLAPSE OF THE RECTUM BEFORE (*Ruta*), OR DURING (*Calc., Dulc., Gamb., Ign., Lyc., Sep.*), OR AFTER STOOL (*Aesc., Cocc., Hep., Lach., Merc., Nit-Ac., Phos., Sulph.*) (K.).

Diarrhœa of dirty water, soaking the napkin through
(*Benz-Ac.*), *with gagging* (A.).

Diarrhœa after taking milk (*Calc., Mag-M.*) *or sour milk*
(K.).

PAINLESS CHOLERA MORBUS, OR CHOLERA INFANTUM (*Kali-P., Ricin., Sulph.*) (A.).

Severe straining during stool, with emission of much
flatulence; mucous stools, with spots and streaks of blood;
thirst, but no appetite (*Sulph.*) (An.)

Dysenteric diarrhœa, depending upon inflammatory irritation of the rectum (*Aloe, Merc., Sulph.*) (Hg.).

Constipation alternating with diarrhœa (*Aloe, Nux-V., Sulph.*) (G.).

Hæmorrhoids, with prolapsus ani and morning diarrhœa (G.).

Clay-coloured stools (*Calc., Hep.*), from *absence of bile* (D.).

Pale, hard, chalky stools (*Calc., Chel., Lyc.*) (B.).

Suppression of urine (*Apis, Bell., Camph., Stram., Tereb.*) (C.).

The whites of the eyes and the face are yellow (D.).

Moaning and whining during sleep (*Ars., Aur., Bell., Cham., Crot-C., Hyos., Ign., Kali-P., Lyc., Mur-Ac., Nux-V., Op., Puls., Sep., Sil., Sulph.*) (B.).

Restless sleep, especially in the forepart of the night (*Phos.*) (C.).

Pain under the right shoulder-blade (*Abies-C., Bry., Card-M., Chel., Chen-A., Lycps., Nat-M., Nux-V., Phos., Pic-Ac., Ruta, Sanic.*) (C.).

Drowsy, half-closed eyes (*Op.*); *rolling the head from side to side* (*Bell., Hell., Hyos., Nux-V., Op., Stram., Tub.*), *with moaning and whining* (*Acon., Bell., Cann-I., Hyos., Kali-C., Phos., Puls., Stram., Sulph., Verat, Zinc.*), *especially children* (N.).

Headache alternates with diarrhœa (*Aloe*) (A.).

Headache in winter, diarrhœa in summer (A.).

Difficult dentition (*Calc., Calc-P., Sil.*) (A.).

Intense desire to press the gums together (*Phyt.*) (A.).

Depression of spirits (*Ars., Kali-P., Puls.*) (A.).

Imagines he is going to die or be very ill (*Ars.*) (A.).

Disgust for life (*Ars., Aur., Nux-V.*) (A.).

Feels fatigued (*Kali-P., Phos-Ac.*) (G.).

Often useful in bilious fever of a remittent type, with pronounced bilious symptoms (*Bry., Chin., Nat-S.*) (C.).

GREAT, EVEN DELIRIOUS LOQUACITY, DUR-
ING CHILL AND HEAT (N.).

Fever paroxysm at 7 A.M. (A.).

Sleep during perspiration (*Ars., Chin., Op., Phos-Ac.,*
Puls., Rhus-T., Sabad.)

Suppressed menses in young girls (*Alum., Calc-P., Cycl.,*
Puls., Tub.) (A.).

Pain and numbness in the right ovary, running down the
thigh of that side (*Lil-T.*) (A.).

In the early months of pregnancy, can lie comfortably
only on the stomach (*Acet-Ac.*) (A.).

Prolapsus uteri: from overlifting or straining; from
constipation; after parturition, with sub-involution (A.).

Weak, bearing down sensation in the abdomen after
parturition (G.).

Pain in the lumbar and sacral region, worse during
stool, and still worse afterward (G.).

Pendulous abdomen, after confinement (G.).

Leucorrhœa, consisting of thick, transparent mucus (G.).

AGGRAVATION: In the early morning; in hot
weather; during dentition; after eating and drinking; while
being bathed or washed; from overlifting or straining;
during stool; and from motion.

AMELIORATION: From bending forward, from
external warmth; from lying on the abdomen; and by
stroking or massaging the liver; and in the evening.

RELATIONSHIP: *Compare*: *Aloe, Berb., Chel.,*
Chin., Collin., Ferr., Gamb., Hep., Ipec., Kali-P., Lach.,
Lyc., Merc., Nat-S., Nux-V., Op., Puls., Sep., Sulph., Tub.,
Verat. and *Zinc.*

Useful after *Ipec.* and *Nux-V.*, in gastric troubles, and
after *Calc.* and *Sulph.* in liver diseases.

Complementaries: *Nat-M.* and *Sulph.*

Antidotes: *Lact-Ac.* and *Nux-V.*

It antidotes the bad effects of mercury.

Pulsatilla.

COMMON NAME: WIND FLOWER.

The weather-cock among the remedies (Br.).

Especially adapted to females, with blue eyes, very affectionate, easily excited to tears (*Sep.*) and of a very yielding disposition (Bt.).

One of the best remedies with which to begin the treatment of a chronic case (*Calc., Nux-V., Sulph.*) (A.).

Ailments from abuse of chamomile, quinine, iron, mercury, sulphur or tea-drinking (A.).

The disposition and mental state are the chief guiding symptoms to the selection of *Pulsatilla.*

The forms of her symptoms are very changeable; she is very well one hour, and very miserable the next (G.).

SHE IS TIMID AND FEARFUL, EXTREMELY MILD AND GENTLE, AND SOMETIMES SILENT AND MELANCHOLIC.

WEEPS VERY EASILY; CAN HARDLY GIVE HER SYMPTOMS WITHOUT WEEPING (*Kali-C., Med., Sep.*) (G.).

VERY TEARFUL; SHE WEEPS AT EVERYTHING, WHETHER IT IS JOYFUL OR SORROWFUL (G.).

EASILY MOVED TO LAUGHTER OR TEARS (*Ign., Nux-M.*) (A.).

Throbbing, pressive headache, relieved by external pressure or by tying up tightly (N.).

Violent pain in the ear, as of something forcing outward (N.).

Affections of ears, as sequelæ of measles (N.).

Is especially called for women who are inclined to be fleshy, with scanty and protracted menstruation (*Graph.*) (A.).

The first serious impairment of health is referred to puberal age; " have never been well since"—anæmia, chlorosis, bronchitis, or phthisis (A.).

The lower limbs go to sleep when sitting (G.).

SECRETIONS FROM ALL THE MUCOUS MEMBRANES ARE THICK, BLAND AND YELLOW-ISH-GREEN (*Kali-S., Nat-S., Stann.*) (A.).

Sick headache, from suppression of the menses, or from some menstrual or gastric disorder (*Bry., Sep.*) (Bt.).

Semilateral headache (*Kali-B., Nat-M., Spig.*) (G.).

Dizzy, when rising from a chair (*Phos.*) (G.).

Obstruction in the nose, especially in the evening (*Sep.*) (K.).

Foul discharge or bad odour from the nose (*Aur., Calc., Hep., Sep.*) (B.).

Coryza, much worse every evening (Bt.).

Cough very loose, with vomiting of mucus (*Ipec.*) (G.).

Hard, racking cough that makes the stomach sore; and water escapes the bladder, during every cough.

Loose cough through the day, but dry at night, worse towards evening, and in the recumbent position (Cl.).

Asthma, from deranged menstruation or suppressed urticaria (Bt.).

Cloudiness of vision, with a kind of flashing fire, as if she had received a slap in the face (N.).

Profuse lachrymation in the wind or open air (N.).

Catarrhal ophthalmia, with profuse lachrymation and secretion of mucus (*Arg-N., Euphr., Nat-M., Rhus-T.*) (Bt.).

Styes, especially on the upper eyelid (*Am-C., Bell., Ferr., Merc., Phos-Ac., Staph.*) (A.).

Agglutination of the lids in the morning (*Arg-N., Calc., Graph.*) (R.).

Rheumatism: Pains shift rapidly from one part to another, unattended with any great swelling or redness;

chronic cases, with weakness, rigidity, coldness and weight in the diseased tissues (Bt.).

Urticaria worse at night, caused by fat, rich food (Bt.). Chlorosis from abuse of iron (Bt.).

CHRONIC OTORRHOEA (*Calc., Hep., Merc., Sil.*) (Bt.).

Much pain in the ears, with deafness; the meatus is red and swollen (*Sulph.*) (Bt.).

Mumps with metastasis to the mammæ or to the testicle (*Ars., Carb-V., Jab., Nat-M., Rhus-T.*) (A.).

Bad taste in the mouth, every morning on awaking (*Bar-C., Bry., Calc-P., Lyc., Merc., Nat-M., Nat-S. Nux-V., Sep., Sulph.*); *she has to wash it out soon; it is so bad she cannot bear it* (*Nux-V.*) (G.).

NOTHING TASTES GOOD TO HER (*Calc., Merc., Nat-S.. Nux-V., Sulph.*) (G.).

TONGUE THICKLY-COATED, WHITE OR YELLOW (*Bry., Kali-M., Nat-S.*) (Bt.).

GREAT DRYNESS OF THE MOUTH (IN THE MORNING), WITHOUT THIRST (*Nux-M.; mouth* moist, with intense thirst—*Merc.*) (A.).

LICKS THE LIPS, BUT DOES NOT DRINK (A.).

TOOTHACHE RELIEVED BY HOLDING COLD WATER IN THE MOUTH (*Bry., Clem., Coff., Ferr-P.*); WORSE FROM WARM THINGS AND HEAT OF THE ROOM (A.).

Toothache on one side of the face; always ceases on going into the open air, but returns in a warm room, and gets worse; the pains are throbbing or shooting, accompanied with much swelling; worse evenings; in mild, tearful females (G.).

Sensation as if the food were lodged undigested above the stomach (*Bhr.*).

Loathing nausea and retchings after greasy food (*Kali-M.*) (G.).

Morning sickness, with vomiting of mucus (G.).

ABSENCE OF THIRST OR THIRSTLESSNESS WITH NEARLY ALL COMPLAINTS (*Cocc., Nux-V., Sep.*) (A.).

Pulsations in the pit of the stomach (*Acon., Ant-T., Calc., Chin., Cic., Ferr., Glon., Kali-C., Nux-V., Phos., Sep., Sil.*) (G.).

REPUGNANCE TO FOOD (*Ant-C., Ars., Bry., Chin., Colch., Sep.*) (G.).

Gastric disturbances from rich or fat food (*Kali-M.*) (G.).

The sight or even the thought of pork causes disgust (A.).

All-gone sensation in the stomach, in tea-drinkers especially (A.).

Distension of the stomach after eating (*Arg-N., Chin., Nux-M.*) (R.).

Rumbling and gurgling especially in the evening (*Lyc.*) (R.).

Incarcerated flatus in the abdomen, pressing here and there (C.).

Pressure in the abdomen and small of the back, as from a stone (*Bry., Nux-V.*) (Ra.).

Colicky pains in the abdomen (*Bry., Coloc.. Nux-V., Verat.*) (G.).

She cannot sit long at a time; must walk about to relieve her (abdominal) pains (G.).

Drawing, cutting pains around the navel (Bt.).

Diarrhœa only or usually at night (*Chin.*); watery, greenish-yellow, very changeable (*Podo., Sulph.*); as soon as one eats; from fruits, cold food or drinks, or ice-cream (*Ars.*) (A.).

Diarrhœa after measles (*Carb-V., Chin., Merc.*) (K.).

Constipation attended with ineffectual desire for stool (Ra.).

Discharge of blood and mucus during stool (*Aloe, Kali-M., Merc., Sulph.*) (G.).

After urinating, spasmodic pain in the neck of the bladder, extending to the pelvis and thighs (G.).

Frequent and almost ineffectual urging to urinate, with cutting pain (Canth.) (G.).

Retention of urine, with redness, heat and soreness of the vesical region externally (Ra.).

INVOLUNTARY EMISSIONS OF URINE WHEN SITTING, COUGHING OR WALKING (*Caust., Sep.*) (J.).

Constant pressure on the bladder without desire to urinate (G.).

Scanty and high coloured-urine (*Apis, Berb., Colch., Lyc., Sep.*) (K.).

Milky leucorrhœa, with swelling of the vulva, particularly after the menses (G.).

Thick, white, albuminous leucorrhœa (Bt.).

Menses: Suppressed from getting the feet wet; too late, scanty, slimy, painful; irregular, intermittent flow, with evening chilliness; with intense pain and great restlessness and tossing about (Mag-P.); flow more during the day (A.).

DELAYED FIRST MENSTRUATION (*Caust., Graph., Kali-C., Senec., Sep.*) (A.).

Morning sickness (*Cycl., Graph., Sep.*) (K.).

Threatened abortion; flow ceases and then returns with increased force; pains spasmodic, excite suffocation and fainting; must have fresh air (A.).

Labour: The pains excite palpitations; suffocating and fainting spells, unless the doors and windows are open; feels as though she must have them open (G.).

Acute inflammation of the testicles (Bell., Ferr-P., Rhod.) (Bt.).

ORCHITIS CAUSED FROM COLD OR SUPPRESSED GONORRHOEA (Bt.).

The testicles and spermatic cord swollen and painful (Clem., Rhod.) (Bt.).

Hæmorrhage from the urethra after suppressed gonorrhœa, or after urination (*Hep., Sars., Thuj.*) (K.).

Gonorrhœal discharge greenish-yellow or yellow-looking (*Merc.*) (K.).

Chordee (*Arg-N., Cann-S., Canth., Caps., Kali-Chl., Tereb., Thuj.*) (K.).

Hydrocele, especially of the boys (*Rhod., Sil.*) (K.).

Sexual passion increased (*Cann-I., Canth., Con., Lyc., Nux-V., Phos., Staph.*) ((K.).

Stricture (*Clem., Con., Staph.*) ; pain and tenesmus in urinating, worse lying on back (Br.).

Acute prostatitis (*Con., Merc., Sep.*) (Br.).

Very useful in intermittent fevers, where chilliness predominates (*Ars., Chin., Nux-V., Rhus-T.*) (Bt.).

Fever just at sunset (*Ign., Thuj.*) (A.).

There is little heat and no thirst (*Ipec.*) (Bt.).

Chilliness even in the summer, when warmly clad, with vertigo, throbbing headache, pressure in the stomach, etc. (G.).

CHILLY, YET AVERSE TO HEAT (B.).

Irregular types of malarial fever (*Nux-V., Psor., Sep.*) (K.).

Anxious heat as if dashed with hot water (C.).

Intolerable, dry, burning heat, evening or night; with distended veins and burning hands that seek out cool places; without thirst (C.).

MOANING DURING HEAT (*Arn., Bell., Eup-P., Ipec., Lach., Nux-V.*) (K.).

Unable to breathe well, or is chilly in a warm room (A.).

CRAVES FRESH, COOL AIR (*Kali-S., Phos., Sulph., Tub.*) (Bt.).

Very sluggish circulation, manifested by constant chilliness, coldness and paleness of the skin (*Graph., Sep., Sil.*) (Ra.).

SYMPTOMS EVER-CHANGING; NO TWO CHILLS, NO TWO STOOLS, NO TWO ATTACKS ALIKE; VERY WELL ONE HOUR, VERY MISERABLE THE NEXT—APPARENTLY CONTRADICTORY (*Ign.*) (A.).

Pains on first motion (*Rhus-T.*) (A.).

Pains: Drawing, tearing, erratic, rapidly shifting from one part to another (*Bell., Ign., Kali-B., Kali-S., Lac-C., Mang.*); are accompanied with constant chilliness; the more severe the pain, the more severe the chill; appear suddenly, leave gradually, or tension much increases until very acute and then lets u; with a snap (A.).

Cannot sleep in the early part of the night, but sleeps late in the morning (G.).

Awakes languid, unrefreshed (A.).

AGGRAVATION: In a warm, closed room; towards evening; from warm things; from rich or warm food; from pork and pastry; from fruits; from lying on the left, or on the painless side; from heat; and during menses.

AMELIORATION: In the open air; from cold things; from lying on the painful side; from cold air or cool room; and from cold application.

RELATIONSHIP: *Silicea* is the chronic of *Pulsatilla* in nearly all ailments.

Follows well after: *Kali-B., Lyc., Sep., Sil.* and *Sulph.*

Follows, and is followed by *Kali-Br.*, which is its chemical analogue.

Complementary: *Kali-M., Lyc., Sil.* and *Sulph-Ac.*

Pyrogen.

COMMON NAME: SEPSIN.

This remedy is employed in typhoid and septic conditions when the well-selected remedy fails to relieve (Bl.).

Diseases originating in ptomaine or sewer gas infection (N.).

Septic conditions following abortions and confinements, when the lochia is thin, acrid, and very fœtid, or suppressed (Bl.).

Chronic complaints that date back to septic conditions (Br.).

Puerperal peritonitis (*Apis, Bell.*) (Br.).

RAPID DECUBITUS (*Ars., Carb-Ac., Lach., Sec.*) (A.).

Post-operative cases, with overwhelming sepsis (Br.).

Great restlessness; must move constantly (*Ars., Phos.*) (A.).

The bed feels hard, parts lain on sore and bruised; must move to relieve the soreness (*Arn., Bapt.*) (N.).

Skin pale, cold, of an ashy hue (*Sec.*) (A.).

BONE-PAINS (*Eup-P., Ipec.*) (B.).

Loquacious (*Bell., Hyos., Lach., Stram.*) (B.).

Excited (*Bell., Stram.*) (B.).

Sense of duality (*Anac., Petr.*) (B.).

Hallucination (*Hyos.*) (B.).

Vomits water, when it becomes warm in the stomach (*Chlf., Phos.*) (Br.)

Full of anxiety and insane notions (Br.).

Thinks he is very wealthy (*Bell., Cann-I., Sulph., Verat.*) (Br.).

Tongue: Large, flabby, clean, smooth, as if varnished; fiery red, cracked; difficult articulation (N.).

Taste: Sweetish, terribly fœtid, pus-like (A.).

Breath horribly offensive (*Bapt., Merc., Sulph.*) (A.).

ALL THE DISCHARGES ARE HORRIBLY OFFENSIVE (*Bapt., Carb-Ac., Nit-Ac., Psor., Sulph.*) (Br.).

Vomiting: Persistent, brownish, coffee-ground like, offensive, stercoraceous (N.).

Vomiting with impacted or obstructed bowels (*Op., Plb.*) (A.).

Constipation with complete inertia (*Bry., Op., Sanic., Sil.*) (A.).

STOOL: LARGE, BLACK, CARRION-LIKE; SMALL BLACK BALLS, LIKE OLIVES (A.).

Diarrhœa: Horribly offensive, brown or black (Ars., Kali-P., Lach.); painless, involuntary (Kali-P., Podo., Sulph.) (N.).

Fever each menstrual period consequent upon latent pelvic inflammation (Br.).

Pulse abnormally rapid, out of all proportion to temperature (Lil-T.) (A.).

Coldness and numbness of hands and feet, of arms and legs (A.).

DISTINCT CONSCIOUSNESS OF A HEART; IT FEELS TIRED, AS IF ENLARGED; PURRING, THROBBING, PULSATING, CONSTANT IN EARS, PREVENTING SLEEP (N.).

Chronic malaria (Ars., Ipec., Nat-M.) (Br.).

Aching in the limbs, or over the entire body as from a severe cold (A.).

Chill begins in the back between the scapulæ (*Caps., Eup-P., Polyp.*) (A.).

Frequent urging to urinate as soon as fever came on; urine profuse and clear as spring water; could tell when fever was coming on from frequent calls to urinate (A.).

Chilly as soon as he touches the cold sheets (*Aran.*) (A.).

Circumscribed redness of the cheeks during the hot stage (A.).

Quickly oscillating temperature (B.).

Cold sweat over the entire body (*Camph.*) (A.).

Sweat without relief (*Bell., Merc.*) (B.).

Menses: Horribly offensive. carrion-like, a rotten odour; last but a day, then a bloody leucorrhœa of the same horrible odour (A.).

Seems to be in semi-sleep; dreams all night (Br.).

Suppression of lochia, followed by chills, fever and pro-fuse, fœtid perspiration (*Sec.*) (A.).

Sapræmia or septicæmia (*Arn., Bry., Chin., Hyos., Kali-P., Lach., Lyc., Op., Phos., Rhus-T.*) (A.).

After-effects of miscarriage (*Chin., Sec.*) (Br.).

Fœtus or secundines retained, decomposed; dead for days; black, horribly offensive discharge (A.).

Cardiac asthenia from septic conditions (*Ars., Kali-P., Lach., Phos., Sec.*) (A.).

Threatening heart failure in zymotic and septic fevers (Br.).

Obstinate, varicose, offensive ulcers of old persons (*Psor., Sec.*) (A.).

Dissecting wounds (*Ars.*) (Br.).

AGGRAVATION: From cold; from passing flatus; and at night.

AMELIORATION: From motion; from heat; and from pressure.

RELATIONSHIP: *Compare*: *Arn., Ars., Bapt., Carb-Ac., Carb-V., Echin., Kali-P., Lach., Op., Rhus-T., Psor., Sec., Sulph,* and *Verat.*

Follows: *Bry., Lach.* and *Rhus-T., well.*

Radium Bromide.

COMMON NAME: BROMIDE OF RADIUM.

General lassitude and tired feeling; wants to lie down and rest (*Gels., Phos-Ac., Stann.*) (C.).

Vivid dreams of fire (*Anac., Hep., Laur., Mag-C., Mag-M., Sulph.*) (B.).

Frontal headache (*Bry., Nux-V., Sep.*) (Br.).

Vertigo, with pain in the back of head (*Cocc., Nux-V., Petr.*) (C.).

Itching all over the body (*Psor., Sulph.*) (Br.).

Dry, bran-like scaly eruptions (*Ars.*) (C.).

ECZEMATOUS ERUPTIONS (*Anac., Rhus-T., Tub.*) (C.).

BURNING OF THE SKIN, AS IF AFIRE (*Ars., Sulph.*) (Br.).

Psoriasis (*Kali-Ars., Sep., Sulph.*) (Br.).

Arthritis with aching pains, worse at night (*Merc., Rhus-T.*) (Br.).

Gout (*Benz-Ac., Colch., Lyc.*) (B.).

ULCERS AND CANCERS (*Ars., Carb-An., Nit-Ac., Sil.*) (Br.).

Apprehensive and depressed (*Kali-P.*) (C.).

Fear of being alone in the dark (*Ars., Phos., Stram.*) (Br.).

Metallic taste in the mouth (*Cocc., Merc., Nat-C., Rhus-T., Seneg.*) (C.).

Tongue bluish white, thick, feels swollen (C.).

Empty feeling in the stomach (*Carb-An., Sep., Sulph.*) (Br.).

Aversion to sweets (*Graph.*) (Br.)

Belching of gas (*Carb-V., Lyc., Nux-M., Puls.*) (C.).

Much flatulence (*Aloe, Carb-V., Lyc., Nat-S., Puls., Sulph.*) (C.)

Pruritus ani and piles (*Aloe, Nux-V., Sulph.*) (Br.).

Craving for, and relief in, open air (*Arg-N., Phos., Puls.*) (C.).

Diabetes mellitus (*Phos-Ac., Sulph.*) (Bl.).

AGGRAVATION: On rising after lying down; after eating; from motion and at night.

AMELIORATION: In open air; from continued motion; and on lying down.

RELATIONSHIP: *Similar to: Ars., Brom., Carb-An., Ferr-P., Gels., Graph., Kali-Ars., Kali-P., Lach., Lyc.,*

Merc., Nux-V., Phos., Rhus-T., Sep., Sil., Sulph., Tub.
and *Urt-U.*

ANTIDOTES: *Rhus-T., Rhus-V.* and *Tell.*

Rananculus Bulbosus.

COMMON NAME: BUTTER CUP.

One of our most effective remedies for the bad effects of alcoholic beverages (A.).

Pleurisy or pneumonia from sudden exposure to cold, while over-heated (Acon., Arn.) (A.).

Shocks through the whole body.

The whole body feels as if beaten (Arn., Bapt., Pyrog.).

Burning and stinging pains (Apis).

Trembling of the limbs after anger (Nit-Ac.).

Muscular pains about the margins of shoulder-blades in women of sedentary employment, often burning in small spots (*Agar., Phos.*); from needle-work, type-writing, and piano-playing (*Act-R.*) (A.).

Blister-like eruptions (eczema) in the palms of the hands (N.).

Burning and itching vesicular eruptions (Canth., Rhus-T.).

Shingles preceded or followed by intercostal neuralgia (Mezer.); vesicles may have a bluish appearance (A.).

Corns: Sensitive to touch; smart and burn (*Salic-Ac.*) (A.).

Day-blindness (*Con., Sil., Stram., Sulph.*) (A.).

Mist before eyes (*Ars., Calc., Caust.*) (A.).

Pressure and smarting in eyeballs (*Phos.*) (A.).

Delirium tremens (Bell., Gels., Hyos., Stram.) (A.).

Pleurodynia, with short and oppressive breathing (*Bry., Phos.*) (Bl.).

INTERCOSTAL RHEUMATISM; CHEST SORE, BRUISED, WORSE FROM TOUCH, MOTION OR

TURNING THE BODY (*Bry.*); IN WET, STORMY WEATHER (*Rhus-T.*) (A.).

Pleurisy dependent upon a sudden exposure to cold while over-heated (Bl.).

PAINS: STITCHES, SHARP, SHOOTING, NEURALGIC, MYALGIC OR RHEUMATIC IN THE WALLS OF THE CHEST, COMING IN PAROXYSMS; EXCITED OR BROUGHT ON BY ATMOSPHERIC CHANGES; INFLAMMATORY DEPENDING UPON SPINAL IRRITATION (*Agar.*) (A.).

Hiccough in drunkards (A.).

Spasmodic hiccough (*Bell., Ign., Mag-P., Nux-V., Sec., Verat.*) (A.).

Hiccough with convulsions (*Bell., Cic., Cupr., Hyos.*) (K.).

HICCOUGH AFTER ALCOHOLIC DRINKS (K.).

Fear in the evening; does not want to be alone; fear of ghosts (R.).

Thoughts vanish (R.).

Confusion in the head (*Bapt., Gels.*) (R.).

ENLARGED SENSATION IN THE HEAD (*Bell., Glon.*). (K.).

Pain in the forehead and into eyes (*Spig.*) (R.).

Ciliary neuralgia (*Bell., Spig.*) (R.).

Iritis (*Merc-C., Sil., Sulph.*) (R.).

Rattling respiration (*Ant-T., Cact., Cupr., Dulc., Hep., Ipec., Kali-S., Lyc., Phos., Puls., Seneg.*) (K.).

AGGRAVATION: In the morning; in the evening; from change of temperature; from motion; from stretching, during stormy weather; from contact; from alcohol; from breathing; and from change of position.

AMELIORATION: From rest; from warm application; and in warm weather.

RELATIONSHIP: *Compare: Acon., Apis, Arn., Bapt., Bry., Canth., Clem., Euphorb., Mezer.*

Incompatible with: *Staph.* and *Sulph.*

Rananculus Scleratus.

COMMON NAME: MARSH BUTTER CUP.

Under this drug the symptoms usually appear on the right side (*Bell., Bry., Lyc.*) (G.).

Gnawing and screwing pains in the evening and before mid-night.

Twitches in the limbs (*Bell.; Cupr., Gels., Hell., Ign., Kali-P., Lach., Mosch., Nux-V., Op., Phos., Sil., Zinc.*).

FAINTING FROM PAIN (*Apis, Cham., Cocc., Hep., Nux-V., Phyt., Valer., Verat.*)

Fainting from pain in the stomach (*Coll., Puls.*) (K.)

The pains are aggravated in the evening and diminish toward mid-night and are followed then by sleeplessness.

Periodical complaints (*Ars., Chin., Kali-B., Nat-M., Sulph.*).

Sensation of enlargement of the head (*Glon., Nux-M., Nux-V., Sil., Spig.*).

Vesicular eruptions, with an acrid exudation that renders the surrounding parts sore (Bl.).

Pain over the liver (*Bry., Chel., Hep., Iod., Kali-M., Lyc., Merc., Nat-S., Pod., Sep., Sulph.*) (Bl.).

A feeling as though diarrhœa would come on (Bl.).

Sensation of cobwebs on the face (*Alum., Bar-C., Bor., Brom., Calc., Con., Graph., Laur., Mag-C., Mezer., Phos-Ac., Plb., Sulph., Sulph-Ac.*) (K.).

Mapped tongue (*Ars., Cham., Kali-B., Lach., Merc., Nat-M., Nit-Ac., Rhus-T., Sulph-Ac., Tarax.*) (K.).

Tongue covered with a white film, which comes off in patches, leaving dark-red, tender and very sensitive spots (*Tarax.*) (A.).

Burning and rawness of the tongue (*Ars., Nat-M., Sulph.*) (Br.).

Ulcers or large sores on the right side of the nose (G.).

Fluent coryza, with sneezing and burning micturition (*All-C.*) (Br.).

Frightful dreams about corpses, serpents, battles, etc. (Br.).

STITCHES IN THE CHEST MUSCLES (*Apis, Bell., Bry., Carb-An., Kali-B., Kali-C., Lach., Merc., Nat-M., Phos., Sil., Sulph.*) (B.).

Bullæ with acrid contents (B.)

Pemphigus (*Apis, Canth., Ran-B.*) (B.).

Gnawing in the knees (*Benz-Ac.,Kali-I., Merc., Nat-M., Zinc.*) (B.).

Sensation as of a plug forced between the ribs, under the navel, in the heart, etc. (B.).

Gout of small joints (*Benz-Ac., Calc-P., Lyc., Nit-Ac.*) (B.).

AGGRAVATION: In the evening; before midnight; from deep breathing; and from motion.

AMELIORATION: After midnight.

RELATIONSHIP: *Similar to:* Apis, Bry., Canth., Ferr-P., Graph., Hep., Kali-B., Lach., Merc., Nat-M., Rhus-T. and Sulph.

Remedies following: Bell., Phos., Puls., Rhus-T. and Sil.

ANTIDOTE: *Camph.*

Ratanhia.

COMMON NAME: RHATANY.

The rectal symptoms are most important, and have received much clinical confirmation (Br.).

GREAT SENSITIVENESS OF THE RECTUM (*Lach., Mur-Ac.*) (A.).

FISSURE OF THE ANUS (*Aesc., Graph., Nat-M., Nit-Ac., Sulph.*) (A.).

EXCRUCIATING PAINS AFTER STOOL (*Ign.,*
Nit-Ac., Thuj.) (A.).

Burning after soft stool (*Aloe, Nit-Ac.*) (A.).

Constipation; bowels inactive; stool hard and expelled
with great straining (A.).

Protrusion of hæmorrhoids, followed by long-lasting
aching and burning in the anus (*Sulph.*) (A.).

PAIN AFTER STOOL AS IF SPLINTERS OF
GLASS WERE STICKING IN THE ANUS AND
RECTUM (*Aesc., Nit-Ac., Thuj.*) (A.).

Dry or itching anus (*Aesc., Sulph.*) (B.).

Fissures of the nipples in nursing women (*Graph., Petr.,*
Sep.) (A.).

Terrible toothache during early months of pregnancy
(*Acon., Bell., Bry., Calc., Cham., Hyos., Lyss., Mag-C.,*
Merc., Nux-M., Puls., Rhus-T., Sep., Staph.; Tab.) (A.).

Tooth feels elongated (*Alum., Am-C., Ant-T., Bor.,*
Bry., Calc., Carb-V., Caust., Cham., Lach., Mag-C., Mezer.,
Nux-V., Phyt., Rhus-T., Staph.) (A.).

. *Toothache, worse from lying, compelling one to rise and*
walk about (*Mag-C., Rhus-T.*) (A.).

Bursting headache when straining at stool (*Ind.*) (B.).

Violent, painful hiccough (*Am-M., Cic., Lyc., Mag-P.,*
Nat-M., Nux-V., Stram., Verat.) (B.).

Hiccough after eating (*Alum., Ars., Bry., Carb-V.,*
Cycl., Graph., Hyos., Ign., Lyc., Mag-M., Nat-C., Nux-V.,
Phos., Sep., Teucr., Sulph., Verat., Zinc.) (K.).

Pin-worms (*Calc., Cina, Merc., Sil., Sulph., Teucr.*)
(Br.).

Pain like knives cutting the stomach (*Abrot., Ars., Bell.,*
Cham., Coloc., Dios., Hydr., Ign., Kali-C., Lyc., Merc.,
Nux-V., Op., Phos., Puls., Sil., Sulph., Thuj., Valer., Zinc.)
(Br.).

Oozing at the anus (*Aloe, Phos., Pæon.*) (Br.).

Fœtid, thin diarrhœa; stools burn (*Aloe, Nux-V., Sulph.*)
(Br.).

Sensation as if the brain would fall out of the forehead (B.).

AGGRAVATION: From lying; during pregnancy; at night; from touch; from heat; during and after stool; and after eating.

AMELIORATION: From walking about, from cool bathing and from washing with hot water.

RELATIONSHIP: *Compare*: *Aesc., Bry., Canth., Carb-Ac., Cycl., Hyos., Ind., Iris, Kali-C., Kali-M.; Lach., Lyc., Mag-C., Nat-M., Nit-Ac., Nux-V., Pæon., Petr., Phos., Rhus-T., Sulph., Thuj.* and *Verat.*

Rheum.

COMMON NAME: RHUBARB.

Especially suitable for children, during lactation and *dentition* (*Calc., Calc-P., Mag-C., Pod., Sil., Sulph*)

We use this remedy most particularly for sour-smelling children; stools, vomit, breath—all smell sour (G.).

Nightly sleeplessness with loping about and crying.

All joints are painful when moving (*Arn., Bry., Cham., Colch., Kali-B., Led., Lyc., Mang., Nux-V., Phyt., Ruta*).

Bubbling sensation, as from small bubbles in the muscles and joints.

The limbs on which one lies go to sleep (*Arn., Bry., Calc., Carb-V., Chin., Kali-C., Lyc., Puls., Rhod., Rhus-T., Sil., Sumb.*).

Debility and heaviness in the whole body as if he was awakened from a heavy sleep.

Cool perspirations (around the mouth and the chin and the palms of the hand).

THE CHILD'S WHOLE BODY SMELLS SOUR (*Calc., Hep.*) (D.).

Very sour smell of the child, which cannot be removed by any amount of washing and care in keeping it clear (G.).

Cholera infantum; stools frequent, uniformly frothy, watery and of a pea-green colour (Sm.).

Diarrhœa, with cutting pains about the navel (*Aloe, Ipec.*) (Bt.).

Colic and diarrhœa during dentition (*Mag-C.*) (N.).

Brown and frothy stools (*Arn., Kali-B., Mag-C., Merc., Nat-S., Sulph.*) (D.).

Diarrhœa of sour, slimy stools, with tenesmus and griping colic (*Merc.*) (D.).

STOOLS ARE SOUR (*Calc., Hep., Mag-C., Merc., Phos., Sulph.*), AND THERE IS TENESMUS (*Nux-V., Merc., Sulph.*).

YELLOW STOOL, TURNING GREEN ON STANDING (*Arg-N.*) (K.).

Screaming of children, with urging and sour stools (A.).

CHILDREN CRY AND TOSS ABOUT ALL NIGHT (*Psor.*) (A.).

Child impatient, desires many things, and cries; dislikes even favourite play-things (*Cham., Cina, Staph.*) (A.).

Its temper is as acrid and acid as are the stools (Bl.).

Loathing after first bite (B.).

Desires many kinds of food, but cannot eat them; becomes repugnant (A.).

Colic: Worse at once by uncovering an arm or leg; with very sour stool; worse when standing; not better by stool (A.).

Difficult dentition; child restless, irritable, peevish, with pale face and sour smell (*Cham., Kreos.*) (A.).

Sweat of the scalp, constant, profuse; whether asleep or awake, quiet or in motion, the hair is always wet; may or may not be sour (*Calc., Sanic.*) (A.).

Perspiration on the upper part of the body (*Asar., Carb-V., Cham., Kali-C., Nit-Ac., Op., Par., Sec., Thuj.,*

Verat.; on the lower part—*Am-C., Apis, Ars., Coloc., Croc., Cycl., Euph., Hyos., Mang., Merc., Nit-Ac., Sep., Thuj.*) (K.).

Colic with cries; ameliorated by doubling up, and aggravated by uncovering any part (B.).

Shivering during stool (*Merc.*) (C.).

Snoring inspiration during sleep (C.).

Vivid, sad, anxious dreams (C.).

May be given after abuse of magnesia, with or without rhubarb, if stools are sour (A.).

Gout with fibrous deposit in great toe-joint (*Colch., Led.*) (A.).

AGGRAVATION: At night; during dentition; from uncovering any part; when standing; during stool; from eating; and during summer.

AMELIORATION: From warmth; from wrapping up; and from doubling up.

RELATIONSHIP: *Compare: Ars., Calc., Cham., Coll., Hep., Ipec., Mag-C., Merc., Nat-M., Pod., Sanic., Staph.* and *Sulph.*

It follows well after *Mag-C.*, when milk disagrees and the child has sour odour.

Remedies following: Bell., Calc., Puls., Rhus-T. and *Sulph.*

Antidotes: Camph., Cham., Coloc., Merc., Nux-V. and *Puls.*

Rheum antidotes *Canth.* and *Mag-C.*

Rhododendron.

COMMON NAME: SNOW ROSE.

Especially suitable for nervous persons who dread a storm and are particularly afraid of thunder (A.).

Sensation of formication in the limbs (*Agar., Camph., Ign., Lyc., Nux-V., Phos-Ac., Phos., Puls., Rhus-T., Sec., Tarant., Zinc.*).

During rest weakness and loss of power in the limbs.

THE PAINS ARE CAUSED AND ARE AGGRAVATED BY WET COLD WEATHER AND DURING A THUNDER-STORM.

During rest the pains are most violent.

Violent rheumatic tearing in the limbs, as if in the periosteum (*Phyt.*).

Rheumatism worse from rest and change of weather (D.).

Rheumatism of the small joints (*Act-S.*) (D.).

Rheumatic gout (*Benz-Ac., Calc-P.*) (D.).

Arthritic nodes (*Caust., Lyc., Mezer.*) (G.).

Tearing jerking faceache or toothache; better from food or warmth (B.).

Drawing pain in the joints, as if they were dislocated, with gouty nodosities and swelling.

Inferior and superior dental neuralgia of an agonizing character, with a marked tendency to retraction of the gums in all cases.

Very curative in severe neuralgic pains of an alarming character.

Toothache, which ceases suddenly, beginning again in two or three hours (G.).

Toothache, every spring and fall during sharp east winds; worse from change of weather, thunderstorm and windy weather (A.).

Sweat, with formication (N.).

Pressing in the stomach from drinking cold water.

Stitches in the spleen from fast walking (*Arn., Chin., Hep., Lach., Nat-C., Nat-M., Sel., Verat.*).

Itchy, sweaty, wrinkled scrotum (B.).

Hydrocele of boys (*Abrot., Calc., Puls., Sil.*) (B.).

Hard, indurated testicle, with tendency to atrophy and a sensation as if it were crushed (D.).

Drawing in spermatic cord, extending to abdomen and thigh (D.).

INDURATION OR SWELLING OF THE TESTICLES, PARTICULARLY OF THE RIGHT ONE (G.).

TESTICLES, ESPECIALLY EPIDIDYMIS, INTENSELY PAINFUL TO TOUCH, DRAWN UP, SWOLLEN AND PAINFUL (N.).

Induration and swelling of the testicle after. gonorrhœa (*Clem., Puls.*) (A.).

Drawing and tearing in the limbs, especially the periosteum, and forearms, and legs; worse in wet weather, or before a storm, and at rest (N.).

Menses with fever (*Bell., Graph., Phos., Sep.*) (B.).

Diarrhœa from eating fruit (*Ars., Bry., Chin., Coloc., Nat-S., Puls., Verat.*), *and from wet, cold weather* (*Calc., Dulc., Nat-S., Nit-Ac., Nux-V., Polyg., Rhus-T.*).

Burning pain and on reading or writing heat in the eyes (R.).

Ears: Pain in the outer ear nearly all day; humming, buzzing, ringing; sensation as if water were rushing into them; loud sounds re-echo for a long time (R.).

Confused and stupid; forgets his subject (*Bar-C.*) (B.).

Nostrils obstructed alternately (*Lac-C.*) (B.).

Scraping and scratching sensation in the throat, as if lined with mucus (C.).

Acute inflammatory swelling of the joints, wandering from one joint to another; severe at night; worse in rest and during rough stormy weather (*Kalm.*) (A.).

Rheumatic drawing, tearing pains in all the limbs, worse at rest and in wet, cold, windy weather (*Rhus-T.*) (A.).

Rheumatic headaches involving the forehead and temples with tearing of the bones of the skull. These pains are always aggravated by cold, wet weather (*Kali-C.*) and wine, and ameliorated by wrapping the head up warm (*Sil.*) (R.).

Symptoms reappear with rough weather (A.).

Stiffness of the nape of the neck in the morning in bed and after rising, with rheumatic pains (R.).

Cannot get asleep, or remain asleep unless legs are crossed (A.).

Urine somewhat increased, pale and of offensive, acrid odour (C.).

Breathless and speechless from violent pleuritic pains running down the anterior chest (B.).

Pain in the back when sitting, better from motion, worse from stooping (B.).

Diarrhœa in damp weather; food passed undigested (R.).

AGGRAVATION: On beginning to move; in stormy, windy weather; from electrical changes in the atmosphere; on approach of thunder-storm; during night; from rest; and from wine.

AMELIORATION: From wrapping the head warmly; from exercise; from dry heat; from motion; and in the sun.

RELATIONSHIP: *Antidotes*: *Bry., Camph., Clem.* and *Rhus-T.*

Compare: *Apis, Bry., Con., Dig., Dulc., Ferr-P., Gels., Led., Lyc., Merc., Nat-S., Puls., Rhus-T., Sil., Sulph.* and *Thuj.*

Rhus Toxicodendron.

COMMON NAME: POISON IVY.

It affects powerfully the skin, mucous membranes and fibrous tissues (viz., aponeuroses, ligaments and tendons of muscles.) (D.).

It affects the right side more than the left (A.).

Headache, as if a board were strapped on the forehead

(as if a rubber band were stretched tightly over the fore-head—*Carb-Ac.*) (D.).

Headache relieved by motion (Bt.).

Aching in the occipital protuberances and soreness of the scalp (D.).

Vertigo while walking (Nat-M., Nux-V., Phos., Puls.) (K.).

Vertigo, with heaviness in the limbs, in the aged (Ambr., Bar-C., Calc-P., Cupr., Sin-N.) (D.).

Pain in the back on attempting to rise; rheumatic pains in the back and stiff neck from sitting in a draught; the lumbago is a condition which may not be relieved by motion and still indicate *Rhus-T.* (D.).

PAINS IN THE BACK COMPELLING TO MOVE CONSTANTLY IN BED (N.).

LUMBAGO, BETTER FROM LYING ON SOME-THING HARD *(Nat-M.)* (K.).

Lameness in the back as if strained or after straining (N.).

RHEUMATIC DRAWING AND TEARING PAINS IN THE LIMBS, WORSE DURING REST, RELIEV-ED BY CONTINUED MOTION.

Tension as from shortening of the muscles (*Cimx., Cupr., Plb., Puls.*)

Powerlessness of the lower limbs; cannot draw them up (N.).

Stiffness of the joints, worse when rising from rest.

Aching pains in the legs; must change position every moment (N.).

Tingling in the feet and other places of the body (*Acon., Cocc., Kali-C., Nit-Ac., Phos-Ac., Rhos., Pub., Rhod.*).

SERIOUS CONSEQUENCES FROM OVER-LIFTING IN SPRAINS AND CONTUSIONS.

Rheumatic paralysis (*Caust.*) (Bt.).

Nervous inflammations—a wide range in this respect.

THE PAIN AND STIFFNESS IS WORSE ON COMMENCING TO MOVE, BUT CONTINUED MOTION RELIEVES (D.).

Patients cannot bear cold air (*Hep.*) (D.).

Swelling around the ankles after sitting too long, particularly in travelling (N.).

SCIATICA (left side) (N.).

Swelling of the whole eye and surrounding parts (N.).

Conjunctivitis and iritis, when of traumatic or rheumatic origin, with severe pains worse at night (D.).

Scrofulous ophthalmia and orbital cellulitis (D.).

Ptosis and stiffness of the lids in rheumatic subjects (D.).

Oedematous swelling of the eyes and acrid discharge (D.).

Lachrymation on forcibly opening the eyes (*Apis, Con., Ipec., Merc-C.*) *or when yawning* (*Ant-T., Calc-P., Ign., Kali-C., Kreos., Nux-V., Sabad., Staph.*) (K.).

Sac-like swelling of the conjunctiva (N.).

THE LOWER JAW CRACKS ON EVERY MOTION (*Am-C., Lach., Nit-Ac.*) AND DISLOCATES EASILY (*Staph.*) (D.).

The tongue takes imprints of teeth (*Ars., Chel., Merc., Sep., Stram.*) (N.).

THE TONGUE IS CRACKED AND COATED, ALL EXCEPT A TRIANGULAR SPACE AT THE TIP, WHICH IS VERY RED (D.).

White coating only on one side of the tongue (N.).

Salivation during sleep (*Bar-C., Carb-An., Kali-C., Lac-C., Merc., Puls.*) (K.).

Sordes on the teeth (*Bapt., Hyos., Mur-Ac.*) (Bt.).

Epistaxis at night, during straining at stool, from bending forward, or from any bodily exertion (N.).

In typhoid fever hæmorrhage from the nose after 4 o'clock in the morning (N.).

Mumps or swelling of the parotid glands (*Bell., Brom., Merc.*), with sticking pains when swallowing (*Phyt.*) (D.).

Catamenia causes violent biting pain in the vulva (N.).

The lochia after having almost ceased, again becomes bloody and offensive (N.).

External genitals inflamed, erysipelatous and œdematous (A.).

Abortion from a strain (G.).

Pain between the shoulders in swallowing (N.).

Membranous dysmenorrhœa, in rheumatic females (G.).

It produces a vesicular eruption, accompanied by œdema, with burning, itching and tingling (D.).

Phlegmonous erysipelas (N.).

Red, shiny swellings and vesicular erysipelas (*Anac., Canth., Tarant.*).

ECZEMATOUS ERUPTIONS, WITH GREAT BURNING AND ITCHING, WITH A TENDENCY TO FORM SCALES (*Ars., Graph., Mezer.*).

Rhagades (*Calc., Carb-S., Graph., Petr., Puls., Sars., Sep., Sulph.*).

CUTANEOUS ERUPTIONS ALTERATING WITH DYSENTERY OR ASTHMA (*Calad., Mezer., Sulph.*) (K.).

Rubbing the affected parts increases the eruption (G.).

Urticaria: In cold weather; from becoming wet; during chill (*Apis, Ars., Ign., Nat-M.*); during fever (*Apis, Chlor., Cop., Cub., Ign., Rhus-V., Sulph.*); during perspiration (*Apis*); during rheumatism (*Urt-U.*); and every spring (K.).

Hydroa on the upper lip (*Ars., Nat-M.*) (D.).

Blistering herpes (*Canth., Rhus-V.*) (D.).

Corners of mouth ulcerated (*Nit-Ac.*) (A.).

Typhus Fever (*Bapt., Hyos., Op., Stram.*).

USEFUL IN INFLUENZA, WITH ACHING IN THE BONES, SNEEZING AND COUGHING; DRY COUGH; BRONCHIAL COUGHS OF OLD PEOPLE; AND TYPHOID PNEUMONIA (D.).

Typhoid fever: Mild delirium, with desire to escape (*Hyos.*); great restlessness, with apparent relief from motion; answers questions slowly (*Phos-Ac.*); frontal headache; dry, brown, cracked or red tongue, with triangular red tip; yellowish, brown, cadaverous and sometimes involuntary diarrhœa; pains in the limbs and a tympanitic abdomen (D.).

Intermittent fever characterized by a dry, teasing cough during the chill (D.).

Easily chilled, worse from least uncovering, with pains in the limbs (B.).

Chill as if dashed with cold water, or as if cold water were in the veins (B.).

It should be given in scarlet fever, when the child is drowsy, restless and has a red and smooth tongue, œdematous fauces and enlarged glands; eruption does not come out and is miliary; great depression and weakness (D.).

Cellulitis and Carbuncle: There is formation of pus, intense pain and dark red swelling, with the general prostration of the remedy (D.).

Pains as if sprained, as if a muscle or tendon was torn from its attachment or as if the bones were scraped with a knife; worse after midnight or in wet weather (A.).

Affected parts feel sore to touch (A.).

GREAT SENSITIVENESS TO OPEN AIR; PUTTING THE HAND FROM UNDER THE BED-COVER BRINGS ON THE COUGH (*Bar-C., Hep.*) (N.).

Has helped many cases of small-pox with the same group of symptoms as in scarlet fever, except that there were black, bloody pustules (R.).

Putrid taste in the mouth (*Puls.*) (G.).

Desire for cold milk (*Phos., Staph., Tub.*) (K.).

After the first mouthful has no appetite (*Lyc.*) (G.).

Great thirst, with dry tongue, mouth and throat (A.).

Dysentery .(*Acon., Aloe, Ferr-P., Merc., Nux-V., Puls., Sulph.*).

A bloody, slimy diarrhœa, or an involuntary stool of cadaverous odour in typhoid fever (*Bapt., Lach*) (D.).

DIARRHOEA, WITH TEARING PAINS DOWN THE LEGS (G.).

Great pain before stool, which is greenish, and contains jelly-like globules or flakes (Bt.).

Jelly-like stools (*Aloe, Kali-B.*) (Bt.).

Red and scanty urine (*Berb., Canth.*) (Bt.).

Discharge of urine too copious, too frequent and involuntary (G.).

Bloody urine discharged in drops (*Canth., Hep., Sars.*) (Bt.).

ERYSIPELAS OF THE GENERATIVE ORGANS, IN BOTH SEXES, ESPECIALLY IN THE MALE (Bt.).

Phimosis or paraphimosis (*Merc., Nat-M., Nit-Ac., Sep., Sulph., Thuj.*) (K.).

Sad, listless (*Phos-Ac., Sep.*) (Br.).

Restless, cannot stay long in one position (Ars.) (A.).

Great restlessness, anxiety and apprehension (*Acon., Ars., Kali-P.*) (A.).

Great apprehension at night; fears he will die of being poisoned; cannot remain in bed (A.).

Thoughts of suicide (*Ars., Aur., Hep., Nit-Ac., Nux-V.*) (Bt.).

Brain feels loose when stepping or shaking the head (A.).

Sensation of swashing in the brain (*Ars., Bell., Carb-An., Hep., Hyos., Lyc., Nux-V., Spig., Sulph-Ac.*) (A.).

Paralysis with numbness of the affected parts, from getting wet, on lying on damp ground, and after exertion, parturition, sexual excesses, ague or typhoid (A.).

Locomotor ataxia (*Alumn., Gels., Zinc.*) (C.).

DREAMS OF GREAT EXERTION—SUCH AS ROWING, SWIMMING, WORKING HARD AT HIS DAILY OCCUPATION, AND ROAMING OVER FIELDS (A).

Yawning, with violent stretching of the limbs (G.).

Pain in the abdomen, ameliorated by lying on the abdomen (*Aloe, Bell., Bry., Coloc., Phos., Plb., Stann.*) (K.).

Weak, rapid, sharp, tremulous or irregular pulse (Bt.).

Colic, compelling one to walk bent (*Coloc., Nit-Ac.*) (Br.).

Swelling of the inguinal glands (*Bell., Calc., Hep., Iod., Merc., Sil.*) (C.).

Humid eruptions on the genitals and between the scrotum and thighs (C.).

Scrotum becomes thick and hard (*Sulph.*), with intolerable itching (*Crot-T., Graph., Sulph.*) (C.).

Uncomplicated hypertrophy of the heart from overexertion, with a sense of numbness of the left arm and shoulder (*Acon., Act-R., Arn., Kalm.*) (D.).

Sensation of weakness and trembling in the heart (N.).

Aching in the left arm, with heart disease (N.).

Tickling under the sternum, that excites cough (Bt.).

Terrible cough, which seems as if it would tear something out of the chest (G.).

Expectoration of brick-dust or bloody sputa, raised with difficulty (*Phos.*), and accompanied with high fever, in the worst cases of pneumonia (Bt.).

Sepia often quickly relieves the itching and burning of *Rhus-T.*, the vesicles drying up in a few days (A.).

AGGRAVATION: During rest; whilst rising from a seat; when entering the room from the open air; from getting wet, especially while perspiring; during the winter season; during the night; after midnight; before storms; on beginning to move after quiet; and in wet, rainy, weather.

AMELIORATION: From continued motion; from walking; from change of position; from lying on something hard; from warmth; in dry air; and from warm or hot things; from wrapping up; and from moving the affected parts.

RELATIONSHIP: *Complementary to*: *Bry., Calc., Mag-C., Med.* and *Phyt.*

Inimical to: *Apis* (must not be used before or after).

Compare: *Acon., Apis, Arn., Ars., Bell., Bry., Calc-P., Cham., Ferr., Gels., Hep., Kali-P., Lach., Merc., Nat-M., Nat-S., Rhod., Sep., Sil., Sulph., Thuj.* and *Zinc.*

Rumex Crispus.

COMMON NAME: YELLOW DOCK.

This remedy is indicated in those of tubercular diathesis, who are extremely sensitive to the open air (Bl.).

Intense itching of the skin when undressing to go to bed (N.).

Itching of various parts, worse by cold, and better by warmth.

It should be remembered in urticaria and prurigo, when there is intense i.ching of the skin; this is made worse from exposure to cold air (Bl.).

The urine passes involuntarily during coughing (*Apis, Bell., Caust., Ferr-P., Kreos., Lyc., Nat-M., Phos., Puls., Squil.*) (Bl.)

Early morning diarrhœa from 5 to 10 A.M. (*Aloe, Nat-S., Podo., Sulph.*) (A.).

The stool is profuse, painless and offensive, and may accompany pulmonary tuberculosis (Bl.).

Brownish diarrhœa, worse in the morning (*Nat-S., Sulph.*) (N.).

Ravenous appetite (*Petr., Sulph.*) (B.).

SUDDEN URGING, DRIVING OUT OF BED IN THE MORNING (*Sulph.*) (A.).

Attacks of sneezing (*Ars., Cycl., Sabad.*) (B.).

VIOLENT INCESSANT COUGH, WORSE ON INHALING THE LEAST COLD AIR (*Hep., Rhus-T.*); COVERS THE MOUTH TO KEEP THE COLD AIR OUT, WITH RELIEF (N.).

Night cough in phthisis (*Con., Hyos., Phos., Puls.* (D.).
Cough caused by tickling in the supra-sternal fossa (D.).
Touching the throat-pit brings on the cough ((G.).

EVERY BREATH OF COLD AIR CAUSES
TICKLING AS FROM A FEATHER OR DUST IN
THE THROAT-PIT AND CONTINUOUS COUGH
(B.).

By covering up all the body and head with the bed-clothes there is no cough (G.).

Cough provoked by change of air, cool or warm, or change in the rhythm of respiration (N.).

Violent, incessant dry cough, fatiguing, with little expectoration, aggravated by pressure, talking, and especially by inhaling cold air (N.).

Cough, worse in the evening, after lying down, especially from lying on the left side (*Phos.*) (A.).

COUGH WORSE FROM CHANGING AIR OR
ROOM (*Phos., Spong.*) (A.).

Raw sensation in the larynx and trachea when coughing (*Caust.*) (A.).

Hawks out much tenacious mucus (*Kali-B., Kali-C.*) (B.).

Hoarseness: Worse evenings and after exposure to cold; voice uncertain (A.).

Complete aphonia (*Am-Caust., Arg-N., Carb-V., Caust., Phos.*) (Bt.).

Sensation of a lump in the throat (*Bell., Ign., Lach.*), which descends on swallowing, but returns immediately (*Ign.*) (A.).

Sense of excoriation behind the sternum (*Phos.*) (Dn.).

The left chest is more often affected than the right (*Phos.*) (Dn.).

Every cold affects the joints (*Calc-P.*) (B.).

AGGRAVATION: From inhaling cold air; in the evening; after lying down; from uncovering; at night; from pressure on trachea; and early in the morning.

AMELIORATION: From warmth; from keeping the mouth covered to exclude cold air; and from wrapping up.

RELATIONSHIP: *Compare*: *Bell., Caust., Dros., Hyos., Merc., Nat-S., Phos., Podo., Psor., Rhus-T., Sang., Sil., Sulph.* and *Tub.*

Ruta Graveoleus.

COMMON NAMES: RUE; BITTER WORT.

Bruises and other mechanical injuries of bones and perios eum (N.).

All parts of the body upon which he lies are painful, as if bruised (N.).

Soreness and lameness, as from a sprain or bruise (Arn., Rhus-T.) (D.).

Wrists feel as if sprained, stiff, worse in cold, wet weather (N.).

Rheumatism of wrists and ankles (Rhus-T.) (D.).

Hamstrings feel shortened (*Graph.*) (Br.).

Scrofulous exostosis (*Calc-F.*) (A.).

Periostitis (*Calc., Calc-F., Calc-P., Merc., Sil.*) **(A.).**

Fractures, and especially dislocations (*Symph.*) (A.).

Eye-strain followed by headache (*Calc-P., Nat-M.***)** (Br.).

Eyes burn like balls of fire (N.).

Asthenopia and amblyopia from fine sewing, or reading with a bad light (Bl.).

EYES ACHE AND FEEL STRAINED, FROM FINE SEWING OR READING, PARTICULARLY BY GAS LIGHT (*Arg-N., Nat-M.*) (N.).

Blurred vision (*Chin., Cycl., Phos.*) (A.).

Misty or dim vision, with complete obscuration at a distance (*Phos.*) (A.).

Spasms of the lower eyelids (A.).

Disturbances of accommodation (*Nat-M.*) (Br.).

Eye diseases after easing the eyes at fine work, such as watch-making, engraving etc. (*Nat-M.*) (A.).

Pressure deep in the orbits (Br.).

Warts with sore pains; flat, smooth on the palms of hands (*Nat-C., Nat-M.; on the back of hands—Dulc.*) (A.).

BACKACHE, RELIEVED BY LYING ON THE BACK (*Kali-C., Nat-M., Nux-V., Phos., Puls., Rhus-T.*) (A.).

Restless, turns and changes position frequently when lying (*Rhus-T.*) (A.).

PROLAPSUS OF THE RECTUM, IMMEDIATELY ON ATTEMPTING A PASSAGE, FROM THE SLIGHTEST STOOPING, AND AFTER CONFINEMENT (N.).

Constipation from inactivity of the rectum, or from impaction following mechanical injuries (*Arn.*) (A.).

Frequent, unsuccessful urging for an evacuation (A.).

Pressure on the bladder, as if constantly full; it continues after urinating (A.).

Could hardly retain urine on account of urging, yet if not attended to it was difficult afterwards to void it (A.).

Scanty, green urine (*Ars., Camph., Merc-C.*) (A.).

Involuntary urination (*Apis, Caust., Nat-M., Puls.*) (A.).

Corrosive leucorrhœa (*Calc., Nit-Ac.*) (B.).

PHTHISIS AFTER MECHANICAL INJURIES TO THE CHEST (*Arn., Ham., Mill.*) (A.).

Cough with copious, thick, yellow expectoration (*Lyc., Puls., Sep., Stann.*) (Br.).

Short breath, with tightness of the chest (Br.).

Frequent waking at night (*Bell., Stram., Sulph.*) (C.).

Dyspepsia resulting from a strain of the abdominal muscles (C.).

Epigastric region sensitive (C.).

AGGRAVATION: In cold, wet weather; after using the eyes at fine work; from eye-strain; from stooping; after mechanical injury; from straining at stool.

AMELIORATION: From lying on the back; from motion; from warmth.

RELATIONSHIP: *Compare*: *Arg-N., Arn., Bapt., Bov., Calc., Calc-F., Calc-P., Con., Dulc., Euphr., Ferr-P., Kali-P., Mill.. Nat-C., Nat-M.. Phyt., Rhus-T., Seneg., Symph.* and *Thuj.*

After *Arn.*, it hastens the curative process in the joints; after *Symph.* in injuries of the bones.

Complementary: *Calc-P.*

Antidote: *Camph.*

Sabadilla.

COMMON NAME: CEVADILLA.

Worm affections of children (*Bell., Bry., Calc., Cina, Merc., Sil., Spig., Sulph.*) (A.).

Twitching, convulsive tremblings and catalepsy from worms (*Cina, Graph., Psor.*) (A.).

Nymphomania from ascarides (*Plat.*) (A.).

Hay fever (*All-C., Ars., Gels.*) (D.).

Chill returning at the same hour (*Ars.*) (C.).

Chilliness from feet to head (A.).

Chill predominates (*Camph., Nux-V., Verat.*) (Br.).

No thirst during chill; heat often internal (G.).

Influenza with violent, spasmodic sneezing (*Ars.*) *and lachrymation on going into open air* (*Calc., Phos., Sil., Sulph., Thuj.*) (D.).

Many symptoms go from right to left (*Lyc., Podo.*) (A.).

Eyes swollen and watery (*Euphr.*) (D.).

Headache from too much thinking, too close application or attention (*Arg-N.*) (A.).

BURNING, WATERY DISCHARGE FROM THE NOSE (*All-C., Ars., Nat-M.*) (D.).

Delirium during intermittents (*Ars., Lach., Nat-M., Podo., Verat.*) (A.).

Nervous, timid, easily startled (*Bor., Gels., Kali-C.*) (Br.).

ILLUSIONS: THAT HE IS SICK; THAT PARTS ARE SHRUNKEN; THAT SHE IS PREGNANT (*Ign., Thuj., Verat.*), WHEN ONLY DISTENDED WITH FLATUS; AND THAT SHE HAS SOME HORRIBLE THROAT DISEASE THAT WILL BE FATAL (A.).

Parchment-like dryness of the skin (*Ars.*) (A.).

Swelling of the throat and tonsils (*Bell., Merc., Sil.*) (D.).

DIPHTHERIA OR TONSILLITIS (*Ars., Bell., Kali-M., Lach., Lyc., Merc-P-I., Nux-V., Phyt., Rhus-T., Sil.*) (A.).

CAN SWALLOW WARM FOOD MORE EASILY, (A.).

Stitches and most symptoms, especially of the throat, go from left to right (*Lach., Lac-C.*) (A.).

Sensation of a skin hanging loosely in the throat; must swallow over it (A.).

Dryness of the fauces and throat (*Aesc., Bry., Sulph.*) (A.).

Tongue feels burnt (*Bell., Iris, Thuj.*) (B.).

Canine hunger (*Lyc., Sulph., Tub.*) (B.).

Craves hot things, sweets or milk (B.).

Crawling, itching at the anus (*Calc., Cina, Sulph., Teuc.*) (B.).

Loss of appetite (*Cycl., Nux-V., Puls.*) (A.).

Sour or rancid eructations (*Alum., Bar-C., Calc., Carb-V., Ferr-I., Graph., Kali-B.*) (A.).

Sneezing in spasmodic paroxysms, followed by lachrymation (*All-C.*) (A.).

COPIOUS, WATERY CORYZA (*All-C., Euphr., Rhus-T.*) (A.).

Face hot and eye-lids red and burning (*All-C., Ars., Sulph.*) (A.).

Great sleepiness in the forenoon (*Ant-C., Bism., Calc., Calc-P., Carb-An., Carb-V., Gels., Mosch., Nat-C., Nux-V., Podo., Sep., Thuj.*) (G.).

Disturbed and unrefreshing sleep at night (*Nux-V., Puls., Sulph.*) (C.).

Confused dreams (*Bry., Calc., Coff., Dulc., Ferr., Glon., Ign., Lyc., Nat-M., Nux-V., Puls., Sep.*) (C.).

Lassitude and weakness (*Gels., Nux-V., Phos., Pic-Ac., Zinc.*) (C.).

AGGRAVATION: In the fore-noon; before midnight; from cold; while resting; from cold drinks; during new and full moon; and from odours.

AMELIORATION: From motion; while swallowing; while getting warm; from warmth; and from warm food and drink.

RELATIONSHIP: It follows *Bry.* and *Ran-B.* well in pleurisy, and has cured after *Acon.* and *Bry.* failed.

Antidotes: *Con., Lach., Lyc.* and *Puls.*

Complementary: *Sep.*

Sabina.

COMMON NAME: SAVINE.

Chronic ailments of women (*Calc., Ferr., Graph., Kali-C., Lach., Lyc., Merc., Nat-M., Nit-Ac., Phos., Puls., Sep., Sulph., Thuj.*) (A.).

Ailments following abortion or premature labour (*Caul., Kali-C., Sep.*) (A.).

DRAWING PAINS IN THE SMALL OF BACK, FROM SACRUM TO PUBES, IN NEARLY ALL DISEASES (from back, going round the body to the pubes —*Vib-Op.*) (A.).

Fig-warts with intolerable itching and burning; exuberant granulations (*Nit-Ac., Thuj.*) (A.).

Craves lemonade (*Bell., Calc., Cycl., Eup-Pur., Jatr., Nit-Ac., Puls., Sec., Sulph-I.*) (B.).

Menses: Too early, too profuse, too protracted; partly fluid, partly clotted (Bell., Chin., Ferr., Ipec., Nux-V., Puls.); in women who menstruated very early in life (Calc., Puls.); flow in paroxysms (Caust., Kreos., Puls., Sep.); with colic and labour-like pains (A.).

Metrorrhagia, with paroxysmal flow of bright colour (Bell.), accompanied by pains in the joints (D.).

Menorrhagia during climacteric, in women who formerly aborted, or with early first menses (*Calc., Ferr., Kali-C., Lach., Murx., Nux-V., Puls., Sec., Sep., Sulph.*) (A.).

HAEMORRHAGE FROM THE UTERUS; FLOW PARTLY PALE RED, PARTLY CLOTTED; WORSE FROM LEAST MOTION (*Bry., Croc., Erig., Helon., Ipec., Sec., Sulph., Tril., Ust.*) ; OFTEN RELIEVED BY WALKING (A.).

Discharge of blood between periods, with sexual excitement (*Ambr., Calc., Cham., Ipec., Phos., Rhus-T., Sil.*) (A.).

Inflammation of ovaries or uterus after abortion, or premature labour (*Sep.*) (A.).

THREATENED ABORTION ABOUT THE THIRD MONTH (*Apis, Cimic., Croc., Eup-Pur., Merc., Sec., Thuj:, Ust.*), WITH PAINS IN THE SMALL OF THE BACK, GOING DOWN THE THIGHS (D.).

Retained placenta from uterine atony (Canth., Caul., Cimic., Croc., Gels., Ipec., Nux-V., Puls., Sec., Sep.) (A.).

INTENSE AFTER-PAINS (*Arn., Cham., Cupr., Hyper., Kali-C., Puls., Rhus-T., Sec., Sep., Vib., Xanth.*) (A.).

Promotes expulsion of moles or foreign bodies from the uterus (*Canth.*) (A.).

PAIN FROM LUMBAR REGION FORWARD TO PUBES OR REVERSE, OR SHOOTING UP TO THE VAGINA (B.).

Foul, acrid leucorrhœa (*Calc., Nit-Ac.*) (B.).

Itching of the genitalia from leucorrhœa (K.).

Suppression of the menses is followed by a thin, fœtid leucorrhœa (G.).

Bruised sensation along the anterior surface of the thighs (D.).

Arthritic pains (*Bell., Caul., Rhus-T.*) (A.).

Much irritability of temper (*Nux-V., Sulph.*) (G.).

MUSIC IS INTOLERABLE; PRODUCES NERVOUSNESS, GOES THROUGH BONE AND MARROW (Causes weeping—*Thuj.*) (A.).

Quivering in the abdomen as if there was something alive in it (*Sabad., Thuj., Verat.*) (G.).

Frequent urging to s.ool; finally a liquid portion is discharged, followed by a hard portion (G.).

Constipation; stools difficult and painful (G.).

Piles, with discharge of bright red or dark, venous blood (G.).

Attacks of shivering chilliness all day (A.).

Burning of the whole body, with great restlessness (*Ars., Canth., Phos., Sec.*) (A.).

Flushes of heat in the face, while the rest of the body is chilly; with icy cold hands and feet (*Sep.*) (A.).

Sweats easily (*Bry., Calc., Chin., Sil.*) (A.).

Night-sweats (*Calc., Chin., Merc.*) (A.).

AGGRAVATION: From least motion; in a warm room; in warm air; after parturition; from music; from taking a deep breath; and during menopause.

AMELIORATION: In cool, open, fresh air; while exhaling; from cold.

RELATIONSHIP: *Compare*: *Apis, Arn., Bell., Bry., Calc., Canth., Caul., Croc., Ferr., Lach., Lyc., Mill., Puls., Sec., Sep., Sulph., Thuj., Ust., Vib-O., Xanth.* **and** *Zinc.*

Complementary to: *Thuj.*

It follows *Thuj.* well in condyloma and sycotic affections. *Antidotes*: *Camph.* and *Puls.*

Sambucus Nigra.

COMMON NAME: ELDER.

We are often led to this remedy, when we find a great deal of perspiration, occurring with any other trouble, which may last all the time, or it may come and go in paroxysms (G.).

Bad effects of violent mental emotions, anxiety, grief, or excessive sexual indulgence (*Kali-P., Phos-Ac.*) (A.).

SNUFFLES IN CHILDREN (*Am-C., Aesc-T., Aur., Aur-M., Elaps, Lyc., Nux-V., Puls.*) (D.).

NOSE DRY AND COMPLETELY OBSTRUCTED, PREVENTING BREATHING AND NURSING (*Am-C., Lyc., Nux-V., Stict.*) (A.).

Child awakes suddenly almost suffocated, face livid, blue, sits up in bed; turns blue, gasps for breath, which it finally gets; attack passes off, but again repeated (A.).

CHILD INSPIRES BUT CANNOT EXPIRE (*Chlor., Meph.*) (A.).

SPASM OF THE GLOTTIS (*Ars., Bell., Cupr., Gels., Ign., Lach., Mag-P., Mosch., Op., Phos., Sil., Spong., Stram., Tab., Tarant., Verat.*) (D.).

Asthma with suffocative attacks of breathing; patient may be well enough while awake, but sleeps into the trouble (G.).

Attacks of suffocation as in last stage of croup (A.).

Cough: Suffocative, with crying children; worse about midnight; hollow, deep, whooping, with spasm of the chest; with regular inhalations but sighing exhalations (A.).

There is much mucus in the bronchi, while expectoration is difficult (Bl.).

Face turns blue with cough (*Coc-C., Cor-R., Dros., Ipec., Mag-P., Verat.*) (Br.).

MILLAR'S ASTHMA (Br.).

Half-open eyes (*Ant-T., Apis, Bell., Cham., Cupr., Dig., Ferr., Gels., Hell., Ipec., Kreos., Lach., Lyc., Merc., Nat-M., Op., Phos., Rhus-T., Stram., Sulph., Verat., Zinc.*) (B.).

Sees images when shutting the eyes (*Arg-N., Bell., Calc., Caust., Graph., Puls., Sep., Sil., Sulph., Tarant., Thuj.*) (Br.).

Fright followed by suffocative attacks (Br.).

Very easily frightened (*Arg-N., Ars., Bar-C., Bor., Graph., Kali-C., Lyc., Nat-Ars., Nat-C., Sep., Stram.*) (Br.).

Constant fretfulness (*Cham., Cina, Lyc., Nux-V., Sulph.*) (Br.).

Trembling, anxiety and restlessness (*Acon., Ars., Hyos., Stram.*) (C.).

Hoarseness, with much tenacious, glutinous mucus in the larynx (*Kali-B., Rumx.*) (C.).

Quick, wheezing respiration (*Ant-T., Brom., Seneg.*) (C.).

Sleepness, without sleep (*Bell., Cham., Lach.*) (C.).

ICY COLD FEET (*Camph., Carb-V., Crot-C.*) (B.).

Scanty urine (*Apis, Ars., Bell., Canth., Colch., Dig., Ferr-P., Lyc., Merc-C., Sep.*) (Br.).

Acute nephritis (*Apis, Bell., Canth.*) (Br.).

Dropsical symptoms with vomiting (*Ars., Dig., Kali-C., Lyc., Nat-S.*) (Br.).

Coldness creeps over the whole body, especially hands and feet, which are cold to the touch (A.).

Dry heat while he sleeps; on falling asleep, after lying down; fever without thirst, dreads uncovering (must be covered in every stage—*Nux-V.*) (A.).

Deep, dry cough precedes the fever paroxysms (A.).

PROFUSE SWEAT OVER THE ENTIRE BODY DURING WAKING HOURS; ON GOING TO SLEEP, DRY HEAT RETURNS (sweats as soon as he closes his eyes to sleep—*Chin., Con.*) (A.).

Most of the pains occur during rest and disappear during motion (*Rhus-T.*) (A.).

Persons formerly robust and fleshy, suddenly become emaciated (*Iod., Tub.*) (A.).

Oedematous swelling in various parts of the body, especially in legs, insteps and feet (A.).

AGGRAVATION: From uncovering; while lying down; while resting; after eating fruit; during midnight, in dry, cold air; from cold drinks; and during expiration.

AMELIORATION: From moving; on rising; while walking; from wrapping up warmly; from sitting up in bed; and from pressure.

RELATIONSHIP: *Antidotes: Ars., Camph.*

Follows well after *Op.* in bad effects of fright.

Relieves ailments from abuse of *Ars.*

Compare: Ars., Bell., Brom., Chin., Chlor., Cupr., Dig., Gels., Hep., Ign., Iod., Ipec., Lach., Lyc., Mag-P., Meph., Mosch., Nux-V., Op., Phos., Sil., Spong., Stram., Sulph., Tab. and *Verat.*

Sanguinaria Canadensis.

COMMON NAME: BLOOD ROOT.

Is pre-eminently a rightsided remedy (*Bell., Lyc.*) (D.).

Acts intensely on the right lung and chest (N.).

Roundish or oval, whitish and raised patches on the mucous membrane of the nose, mouth, prepuce and anus (Bt.).

Burning in the palms and soles (Ars., Lach., Phos., Sep., Sulph.) (D.).

Jaundice, with nausea and vomiting (*Ars., Bry., Card-M., Chel., Dig., Kali-M., Lach., Lyc., Merc., Nat-M., Nat-S., Phos., Sep.*) (Bt.).

Circumscribed redness of the cheeks (*Chin., Ferr., Lachn., Phos., Stann., Sulph., Tub.*) (D.).

Headache during the climacteric (*Graph., Lach., Sep., Sulph.*) (A.).

Determination of blood to the head and chest (*Bell., Cact., Ferr-P.*) (D.).

PERIODICAL SICK HEADACHE; BEGINS IN THE MORNING, INCREASES DURING THE DAY, AND LASTS UNTIL EVENING (*Nat-M., Spig.*) (A.).

Head feels as if it would burst (*Bell., Bry., Calc., Chin., Con., Glon., Lach., Lyss., Merc., Nat-M., Phos., Sep.*) (A.).

Sensation as if the eyes would be pressed out during headache (A.).

Distension of temporal veins (*Bell., Glon., Verat-V.*) (D.).

Headache relieved by sleep (*Bell., Chel., Ferr., Gels., Glon., Graph., Hyos., Lac-C., Pall., Phos., Pic-Ac., Puls., Sep.*) (A.).

HEADACHE BEGINS IN THE OCCIPUT, SPREADS UPWARDS AND SETTLES OVER THE RIGHT ORBIT (*Sil.:* over the left orbit—*Spig.*)

Headache every seventh day (*Ars., Gels., Iris, Lac-D., Lyc., Nux-M., Phos., Psor., Sil., Sulph., Tub.*) (A.).

PAINS IN THE HEAD INCREASE AND DE-CREASE WITH THE SUN (*Acon., Glon., Kalm., Nat-M., Phos., Spig., Stann., Stram.*) (R.).

Headache ameliorated by voiding a large amount of urine (*Acon., Ferr-P., Gels., Ign., Kalm., Meli., Sil., Tereb., Verat.*) (R.).

The pains in the head are so severe that the patient can neither tolerate noise nor light and vomits everything, and buries the head in the pillow, or presses it on something hard (D.).

9

Facial neuralgia ameliorated by kneeling down and pressing the head firmly against the floor; pain extends in all directions from the upper jaw (A.).

Burning and rawness in the nose, with fluent coryza (*All-C., Arum-T., Ars., Nat-M., Rhus-T.*) (D.).

Humming and roaring in the ears (*Bell., Carb-S., Carb-V., Caust., Chin., Chin-S., Graph., Lyc., Nux-V., Phos., Puls., Sep., Sil., Spig., Sulph., Tab., Verat.*) (R.).

Nasal polypi (*Calc., Phos., Sil.*), *which tend to bleed easily* (D.).

Eruption on the face of young women, especially during scanty menses (*Bells, Calc., Eug-J., Psor.*) (A.).

Burning in the pharynx and œsophagus (*Asaf., Canth., Kreos., Merc-C.*) (A.).

Dyspnœa and desire to breathe deeply (*Bry., Cact., Calc., Ign., Lach., Nat-S., Sel., Sulph.*) (R.).

EXCESSIVE DYSPNOEA (*Ant-T., Ars., Brom., Carb-V., Dig., Hydr-Ac., Lach., Lyc., Nat-P., Phos., Samb., Sulph., Verat.*) (Bt.).

Tough, rusty-coloured sputa, in the second and third stages of pneumonia (*Phos.*) (Bt.).

BREATH AND SPUTA SMELL BAD, EVEN TO THE PATIENT (*Ars., Caps., Chin., Lach., Puls.*) (Bt.).

Hacking cough, evenings after lying down, from tickling in the throat (*Ars., Hyos., Rumx.*) (R.).

Cough with expectoration of thick, blood-streaked mucus (*Ars., Bry., Ferr., Phos., Sabin., Sep., Sulph-Ac., Zinc.*) (R.).

Cough day and night with great emaciation (N.).

Dry cough, ameliorated by sitting up in bed and discharging flatus upward and downward (R.).

Hæmoptysis (*Bell., Cact., Ferr-P.*) (R.).

Phthisis florida (*Ferr-P., Phos.*) (D.).

Asthma after the " rose cold," aggravated from odours (A.).

The cough returns every-time the patient takes cold (*Hep., Tub.*) (A.).

Burning in the chest (*Phos., Sulph.*) (D.).

Heat and tension behind sternum (N.).

Congestion of the lungs with bright red face and flushing of one or both cheeks (*Ferr-P.*) (D.).

Sharp, stitching pains through the right lung (*Bry.*) (D.).

RHEUMATIC PAIN IN THE RIGHT ARM AND SHOULDER (*Fluor-Ac.;* left arm and shoulder—*Rhus-T.*); CANNOT RAISE THE ARM (*Bry., Calc., Ferr.*); WORSE AT NIGHT (*Bell., Calc., Caust., Kali-B., Merc., Phos., Sil.*) (A.).

Great susceptibility to odours, which causes the patient to faint (*Ign., Nux-V., Phos.*) (D.).

Faintness from odours of flowers (*Phos.;* from odours of fish—*Colch.;* from odours of cooking food—*Colch., Ipec.*) (K.).

Flatulent distension of the stomach (*Carb-V., Chin., Lyc., Nux-V., Puls.*) (D.).

Flushes of heat and leucorrhœa, during the climacteric (*Lach., Sep., Sulph.*) (A.).

Painful enlargement of breasts (*Bry., Puls.*) (A.).

Sharp, stitching pains (*Kali-B., Kali-C., Nit-Ac., Sil.*), with soreness and stiffness of muscles (*Rhus-T.*) (D.).

Sudden stopping of catarrh of the respiratory tract followed by diarrhœa (*Sel.*) (Br.).

Afternoon fever with circumscribed red cheeks, 2 to 3 P.M. daily; burning of palms and soles; cough and expectoration (N.).

Ozæna, with profuse, offensive, 'yellowish discharge (*Hydr., Kali-I., Sep., Sil.*) (Br.).

Aversion to butter (*Ars., Carb-V., Chin., Cycl., Mag-C., Merc., Phos., Ptel., Puls.*) (Br.).

Craving for piquant things (Br.).

Unquenchable thirst (*Ars., Eup-P., Phos., Sulph., Verat.*) (Br.).

Deathly nausea, in paroxysms (*Ant-T.*), with much salivation (C.).

Vertigo: In the morning on rising from a sitting or stooping position, on quickly turning the head, or from looking upward (C.).

AGGRAVATION: During the climacteric; periodically; every week; from lying down; from motion; at night; with the sun; from odours; from light; from looking up; and from raising the arm.

AMELIORATION: From sleep; from voiding a large amount of urine; from vomiting; in the darkness; from sitting up; from eructation; in the cool air; and from passing flatus.

RELATIONSHIP: *Sang.* is the chronic of *Bell.* and may be used after *Bell.* when it fails in scarlatina.

Complementary: *Ant-T.* and *Phos.*

Sanicula.

COMMON NAME: MINERAL SPRING WATER.
Especially useful in sweaty-headed children with defective assimilation (*Calc., Sil.*).

Marasmus (*Abrot., Calc-P., Lyc., Nat-M., Op., Sil., Sulph.*) (B.).

Progressive emaciation (*Iod., Nat-M.*) (A.).

Child kicks off covers at night (*Sulph.*) (B.).

Profuse, scaly dandruff on the scalp, eyebrows and in the beard (A.).

LOOKS OLD AND THIN (*Arg-N., Lyc., Op.*) (B.).

Child looks dirty, greasy and brownish; skin about neck wrinkled, hangs in folds (*Abrot., Iod., Nat-M., Sars.*) (A.).

Soreness behind ears, with discharge of white, gray, viscid fluid (*Graph., Psor.*) (A.).

Ringworm on the tongue (*Nat-M.*) (A.).

Tongue large, flabby, burning; must protrude it to keep it cool (A.).

Body smells like old cheese (*Psor.*) (B.).

The odour of stool follows despite bathing (*Sulph.*) (A.).

Stubborn and touchy (*Ant-C., Bry., Cham., Cina, Nat-M.*) (B.).

Dread of downward motion (*Bor., Gels., Stram.*) (A.).

Child headstrong, obstinate, cries and kicks (*Bell., Lyc., Stram., Verat-V.*); *cross, irritable, does not want to be touched* (*Ant-C., Bell., Bry., Cham., Cina, Kali-C., Lach., Nux-V., Sil., Stram., Tarant.*) (A.).

Alternately laughing and crying (*Ign., Nux-M., Puls.*) (A.).

Constantly changing his occupation (A.).

SYMPTOMS CONSTANTLY CHANGING (*Lac-C., Puls.*).

Nausea and vomiting from riding in a car (*Cocc., Nux-M., Petr., Sulph., Tab.*) (Bl.).

Sea-sickness (*Cocc., Colch., Con., Kreos., Nux-V., Petr., Sep., Tab., Ther.*) (Bl.).

Water is vomited as soon as it reaches the stomach (*Ars., Phos.*) (A.).

Drinks little and often (*Ars.*) (A.).

Craves bacon (*Calc-P., Ench., Mezer., Tub.*), *or ice-cold milk* (*Phos., Rhus-T., Tub.*) (B.).

LOSES FLESH WHILE EATING WELL (*Acet-Ac., Abrot., Iod., Nat-M., Tub.*).

The stool is of such immense size that it cannot be discharged without mechanical aid (*Sel.*) (N.).

The little fellow strains and strains, the stools partly protruding and then slipping back again (*Sil., Thuj.*) (N.).

NO TWO STOOLS ALIKE (*Podo., Puls., Sulph.*) (N.).

The stools are large and painful, as though they would rupture the perineum (*Bry., Nat-M., Sulph.*) (Bl.).

Cold clammy hands and feet (*Bar-C., Calc., Carb-V., Sil.*) (B.).

Head and neck sweat profusely during sleep, wetting the pillow far around (*Calc., Sil.*) (A.).

FOUL FOOT-SWEAT (*Bar-C., Graph., Kali-C., Lyc., Nit-Ac., Puls., Sil., Tell., Thuj.*) (B.).

Excoriation of skin about the anus (*Sulph.*), covering perineum and extending to genitals (A.).

No desire for stool until a large accumulation (*Anac., Bry., Nat-M., Op., Sulph.*) (A.).

Stool hard, impossible to evacuate; of grayish-white balls, like burnt lime; crumbling from the verge of anus (*Mag-M.*) (A.).

Diarrhœa, changeable in charac.er and colour; like scrambled eggs; frothy, grass-green; turns green on standing; like scum of a frog pond; after eating, must hurry from the table (A.).

Incontinence of urine and fæces; sphincter unreliable (*Aloe, Sulph.*); urging from flatus; must cross the legs to prevent fæces escaping (A.).

BURNING OF THE SOLES OF FEET; MUST UNCOVER OR PUT THEM IN A COOL PLACE (*Lach., Med., Sang., Sulph.*) (A.).

Leucorrhœa with strong odour of fish-brine (A.).

Weakness, with bearing down, as if contents of the pelvis would escape; worse from walking, misstep or jar, and ameliorated by rest or lying down; desire to support parts by placing hand against the vulva (*Lil-T., Murx.*) (A.).

Soreness of the uterus (*Arn., Bell., Lach.*) (A.).

AGGRAVATION: At night; from downward motion; from touch; from riding in a carriage; from drinking; after eating and from walking.

AMELIORATION: From cold; from uncovering; from rest; and from lying down.

RELATIONSHIP: *Similar to: Abrot., Aloe, Alum., Ars., Bor., Calc., Graph., Lac-C., Lach., Lyc., Murx., Nat-M., Psor., Sil., Sulph., Tell., Thuj., Tub.*

Sarracenia Purpurea.

COMMON NAME: PITCHER PLANT.

This remedy is indicated in variola; it aborts the disease and prevents pustulation (Bl.).

Photophobia (*Acon., Bell., Euphr., Nat-M., Phos., Sulph.*) (Br.).

Black objects move with the eye (*Cocc., Phos., Stram.*) (Br.).

Pain in the orbits (*Ruta*) (Br.).

Eyes feel swollen' and sore (*Arn.*) (Br.)

Bruised pain in the knees and hip-joints (*Arn.*) (Br.).

The head is congested (Bell., Glon., Stram.) (Bl.).

Sick headache (Bry., Nux-V., Sang.) (Br.).

Throbbing in various parts, especially in neck, shoulders and head, which feels full to bursting (Br.).

The limbs are weak (*Kali-P., Nat-M., Nux-V., Rhus-T.*) (Bl.).

Bad taste in the mouth, with loss of appetite (*Nux-V., Puls.*) (A.).

Brownish-white coating on the tongue (*Ant-T., Bapt., Bry., Chin-A., Hyos., Kali-P., Lach., Phos., Plb., Rhus-T., Sec.*) (A.).

Hungry all the time, even after a meal (Chin-S., Cina, Iod., Lyc., Phos.) (Br.).

Copious, painful vomiting (*Ant-T., Ars., Cup-S., Phos., Verat.*) (Br.).

Horripilations between shoulder-blades in the afternoon or evening (A.).

General chills between the shoulder-blades (*Caps., Eup-Purp., Led., Polyp.*) (A.).

Fever with heat and redness of the face, burning in the stomach, great prostration, delirium and loss of consciousness (A.).

Copious night-sweat (*Chin.*) (A.).

AGGRAVATION: From light; at night; in the evening; and after meals.

AMELIORATION: From lying down.

RELATIONSHIP: *Compare*: *Ant-T., Bell., Bry., Cocc., Glon., Hyos., Maland., Nux-V., Rhus-T., Sil., Sulph.,* and *Variol.*

Sarsaparilla.

COMMON NAME: SARSAPARILLA.

Useful in periosteal pain due to syphilis (*Asaf., Aur., Mezer.*) (Bl.).

Headache and periosteal pains from mercury, syphilis, or suppressed gonorrhœa (A.).

Dry, itch-like eruptions, prone to appear in the spring; become crusty (A.).

Herpetic eruptions on all parts of the body (A.).

Eruptions following vaccination (*Sil.*) (Bt.).

Eruptions looking like the roseola of syphilis and itching intolerably (*Merc.*) (D.).

Eruptions exuding an irritating pus (*Calc-S., Merc., Rhus-T.*) (D.).

USEFUL IN MARASMUS; THE NECK IS GREATLY EMACIATED AND THE SKIN ALL OVER THE BODY LIES IN FOLDS (D.).

Itching eruption on forehead during menses (*Eug-J., Psor., Sang.*) (A.).

Skin hard, indurated (*Ant-C., Ars., Graph., Rhus-T., Sep.*) (A.).

Skin cracked on hands and feet (*Graph.*, *Petr.*) (A.).

RETRACTION OF NIPPLES (*Carb-An.*, *Con.*, *Cund.*, *Nux-M.*, *Sil.*) (K.).

Nipples are small, withered, unexcitable (*Sil.*) (A.).

Intolerable *stench* on genital organs (A.).

Bloody seminal emissions (*Led.*, *Merc.*) (A.).

Excruciating pains from the right kidney downwards (*Lyc.*) (A.).

Gonorrhœa checked by cold, wet wea.her, or mercury, followed by rheumatism (A.).

Child screams before and while passing urine (*Bor.*, *Lyc.*) (A.).

Hæmorrhage from the urethra after urination (*Hep.*, *Mezer.*, *Puls.*, *Sulph.*, *Thuj.*, *Zinc.*) (K.).

URINE DRIBBLES WHILE SITTING, PASSES FREELY WHILE STANDING (*Con.*) (A.).

CAN ONLY PASS URINE WHILE STANDING (*Hyper.*) (K.).

Painful distension and tenderness in the bladder (*Apis*, *Bell.*, *Canth.*) (A.).

Urine deposits white sediment (*Berb.*, *Graph.*, *Kreos.*, *Phos.*, *Rhus-T.*, *Sep.*) (A.).

Excessive pain in the urethra, which may run back into the abdomen (G.).

Urine passes, toward the end, mingled with blood, after which the pain abates (G.).

IS INDICATED IN RENAL COLIC, WHEN THERE IS A SHOWER OF SMALL, LIGHT COLOURED CALCULI, AND MOST EXCRUCIATING PAIN AT THE CLOSE OF URINATION (Bl.).

Frequent discharge of pale copious urine (*Kali-P.*, *Merc.*, *Nat-M.*, *Phos-Ac.*, *Sulph.*) (Bt.).

Urine passes in thin, feeble stream (*Clem.*) (Br.).

MUCH PAIN AT THE CONCLUSION OF PASSING URINE; ALMOST UNBEARABLE WITH WOMEN (*Berb.*, *Equis.*, *Med.*, *Thuj.*) (G.).

Turbid, scanty, slimy, clayey, and sandy urine (Bt.).

He has to get up two or three times in the night to urinate (*Bar-C., Lyc., Merc., Phos-Ac., Sulph.*) (Hr.).

Bloody urine (*Canth., Merc-C.*) (A.).

WHITE SAND IN THE URINE (*Am-C., Aspar., Bell., Benz-Ac., Calc., Canth., Carb-V., Chin., Chin-S., Eup-Pur., Nat-M., Nat-S., Nit-Ac., Phos., Sec., Zinc.*) (N.).

Cystitis (*Bell., Canth., Merc-C.*) (C.).

Moist eruption about genitals (*Crot-T., Graph., Petr., Rhus-T.*) (D.).

Herpes preputialis (*Graph., Petr.*).

Rheumatic pain, worse at night (*Aur., Merc., Nit-Ac.*), *in damp weather* (*Dulc., Nat-S., Rhus-T.*), *or after taking cold water* (A.).

Sensation as of tight band around the head and forehead, which is pery painful (G.).

Belching of wind (*Carb-V., Lyc., Nux-V., Puls.*) (G.).

Very sore, gouty nodes (*Colch.*) (B.).

Backache with colic (*Lyc., Nux V.*) (B.).

Chill starts from the region of bladder (B.).

Desponden., sensitive, easily offended, ill-humoured and taciturn (Br.).

Aphthæ (*Bor., Kali-M., Lach., Merc., Nat-M., Nux-V., Rhus-T., Sil.*) (Br.).

Salivation (*Kali-B., Merc., Nat-M.*) (Br.).

Metallic taste in the mouth (*Merc., Plb.*) (Br.).

AGGRAVATION: In spring; at conclusion of urination; at night; in damp weather; during menses and from yawning.

AMELIORATION: From standing and from uncovering neck or chest

RELATIONSHIP: Frequently called for after the abuse of mercury.

Compare: *Abrot., Bar-C., Berb., Bor., Canth., Eug-J., Equis., Iod., Led., Lyc., Med., Merc., Psor., Nat-M., Op., Phos., Sang., Sep., Sil., Sulph., Thuj.*

Complementary: *Merc.* and *Sep.* (either of this follows it well).

Antidotes: *Bell.* and *Merc.*

✗ Secale Cornutum.

COMMON NAME: ERGOT.

Particularly useful in tall, scrawny women of lax muscular fibre, feeble, cachectic, or very old decrepit persons (N.).

Varicose ulcers wonderfully cured by the action of this medicine.

Spasmodic tension in the limbs, relieved by violent stretching of them.

Burning in all parts as from sparks falling on them (*Ars.*).

Convulsive twitching of the limbs mostly at night (*Ars., Calc., Phos.*).

Limbs feel as if beaten (*Arn., Bapt.*).

Drawing and tearing in the limbs with tingling (*Acon., Bell., Carb-V., Cupr., Graph., Lyc., Rhus-T.*).

Numbness of the limbs (*Agar., Arg-M., Arg-N., Carb-S., Carb-V., Cocc., Gels., Graph., Guai., Lyc., Nux-M., Op., Ox-Ac., Rhus-T.*).

Great debility (*Ars., Chin., Kali-P.*).

Spasms after fright (*Acon., Arg-N., Bufo, Calc., Cupr., Hyos., Ign., Indg., Kali-Br., Lyss., Op., Plat., Stram., Sulph., Verat., Zinc.*).

Senile, dry gangrene, aggravated by external heat (A.).

Anæmic conditions (*Chin., Ferr., Graph., Nat-M., Phos., Puls.*) (D.).

GANGRENE (*Ars., Carb-V., Kali-P., Lach.*).

Petechiæ (*Arn., Bapt., Ham.*) (D.).

Skin shrivelled, dry and brittle. Formication, black suppurating blisters, petechiæ; feels better from cold applications (D.).

Sensation of something creeping under skin (*Acon., Phos.*) (N.).

Heat applied to any part of the body aggravates his pains; extreme aversion to being covered (N.).

GREAT OBJECTIVE COLDNESS, BUT GREATLY AGGRAVATED BY COVERING (*Carb-V.*) (N.).

Passive hæmorrhage; everything open and loose; no action; in thin, scrawny, cachectic, women (N.).

Complains of an empty feeling in the abdomen (*Phos., Sep., Sulph.*) (D.).

Cold, dry and livid tongue (*Carb-V.*) (Ra.).

HICCOUGH (*Cic., Cycl., Hyos., Ign., Iod.*) (K.).

Disgust for food, meat and fats (A.).

Craves lemonade (*Bell., Calc., Cycl., Eup-Pur., Jatr., Nit-Ac., Puls., Sab., Sulph-I.*) *and acids* (*Ant-T., Ars., Bry., Calc., Ferr-P., Hep.*) (A.).

UNNATURAL, RAVENOUS APPETITE; EVEN WITH EXHAUSTING DIARRHOEA HE IS HUNGRY (*Aloe, Iod., Petr., Sulph., Verat.*) (A.).

Anus wide open with diarrhœa (*Apis, Phos.*)

Profuse, watery, putrid, brown stools, discharged with great force (*Gamb., Grat.*) (A.).

Putrid, fœtid, and colliquative diarrhœa (*Ars., Bapt., Carb-V., Kali-P., Lach.*) (G.).

Involuntary diarrhœa (*Aloe, Kali-P., Nat-S., Podo., Sulph.*) (Bt.).

Asiatic cholera (*Acon., Ars., Bism., Camph., Canth., Carb-V., Cic., Cupr., Ipec., Kali-P., Lach., Phos., Podo., Sulph., Tereb., Verat.*).

Retching and vomiting of undigested food, body wasted and cold, cramps, tingling in the limbs, face sunken, mouth distorted; profuse painless discharge from the bowels, ejected with violence; cold clammy sweat (D.).

Cholera infantum; great debility; vomiting and diarrhœa; much thirst; pale face; sunken eyes; dry heat; quick pulse; restless and sleepless, don't want to be covered (N.).

Suppression of urine (*Apis, Bell., Canth., Merc-C., Stram., Tereb.*) (Ra.).

Enuresis of old people (*Lyc., Op., Sep.*) (A.).

Quiet delirium, or grows wild with great anxiety, and a constant desire to get out of bed (*Hyos., Stram.*) (G.).

Laboured and anxious respiration (*Ant-T., Ars., Kali-P., Lach., Naja*) (G.).

Paralysis of the limbs, with convulsive jerks and shocks in the paralyzed limbs (Hm.).

Moles, polypi, and morbid growths in the uterus, with prolonged forcing pains (Bt.).

Prolapsus uteri (*Nat-M., Nux-V., Puls., Sep.*) (Bt.).

EXCESSIVE MENSTRUATION (*Calc., Chin., Ferr., Lach.. Phos., Sab., Sep.*) (Bt.).

Green, brown and offensive leucorrhœa (*Nit-Ac.*) (A.).

Leucorrhœa, jelly-like, alternating with metrorrhagia (Bt.).

After-pains too long and too painful, with hour-glass contraction (A.).

Threatened abortion, especially at the third month (*Apis, Cimic., Croc., Eup-Pur., Merc., Sabin., Thuj., Ust.*) (A.).

Continuous discharge of watery blood until the next menstrual period (A.).

IS INDICATED IN LABOUR WHEN THE PAINS ARE PROLONGED, CONTINUED AND INEFFECTUAL, OR ENTIRELY WANTING (D.).

LABOUR-PAINS ARE WEAK, SUPPRESSED, OR DISTRESSING IN WEAK, CACHECTIC WOMEN (N.).

Uterine hæmorrhage; passive painless flow of dark liquid blood; the patient is wrinkled and scrawny, is often unconscious and cold; hæmorrhages preceded by formication and tingling (D.).

Copious flow of black liquid blood, worse from the slightest movement, with convulsive motions (*abortion*) (N.).

Hæmorrhage, with spasmodic contractions; every discharge of blood is preceded by a violent, painful contraction of the u.erus, or by distressing bearing down pains (G.).

METRORRHAGIA (*Bell., Calc., Chin., Croc., Crot-H., Ferr., Ham., Ipec., Kali-Fer., Lach., Mill., Murx., Nit-Ac., Nux-V., Phos., Plat., Psor., Puls., Rat., Sab., Tril., Ust.*).

Metritis; great prostration, extremities cold; frequent vomiting; the blood discharged from the uterus is fluid, mingled with dark, badly-smelling coagula (Bt.).

Lochia very offensive and thin; discharge scanty or profuse; may be painless, or accompanied by prolonged bearing down pains (G.).

Failure of lactation (*Agn., Calc., Caust., Dulc., Ign., Lac-C., Lac-D., Puls., Urt-U.*) (G.).

Puerperal convulsions in scrawny, ill-nourished women, with too feeble labour-pains (Bt.).

INSUFFICIENT LABOUR-PAINS (*Caul., Puls.*).

Risus sardonicus (*Phyt.*) (C.).

Boils small, painful, with green contents; mature very slowly and heal in the same manner (*Merc.*) (A.).

HAEMORRHAGIC DIATHESIS; THE SLIGHTEST WOUND CAUSES BLEEDING FOR WEEKS (*Lach., Phos.*) (A.).

Discharge of sanious, liquid blood, with a strong tendency to putrescence (A.).

WANTS ABDOMEN TO BE UNCOVERED (*Tab.*) (B.).

Burning in the stomach and abdomen (*Ars., Carb-V., Lach., Lyc., Phos., Sulph.*) (Br.).

Locomotor ataxia; trembling staggering gait (*Alum., Nux-V., Zinc.*) (Br.).

Roaring in the ears, with great difficulty in hearing (*Calc., Merc., Phos-Ac., Sulph.*) (C.).

Violent, shaking chill followed by violent heat with anxiety, delirium and almost unquenchable thirst. *Intense icy coldness of the skin, particularly of the face and extremities. Cold limbs, cold skin, with shivering* (A.).

Severe, long-lasting dry heat, with great restlessness and violent thirst (Ars., Nat-M., Rhus-T.) (A.).

Cold, clammy sweat over the whole body (A.).

Pulse small, rapid, contracted, and often intermittent (A.).

Congestive headache, the pain extending from the back of the neck and occiput all over the head (*Sil.*) (Bl.).

CRAMPS IN HANDS, LEGS AND FEET (*Cupr., Verat.*) (B.).

FINGERS SPREAD APART (reverse of *Cupr.*) (B.).

AGGRAVATION: From warm covering; from hot application; from drawing up the limbs; during pregnancy; during menses; and from loss of fluids.

AMELIORATION: From uncovering; from rubbing; in the cold air; from stretching out the limbs; after vomiting; from cold; and from bathing.

RELATIONSHIP: Resembles *Ars., Carb-V., Colch., Kali-P., Phos., Sulph.* and *Verat.* in cholera morbus, and Cholera Asiatica.

Similar to: Ars., but cold and heat are opposite.

Compare: Cinnamon. in post-partum hæmorrhage; it increases labour-pains, controls profuse or dangerous flooding, is always safe, while *Ergot* is not infrequently dangerous.

Antidotes: Camph., Op. and *Sol-N.*

Selenium.

COMMON NAME: SELENIUM.

Great aversion to air draughts, and from the same easily catching cold (also tearing in the limbs).

Pruritus of the hands, with violent itching in the palms (*Anac., Caust., Sulph.*).

Great emaciation, especially of hands, face and thighs (*Abrot., Sars., Sil.*).

WEAKNESS FOLLOWING PROLONGED FEVER (K.).

Easy fatigue from any exertion or labour (*Ars., Calc., Kali-P.*) (D.).

Easily debilitated by the heat of the sun (*Lach., Nat-C., Nat-M.*) (B.).

Nervous exhaustion caused by seminal loss (*Con., Gels., Kali-P., Lyc., Phos-Ac., Sulph., Zinc.*) (D.).

Paralytic weakness of the spine (*Cocc., Gels., Kali-P., Pic-Ac., Sep.*) (D.).

Giddiness with nausea and vomiting and faintness, worse when moving (*Bry.*).

Hungry at night (*Cina, Phos., Psor.*) (A.).

After sleep, especially on warm days when he is most inclined to it, an aggravation of the symptoms.

A little mental or physical exertion makes him sleepy (B.).

Irresistible desire for stimulants; wants to get drunk, but feels worse after it (N.).

PULSATION IN THE ABDOMEN AFTER EATING (*Cahin.*) (K.).

Irresistible longing for spirituous liquors (*Ars., Asar., Caps., Crot-H., Lach., Nux-V., Sulph.*) (N.).

DESIRE FOR ALCOHOLIC DRINKS, BEFORE MENSES (K.).

Bad effects from drinking too much tea (*Puls.*); all complaints are aggravated by it (N.).

Coryza ending in diarrhœa (*Sang.*) (B.).

CONSTIPATION (*Anac., Bry., Calc., Graph., Hydr., Ign., Kali-M., Lyc., Mag-M., Nat-M., Op., Phos., Sep., Sulph., Thuj., Verat.*).

VERY LARGE STOOL (*Bry., Nat-M., Sulph.*) (B.).

Constipation after serious illness, especially enteric fever (A.).

Stool is of such immense size that it cannot be discharged without mechanical aid (*Sanic.*); it must be picked away with the fingers (N.).

Involuntary dribbling of urine while walking, or after urinating or stool (Urine dribbles while sitting—*Sars.*) (N.).

Hard stools, with blood at end (*Nat-M.*) (C.).

Sediment in the urine of red sand (*Arn., Ars., Arund., Berb., Caust., Dig., Lob., Lyc., Merc-C., Ocim., Pareir., Phos., Plan., Senec., Sep., Tarant*).

Nocturnal pollutions (*Calc., Dios., Gels., Kali-P., Lyc., Nux-V., Phos-Ac.*) (G.).

Spermatorrhœa (*Agn., Calc., Gels., Graph., Kali-P., Lyc., Merc., Nat-M., Phos., Phos-Ac., Sep., Sulph.*) (G.).

IMPOTENCE WITH VOLUPTUOUSNESS (*Ign., Lyc., Phos., Sulph.*).

Secondary gonorrhœa (*Agn., Calc., Dig., Graph., Hep., Kali-S., Lyc., Merc., Nat-S., Puls., Sep., Thuj.*).

ESCAPE OF SEMINAL FLUIDS, PARTICULAR-LY WHEN STRAINING AT STOOL (*Anac., Carb-V., Caust., Con., Gels., Nat-M., Petr., Phos-Ac., Sep., Sil., Sulph.*) (G.).

The system is so relaxed that the semen dribbles away (*Gels.*) (D.).

Watery semen (*Nat-M., Sulph.*) (B.).

ERECTIONS ARE SLOW AND WEAK, EMIS-SIONS OF SEMEN TOO RAPID IN COITION AND HE IS CROSS AND WEAK AFTERWARDS (N.).

SEXUAL DESIRE STRONG, BUT HE IS PHYSI-CALLY IMPOTENT (*Con., Phos.*) (N.).

Has seminal emission two or three times a weak (*Nux-V., Phos., Phos-Ac., Sulph.*), and gets up with weak, lame back after them (N.).

10

Prostatic fluid oozes while sitting, during sleep, when walking, or at stool (N.).

Headache: Of drunkards; after debauchery; after lemonade or wine; every afternoon (A.).

Hair falls off from the head, eye-brows, whiskers, or genitals (A.).

After typhoid great weakness of the spine; fears paralysis (*Kali-P.*) (A.).

Weak, easily exhausted; from either mental or physical labour; after typhoid, typhus, or debauchery (A.).

IRRESISTIBLE DESIRE TO LIE DOWN AND SLEEP; STRENGTH SUDDENLY LEAVES HIM; ESPECIALLY IN HOT WEATHER (A.).

Vertigo, as if intoxicated (*Agar., Gels., Nux-V., Stram.*) (C.).

Extreme sadness (*Aur., Ign., Nat-M., Puls., Sep., Stann.*) (Br.).

Abject despair (*Ars., Aur., Psor.*).

Hiccough while smoking (*Ambr., Arg-M., Calad., Ign., Lach., Puls., Sep., Staph., Sulph-Ac., Verat.*) (Br.).

Forgetful, especially in business; but when lying half asleep, everything recurs to him (C.).

Liver painful and enlarged (*Chel., Chin., Hep., Nux-V., Sep.*) (Br.).

Greasy, shining skin of face (*Bar-C., Bry., Chin., Mag-C., Merc., Nat-M., Plb., Psor., Rhus-T., Tub.*) (C.).

STITCHES OVER THE LEFT EYE (*Lac-F., Kali-I., Ptel., Sep.*).

Headaches due to excessive use of tea (*Chin., Lach., Sep., Thuj., Verat.*; tea ameliorates headache—*Cimic., Ferr-P., Kali-B.*) (D.).

Headache over the left eye, worse from the heat of the sun (heat of stove aggravates—*Arn.*) (D.).

Falling off of hair (*Lyc., Nat-M., Sulph.*) (B.).

Aphonia after long use of voice (*Phos.*) (A.).

Voice hoarse, as soon as he sings. (*Agar.*, *Arg-N.*, *Arum-T.*, *Caust.*, *Stann.*) (B.).

Tubercular laryngitis (*Calc.*, *Phos.*) (A.).

Hawks up clear mucus (*Arg-M.*, *Nat-M.*, *Stann.*) (B.).

Hoarseness, must often clear the throat of mucus, especially at the beginning of singing (N.).

Sweats profuse, yellow; leaves a salty deposit; stiffens the linen, or makes the hair stiff (B.).

Throbbing in vessels of the whole body (*Glon.*, *Nat-M.*, *Sep.*) (C.).

AGGRAVATION: After stool; while or after talking; from walking in the open air; from taking lemonade; while drinking tea; from taking wine; during hot days; in the sun; from sexual excesses; from loss of sleep; from draughts; after sleep; every afternoon; and from singing.

AMELIORATION: After sunset; from inhaling cool air; and from taking cold water in the mouth.

RELATIONSHIP: *Chin.* aggravates the symptoms greatly—makes them insupportable.

Antidotes: *Ign.* and *Puls.*

Follows well after: *Calad.*, *Nat-M.*, *Phos-Ac.* and *Staph.* in sexual weakness.

Itch checked by mercurials or sulphur often requires *Selen.*

Senega.

COMMON NAME: SNAKE ROOT.

Especially valuable with old people, but works well with others (N.).

Great bodily and mental debility, with stretching of the limbs and accompanied with heaviness and dullness of the head (*Rhus-T.*).

Great weakness, which seems to come from and of the chest.

Many symptoms, especially those of the chest, are aggravated during rest, and are relieved by walking in the open air.

Fainting while walking in the open air (*Lycps., Sep.*; while in close room—*Acon., Asaf., Ipec., Lach., Tab.*).

Wounds from the bites of poisonous animals (*Ars., Led.*).

Diseases of the mucous membranes (*Bry., Carb-V., Hydr., Nat-S., Puls.*).

Angina mucosa.

BRONCHITIS (*Ant-T., Bry., Hep., Kali-C., Kali-M., Lyc., Nat-S., Phos., Rhus-T., Sil.*).

Inflammation of the lungs (*Ant-T., Bry., Chel., Ferr-P., Lyc., Phos.*).

Hoarseness (*Arg-N., Calc., Carb-V.*).

Dry, scraping sensation in the pharynx (*Aesc., Nux-V.*).

Throat so dry that it hurts to talk (*Phos.*) (D.).

GREAT ACCUMULATION OF ALBUMINOUS MUCUS ON THE CHEST, WHICH IS DIFFICULT TO EXPECTORATE (*Ant-T., Kali-M.*) (D.).

MUCH RATTLING, WHEEZING AND DIFFI-CULT BREATHING (*Ant-T., Carb-V., Nat-S.*) (N.).

Cough: Incessant; strangling; choking; ends in sneezing; worse from lying on the right side, or in the evening (B.).

Sneezes, until dizzy (B.).

Nausea continuously (*Ant-T., Ipec., Tab.*).

Dullness of the head, with pressure and weakness of the eyes (*Nat-M.*) (N.).

Feeling as though the thorax were too narrow, with constant inclination to widen it (*Cact., Ign., Phos.*) (N.).

Emphysema (*Am-C., Ant-Ars., Ant-T., Hep.*) (Bl.).

Great burning in the chest, either before or after coughing (G.).

Sensation as of a crushing weight on the chest (B.).

Soreness of the walls of the chest on moving the arms, particularly the left, with much rattling of mucus in the chest (Be.).

Bronchiectasis (*Caps., Chin., Sang.*) (Bl.).

Adynamic pneumonia (*Ant-T., Carb-V., Lyc.*) (Bt.).

Useful in sub-acute or chronic exudations of the pleura, and in catarrhal pleuro-pneumonia, where *Bry.* has failed **(Ha.).**

Boring pain about the heart (Bc.).

Blood-tinged or albuminous expectoration (B.).

Vocal cords partially paralyzed (*Caust., Phos.*) (Br.).

Menses come too soon (*Calc., Ferr., Mill., Sab.*).

Has been administered with great success in hydrothorax ascites and anasarca, after primary or secondary albuminuria (Ha.).

Sensation of trembling, with no visible trembling (*Sulph-Ac.*) (Bt.).

Watery diarrhœa, with griping pains in the bowels, nausea and vomiting (*Coloc., Dios., Nux-V.*) (Bt.).

Watery stools, spurting from the anus (*Crot-T., Grat., Thuj.*) (C.).

The urinary secretions are diminished (*Apis, Berb., Canth., Dig., Eup-P., Ferr-P., Gels., Lyc., Merc.*)

Urine at first mixed with mucous filaments; afterwards it becomes thick and cloudy (J.).

Frequent urination, with greenish tinge, depositing a cloudy sediment (Hn.).

Gnawing pain in the left side at the waist.

Iritis and specks on the cornea (Hg.).

Is of service in muscular asthenopia and opacities of the vitreous humour (Bl.).

Objects look shaded (*Chin., Cycl., Gels., Merc., Phos., Puls., Sulph., Zinc.*) (Bl.).

Double vision (*Bell., Gels., Stram.*) (Bl.).

Eyeballs feel distended (B.).

Burning in the eyes when reading or writing (*Cob., Lil-T., Nat-Ars., Nat-C., Nat-M., Rhod., Zinc.*) (C.).

Blepharitis (*Bor., Caust., Graph., Petr.*) (C.).

Cilia hang full of hard mucus (C.).

Paralytic feeling in the left half of the face (*Rhus-T.*) (C.).

Pressure below the pit of the stomach (C.).

Deranged digestion (*Carb-V., Chin., Ferr., Graph., Hep., Iris, Kali-C., Lyc., Nux-M., Nux-V., Puls.*) (C.).

AGGRAVATION: In the evening; during rest; from looking fixedly at an object for a long time; in the open air; from inhaling cold air; from pressure; from touch; and at night.

AMELIORATION: From motion; from bending head backwards; and from sweat.

RELATIONSHIP: *Antidotes*: *Arn., Bell., Bry.,* and *Camph.*

Remedies following: *Calc., Lyc., Phos.,* and *Sulph.*

Sepia.

COMMON NAME: CUTTLE FISH.

Adapted to women with dark hair, rigid fibre, but mild and easy disposition, particularly during pregnancy, child-bed, or while nursing (N.).

Want of animal heat (*Sil.*).

The symptoms are relieved from violent exertions, but reappear most violently when sitting quietly in the forenoon and evening.

Painful sensitiveness of all parts of the body (*Bell., Lach.*).

Great sensitiveness to cold air (*Bell., Hep., Sil.*).

After getting wet, afterwards fainting spells and finally coryza.

General relaxation; weak; faints while kneeling at church (N.).

Dyspnœa, worse from sitting, after sleep, and in room, ameliorated by dancing or walking rapidly (N.).

Involuntary fits of laughter (*Bor., Cann-I., Ign., Nat-M., Phos.*) (G.).

Anxiety about real or imaginary evils (A.).

Greedy, miserly (*Ars., Lyc.*) (A.).

DULLNESS AND WANT OF INTEREST, ESPECIALLY IN THE FAMILY; ALSO LACK OF INTEREST IN HIS OCCUPATION (*Phos-Ac.*).

Irritable and easily offended (*Cham., Nux-V., Puls.*) (N.).

Weak memory (*Calc., Kali-P., Lyc., Nat-M., Phos., Sil.*) (N.).

Great sadness and weeping during menses, pregnancy or lactation (N.).

Dread of being alone (*Ars., Stram.*) (N.).

Bad effects from anger (*Bry., Ign., Nux-V., Staph., Stram.*).

Dread of meeting friends (N.).

Sense of helplessness and great susceptibility to excitement, and still more to terror (D.).

She dreads to be alone, wants company, but has an aversion to her own friends, and is indifferent to her household affairs (D.).

Indolent: Does not want to do anything, either work or play; even an exertion to think (A.).

The pain comes on in terrific shocks or jerks in the head (*Glon.*) (N.).

Pressing or bursting headache, worse from motion, stooping, and mental labour; ameliorated by pressure, or from continued fast motion (N.).

Headaches, commencing in the morning and, relieved by sleep or violent motion (D.).

Menstrual headache with scanty flow (*Bry., Graph., Kreos., Lyc., Nat-M.*) (B.).

Coldness of the vertex with headache (*Verat;* heat of the vertex—*Calc., Graph., Sulph.*) (A.).

Great falling off of the hair, after chronic headaches **or at** the climacteric (A.).

At night palpitation of the heart and pulsation through the whole body.

Loose cough in the morning, with efforts to vomit (G.).

Toothache after sweets (*Am-C., Nat-C., Phos.*) and from tea-drinking (*Chin., Coff., Ferr., Ign., Lach., Selen., Thuj.*) (K.).

Swelling and cracking of the lower lip (A.).

Coryza of a profuse character (*All-C., Ars., Nat-M., Puls., Sabad.*).

Paroxysms of spasmodic cough, ending in gagging or vomiting (*Ipec.*) (N.).

Affection of the middle right lung (N.).

Cough seeming to come from the stomach or abdomen (D.).

Cough with salty expectoration, and attended by stitches in the epigastrium (D.).

YELLOW SPOTS (MOTH SPOTS) IN THE FACE, AND A YELLOW SADDLE ACROSS THE UPPER PART OF CHEEKS AND NOSE (N.).

Drooping of the eye-lids (*Caust.*) (N.).

All the coverings of the neck felt too tight and were constantly loosened (*Lach.*) (A.).

Sour or putrid taste in the mouth (*Nux-V., Puls.*) (D.).

Toothache during pregnancy (*Lyss., Mag-C.*) (K.).

White coating on the root of the tongue only, strongly marked (N.).

Tongue foul, but becomes clear at each menstrual nisus, returns when flow ceases (A.).

Sensation of emptiness and debility in the stomach and abdomen (*Phos., Sulph.*).

Pulsation in the pit of the stomach (*Acon., Ant-T., Calc., Chin., Cic., Ferr., Glon., Kali-C., Nux-V., Phos., Puls., Sil.*).

Painful sense of emptiness or goneness at the pit of the stomach (*Carb-An.*) (N.).

NAUSEA AT THE SIGHT OR SMELL OF FOOD (*Colch.*) (D.).

Great longing for acids or pickles (*Hep.*) (D.).

Sensation of a lump in the stomach (D.).

Heaviness or sensation of a load in the abdomen, especially during motion (N.).

Pot-belliedness of mothers (of children—*Sulph.*).

Eructations like spoiled eggs or manure, with aversion to meat (G.).

Vomiting of bile (*Ars., Bry., Nat-S.*) (G.).

Inclination to vomit in the morning, when rinsing her mouth out (G.).

Morning sickness (*Nux-V., Puls.*) (G.).

CONSTIPATION DURING PREGNANCY (*Alum., Bry., Coll., Dol., Hydr., Lyc., Nat-S., Nux-V., Op., Plb., Plat., Podo., Puls., Sulph.*) (K.).

Pain in the rectum during and long after stool (*Nit-Ac., Sulph.*) (A.).

Constipation: Stools hard, difficult and knotty, with sense of weight or a lump in the anus, not relieved by an evacuation (N.).

No desire or urging for days and days; the stools are hard and large; inactivity of the rectum, and a sensation of a ball in it; patient cannot strain and consequently cannot expel stool (D.).

Diarrhœa from boiled milk (*Nux-M.*) (B.).

Intermittent fever with thirst during the chill only (*Apis, Ign.*).

Flushes of heat; heat ascends (N.).

Flushes of heat from least motion, with anxiety and faintness, followed by perspiration over the whole body (*Lach., Sang., Sulph.*) (A.).

Flushes of heat ascends from pelvic organs (A.).

Internal chilliness with external heat (*Ars., Nux-V.*) (G.).

COLDNESS OF THE EXTREMITIES DURING FEVER (*Carb-An., Kali-Ars., Stram.*) (K.).

Perspires easily (*Bry., Calc., Chin.*) (G.).

Single parts perspire profusely (*Puls.*) (G.).

Icy cold and damp feet all day, like standing in cold water up to ankles (*Lyc., Puls.*) (A.).

Feet hot at night (*Sulph.*) (A.).

Pains extend from other parts to the back (reverse of *Sab.*) *and are attended with shuddering* (with chilliness— *Puls.*) (A.).

Twitching in the muscles (*Cupr., Gels., Hyos., Kali-P., Lach., Nat-M.*).

Restlessness in all the limbs with anxiety, which does not permit him to remain quiet anywhere (*Ars., Kali-P., Phos., Rhus-T.*).

Twitching and jerking of the limbs night and day (*Tarant*).

Tension in the limbs, as if too short (*Am-M.*).

Restlessness and pulsation in all the limbs (*Ars., Chin-Ars., Ferr., Kali-C., Nat-Ars., Rhus-T., Sep., Zinc.*).

Stinging pain in the limbs (*Apis*).

Stiffness of the joints (hands, feet and knees).

Coldness of the legs and feet (*Calc., Dig., Lach.*).

Cold knees or heels (B.).

As the feet becomes hot the hands become cold (Bl.).

"The washer-woman's remedy," that is to say, com- *plaints are brought on by or aggravated after laundry work* (A).

Faints easily—after getting wet, from extremes of heat or cold, from riding in a carriage, or while kneeling at the church (A.).

Loud talking in sleep (*Bell., Hyos., Kali-C., Sulph.*) (B.).

Great sleepiness in the day-time, especially in the fore- noon (*Ant-C., Bism., Calc., Calc-P., Cann-S., Carb-An., Carb-V., Graph., Mag-M., Merc-Sulph., Mosch., Nat-C., Nat-P., Nux-V., Phos., Podo., Sabad., Thuj.* (C.).

Restless, unrefreshing sleep (C.)

Wakes at night in a fright, and screaming (*Bell., Stram.*) (C.).

Vesicular eruptions around mouth and chin (*Nat-M., Rhus-T.*) (D.).

Ringworms (*Ars., Nat-M., Sulph.*) (D.).

Liver spots on the chest and abdomen (D.).

Herpetic eruptions about the knees and ankles (*Petr.*) (D.).

Herpes circinatus in isolated spots on upper part of the body (in intersecting rings over the whole body—*Tell.*) (A.).

Itching of the skin, of various parts, of external genitals.

Skin yellow, like jaundice (*Chel., Iod., Merc., Nat-M., Phos., Sulph.*) (G.)

Salt-rheum (*Ars., Nat-M., Rhus-T.*) (G.).

Indolent ulcers, with itching, stinging and burning (C.).

SUPPRESSED MENSTRUATION (*Cycl., Ferr., Graph., Kali-P., Lach., Nat-M.*).

Prolapsus uteri complicated with indurations, ulcerations and profuse leucorrhœa (*Aur., Nat-M.*) (N.).

Yellowish leucorrhœa, with bearing down in the pelvic region (*Nat-M.*) (N.).

Pressure in the uterus downward, as if everything would fall out, with pain in the abdomen; feels as though she must cross her legs to prevent everything coming out (N.).

Left ovarian soreness and bearing down sensation in the uterus (*Lach.*).

Bearing down pains in the uterus, with a sense of lump or ball in the anus, not ameliorated by evacuation (N.).

Sense of fullness in the pelvic organs, and pressure down into the anus, as of a ball or weight; oozing of moisture (N.).

Violent stitches upward in the vagina (N.).

Discharge of a green-red fluid from the vagina during pregnancy (G.).

Ailments during pregnancy (Ars., Bry., Calc., Kali-C., Lyc., Merc-C., Nat-M., Phos., Sil.).

TENDENCY TO ABORT FIFTH TO SEVENTH MONTH (G.).

FLUSHES OF HEAT AND PERSPIRATION AT THE CLIMACTERIC (*Amyl-N., Graph., Lach., Sulph.*) (N.).

Flushes of heat over face and head (A.).

Enlargement and hardening of the uterus (*Aur., Am-M., Calc-F., Sil.*) (D.).

Offensive, excoriating lochia (*Kreos.*) (G.).

Lancinating pains from the uterus to the umbilicus (A.).

Sharp, clutching pains (in the uterus), as if clutched with a hand (D.).

Troublesome and severe itching of the vulva, with pimples all around (G.).

MENSES TOO LATE AND TOO SCANTY; OR TOO EARLY AND TOO PROFUSE (K.).

Weakness and tired pain in the small of back when walking (N.).

Aching and dull pain in the lumbar and sacral regions, extending to thighs and legs (N.).

Pain in the back and small of back, particularly with stiffness, improved by walking (N.).

Intense burning and cutting pain when urinating (*Canth.*) (Bt.).

URINE THICK, SLIMY, VERY OFFENSIVE, DEPOSITING A YELLOW OR PASTY SEDIMENT, WHICH SOMETIMES ADHERES TO THE VESSEL LIKE BURNT CLAY (N.).

CHILD ALWAYS WETS THE BED DURING THE FIRST SLEEP (*Benz-Ac., Caust., Cina, Kreos., Phos-Ac.*) (N.).

Irritable bladder (*Apis*, *Bell.*, *Canth.*, *Nux-V.*, *Puls.*) (D.).

Red sediment in the urine (*Lyc.*), which is acid and fetid (D.).

Weakness of sexual organs (*Calad.*, *Dig.*, *Gels.*, *Phos.*) (D.).

Discharge of prostatic juice (*Nat-M.*, *Nux-V.*, *Phos-Ac.*, *Sel.*, *Sulph.*) (G.).

Nocturnal pollutions (*Dios.*, *Gels.*, *Nux-V.*, *Phos-Ac.*) (G.).

GLEET, WITH SCANTY DISCHARGE IN THE MORNING ONLY (D.).

MEATUS GLUED TOGETHER IN THE MORN-ING (*Canth.*, *Phos.*, *Thuj.*) (A.).

Painless, yellowish, gleety discharge, staining the linen; obstinate gonorrhœa, of long standing (A.).

AGGRAVATION: During and right after eating; in the forenoon; in the afternoon; in the evening; when sitting quietly; from standing; from mental labour; from sexual excesses; from jar; after sleep; from laundry work; from milk; during climacteric; while kneeling at church; in the cold air; and before a thunder-storm.

AMELIORATION: From external heat; from violent exertions; from sitting with legs crossed; from loosening clothes; in open air; and from warmth of bed.

RELATIONSHIP: It antidotes mental effects of over-use of tobacco in patients of sedentary habits, who suffer from overmental exertion.

Complementary: *Nat-M.*

Frequently indicated after *Nux-V.*, *Sil.* and *Sulph.*

Similar to: *Lach.*, *Sang.*, and *Ustil.*, in climacteric irregularities of the circulation.

Inimical to: *Lach.* (should not be used before or after), and *Puls.* (with which it should never be alternated).

Silicea.

COMMON NAMES: SILICA; PURE FLINT.

Want of animal heat; always chilly, even when exercising (N.).

Ailments following vaccination, abscesses, etc., even convulsious (N.).

Many complaints in those of the scrofulous habit favourably affected.

He catches cold easily, especially when he uncovers his feet and head (Psor.).

Lameness in the limbs in the evening (at night—Cham.).

Stitches in all the joints at night (Cedr., Kali-I.).

FEET SWEAT, WITH RAWNESS BETWEEN THE TOES, OR A BAD ODOUR; ALSO COMPLAINTS AFTER CHECKING IT (N.).

Small foreign bodies in the skin or larynx (N.).

Scrofulous children, large bellies and weak ankles, and much sweat about the head (Calc-P., Nat-M.) (N.).

Over-sensitive; imperfectly nourished, not from want of food taken, but from imperfect assimilation (N.).

Complaints worse during new moon or from uncovering the head (N.).

Weakness with associated sleepiness (Gels., Nux-V., Op.).

Restlessness consequent upon physical inactivity.

Great weakness of the nerves and states of emaciation (Lyc., Nat-M., Phos.).

Painless swelling of the glands with troublesome itching (Merc., Rhus-T.).

SUPPURATION OF THE GLANDS AND SUPPURATION OF ALL KINDS, ESPECIALLY IN THE MEMBRANOUS PARTS (Nit-Ac.).

Psoas abscess (Arn., Cupr., Phos-Ac., Staph., Symph., Syph.).

Hip-joint disease (*Calc., Merc., Sulph.*) (D.).

Fistula (Fluor-Ac., Hep., Merc.).

Inflammation and swelling of the bones and caries in any part (Asaf., Aur., Calc., Fluor-Ac.).

Non-tuberculous curvation of the spine (Calc., Calc-P.).

Little perspiration, illy smelling on the head and malodorous foot-sweats (*Bar-C.*).

ENLARGEMENT OF THE HEAD WITH OPEN FONTANELLES (*Calc.*).

DAILY HEADACHE BEGINNING IN THE NECK (*Bell., Calc., Con., Lyc., Mag-C., Sulph.*).

Headache rising from the nape of the neck to the vertex (Gels., Glon., Sang.) (N.).

Chronic suppuration of joints (*Merc., Sulph.*) (Bt.).

Induration and suppuration of the lymphatic or glandular system in any part of the body (Hg.).

Chronic sick headache; as if coming from the spine and locating in one eye, especially the right (left—*Spig.*); worse from draught of air or uncovering the head and better by profuse urination (A.).

MUCH PERSPIRATION IN CHILDREN ABOUT THE HEAD, IS VERY CHARACTERISTIC OF SILICEA (Bt.).

THE HEAD IS WET FROM SWEATING (*Calc.*), PARTICULARLY AT NIGHT (Hr.).

Of marked usefulness in running ears and fistula lachrymalis (Nat-M., Puls., Sulph.).

Styes or pustular affections about the eyes (*Puls.*) (D.).

Swelling in the region of the right lachrymal gland and sac. (N.).

Ophthalmic troubles with great sensitiveness to cold and a desire to be warmly wrapped, especially about the head (N.).

Headaches are worse from noise, mental exertion, jarring; better by binding the head tightly (Arg-N., Puls.), or wrapping the head warmly (N.).

Suppurative ear troubles, accompanied by caries in the mastoid cells (*Aur.*) (D.).

Stoppage of the ears, which open at times with a loud report (N.).

Difficult hearing of human voice (*Phos., Sulph.*) (N.).

Vertigo: Falling forward after stooping, riding, or looking up; rises from the neck into the head with nausea (Hr.).

Sensation as if a hair were lying on the forepart of the tongue (A.).

Congestion and thirst after drinking but little wine.

Water tastes badly; vomits after drinking (N.).

ULCERS ON THE LIPS (*Ars., Caust., Graph., Kali-B., Merc., Nat-M., Nit-Ac., Stram.*) (K.).

Scrofulous children during dentition keep grasping at their gums continually (G.).

Abscesses about the roots of the teeth (D.).

Dental fistula (*Fluor-Ac.*) (D.).

Spongy, readily bleeding ulcers, with torpid, callous edges (Frn.)

FISTULOUS ULCERS, SECRETING A THIN, ICHOROUS, FETID, YELLOW FLUID (*Fluor-Ac.*) (Frn.).

CARIES OF BONES, WITH FISTULOUS OPEN-INGS, AND DISCHARGE OF THIN PUS AND BONY FRAGMENTS (Frn.).

Is a specific for whitlow (*Apis, Hep., Lach.*) (Bt.).

RAVENOUS APPETITE (*Am-C., Arg-M., Ars., Ars-I., Calc., Calc-P., Calc-S., Ferr., Graph., Iod., Lyc., Nat-M., Olnd., Petr., Phos., Psor., Sulph.*) (K.).

Hungry, but cannot get down the food (G.).

Averse to warm food: desire only for cold things (*Puls.*) (A.).

After a meal, load as of a stone in the stomach, or like lead (*Bry., Nux-V., Puls.*) (Py.).

Disgust for meat (*Graph.*) (A.).

Abdomen distended, hard and tense; excessive distension of the abdomen with meteorism (*Carb-V., Lyc.*) (N.).

Colic from worms and from constipation (Calc., Merc., Nux-V., Plb., Stann., Sep.).

Constipation (*Alum., Bry., Graph., Nat-M.*).

Stools very offensive (*Lach., Nit-Ac., Sulph.*).

Stool scanty, or composed of hard lumps, light coloured; expulsion difficult, as from inactivity of the rectum (Alum., Bry., Op.); *when partly expelled it slips back again (Sanic., Thuj.)* (N.).

Fistula in ano alternates with chest symptoms (Berb., Calc-P.) (A.).

Fissura ani (*Aesc., Nat-M., Petr., Sulph.*); great pain after stool (*Ign., Nit-Ac., Thuj.*) (A.).

Catamenia insufficient (Alum., Bry., Ferr., Graph., Nat-M., Puls., Sep.).

Always great costiveness immediately before and during catamenia; also cold feet (N.).

Paroxysms of icy coldness over the whole body at the appearance of the menses (Bt.).

Discharge of white water from the uterus instead of the menses (G.).

PURE BLOOD IS CAUSED TO FLOW FROM THE UTERUS, EVERY TIME THE BABE NURSES (G.).

Fistulous ulcers of the mammæ; the substance of the mammæ seems to be discharged in the pus; one lobe after another seems to ulcerate and discharge into one common ulcer, often with great pain, or there may be several orifices, one for each lobe (G.).

Nipples ulcerate easily (*Sulph.*) (G.).

Nipple is drawn in like a funnel (*Sars.*) (A.).

The mother's milk is so bad that the child refuses it, or vomits it soon after nursing (N.).

11

Chill without thirst, on every movement (*Arn., Nux-V.*) (A.).

Very chilly even in a warm room (A.).

Intermittent fever with heat predominating (*Ars., Phos., Sulph.*).

Fever in evening, worse at night (A.).

Debilitating night-sweats (*Chin., Merc., Nit-Ac., Psor., Sulph.*) (Bt.).

PROFUSE NIGHT-SWEATS (*Ars., Calc., Chin.*) (Ho.).

Great heat all night, with catching respiration (A.).

Unhealthy skin; every little injury suppurates (*Graph., Hep., Merc., Petr., Sulph.*) (A.).

Sweat only on the head, or head and face (A.).

SWEAT OF HANDS, TOES, FEET AND AXILLAE; OFFENSIVE (A.).

Ingrowing toe-nails (*Graph.*) (A.).

Crippled nails on fingers and toes (*Ant-C., Graph., Thuj.*) (A.).

Panaritium (*Apis, Hep., Nit-Ac.*) (A.).

Carbuncles (*Apis, Ars., Lach., Rhus-T.*) (A.).

Promotes expulsion of foreign bodies from the tissues, such as fish-bones, needles, etc. (A.).

NIGHT WALKING; GETS UP WHILE ASLEEP, WALKS ABOUT AND LIES DOWN AGAIN (*Kali-Br.*) (A.).

Dreams about corpses and dead persons generally (*Anac., Aur., Calc., Calc-Sil., Elaps, Iris, Mag-M., Mag-S., Thuj.*) (J.).

Yielding mind, faint-hearted, anxious mood (*Puls.*) (N.).

She is occupied with pins, counts them, hunts for them, and is always worse during the increase of the moon (Bt.).

Mental labour difficult; reading and writing fatigue; cannot bear to think (*Kali-P.*) (A.).

Restless, fidgety, starts at the least noise (*Bor., Kali-C., Phos.*) (A.).

Exhaustion with erythism, from hard work and close confinement; may be overcome by force of will (A.).

Nervous debility (*Ambr., Kali-P., Lyc., Phos-Ac.*) (A.).

Children are obstinate, head strong, cry when spoken to kindly (*Iod.*) (A.).

The patient is over-sensitive to noise (*Bell., Nux-V.*), is despondent, and has a disgust for life (D.).

Rattling in the chest (*Ant-T., Hep., Nat-S.*) (B.).

Cough with expectoration thick, yellow, lumpy, purulent, profuse and greenish (N.).

Chronic bronchitis; the cough is loose, racking and suffocating (*Kali-C., Phos.*) (Bl.).

Pneumonia in stage of suppuration (D.).

Suppurative stage of pulmonary tuberculosis (*Hep., Merc., Nit-Ac., Phos.*) (Bl.).

EMPHYSEMA (*Dros.; Hep., Ipec., Lach., Lob., Merc., Nat-M., Phel., Phos.*) (Bl.)

Dry, nocturnal cough, waking the patient from sleep (*Graph., Puls., Sulph.*) (K.).

Dry cough, worse from cold drinks (K.).

Dust complaints of stone-cutters, with total loss of strength (N.).

Hectic fever accompanied by debility and profuse night-sweats (*Nit-Ac.*) (Bl.).

All the symptoms except gastric are ameliorated by warmth; while the gastric symptoms are relieved by cold food (reverse of *Lyc.*, which likes warmth inside and cold outside) (A.).

Desire to be magnetized, which relieves (*Bar-C., Bell., Calc., Cupr., Graph., Nux-V., Phos., Sep., Sulph., Viol-O.*) (A.).

Inflammation and suppuration of the inguinal glands (D.).

Epilepsy recurring at night, with the aura beginning in the solar plexus (D.).

Chronic gonorrhœa with thick fetid discharge (*Hyos., Nat-S., Puls.*) (Br.).

Itching and swelling of the scrotum (*Graph., Rhus-T., Sulph.*) (R.).

Violent erections (*Canth., Phos., Sulph.*) (R.).

Seminal emission at night (*Nux-V., Phos-Ac.*) (R.).

Hydrocele (*Apis, Puls., Sulph.*) (Br.).

Elephantiasis of the scrotum (Br.).

AGGRAVATION: From cold; during menses; at new moon; from uncovering, especially the head; from lying down; after vaccination; from a draught; from motion; in the open air; at night.

AMELIORATION: From warmth, especially from wrapping up the head; in a warm room; from magnetism and electricity.

RELATIONSHIP: *Complementary*: *Fluor-Ac., Sanic.* and *Thuj.*

Compare: *Bar-C., Calc., Calc-P., Dios., Ferr., Gettysburg, Graph., Hep., Hyper., Iod., Kali-P., Lyc., Merc., Nat-M., Nat-S., Op., Petr., Phos., Pic-Ac., Puls., Ruta, Sanic., Sep., Sulph., Thuj., Verat.*

Follows well after: *Calc., Graph., Hep., Nit-Ac., Phos.*

Is followed well by: *Fluor-Ac., Hep., Lyc.,* and *Sep.*

Sil. is the chronic of *Puls.*

Merc. should not be given before or after *Sil.*

Its action is deep and long-lasting.

Difference between *Sil.* and *Calc-S.*, in suppurative process:—*Silicea* promotes suppuration and brings the suppurative process to maturity. *Calc-Sulph.* checks suppuration and promotes healthy granulation.

Spigelia Anthelmintica.

COMMON NAME: PINK ROOT.

Heaviness and soreness of the whole body (*Bry., Gels., Nux-V.*).

Painful sensitiveness of the whole body to contact, with shivering of those parts that have been touched, or with formication through the whole body.

Stinging, tearing pains in association with twitchings of the affected areas.

Tearing near the joints, as from scraping of a knife.

Spasmodic pains in the limbs, especially the joints.

LEFT-SIDED NEURALGIAS (OF THE HEAD, FACE AND EYES); PAINS INCREASE AND DECREASE WITH THE RISING AND SETTING SUN; WATERING OF THE EYE, ON THE AFFECTED SIDE (N.).

Intolerable pressive pain in the eye-balls; could not turn the eyes without turning the whole body; worse especially on making a false step (A.).

Prosopalgia, left-sided; tearing, shooting, burning pains, especially in cheek bones, lower jaw, about eye-brows and in the eye-ball; periodical from morning until sunset; worse at noon, from noise or motion (N.).

Rheumatic sclerotitis; pains are sharp and tearing with pressure in the eye-balls (Bt.).

Disposition to squint (Apis, Bell., Cic., Cycl., Gels., Hyos., Kali-I., Lyc., Mag-P., Merc., Nat-M., Nux-V., Puls., Spig., Stram., Sulph., Tab., Verat., Zinc.).

Eyes hurt on motion, as if too large for the orbit (N.).

Ciliary neuralgia; pains radiate; cold feeling in the eye (D.).

JERKING, TWITCHING, OR SPASMODIC MOVEMENTS OF THE EYE-LIDS (*Agar., Ars., Bell., Cic., Cupr., Ign., Mag-P., Nux-V., Phys., Puls., Rheum, Sulph.*).

Intense pressing pains in the eye-balls, especially on turning them (N.).

Hemicrania; pain increased by motion, noise, and especially by stooping; one or both eyes are involved (N.).

The headaches are generally onesided, beginning in the occiput and extending forward, and settling over the left eye (right eye—*Sang., Sil.)*. They are aggravated by the least noise or jar.

THEY INCREASE WITH THE RISING OF THE SUN AND DECREASE WITH ITS GOING DOWN (*Nat-M., Tab.*) (N.).

Sensation as if the head was open along the vertex (D.).

Sensation as of a band around the head (*Cact., Carb-Ac., Sulph.*) (A.).

Paleness of the face (*Cina, Ferr., Nat-M., Puls., Sep.*) (D.).

Blue rings around the eyes (*Cina, Staph.*) (D.).

Afraid of sharp, pointed things, pins, needles, etc. (A.).

Heart disease, when the same are characterized by violent and visible and audible palpitations (*Ars., Iod., Thuj.*).

PALPITATION OF THE HEART, WORSE WHEN BENDING THE CHEST FORWARD (*Kalm.*) (N.).

Violent beating of the heart, especially at night; visible and audible, with anguish (N.).

Stitch or darting-like pain in the heart (*Apis, Bry., Caust., Kalm., Lach., Mag-M., Naja, Petr., Psor., Spong., Staph., Sulph.*).

Valvular affections with loud, blowing sounds and attacks of violent palpitation. The patient can only lie on the right side (*Nat-M., Phos.*), *or with the head very high; least motion aggravates* (*Naja*) (N.).

Aneurism (*Bar-C., Cact., Calc., Carb-V., Lyc., Lycps., Ran-S.*) (A.).

Sharp, stitching pains in the left chest, shooting into arm and neck, worse by motion; pulse not synchronous with heart-beat (D.).

On placing hand over the cardiac region there is a purring feeling, as when stroking a cat's back (D.).

Dyspnœa: Can lie only on the right side, with trunk raised; the least motion produces great suffocation; with anxiety and palpitation of the heart (G.).

Rheumatic pericarditis, with violent palpitation of the heart and anxiety (Bt.).

Trembling carotids (Ra.).

Rheumatic affections of the heart (*Kali-C., Led., Naja, Phos., Rhus-T.*) ; *systolic blowing at the apex* (A.).

Faint, nauseated feeling (*Ant-T., Ipec., Lob., Tab., Verat.*) (D.).

Colic around the navel (*Aloe, Bell., Coloc., Dios., Ipec., Merc., Nat-S., Nux-V., Plb., Rhus-T., Stann., Sulph., Thuj., Verat.*) (D.).

Nausea every morning before breakfast (*Alum., Alumn., Anac., Bar-C., Berb., Bov., Calc., Fago., Lyc., Petr., Sep., Tub.*) (Bt.).

Desire for alcoholic drinks (*Lach., Led., Lyc., Med., Merc., Mur-Ac., Naja, Nux-V., Op., Phos., Puls., Sel., Sep.*) (A.).

Ravenous hunger with nausea and thirst (*Sulph.*) (A.).

Scrofulous children afflicted with ascarides and lumbrici (*Calc., Merc., Sulph.*) (Bt.).

Itching and tickling in the anus and rectum (C.).

Scirrhus of the sigmoid flexure or rectum, with atrocious unbearable pain (*Alumen*) (A.).

Copious, offensive mucus from the posterior nares drops into the throat, causing choking at night (*Hydr.*) (A.).

Stammering; repeats the first syllable three or four times; with abdominal ailments; with helminthiasis (A.).

Masked intermittents, appearing as periodical; face and head aches.

Chill spreads from the chest (*Apis, Carb-An., Sep.*) (A.).

Least movement of the body causes chilliness (*Apis, Bry., Caps., Coff., Merc-C., Nux-V., Rhus-T., Sep., Sil., Squil.*) (A.).

Heat in back, hands, abdomen, gradually increasing until he becomes hot all over (A.).

Night-sweat, putrid smelling (A.).

Toothache from tobacco-smoking; ameliorated only on lying down and while eating (*Plant*); worse from cold air and water; returns from thinking about it (A.).

AGGRAVATION: When stooping; from touch; while moving; after sexual excitability; from inspiration; from noise; from moving eyes; in cold, damp, and rainy weather; from rising sun; from tea; and from cold water.

AMELIORATION: From quiet; in dry air; from setting sun; and from lying on the right side with the head high.

RELATIONSHIP: *Compare: Acon., Ars., Bell., Cact., Calc., Dig., Euphr., Gels., Hep., Ipec., Kali-B., Kali-C., Kalm., Lach., Lyc., Merc., Naja, Nat-M., Nux-V., Phos., Puls., Rhus-T., Sep., Sil., Spong., Stann., Sulph., Thuj., Verat., Zinc.*

It follows *Acon.* well.

Complementary: Spong.

Antidotes: Aur., Camph., Cocc., and *Puls.*

Spigel. antidotes Merc.

Spongia Tosta.

COMMON NAME: ROASTED SPONGE.

Sorethroat, worse after eating sweet things (A.).

Stiffness in the extremities; arms and legs feel as if they were broken.

Swelling and induration of the glands (*Calc., Merc-I-F., Phyt.*).

Struma (*Calc., Sil., Sulph.*).

Itching in the swollen glands.

Sensation of numbness of the lower half of the body.

Chronic hoarseness and cough; the voice frequently giving out when talking or singing (*Arg-N.*) (G.).

Great dryness of the mucous membranes of the air passages—throat, larynx, trachea, bronchi—" dry as a horn" (A.).

Every mental excitement increases the cough (A.).

COUGH AGGRAVATED BY SWEETS, COLD DRINKS, SMOKING, LYING WITH HEAD LOW, AND DRY COLD WINDS; AND AMELIORATED BY EATING OR DRINKING WARM THINGS (A.).

Watering of eyes; latterly gummy or mucous discharge, with obscured vision (*Kali-B., Kali-S., Nat-M.*).

Goitre, swollen and hard; suffocative at night; in persons who live in villages (N.).

Cough aggravated by talking, reading, singing, swallowing and lying with head low (N.).

Croupy cough, worse on awakening out of sleep (N.).

Bronchitis and inflammation of the larynx (*Brom., Phos., Sil.*).

Clearing of throat constantly (*Arg-N., Kali-B., Phos.*).

Of great value in hoarseness (*Arg-M., Caust., Kali-B., Phos., Sil.*).

Cough dry and sibilant, sounds like a saw driven through a pine-board (croup) (N.).

Great dryness of the larynx, with hoarse, hollow, wheezing cough (*Phos.*) (N.).

BARKING COUGH (*Acon., Dros., Hep., Stram.*), DAY AND NIGHT (K.).

Awakens out of sleep with a sense of suffocation, with violent loud cough, great alarm, agitation, anxiety and difficult respiration.

Palpitation of the heart before the catamenia (*Alum., Cact., Cupr., Ign., Iod., Nat-M., Sep., Zinc.*).

Attacks of severe oppression and pain in the region of the heart; all the symptoms aggravated by lying with the head low; inability to lie down at night (Be.).

CROUP: ANXIOUS, WHEEZING; WORSE DURING INSPIRATION (worse during expiration— *Acon.*); AGGRAVATED BEFORE MIDNIGHT (aggravated before morning—*Hep.*) (A.).

Valvular insufficiency (*Spig.*) (A.).

Angina pectoris; contracting pain, heat, faintness, suffocation, anxiety and sweat; worse after midnight (A.).

Constipation (*Alum., Bry., Caust., Graph., Hep., Kali-M., Lyc., Nat-M.*).

Frequent urging to urinate (*Bell., Canth., Ferr-P., Kali-P., Lyc., Nux-V., Puls., Sep.*) (C.)

Coldness in the back, not relieved by warmth of stone (C.).

Feverish heat, with hot, dry skin (*Acon., Ars., Sulph.*) (C.).

Congestion of blood to the head (*Acon., Bell., Ferr-P., Glon., Lach., Meli., Nat-M., Op., Sep., Sulph.,Verat-V.*) (C.).

Sharp stitches in the left temple extending to the forehead (C.).

Fluent coryza, with much sneezing (*Acon., All-C., Sabad.*) (C.).

Dry coryza; nose stopped up (*Alum., Nux-V., Sep., Sil.*) (C.).

Sleep interrupted by dreams (*Nux-V., Sulph.*) (C.).

Useful for pulmonary tuberculosis following pneumonia, with chronic hoarseness, profuse expectoration and suffocative attacks at night (R.).

TESTICLES SWOLLEN, BRUISED, SQUEEZED, AFTER SUPPRESSED GONORRHOEA OR MAL-TREATED ORCHITIS (*Puls.*) (A.).

Swelling of the testicles (*Clem., Con., Puls., Rhod., Rhus-T., Sil.*).

Inflammation and induration of the testicles (Hm.).

Spermatic cord swollen, painful (*Clem., Puls., Rhod.*) (A.).

Menses preceded by colic, soreness in the sacrum, and craving in the stomach (G.).

Violent drawing in the upper and lower extremities during the menses (G.).

Catamenia too early and too profuse (*Calc., Chin., Kali-P., Nit-Ac., Puls., Sab., Sec.*).

Induration and enlargement of the ovaries (*Aur., Iod., Merc.*) (Bt.).

AGGRAVATION: After sleep; in dry, cold wind; when roused from sleep; from exertion; from raising arms; before midnight; from lying with the head low; from sweets; and from cold drinks

AMELIORATION: Many symptoms (with the exception of those of the respiratory organs) are relieved by rest; by eating or drinking warm things; and when descending.

RELATIONSHIP: *Spongia follows well after*: Acon. and Hep., in cough and croup when dryness prevails; after Spong., Hep., when mucus commences to rattle.

Compare: *Arn., Caust., Iod., Lach.* and *Nux-M.* (sputa loosened, but must be swallowed again).

Antidote: *Camph.*

✗ Stannum Metallicum.

COMMON NAME: TIN.

Burning in the palms of the hands and soles of the feet (*Lach., Sulph.*).

Weakness in the extremities (*Ars., Bry., Calc., Gels., Kali-P., Lyc.*).

Pressing, drawing and burning heat in the limbs.

Marked weakness with trembling, which is felt more when moving slowly.

So weak she drops into a chair instead of sitting down (N.).

While dressing in the morning has to sit down several times to rest (Carb-An.) (N.).

Pressive, stupefying headache (B.).

Headache, usually neuralgic, which comes on gradually and grows steadily worse till it reaches its height or severest point, when it begins to grow easier and goes away just as gradually as it came on (G.).

Pale face, with sunken eyes (*Cina, Ferr., Staph.*) (B.).

When singing or using voice, aching and weakness in the deltoid arms (A.).

Anxious sensation of heat from the least motion.

Fainty sensation because of goneness in the epigastric region (Phos.).

Hoarseness, with deep, husky or hollow voice, relieved for the time by coughing or by expectorating mucus (A.).

Tongue coated with yellow mucus (A.).

Continued use of the voice proves enervating (Phos.).

Hysterical and hypochondriacal spasms, with pain in the abdomen and in the region of the diaphragm.

Rest aggravates, whilst motion relieves; only the debility is felt while walking.

THE PAIN BECOME SLOWLY WORSE AND DIMINISH SLOWLY (*Kalm., Nat-M., Phos., Plat., Spig., Sulph-Ac.*).

Fetid odour from the mouth (*Nux-V., Puls.*) (A.).

EVERYTHING TASTES BITTER BUT WATER (*Acon.*) (A.).

Emaciation, with a gone feeling at the epigastrium (Sep., Sulph., Zinc.).

Sinking, empty, all-gone sensation in the stomach (Chel., Phos., Sep.) (N.).

A FEELING OF HUNGER, BUT HE CANNOT EAT (*Lyc.*).

Gastralgia or gastric ulcer; the pains begin lightly and increase gradually to the highest point, and then gradually decline (N.).

INSATIABLE HUNGER (*Ars., Chel., Iod., Tub.*) (Bt.).

COLIC RELIEVED BY HARD PRESSURE, OR BY LAYING ABDOMEN ACROSS THE KNEE OR ON THE SHOULDER (*Coloc.*) (N.).

Colic with a sensation of hunger, bitter eructations, and diarrhœa.

Nausea and vomiting, especially in the morning (A.)

NAUSEA OR VOMITING FROM THE ODOUR OF COOKING FOOD (*Ars., Colch., Sep.*) (A.).

Lumbrici; passes worms (*Calc., Sulph.*) (N.).

Vomiting of blood (*Acon., Ipec., Phos.*) (Bt.).

Diarrhœa consisting of mucus (*Aloe, Merc., Nux-V., Sulph.*).

Prolapsus, worse during stool (*Calc-P., Con., Nux-V., Podo., Puls.*) (N.).

Leucorrhœa, with great debility; weakness seems to proceed from the chest (N.).

Before menses, mania erotica (*Calc-P., Phos., Stram., Verat.*) (B.).

Gushes of debilitating leucorrhœa (*Calc., Graph., Lyc., Sep., Sil.*) (B.).

Menses too early and too profuse (*Calc., Kali-C., Nit-Ac.*) (A.).

SADNESS BEFORE MENSES (*Calc., Caust., Con., Ferr., Lac-C., Lyc., Murx., Nat-M., Nit-Ac., Puls., Sep., Verat.*) (A.).

Pain in the malar bones, during menses (A.).

Atony of the bladder (*Ars., Caust., Con., Gels., Lyc., Nux-V., Op., Parier., Tereb.*) (B.).

Want of desire to urinate (Caust.).

Diseases of the mucous membranes (*Bry., Kali-B., Nat-M., Puls., Rhus-T.*).

Distressing cough of a constant nature (Bry., Phos.).

Bronchitis (*Acon., Bry., Calc-S., Ferr-P., Kali-M., Nat-S., Phos., Puls.*)

LOOSE COUGH, WITH HEAVY, GREEN, SWEET EXPECTORATION (*Puls.*) (N.).

GREAT WEAKNESS IN THE CHEST; CAN HARDLY TALK; WITH GENERAL DEBILITY, WHICH CENTERS IN THE CHEST (N.).

Faint and weak, especially when going downstairs; can go up well enough (reverse of Calc.) (N.).

It should be remembered in pulmonary tuberculosis, when the pulmonary changes are rapid and persist inspite of the well-directed efforts to check them. The character of the expectoration and the sensation of great weakness, referred to the chest, are characteristic (Bl.).

Empty sensation in the chest (Cocc., Phos.) (A.).

Short breath, from every effort; must loosen clothes (B.).

Catarrhal phthisis; chest feels raw or hollow (*Phos.*) (B.).

Easily expectorates quantities of sweet, or bright yellow pus or balls of mucus (B.).

Expectoration profuse, like the white of an egg; sweetish or salty; sour, putrid, or musty; during the day (A.).

Extreme exhaustion of mind and body (*Kali-P.*) (A.).

Sad, despondent; feels like crying all the time, but crying makes her worse (N.).

Cannot answer questions, feels so weak (Gels., Phos-Ac.) (G.).

Child wants to be carried over shoulder (B.).

Dread of seeing people (*Puls.*) (Br.).

Cough: Deep, hollow, shattering, strangling; concussive, in paroxysms of three coughs (of two coughs—*Merc.*) ; dry, while in bed, in the evening (A.).

Worm fevers (Bry., Cina, Nat-P., Phos., Sil.).

Answers unwillingly and abruptly (C.).

Seminal emissions without dreams (*Anac., Camph., Con., Dios., Graph., Ham., Pic-Ac.*) (C.).

Sexual desire increased (Canth., Con., Graph., Kali-P., Nux-V., Phos., Pic-Ac.).

Easy sexual organs (*Nux-V., Phos., Sulph.*) (B.).

Sleeps with one leg drawn up, the other stretched out (*Lac-C.*) (Br.).

Sleeps, lying on the abdomen (*Bell., Cina, Coloc., Podo., Puls., Stram.*) (K.).

Chilliness over the whole body (Ars., Nux-V., Sil.) (C.).

Hectic fever (Ars-I., Ferr., Phos., Puls.) (A.).

Low fever, with bronchial or pulmonary complications (Phos., Sil.) (A.).

Chill at 10 A.M., with numb fingertips (B.).

Sweat: Mouldy, musty odour; after 4 A.M., every morning; on neck and forehead; very debilitating (A.).

AGGRAVATION: From using voice; at 10 A.M.; from lying on the right side; ascending steps; from laughing; from singing; by drinking anything warm; and after motion.

AMELIORATION: From hard pressure; after expectoration and by rapid motion.

RELATIONSHIP: *Antidotes: Hep.* and *Puls.*

It follows well after *Caust.* and is followed by *Calc., Phos., Sil., Sulph.* and *Tub.*

Complementary: Puls.

Staphisagria.

COMMON NAME: STAVESACRE.

Drawing and tearing in the muscles (*Carb-V., Nit-Ac., Valer.*).

Painfulness of the muscles to contact and of the joints when moving (*Bry.*).

INJURIES FROM SHARP INSTRUMENTS (*Hyper., Led.*).

Coxalgia with pulsating pain, as from suppuration.

One-sided paralysis from anger.

In the morning great debility and stiffness of all the joints (mostly in the shoulder, small of the back and hip).

Nightly twitchings (*Ambr., Calc., Nat-C., Phos., Sep., Stront.*).

Deep, penetrating, sharp stitches (*Nit-Ac.*).

Gouty nodosities in the joints (*Benz-Ac.*) and swelling of the bones or periosteum with suppuration (*Calc., Merc., Sil.*).

Itching and burning tettery eruptions quickly helped (*Ars., Sep., Sulph.*).

Tinea capitis (*Calc., Graph., Mezer., Sep., Sulph., Viol-T.*).

Excrescences on the gums and sycotic excrescences behind the glans penis (*Thuj.*).

SEXUAL EXCESSES AND ONANISM (*Nux-V., Phos-Ac., Zinc.*) (D.).

Crawling on the external genitals as from insects; parts very sensitive (D.).

Eruption with violent itching, and when scratched it changes place and itches somewhere else (D.).

Effects of onanism: hypochondriacal: face sunken: abashed look; nocturual emissions; backache; weak legs; organs relaxed (N.).

Bad effects from the abuse of mercury (*Aur., Chin., Dulc., Hep., Nit-Ac., Podo., Sil.*).

Flaccidity of the skin (*Abrot.*, *Arg-N.*, *Lyc.*, *Op.*).
Puffiness (*Apis*, *Ars.*, *Bry.*, *Merc.*, *Phos.*, *Sulph.*).

BLOATEDNESS OF THE BODY AND FACE, WITH SWOLLEN ABDOMEN IN CHILDREN.

Inclination to become fat (in children and young persons).

CHEWING MOTION OF THE JAW DURING SLEEP (*Podo.*, *Sep.*, *Zinc.*) (K.).

Cutting pains (*Bell.*, *Dros.*, *Nat-C.*, *Petr.*, *Rhus-T.*, *Sil.*, *Viol-T.*).

Pricking in outer parts and in the bones.

Sensation of dryness, or of trembling in inner parts (*Sulph-Ac.*).

Tearing in the muscles (*Carb-V.*, •*Caust.*, *Kali-C.*, *Lyc.*, *Merc.*, *Nit-Ac.*, *Rhod.*, *Sep.*, *Sil.*, *Staph.*, *Zinc.*).

ARTHRITIC TEARING AND ARTIFICIAL NODOSITIES (*Amm-M.*, *Calc-F.*, *Sil.*).

Cramps in single parts, which draw the limbs crookedly, especially in the toes and fingers (*Cupr.*, *Mag-P.*, *Sec.*).

Bleeding from inner parts (*Crot-H.*, *Ferr.*, *Lach.*, *Nit-Ac.*, *Phos.*, *Sec.*).

PAINFUL SWELLING OF THE GLANDS (*Bell.*, *Carb-An.*, *Hep.*, *Kali-M.*, *Lach.*, *Lyc.*, *Merc.*, *Nit-Ac.*, *Rhus-T.*, *Sil.*).

Hardness of hearing ; deafness (*Phos.*) (G.).

OTORRHŒA, WITH MUCO-PURULENT DISCHARGE (*Calc-S.*, *Hep.*, *Merc.*) (Br.).

12

Bones swollen with softening (*Aur.*, *Calc.*, *Merc.*, *Sil.*).

CARIES (*Asaf.*, *Calc-F.*, *Calc-S.*, *Hep.*, *Merc.*, *Nit-Ac.*, *Phos.*, *Sil.*).

It is of service in cases of rachitis.

The teeth appear late ; the child does not learn to walk as early as is normal, and the fontanelles are late in closing. When the child is sleeping, the head perspires, so that the pillow is wet far around it (Bl.).

Acidity of the digestive tract : *sour eructation, sour vomiting, and sour stool* (*Hep.*, *Mag-C.*, *Rheum*, *Sulph.*) (A.).

VOMITING OF SOUR SUBSTANCES (*Chin.*, *Ferr-P.*, *Iris*, *Mag-C.*, *Nux-V.*, *Phos.*, *Sulph-Ac.*).

GREAT LONGING FOR EGGS (*Hydr.*, *Nat-P.*, *Ol-An*) (A.).

Craves indigestible things (*Alum.*, *Alumn.*, *Bell.*, *Bry.*, *Calc-P.*, *Cycl.*) (A.).

Desire for clay, chalk, lime, slate pencils, etc. (*Alum.*, *Cic.*, *Ferr.*, *Nat-M.*, *Nit-Ac.*, *Nux-V.*) (K.).

Aversion to milk and meat (*Amm-C.*, *Arn.*, *Bry.*, *Calc-S.*, *Carb-S.*, *Carb-V.*, *Ferr-P.*, *Ign.*, *Mag-C.*, *Nat-C.*, *Nat-P.*, *Nat-S.*, *Nux-V.*, *Phos.*, *Puls.*, *Sep.*, *Sil.*, *Sulph.*) (A.).

The least mental excitement causes profuse return of menstrual flow (*Sulph.*, *Tub.*) (A.).

THICK, MILKY, GUSHING LEUCORRHŒA (*Amm-C.*, *Bor.*, *Calc-P.*, *Cop.*, *Ferr.*, *Kali-Chl.*, *Puls.*, *Sep.*) (B.).

CATAMENIA TOO EARLY AND TOO PRO-FUSE (*Chin., Ferr., Ham., Phos., Sep., Sulph.*).

UTERINE POLYPI (*Ars., Aur., Bell, Calc-P., Con., Lyc., Phos., Sang., Sep., Staph., Teucr., Thuj.*) (B.).

Chlorosis, with scanty or suppressed menses (*Alum., Ferr., Graph., Puls., Sep.*) **(A.)**.

Inflammation, redness and swelling of the vulva, with purulent discharge (*Ars., Bor., Calc-S., Kreos., Merc., Sep.*) (G.).

LEUCORRHŒA OF LITTLE GIRLS (*Cann-S., Merc., Puls., Sep.*) (D.).

DIFFICULT AND DELAYED DENTITION (*Calc-P., Sil.*). (A.).

Grinding of teeth during sleep (*Ars., Bell., Bry., Cann-I., Cina, Hyos., Ign.*) (K.).

Sour odour of the whole body (*Hep., Rheum.*) (A.).

Sweat: of single parts; head, scalp wet, cold; nape of neck; chest, axillæ, sexual organs; hands, knees; feet (*Sep.*) (A.).

Rawness of soles of feet from perspiration (*Graph., Sanic., Sil.*) (A.).

Smell before nose as of bad eggs or gun-powder (R.).

Feet habitually cold and damp, as if they had on cold, damp stockings (A.).

Feet continually cold in bed (A.).

Nasal polypi (*All-C., Aur., Calc-S., Con., Hydr., Kali-B., Lem-M., Merc., Phos., Sang., Sil., Sulph., Teucr., Thuj.*) (R.).

Painless hoarseness, worse in the morning (*Carb-V.*, *Caust.*) (A.).

Nocturnal enuresis (*Apis*, *Bell.*, *Caust.*, *Ferr.*, *Graph*, *Kreos.*, *Mag-P.*, *Nat-M.*, *Puls.*) (K.).

Much crawling and itching in the anus (*Calc-S.*, *Graph.*, *Lyc.*, *Nux-V.*, *Phos.*) (G.).

WHITE, CHALK-LIKE STOOLS (*Aur-M-N.*, *Chel.*, *Podo.*) (G.).

Chronic diarrhœa ; clay-like stools (*Dig.*, *Mag-C.*, *Podo.*, *Sil.*) (Hg.).

Feels better in every way when constipated (A.).

Obstinate constipation ; stool has to be removed mechanically (*Aloe*, *Alum.*, *Plat.*, *Sanic.*, *Sel.*, *Sep.*, *Sil.*) (A.).

CHOLERA INFANTUM : MILK DISAGREES ; THE CHILD VOMITS IT IN SOUR CAKES OR CURDS ; THERE IS A DIARRHŒA WHICH IS WORSE TOWARDS EVENING ; IT IS GEENISH, WATERY, UNDIGESTED AND SOUR (D.).

AGGRAVATION : In the morning ; on awakening ; from exertion of the mind ; after eating ; in cold and wet weather ; from fasting ; in the evening ; after mid-night ; from cold water ; from washing ; and during full moon.

AMELIORATION : From rubbing ; from drawing the limbs up ; whilst lying on the back ; in the dark ; in dry weather ; and from lying on the painful side.

RELATIONSHIP. *Similar to* : *Alum.*, *Bell.*, *Calc-S.*, *Chin.*, *Dut.*, *Ferr.*, *Graph.*, *Hep.*, *Kali-C.*, *Lyc.*, *Nat-S.*, *Sep.*, and *Thuj.*).

According to Hahnemann, *Calc.* must not be used before *Nit-Ac.* and *Sulph.* ; may produce unnecessary complications.

Calc. acts best before *Lyc., Nux-V., Phos.* and *Sil.*

Complementary to : *Bell.*, which is the acute of *Calc.*

It follows : *Nit-Ac., Puls.* and *Sulph.*, and is followed by *Kali-B.*

Note. In children it may be often repeated. In aged people, it should not be repeated ; especially if the first dose benefitted, it will usually do harm.

Calcarea Phosphorica

COMMON NAME : PHOSPHATE OF LIME.

Useful during first and second dentition of scrofulous children ; diarrhœa and great flatulence (A.).

Children : *emaciated, unable to stand* ; *slow in learning to walk* (*Calc., Sil.*).

SUNKEN, FLABBY ABDOMEN (A.).

Hydrocephalus (*Apis, Bry., Hell., Lyc., Op Phos-Ac , Sulph.*) (B.).

SLOW OSSIFICATION ; NON-UNION (*Calc., Sil*) (B.).

HEADACHE OF SCHOOL GIRLS (*Nat-M.*) (Bl.).

Perspiration on the scalp during sleep (*Calc.*, *Merc.*, *Sil.*).

Feels complaints more when thinking of them (*Helon.*, *Ox-Ac.*).

Difficulty in performing intellectual operations. (C.).

Wants to go away from home, and when away, wants to come back again (F.).

Ailments from disappointed love (*Caust.*, *Ign.*, *Nat-M.*) (G.).

Involuntary sighing (*Cimic.*, *Ign.*, *Kali-P.*, *Nat-M.*, *Puls.*, *Stram.*) (Bl.).

Peevish and fretful (*Bry.*, *Cham.*, *Cina*) (C.).

Oozing of bloody fluid from navel of infants (*Sil.*) (A.).

Pott's disease or hip-joint disease (*Calc.*, *Phos.*, *Rhus-T.*, *Sil.*) (B.).

Can't use the eyes by gas-light (G.).

IT AIDS FORMATION OF CALLUS IN FRACTURES (D.).

RACHITIS : CRANIAL BONES THIN AND BRITTLE ; FONTANELLES AND SUTURES REMAIN OPEN TOO LONG, OR CLOSE AND REOPEN ; DELAYED OR COMPLICATED TEETHING (A.).

MAL-ASSIMILATION (*Alum.*, *Calc.*, *Nat-M.*, *Sanic.*, *Sil.*) (B.).

THE CHILD SUFFERS FROM COLIC AFTER EVERY FEEDING (F.).

Useful as a restorative after acute diseases (*Ars.*, *Chin.*, *Phos.*, *Sel.*) (D.).

Pain in the sacro-iliac symphyses (that is, the places where the sacrum unites with the iliac bones) (F.).

Pains along the sagittal suture (F.).

Spine weak, disposed to curvatures, especially to the left ; unable to support the body (A.).

Neck weak, unable to support the head (A.).

DIARRHŒA : STOOLS FOUL, HOT, LIENTERIC, SPLUTTERING AND WATERY (*Aloe*, *Podo.*, *Sulph.*) (B.).

Sunken, flabby abdomen (D.).

Slow development and rapid decay of the teeth (*Kreos.*, *Staph.*) (D.).

Excessive flatulence (*Carb-V.*, *Lyc.*) (D.).

Anal fistula, alternating with chest symptoms (B.).

CRAVES HAM, BACON, SALTED OR SMOKED MEAT (D.).

Pain in the stomach after a small quantity of food (D.).

Rheumatism appearing in any change of weather. On exposure to dampness, we find stiffness of the neck, aching and soreness in the limbs and wandering pains through the limbs, particularly around the sacral region and down the legs (F.).

Child loses its breath on being lifted up (*Bor.*) (B.).

Persistently vomits milk (*Æth.*, *Ant-C.*, *Calc.*, *Mag-C.*, *Sep.*, *Sil.*) (B.).

Acne in anæmic girls at puberty (A.).

Rheumatic affections, worse in spring and fall, especially when air is cold and damp from melting snow (N.).

Bones affected along sutures or at symphyses (N. .

Soreness in the sacro-iliac symphysis, as if broken or separated (N.).

Menses : early, scanty ; every two weeks (*Bry.,* *Puls., Sep.*) (B.).

Uterine displacement, aggravated by the passage of stool or urine (G.).

Leucorrhœa, like white of an egg (Br.).

Nymphomania (*Apis, Canth., Lach., Phos., Plat.,* *Puls., Stram.*) (Br.).

Excoriating discharge from the ears (*Calc., Merc., Sil.*) (C.).

Hoarseness : must hawk or hem to clear the voice (C.).

AGGRAVATION : From exposure to damp, cold and changeable weather ; from east wind ; from melting snow ; and from mental exertion.

AMELIORATION : In summer : and in warm, dry atmosphere.

RELATIONSHIP. Complementary : *Ruta.*

Similar to : *Calc., Calc-F., Carb-An., Kali-C.,* *Kali-P., Merc., Psor., Sil.,* and *Sulph.*

Acts best : *before Iod., Psor., Sanic.* and *Sulph.* ; and *after Ars., Iod.,* and *Tub.*

Calcarea Sulphurica.

COMMON NAMES: SULPHATE OF LIME;
PLASTER OF PARIS; GYPSUM.

It corresponds to the suppurative processes, abscesses, etc. (D.).

Glandular swellings (*Bad., Bell., Brom., Calc., Carb-An., Graph., Hep., Iod., Kali-M., Lyc., Merc., Nit-Ac., Phos., Rhus-T., Sil., Sulph.*) (Bl.),

When the abscess has broken or has been lanced and is discharging, then Calc-S. comes in ; the presence of pus with a vent is the characteristic indication (D.).

Pus : thick, yellow, lumpy and bloody (B.).

Glands are enlarged and hard (*Bad., Carb-An., Merc-I., Phyt.*) (Bl.).

Fistulæ (Fluor-Ac., Hep., Sil.) (B.).

Deafness, with discharge of matter from the middle ear, sometimes mixed with blood (Br.).

Pimples around ear (*Rhus-T., Tell.*) (Br.).

Edges of nostrils sore (*Ars., Bor., Graph., Hep., Kali-Ars, Nit-Ac.*) (C.).

Yellowish discharge from the posterior nares (*Hydr., Kali-B., Lyc., Nat-S.*) (Br.).

One-sided discharge from the nose (*Alum., Aur., Bell., Hep., Kali-C., Nux-V., Phos., Phyt., Plat., Rhod., Stann., Staph.*) (C.).

Yellow coating at the base of the tongue (*Nat-P.*) (Br.).

Pain in the region of the liver (*Bry.*, *Chel.*, *Dig.*, *Hep.*, *Iod.*, *Lach.*, *Merc.*, *Podo.*, *Sep.*, *Sulph.*) (C.).

Pus-like, slimy discharge from the bowels (*Merc.*, *Sil.*) (Br.).

Unhealthy skin ; ulcers do not heal rapidly (*Hep.*, *Sil.*, *Sulph.*) (C.).

Profuse perspiration, especially with hectic rise of temperature (*Chin.*, *Hep.*, *Kali-I.*, *Merc.*, *Nat-M.*, *Sil.*).

Suppuration of the tonsils (*Bell.*, *Hep.*, *Merc.*, *Sil.*) (D.).

Eczema : the eruption has yellowish scales, and there are many pimples and points of suppuration (*Crot-T.*, *Kali-S.*, *Rhus-T.*) (Bl.).

Cough with purulent and sanious sputa and hectic fever (*Hep.*, *Lach.*, *Nit-Ac.*, *Phos.*, *Puls.*, *Sep.*, *Sil.*) (Br.).

Inflammation of the eyes, with discharge of thick, yellow matter (Br.).

Absc:ss of the cornea (*Hep.*, *Merc-C.*, *Sil.*) (D.).

Ophthalmia neonatorum (*Arg-N.*, *Hep.*, *Puls.*, *Sil.*) (Br.).

Sees only one half of an object (*Ars.*, *Aur.*, *Bov.*, *Calc.*, *Caust.*, *Dig.*, *Gels.*) (C.).

Burning of the soles of the feet (*Ars.*, *Calc.*, *Carb-V.*, *Graph.*, *Lach.*, *Lyc.*, *Phos.*, *Sep.*, *Sulph.*, *Sulph-I.*, *Zinc.*) (K.).

Inside of lips sore (*Sil.*) (C.).

Suppurative processes in the lungs (*Ars-I.*, *Calc.*, *Ferr-P.*, *Hep.*, *Kali-I.*, *Lach.*, *Lyc.*, *Merc.*, *Nit-Ac.*, *Phos.*, *Sil.*, *Sulph.*) (D.).

Rattling of mucus in the chest (*Ant-T., Carb-V., Hep., Lyc., Nat-S., Puls., Seneg., Stann., Sulph.*).

Difficulty of breathing worse in the evening and during night ; also when ascending, during cough and on lying.

AGGRAVATION : In the evening ; during night ; when walking ; during sleep ; after dinner ; during menses ; and on rising from sitting.

AMELIORATION : In the morning ; after washing ; from doubling up ; and after scratching.

RELATIONSHIP. It is deeper acting than *Hepar*, and acts after that remedy ceases to act ; *Silicea* comes in before this remedy to favour or to prevent the suppuration.

COMPARE : *Calc., Calend., Hep., Kali-M., Nux-V., Sil.* and *Sulph.*

Calendula Officinalis.

COMMON NAME : MARIGOLD.

It seems to have some specific action upon mucous membranes, for no remedy can equal it as an injection in vaginal and uterine leucorrhœa (Bt.).

It is to be thought of when the injury causes a torn or ragged wound, possibly with loss of substance. It removes the inflammatory condition of the part, and so permits of healthy granulation (F.).

EXTERNAL WOUNDS AND LACERATIONS, WITH OR WITHOUT LOSS OF SUBSTANCE.

It has a reputation as a hæmostatic following the extraction of a tooth (*Alumn., Arn., Ham., Kreos., Lach., Phos.*) (Bl.).

The wound is raw and inflamed ; is painful, as if beaten ; the parts around the wound become red, with stinging in the wound during the febrile heat.

It removes pain and soreness and favours phagocytosis and healing (Bl.).

Traumatic affections (*Arn., Ham., Hyper., Sulph-Ac*) ; to secure union by first intention and prevent suppuration (A.).

Jaundice : curdy stools ; bruised pain at the angle of the right scapula ; yellowish vision (*Cina*) (B.).

ULCERS : IRRITABLE ; INFLAMED ; SLOUGH-ING ; VARICOSE ; PAINFUL AS IF BEATEN ; EXCESSIVE SECRETION OF PUS (A.).

Superficial burns and scalds (*Canth.*) (Br.).

Exhausted from loss of blood and excessive pain (*Arn., Chin , Hyper.*) (A.).

Cough, with green expectoration and hoarseness (*Arg-N., Stann.*) (Br.).

Great disposition to take cold, especially in damp weather (*Dulc , Hep., Nat-S.*) (Br.).

AGGRAVATION : In damp weather ; in the evening.

AMELIORATION : From warmth.

RELATIONSHIP. *Compare* : *Arn., Ham., Hyper., Sulph-Ac., Symph.*

Complementary: *Hep.*, *Sulph-Ac.*

Similar to: *Hyper.*, in injuries to parts rich in sentient nerves, where pain is excessive and out of all proportion to injury; *Arn.*, in traumatism with or without laceration of soft tissue; *Calc-P.* and *Symph.*, for non-union of bones; and *Rhus-T.* and *Ruta*, for strains or injuries of single muscle.

NOTE. Particularly useful in the dressing of torn or cut wounds, the parts being kept wet constantly with a weak solution. For concomitant complaints administer *Calendula* internally.

Camphora.

COMMON NAME : CAMPHOR.

Great faintness and prostration (*Ant-T.*, *Kali-P.*, *Laur.*, *Sep.*, *Verat.*) (Ra.).

Diminished circulation of the blood to parts most distant from the heart (coldness of the external body).

Throbbing pains in the cerebellum, like the pounding of a hammer (*Bell.*, *Glon.*, *Nat-M.*, *Psor.*), *synchronous with the beat of the heart* (N.).

Pulse : weak, extremely small, and scarcely perceptible (*Carb-V.*, *Laur.*) (A.).

BURNING IN THE STOMACH (*Ars.*, *Carb-V.*, *Phos.*, *Sec.*) (Ra.).

Sudden attacks of vomiting and diarrhœa (*Ars.*) (A.).

ASIATIC CHOLERA (*Ars.*, *Carb-V.*, *Cupr.*, *Hydr-Ac.*, *Kali-P.*, *Lach.*, *Naja*, *Phos.*, *Sec.*, *Verat.*).

COLOUR OF THE FACE BLUISH (*Ars.*, *Carb-V.*, *Cupr.*, *Dig.*, *Hyos.*, *Ipec.*, *Lach.*, *Op.*, *Verat.*).

SUDDEN SINKING OF STRENGTH (*Acon.*, *Ars.*, *Carb-V.*, *Colch.*, *Crot-H.*, *Graph.*, *Hydr-Ac.*, *Laur.*, *Phos.*, *Sec.*, *Sep.*, *Verat.*).

Face : livid, pale, haggard ; *pale and anxious ; distorted, bluish and cold* (N.).

GREAT COLDNESS OF THE SKIN, YET THE CHILD CANNOT BEAR TO BE COVERED (*Sec.*) (G. .

Extremities cold and blue, with cramps (*Ars.*, *Carb-V.*, *Cupr.*, *Kali-P.*, *Verat.*) (Bt.).

Tongue : cold, flabby, trembling (*Lach.*). (A.).

Pernicious intermittent (*Ant-T.*, *Ars.*, *Verat.*) (A.).

Long-lasting chills (*Ars.*, *Caust.*, *Chin.*, *Colch.*, *Ferr.*, *Hep.*, *Ign.*, *Lyc.*, *Nat-M.*) (Bt.).

ICY COLDNESS ALL OVER ; FACE DEATHLY PALE (*Carb-V.*, *Sec.*, *Verat.*) (N.).

Involuntary diarrhœa (*Aloe*, *Kali-P.*, *Sulph.*) ; stools blackish (*Ars.*, *Bapt.*, *Sulph.*) (Bt.).

Pains, as if bruised in inner parts (*Apis*, *Arn.*, *Bapt.*, *Bell.*, *Eup-P.*, *Ipec.*, *Nat-M.*, *Nux-V.*, *Pyrog.*, *Rhus-T.*).

Half stupid and senseless (*Ars.*, *Bapt.*, *Bell.*, *Bry.*, *Canth.*, *Hyos.*, *Lach.*, *Lyc.*, *Op.*, *Phos-Ac.*, *Stram.*, *Verat*) (Ra.).

Urine : deep red and depositing a thick sediment (*Apis*, *Berb.*, *Canth.*, *Lyc.*, *Sep.*) (G.).

Great sensitiveness to cold and cold air (*Hep.*).

Retention of urine during cholera (*Canth., Lach., Op , Verat.*) (K.).

Strangury, not relieved by urinating (Bt.).

Loss of sensation (*Anac., Ars., Carb-Ac., Caust., Chin., Cocc., Con., Kali-Br., Merc., Nux-V., Olnd., Op., Petr., Phos., Plb., Puls., Rhus-T., Zinc.*).

IMPOTENCE : WITH COLDNESS, WEAKNESS, AND ATROPHIED CONDITION OF THE SEXUAL ORGANS (*Agn., Calad., Lyc., Sulph.*) (Bt.).

Cracking of the joints (*Ang., Calc., Caps., Cocc., Kali-B., Led., Nat-M., Nit-Ac., Petr., Rhus-T., Sulph*).

Epilepsy, with much congestion of blood to the brain (Max Ht.).

Rheumatic stitches in the muscles (*Asaf., Bell., Bry., Calc., Kali-C., Merc., Puls., Rhus-T., Spig., Staph , Sulph., Tarax., Thuj.*).

STAGE OF COLLAPSE : NOSE COLD AND POINTED ; ANXIETY AND RESTLESSNESS ; SKIN AND BREATH COLD (*Ars., Carb-V., Jatr., Verat.*) (A.).

Rattling in the throat (*Ant-T., Brom., Phos., Puls.*) (G.).

Great anguish, as though he would suffocate (*Apis, Arg-N., Ars., Cupr., Lach., Phos., Sulph.*) (Ra.).

Hoarse, husky voice (*Carb-V., Phos.*) (Ra.).

Pains disappear when thinking of them (*Hell.*; pains worse when thinking of them—*Calc-P., Helon., Ox-Ac.*). (N.).

THE PATIENT OBJECTS TO BEING COVERED, NOTWITHSTANDING THE OBJECTIVE COLDNESS.; THROWS OFF ALL COVERINGS (*Carb-V., Sec., Sulph.*) (N.).

Coryza : first stage, when the nose is stuffed up and the inspired air feels cold ; the patient feels chilly (D.).

CHOLERA SICCA : COLLAPSE, WITH SCANTY OR ABSENT DISCHARGES. *Body cold as ice* ; *great prostration* ; *voice squeaky or husky* ; *upper lip retracted* (D.).

Sexual desire increased. Chordee or priapism (*Cann-S., Canth., Phos., Pic-Ac., Sulph.*). Nightly emissions (Br.).

Satyriasis (*Bell., Canth., Hyos., Phos., Plat., Stram.*) (B.).

Asphyxia neonatorum (*Ant-T., Laur.*) (B.).

Eyes fixed, staring, distorted (*Bell., Hyos., Stram.*) (C.).

Foam at the mouth, during convulsions (*Art-V., Bufo, Cupr., Hyos.*) (K.).

Sleeplessness, from nervous overexcitability (*Coff., Kali-P., Nux-V., Phos., Stram.*).

GREAT PRÆCORDIAL ANXIETY AND DISTRESS (*Acon., Arg-N., Ars., Hydr-Ac., Lach., Phos., Verat.*) (C.).

Camphor, topically, causes an erysipelatous dermatitis, with bright redness, and, eventually, blisters (from concentrated solution) (F.).

WEAK, EMPTY, GONE, FAINT FEELING AT THE PIT OF THE STOMACH AT 11 A.M. (*Sep.*) (N.).

Cannot wait for lunch (A.).

Putrid eructations (*Acet-Ac., Arn., Bell., Cocc., Graph., Mag-S., Merc., Mur-Ac., Nux-V., Psor., Puls., Sep.*) (D.).

Feeling of satiety after a small quantity of food (*Chin., Lyc., Plat., Sil.*) (D.).

Desires for sweets, which make him sick, causing a sour stomach and heart-burn (*Merc.*) (D.).

Rumbling and rolling in the bowels (*Aloe, Gamb., Podo.*) (G.).

There is a craving for spirits (*Nux-V.*) (D.).

Fullness and distension of the abdomen, pressing downward towards the anus (N.).

Painful sensitiveness of the abdominal walls to touch (*Apis, Arn., Bell., Lach.*) (N.).

Movement in the abdomen as of a child (*Croc., Thuj.*) (A.).

Much pain and soreness of the liver (*Lach., Merc.*) (D.).

Useful in hæmorrhoids when the bowels, prove inactive (*Anac., Ign., Sep.*).

Both the flow of urine and discharge of fæces are painful to the parts over which they pass (N.).

DIARRHOEA SOME HOURS AFTER MIDNIGHT, OR DRIVING OUT OF BED EARLY IN THE MORNING, 5 A.M. (*Aloe*) (N.).

Constipation usually alternating with diarrhœa (*Aloe, Nux-V.*) (D.).

Exudations into serous sacs following acute inflammations (N.).

Dropsy and other ailments of drunkards (*Lach., Lyc., Mur-Ac.*) (A.).

Nightly suffocative attacks, wants the doors and windows open (A.).

Weakness in the chest when talking (*Calc., Phos-Ac., Rhus-T., Stann., Sulph-Ac.*), and in the evening when lying down (N.).

Useful in cases of pneumonia where there is no tendency to recuperation and resolution; the lungs tend to break down; there are rales all over the chest, muco-purulent expectoration, and symptoms of hectic fever; all the symptoms being worse at night (D.).

Fan-like motion of the alæ nasi in pneumonia (*Am-C., Ant-T., Kreos., Lyc., Phos.*) (K.).

May be given in the beginning of pulmonary tuberculosis, with pain through the left chest (*Phos.*), heat on the head, cold feet, frequent flushes, etc. (D.).

Weeping during stool (*Aeth., Bor., Cham., Cina, Phos., Rhus-T., Sil.*) (K.).

Child falls asleep as soon as the tenesmus ceases, after the stool (N.).

Diarrhœa, with sensation as if the bowels were too weak to retain their contents (*Aloe, Phos.*) (A.).

CONSTIPATION: STOOLS HARD, KNOTTY, DRY AS IF BURNT (*Bry.*); LARGE, PAINFUL. (A.).

Child is afraid to have the stool on account of pain, or pain compels to desist on first effort (A.).

Bloody stools (*Merc., Nit-Ac.*) (G.).

Much itching about the anus (*Aloe, Calc., Cina, Merc., Staph.*) (G.).

Diabetes mellitus; passes large quantities of colourless urine (*Kali-P., Lyc., Merc.*) (A.).

Incontinence of urine (*Caust., Sep.*) (G.).

Tenesmus for an hour after stool (*Merc.*) (G.).

Piles, either blind or flowing; with discharges of dark, venous blood and violent bearing down pains in the small of back, towards the anus (Ra.).

Weak and slow stream of urine (*Thuj.*) (Bt.).

Yeasty urine (*Caust., Raph.*).

Cloudy urine with penetrating odour (*Nit-Ac.*) (Bt.).

THE DIARRHOEIC STOOLS ARE CHANGE-
ABLE IN COLOUR (*Cham., Colch., Dulc., Podo., Puls.,
Sanic.*) AND MAY CONTAIN UNDIGESTED FOOD
(*Arg-N., Crot-T., Ferr., Nat-M., Podo.*) (D.).

Sour diarrhœa (*Calc., Hep., Mag-C.*) (Bt.)

The odour of the stool clings to the patient for a long
time (D.).

Much soreness at the anus (*Aloe, Lach., Merc., Nit-Ac.*)
(D.).

Pulsation in the anus after stool, which continues all
day (Ra.).

PARTS AROUND THE ANUS RED, EXCORIAT-
ED (*Ars., Cham., Nat-M., Petr.*) (A.).

Emission of prostatic fluid with difficult stools (*Nit-Ac.,
Phos-Ac., Sep., Sil., Staph.*) (K.).

REDNESS OF THE MEATUS URINARIUS
(*Cann-S., Gels., Led., Nit-Ac., Thuj.*) (K.).

BURNING IN THE MEATUS URINARIUS
(*Berb., Cann-S., Kali-S., Nat-M.*) (K.).

BURNING IN THE URETHRA AFTER COITION
OR WHEN SEMEN IS DISCHARGED (*Berb., Canth.,
Sep., Sulph-Ac.*) (K.).

Seminal emissions and irritability (*Nat-M., Nux-V.,
Phos.*).

Such burning in the vagina that she is scarcely able to
keep still (*Ars.*) (N.).

Menses too early, too profuse, protracted (*Calc., Sab.,
Sec.*) (A.).

Menorrhagia; has not been well since her last miscarriage
(*Sep.*) (A.).

Seminal discharge too quick (*Berb., Calad., Calc., Con.,
Graph., Lyc., Nat-M., Phos., Zinc.*), *shortly after an erection* (*Phos-Ac.*) (K.).

Chronic gonorrhœa, with discharge of white mucus
(*Cop., Nat-M., Sep.*) (Bt.).

Menses thick, black, and so acrid as to make the vulva and thighs sore (*Kreos.*) (G.).

Despondent; out of humour; weeps much (Bt.).

Peevishness and fantastic illusions (*Nux-V.*).

MELANCHOLIC MOOD; DWELLING ON RELIGIOUS THINGS; ANXIOUS TO SAVE HIS SOUL (*Aur., Puls., Verat.*) (N.).

The most ordinary objects awake extraordinary admiration (N.).

Everything looks pretty which the patient takes a fancy to; even rags seem beautiful (A.).

Dresses up in rags and imagines that they are the finest silk (D.).

"*A rugged philosopher,*" *life having been a failure* (D.).

A chronic, constitutional grumbler (*Nux-V.*) (D.).

Too lazy to rouse himself; too unhappy to live (*Aur.*) (A.).

Chronic vertigo (*Calc., Calc-P., Con., Kali-P., Lyc., Phos., Puls., Sep.*) (Bt.).

Congestion to single parts (eyes, nose, chest, abdomen, ovaries. arms, legs, or any organ of the body, marking the onset of tumours or malignant growths, especially at climacteric (A.).

Sick headache periodically once a week or two weeks (N.).

BURNING HOT DISTRESS ON THE TOP OF THE HEAD (*Graph., Lach., Phos.*); THIS CONSTANT HEAT ON THE TOP OF THE HEAD IS ONE OF THE MOST PROMINENT SYMPTOMS WE HAVE FOR SULPHUR (Bt.).

Pressive pain in the vertex, as from a weight on the top of the brain (N.).

FRONTAL HEADACHE IN THE MORNING (*Calc., Calc-S., Kali-B., Lach., Nux-V.*).

Of great utility in the cure of idiopathic epilepsy and convulsions of both sexes (*Calc., Cupr., Hyos., Lach., Nat-M., Op., Sil.*).

Chills and fever; no reaction; stupid; constantly sinking (N.).

Sensation of burning in many parts (*Ars., Graph., Lach., Phos., Sec., Sep.*) (N.).

During fever the patient is drowsy (*Apis, Bry., Gels., Nux-M.,*), *the skin is dry and hot, and there is no sweat* (it comes in generally after *Acon.*) (D.).

Hot flushes during the day with weak, faint spells, passing off with a little moisture (A.).

An excellent remedy in chronic cases of ague (*Ipec., Nat-M., Puls.*) (Bt.).

Sorethroat with great burning and dryness (*Ars.*); soreness begins on the right side and goes to the left (N.).

Chronic hæmorrhages; she seems to get almost well, when it comes again and again, for weeks, with weak faint spells (*Chin., Ferr.*) (G.).

STANDING IS THE MOST DISAGREEABLE POSITION (N.).

Acrid leucorrhœa, making the vulva sore (*Kreos., Nat-M., Nit-Ac.*) (G.).

Burning in the vagina, during coition (*Kreos., Lyc., Nat-M.*) (K.).

After nursing, the nipple chaps and bleeds, with much smarting and burning (G.).

Does not walk erect; stoops or bends over forward in walking or sitting (N.).

SEXUAL ORGANS COLD, RELAXED AND POWERLESS (*Calad., Lyc., Nat-M.*) (Br.).

Itching of the genitals on going to bed (Br.).

Paraplegia of the lower limbs (*Caust., Merc., Phos.*) *and paralysis of other parts* (*Alum., Arg-N., Calc., Caust., Nat-M., Op., Phos.*).

Cold feet (*Bell., Calc., Sep.*) (N.).

HEAT IN THE SOLES OF FEET, OR COLD FEET WITH BURNING SOLES; WISHES TO FIND A COOL PLACE FOR THEM, OR PUTS THEM OUT OF BED (N.).

Cramps in the calves and soles (*Ars., Camph., Podo., Sec., Verat.*), particularly at night, also with looseness of the bowels (N.).

Unsteady gait, tremor of the hands or great debility and trembling, weariness, weakness and prostration (*Nux-V.*) (N.).

Violent, bruised pain in small of the back and in coccyx, especially when stooping, or rising from seat (N.).

Intense, persistent, long-continued fever; skin dry, hot, burning; little or no remission, day or night; patient literally been consumed with fever (A.).

Ailments from abuse of metals generally (*Hep.*) (A.).

Happy dreams, wakes up singing (A.).

Drowsy in the afternoon after sunset, wakefulness the whole night (*Coff., Op.*) (A.).

Child is restless, hot, kicks off the clothes at night (*Sanic.*) ; has worms, but the best remedy fails (A.).

Becomes suddenly wide awake at night (A.).

Finds himself at night lying on the back (N.).

" CAT-NAP " SLEEP (D.).

The slightest noise awakens (*Bor.*) (D.).

Vivid, frightful, vexatious, anxious dreams (*Arn., Aur., Puls.*) (C.).

Talks much in sleep (*Puls.*) (Bt.).

Jerks one limb on dropping to sleep (B.).

Slight cuts and injuries inflame and suppurate (*Bor., Graph., Hep., Sil.*) (C.).

Crops of boils (*Kali-I., Merc., Sil.*) (B.).

Sweat in the axillæ, on hands and feet (B.).

Milk disagrees (*Carb-V., Sep.*) (Br.).

AGGRAVATION: In the evening; after midnight **in** the early morning; at 11 A.M.; from warmth of bed; when standing; from touch; from bathing or washing; during rest; in changeable weather; during climacteric; after taking milk; periodically; from alcoholic stimulants; and in a closed room.

AMELIORATION: During motion; on walking; in dry, warm weather; from lying on the right side; from drawing up the affected limbs; and in the open air.

RELATIONSHIP: *Compare*: *Aloe, Apis, Ars., Bell., Bry., Calc., Chin., Colch., Ferr-P., Graph., Hep., Iod., Kali-P., Lach., Lyc., Merc., Nat-M., Nux-V., Phos., Psor., Puls., Rhus-T., Sep., Sil., Thuj., Urt., Verat., Zinc.*

ANTIDOTES: *Acon., Camph., Cham., Chin., Merc., Puls., Rhus-T., Sep.* and *Sil.*

Sulphur antidotes: *Chin., Iod., Merc., Nit-Ac., Rhus-T.* and *Sep.*

Complementary: *Aloe, Calc.* and *Psor.*

N.B.—*Calc.* must not be used before *Sulph.*

Sulph., Calc., Lyc., or *Sulph., Sars.* and *Sep.* frequently follow in given order.

Sulphuric Acid.

COMMON NAME: SULPHURIC ACID.

In contusion and laceration of soft parts it vies with *Calend.* (A.).

Perspiration from every motion (*Bry., Calc., Chin.*).

Variableness (*Ign., Kali-S., Puls.*).

Stitches in the joints (*Berb., Bry., Kali-B., Nit-Ac., Sil.*).

Small, weak, pulse (*Verat.*).

Tight, dry, cough with slight hacking (*Bry.*).

*Very effective in curing bronchitis in children **with short,** teasing cough* (*Dros., Ipec.*).

Child smells sour all over, despite the actual cleanliness (*Hep., Mag-C., Rheum*) (N.).

Bad effects from mechanical injuries, with bruises, chafing and livid skin (N.).

Small, bluish spots as from suggilation (*Arn., Ham.*), *or red itching spots* (*Merc.*).

Purpura hæmorrhagica (*Crot-H., Lach.*) (A.).

Concussion of brain from fall or blow, where the skin is cold and body bathed in cold sweat (A.).

Tendency to gangrene following mechanical injuries, especially of old people (A.).

Cicatrices turn blood-red, or blue, and are painful (A.).

The left side is more affected (*Lach., Rhus-T.*).

The pains are felt during sleep (*Lach.*).

HAEMORRHAGES FROM EVERY OUTLET OF THE BODY (*Crot-H., Ferr-P., Lach., Nit-Ac., Phos.*) (N.).

Prostration (*Ars., Camph., Carb-V., Kali-P., Lach., Phos., Sep., Sulph.*) (N.).

SENSATION AS IF THE BRAIN WAS LOOSE IN THE FOREHEAD AND FALLING FROM SIDE TO SIDE (*Bell., Bry., Rhus-T., Spig.*) (N.).

PAIN OF GRADUAL AND SLOWLY INCREASING INTENSITY WHICH CEASES SUDDENLY WHEN AT ITS HEIGHT, OFTEN REPEATED (*Puls.*).

Weakness of the whole body, with sensation as if from trembling (*Kali-P.*).

SENSATION OF TREMBLING ALL OVER, WITHOUT ACTUAL TREMBLING (N.).

Internal trembling of drunkards (A.).

Drawing and tearing in the body, even in the face.

Aggravation, then sudden relaxation of the pains.

Catamenia too early and too profuse (*Calc., Chin., Ferr.*).

Menses are followed by bloody leucorrhœa (*Ars., Caust., Chin., Pyrog., Zinc.*) (Bl.).

Flushes of heat in climacteric years (*Amyl-N., Graph., Sep.*) (N.).

Fever with great disposition to hæmorrhages from capillaries and rapid sinking of the vital forces, oozing of dark, liquid blood; face deathly pale (*Carb-V., Ferr.*); tendency to collapse and gangrene (A.).

Involuntary urine (*Nat-M., Sep.*) (A.).

Weak and exhausted from some deep-seated dyscrasia; no other symptoms (*Psor., Sulph.*) (A.).

Nose-bleed (*Ferr-P., Ham., Phos.*) (A.).

APHTHAE (*Bor., Kali-M., Nat-M.*).

ULCERATION OF MOUTH, GUMS, OR ENTIRE BUCCAL CAVITY (*Kali-M., Merc., Nit-Ac., Sulph.*) (N.).

GUMS BLEED READILY (*Carb-V., Crot-H., Hep., Kreos., Lach., Merc-C., Nat-M., Phos.*) (N.).

Offensive breath (*Bapt., Carb-V., Kali-P., Lach., Nux-V., Puls.*) (N.).

Aphthous ulcers; painful (*Ars., Bor., Nat-M.*) (N.).

Relaxed feeling in the stomach (*Carb-An., Ipec., Sep.*) (Br.).

Hiccough (*Ars., Bell., Carb-V.*) (Br.).

Nausea with chilliness (*Ars., Cocc., Eup-P., Ipec., Kali-Ars., Nat-M.*) (Br.).

Averse to smell of coffee (Br.).

Often very useful in the stomach troubles of old whisky topers (*Carb-V.*) (N.).

Ailments from brandy drinking (*Nux-V.*) (A.).

HYPERCHLORHYDRIA (*Mag-C., Nat-P., Nux-V.*) (Bl.).

Eructations, after eating (*Carb-V., Nux-V., Puls., Sep., Sulph.*).

The ingesta rise up again (*Chin., Ferr., Nux-V.*).

After eating warm food, cold perspiration.

Sour, acid vomiting (*Calc., Hep., Nux-V., Sulph.*) (N.).

CHRONIC HEART-BURN, SOUR ERUCTA-TIONS; SETS TEETH ON EDGE (*Rob.*) (A.).

Gastralgia; the pains are either violent and contractive, or are of a dull, heavy aching character (Bl.).

Pyrosis (*Nat-P., Nux-V., Puls.*).

Loss of appetite (*Arg-N., Chin., Puls.*) (Bl.).

WATER DRUNK CAUSES COLDNESS OF THE STOMACH, UNLESS MIXED WITH ALCOHOLIC LIQUOR (A.).

Flatulence (*Carb-V., Coloc., Mag-P., Nux-V., Puls.*) (Bl.).

Diarrhœa, fetid, black, with sour odour of the body and faint, empty feeling in the abdomen (Br.).

SAFFRON-LIKE OR ORANGE-LIKE YELLOW STOOL (*Coloc., Merc.*) (K.).

Oozing piles (*Aloe, Graph., Kali-B., Merc., Pæon.*) (B.).

Itching, burning and sticking in the anus (*Ars., Sulph.*) (C.).

Dry coryza, with loss of smell and taste (*Ant-T., Nat-M., Puls.*) (C.).

Hardness of hearing (*Calc., Phos., Sulph.*) (C.).

Profuse hæmorrhage from the lungs (*Ferr., Ipec., Phos.*) (C.).

Hectic fever (*Ars-I., Calc., Ferr., Iod., Lach., Nat-M., Sep.*) (C.).

Feels in a great hurry; everything must be done quickly (*Arg-N.*) (A.).

Unwilling to answer questions not from obstinacy, but inaptness (A.).

Cough with expectoration in the morning, without expectoration in the evening (*Hep., Puls., Squil.*) (G.).

ERUCTATIONS AFTER COUGHING (*Ambr., Ang., Verat.*) (K.).

Bloody expectoration (*Bry., Ferr-P., Phos., Sulph.*) (B.).

Fingers jerk when writing (B.).

Drenching sweats (*Chin., Merc., Nat-M., Verat.*) (B.).

Sensation as if the white of an egg had dried on the face (D.).

AGGRAVATION: After eating; during sleep; in the open air; from excess of heat or cold in the forenoon and evening; during menopause; after traumatism; from spirits; and from odour of coffee.

AMELIORATION: From warmth; from lying on the affected side; from hot drinks; and from putting hands near the head.

RELATIONSHIP: *Compare*: *Ars., Bor., Calend., Carb-V., Chin., Ferr-P., Hep., Ipec., Kali-P., Lach., Led., Lyc., Mag-C., Merc., Nat-M., Nit-Ac., Puls., Rheum, Ruta, Sep., Sulph., Symph.* and *Thuj.*

Follows well after: *Arn.,* with bruised pain, livid skin, and profuse sweat; and *Led.* in ecchymosis.

COMPLEMENTARY: *Puls.*

N. B. *Sulphuric Acid,* one part, with three parts of alcohol, 10 to 15 drops, three times daily for three or four weeks, has been successfully used to subdue the craving for liquor (Hr.).

Symphytum.

COMMON NAME: COMFREY.

Comminuted fractures (B.).

Is an excellent remedy for broken bones where the bones refuse to knit (*Calc-P.*) (N.).

It facilitates union of fractured bones, lessens peculiar pricking pain, and favours production of callus (*Calc., Calc-P.*) (A.).

Irritability at the point of fracture (*Hyper.*) (A.).

In injuries of the eye if there is great pain in the eye-ball itself from the blow, it may have to be used (Arn., Led.) (N.).

Irritable stumps after operations (*Hyper.*) (Bl.).

Periosteal pains after wounds have healed (Calc-P., Sil.) (A.).

Psoas abscess (*Arn., Asaf., Chin., Cupr., Phos-Ac., Sil., Staph., Sulph., Syph.*) (Br.).

Inflammation of inferior maxillary bone with hard, red swelling (Br.).

Neuralgia of knee (*Bell.*) (Br.).

Pain in the occiput (*Cocc., Petr., Sil.*) (Br.).

Injuries to sinews and tendons (Br.).

AGGRAVATION: From touch; from motion; and from pressure; after mechanical injury.

AMELIORATION: From warmth.

RELATIONSHIP: *Compare: Arn., Calend., Calc-P., Fluor-Ac., Hep., Merc., Nit-Ac.,* and *Sil.*

Follows well after *Arn.* for soreness of the periosteum after an injury.

Syphilinum.

COMMON NAME: SYPHILITIC VIRUS.

Is indicated in affections that are dependent upon a latent syphilitic taint (Bl.).

Is of great service in children with congenital syphilis, who show the effects of the disease (*Aur., Bar-C., Nit-Ac.*) (Bl.).

Rheumatism in syphilitic constitutions (*Aur., Kali-B., Nit-Ac., Phos-Ac., Sil.*) (D.).

Rheumatism of the shoulder-joint, or at the insertion of the deltoid; worse from raising the arm laterally (*Rhus-T.*) (A.).

Sciatica, worse at night, better about day-break (B.).

Carious ulcers (Asaf., Fluor-Ac., Sil.); **pains worse from sun down to sunrise** (N.).

Caries of the spine (*Calc., Lyc., Merc., Nit-Ac., Sil.*) (N.).

Severe pain in long bones (Br.).

ALL THE SYMPTOMS ARE WORSE AT NIGHT; THE PAIN BEGINS IN THE EVENING AND END AT DAYLIGHT (Bl.).

Ophthalmia neonatorum (*Arg-N., Calc.; Hep., Kali-S., Sulph.* (A.).

Pain in the eyes intensified at night and are relieved by cold bathing (*Puls.*) (A.).

Falling of the hair (Lyc., Nat-M., Phos-Ac.) (A.).

Chronic syphilitic headaches (Aur., Kali-B., Nit-Ac., Sil.) (D.).

Headache causing sleeplessness and delirium at night (A.).

Deep, crushing head pains (B.).

Profuse lachrymation (*All-C., Euphr., Nat-M., Rhus-T.*) (R.).

Top of the head feels as if coming off (C.).

Eyes glued together in the morning (*Arg-N., Calc., Carb-S., Clem., Graph., Med., Rhus-T., Sulph.*) (R.).

Diplopia; one image seen below the other (C.).

Ptosis (Arg-N., Caust., Sep.) (A.).

Photophobia (Con., Nat-M., Phos.) (C.).

Recurrent phlyctenular inflammation of the cornea (C.).

Otorrhœa with acrid, watery or purulent discharge (*Kali-S.*) (R.).

Abscesses or boils coming in succession (*Sulph.*) (R.).

Copper-coloured, reddish-brown eruptions over the body, with a disagreeable odour (B.).

Pustular eruption on different parts of the body (*Ant-C., Merc., Rhus-T., Sulph.*) (R.).

Pains increase and decrease in severity gradually (*Plat.,* *Stann.*) (Bl.).

Offensive, thick, yellow-green nasal discharge (*Kali-B.,* *Puls.*) (R.).

Scabs form in both nostrils during sleep (*Nux-V., Puls.*) (R.).

Ozæna (*Aur., Calc., Kali-B., Lach.*) (C.).

Caries of nasal bones (*Aur., Kali-I.*) (C.).

Face drawn to one side, with difficult speech and mastication (*Caust.*) (R.).

HEREDITARY TENDENCY TO ALCOHOLISM (N.).

CRAVING ALCOHOL IN ANY FORM (*Sulph-Ac.*) (N.).

Extreme emaciation of the entire body (*Abrot., Iod.,* *Nat-M., Sanic., Sil.*) (A.).

Lancinating pains from the base to the apex of the heart at night (from the apex to the base of the heart—*Med.;* from the base of the heart to the clavicle or shoulder—*Spig.*) (A.).

Salivation at night (*Merc., Rhus-T.*) (B.).

Vomiting of food, or dark, grumous matter (*Con.,* *Lach.*) (R.).

Heart-burn with pain and rawness from the stomach to the throat-pit (*Iris*) (R.).

Teeth decay at the edge of the gum and break off; are cupped, edges serrated; dwarfed in size, converge at their tips (*Staph.*) (A.).

Stools dark, bilious and offensive (*Bapt., Nat-S.,* *Sulph.*) (R.).

Fissure in the anus and rectum (*Graph., Nat-M., Nit-Ac.,* *Petr., Thuj.*) (A.).

Prolapse of the rectum (*Merc., Podo., Sulph.*) (A.).

Thick, yellow and offensive leucorrhœa, with constant pain across the back (*Sep.*) (R.).

Obstinate constipation for years; rectum seems tied up with strictures; when enema was used the agony of passage was like labour (*Lac-C., Tub.*) (A.).

Ulcers on the labia (*Merc., Nit-Ac.*) (C.).

Leucorrhœa profuse, soaking through the napkins and running down to the heels (*Alum., Calc., Graph., Sep., Sil., Stann.*) (N.).

Menses have odour of rotten meat (B.).

Fears the terrific suffering from exhaustion on awakening (*Lach.*) (A.).

Terrible dread of night on account of mental and physical exhaustion on awakening; it is intolerable, death is preferable (A.).

Sensation, as if going insane, as if about to be paralyzed (A.).

Sensation of apathy and indifference (*Phos-Ac., Sep.*) (A.).

Loss of memory (*Kali-P., Lyc., Nat-M.*) (A.).

Cannot remember names of books, persons or places *Merc., Nux-M., Psor.*) (A.).

Hopeless, despair of recovery (*Psor.*) (C.).

Always washing her hands (K.).

AGGRAVATION: At night; from sundown to sunrise; from extreme cold or heat; in damp weather; from raising the arm laterally; during thunder-storm; every alternate full moon.

AMELIORATION: From change of position; from slow motion; by cold bathing; in high altitude; and during the day.

RELATIONSHIP: *Compare*: *Asaf., Aur., Calc., Fluor-Ac., Graph., Kali-I., Lach., Lyc., Merc., Nat-M., Phos-Ac., Phyt., Plat., Rhus-T., Sep., Sil., Thuj.* and *Zinc.*

Tabacum.

COMMON NAME: TOBACCO.

Symptoms occur in paroxysms (asthma, sick headache, vertigo and sneezing) (A.).

Icy coldness of the surface, covered with cold sweat (*Camph., Colch., Carb-V., Sec., Verat.*) (N.).

Death-like pallor (*Ars., Carb-V., Sec.*) (D.).

Nervous tremor and debility (*Gels., Kali-P., Lach., Tarant.*) (D.).

Intermittent pulse (*Dig., Nat-M.*) (D.).

Feeble, irregular pulse (*Carb-V., Verat.*) (G.).

Præcordial oppression with palpitation (*Acon., Amyl-N., Lach., Naja*) (D.).

VERTIGO, ON OPENING THE EYES (on closing the eyes—*Lach., Therid., Thuj.*) (N.).

Headaches increase with the rising of the sun and decrease with its going down (*Nat-M., Spig.*) (N.).

Sick headache, with deathly nausea and violent vomiting, greatly aggravated by noise and light (Bt.).

Paralysis and sudden hyperæmia of the brain, with violent nausea, vomiting and great prostration (Bt.).

VERTIGO, INCREASING TO LOSS OF CONSCIOUSNESS (*Kali-P.*); RELIEVED IN THE OPEN AIR AND BY VOMITING (A.).

VERTIGO, ON RISING OR LOOKING UPWARD (*Puls.*) (A.).

Periodical sick headache, lasting one or two days (A.).

Sudden pain on the right side of the head, as if struck by a hammer or a club (A.).

Renal colic (*Berb., Canth., Lyc., Nux-V., Puls.*); *violent, spasmodic pains along the ureter, left side* (*Berb., Nux-V.*); *with deathly nausea and cold perspiration* (*Ipec.*) (A.).

Constipation of years' standing (*Alum., Plb., Sep., Sulph.*) (A.).

Inactivity of the bowels (*Alum., Bry., Sep.*) or paralysis of the rectum (*Op.*) (A.).

Spasms of the sphincter ani muscle (*Bell., Caust., Ferr., Lach.*) (A.).

Prolapsus ani (*Aloe, Merc., Podo., Sep., Sulph.*) (A.).

Strabismus, depending upon brain troubles (*Stram.*) (A.).

Dim-sightedness (*Cycl., Ferr., Gels.*) (A.).

Sees as through a veil (*Phos., Sep., Sulph.*) (A.).

AMAUROSIS, FROM ATROPHY OF THE RETINA OR OPTIC NERVE (*Phos.*) (A.).

Diplopia (*Aur., Gels., Hyos., Nat-M., Nit-Ac.*) (K.).

Seminal emissions (*Calc., Lyc., Nux-V., Phos., Puls.*) (B.).

Impotency (*Agn., Calad., Gels.*) (B.).

Backache, worse from lying, and better from walking (*Rhus-T.*) (B.).

HICCOUGH AFTER COUGH (K.).

Much spitting (*Ipec., Lob., Sep.*) (B.).

SEA-SICKNESS, BETTER ON DECK, IN FRESH COLD AIR (*Phos.*) (N.).

DEATHLY NAUSEA, GIDDINESS, AND VOMITING (*Ant-T., Ars., Cocc., Colch., Cupr., Dig., Ipec., Lobel., Phos., Sec., Verat.*) (D.).

Dreadful faint feeling at the stomach (*Carb-A., Sep., Zinc.*) (Gr.).

UNCOVERING THE ABDOMEN RELIEVES THE NAUSEA AND VOMITING (G.).

SENSATION AS IF THE STOMACH WERE HANGING DOWN RELAXED (*Ipec., Staph., Sulph.*) (N.).

Violent vomiting (*Ars., Cupr., Ipec., Phos., Verat.*) (Bt.).

Vomiting during pregnancy (*Puls., Symphori.*) (A.).

Diarrhœa of yellowish or greenish slime (*Merc., Puls.*)
(G.).

SUDDEN URGING WITH NAUSEA, VOMITING, PROSTRATION AND COLD SWEAT (*Ars., Camph., Verat.*) (A.).

Vomiting, as soon as he begins to move (or from the
least motion) (*Ant-T., Ars., Bry., Cadm., Colch., Cupr.,
Ferr., Lac-D., Lob., Nux-V., Petr., Theri., Verat.*) (A.).

Diarrhœa, with extreme faintness (*Ars.*) (A.).

Complete prostration of the entire muscular system
(*Ars., Gels., Kali-P., Nux-V.*) (A.).

Sensation of excessive wretchedness (A.).

Great despondency with indigestion, palpitation and
intermittent pulse (A.).

Mental faculties much impaired (*Kali-P., Lyc., Nat-M.,
Phos-Ac., Sil.*) (G.).

Cannot read or study (*Nat-M.*) (G.).

Sudden attacks of extreme faintness (*Ars., Camph.*)
(G.).

Strangulated hernia (*Cocc., Lyc., Nux-V., Op.*) (Bt.).

Complete marasmus (*Abrot., Arg-N., Calc-P., Nat-M.,
Op., Sars., Sil.*) (Bt.).

Emaciation of cheeks and back (A.).

Violent pain in the small of the back during soft stool,
with tenesmus and burning (J.).

STATE OF COLLAPSE, AS IN CHOLERA (*Ars., Camph., Carb-V., Kali-P., Laur., Phos., Sec., Sulph., Verat.*) (Bt.).

Icy coldness of the legs from the knees down (*Carb-V.*)
(Smi.).

Continual paroxysms of sneezing for weeks (*Ars.*) (G.).

During pregnancy an insupportable pruritus over the
whole body, with pyrosis and other gastric symptoms (G.).

Pain between the shoulders (Bl.).

Hands icy cold, body warm (*Sep.*) (A.)

Trembling of the limbs (*Ambr., Gels., Kali-Br., Lach., Merc., Phos.*) (A.).

Palpitation, due to tobacco (N.).

VIOLENT PALPITATION WHEN LYING ON THE LEFT SIDE (*Cact., Lach., Nat-M., Phos., Psor., Puls.*), GOES OFF WHEN TURNING TO THE RIGHT (*Glon., Lach., Phos., Psor.*) (A.).

Angina pectoris, with nausea, cold sweat and collapse (B.).

Tightness of the chest, ameliorated by taking inspiration (N.).

Cough, followed by hiccough (Br.).

Breathlessness (*Acon., Apis., Ign.*) (Br.).

Dry, teasing cough; must take a swallow of cold water (*Caust., Phos.*) (Br.).

AGGRAVATION: From motion; from lying on the left side; from riding in a carriage; from heat; from opening the eyes; in the evening; in a warm room; and from walking.

AMELIORATION: In the fresh, open air; from uncovering the abdomen; in twilight; from vomiting; from vinegar; and from cold application.

RELATIONSHIP: *Complementary*: *Op.*

Antidotes for abuse of tobacco are:—

For ailments from tobacco-chewing—*Ars.*

For dyspepsia caused by tobacco—*Ign.* and *Sep.*

For impotence caused by tobacco—*Lyc.*

For bad taste and headache in the morning from smoking—*Nux-V.*

For tobacco heart, palpitation and sexual weakness—*Phos.*

For excessive nausea and vomiting—*Ipec.*

For annoying hiccough from tobacco-chewing—*Ign.*

For neuralgic affections of the right side of the face, and chronic nervousness, especially in sedentary occupations—*Sep.*

For spasms and cold sweat from excessive smoking—*Lyc.*

For occipital headache and vertigo from excessive use of tobacco (especially from smoking)—*Gels.*

N.B.—*Caladium* and *Plantago Major* cause a disgust for tobacco.

Tabacum antidotes: *Cic.* and *Stram.*

Tarantula Hispania.

COMMON NAMES: LYCOSA TARANTULA: SPANISH SPIDER: A LARGE, HAIRY AND VENOMOUS, TROPICAL SPIDER, of South America).

This spider poison has, like other spider poisons, very positive nervous symptoms (N.).

It acts upon the uterus and ovaries, and upon the female sexual organs generally (N.).

Especially indicated in choreic affections, where the whole body or the right arm and left leg are principally affected (left arm and right leg principally affected—*Agar.*) (Bt.).

Lasciviousness; moral relaxation (*Phos.*) (Br.).

EXTREME RESTLESSNESS; THE PATIENT MUST BE IN CONSTANT MOTION, THOUGH MOTION AGGRAVATES (*Phyt.*) (D.).

Sensitive to music (*Nat-C., Nux-V., Sep.*) (Br.).

Must be doing something all the time (*Kali-Br.*) (D.).

Destructive impulses (*Ars., Stram.*) (Br.).

Hysterical affections (*Apis, Ign., Sep.*) (D.).

Sudden alteration of mood (*Bell., Ign., Puls.*) (Br.).

Twitching and jerking of the muscles (*Bell., Hyos., Ign., Lach.,*) (A.).

Constant movement of the legs, arms, trunk, with inability to do anything (A.).

Seminal emissions (*Phos., Sep.*) (Br.).

Neuralgia of the uterus, accompanied with sadness and despair (Bt.).

Spasms of the uterus (*Bell., Sec.*) (A.).

Kleptomania (Br.).

Wants hair brushed or head rubbed (Br.).

SYMPTOMS APPEAR PERIODICALLY (*Ars., Cedr., Chin., Kali-B., Lach., Lyc., Nat-M., Spig.*) (A.).

Neuralgic headache, aggravated by the least noise, touch, strong light (Bell., Coff., Nux-V.), and ameliorated by rubbing the head against the pillow (A.).

Restless legs, impulse to walk (Br.).

At every menstrual nisus, the throat, mouth and tongue become intolerably dry, especially when sleeping (*Nux-M.*) (A.).

Cough at night, ameliorated by smoking (K.).

Termini of nerves become so irritated and sensitive that some kind of friction is necessary to obtain relief (A.).

Menstrual irregularities (*Ign., Puls., Sep.*) (C.).

Dysmenorrhœa (*Bry., Caul., Vib-O.*) (C.).

Food tastes sour (*Am-C., Calc., Lyc., Puls.*) (K.).

Craves raw food (*Ail., Sil., Sulph.*) (B.).

Extreme sexual excitement (*Plat., Stram.*) (A.).

Nymphomania and pruritus vulvæ; the parts are dry and hot, with much itching and frequent erotic paroxysms (D.).

Sensitiveness of the ovaries (*Apis, Bell., Lach., Plat., Murx.*) (D.).

Hyperæsthesia, least excitement irritates, followed by languid sadness (A.).

Extreme hyper-sensitiveness of the tips of the fingers (A.).

Slight touch along the spine provokes spasmodic pain in the chest and cardiac region (A.).

Alternate chill and heat (*Ars.*) (B.).

Intense headache (*Bell., Glon., Lach., Nat-M.*), as if thousands of needles were pricking in the brain (as though a thousand little hammers were knocking in the brain— *Nat-M.*) (A.).

Intermittent fever, with choreic convulsions (C.).

AGGRAVATION: From motion; from touch of the affected parts; from noise; from change of weather; periodically the same hour; in the evening; and after menses.

AMELIORATION: In the open air; from music; from bright colours; from massaging the affected parts; from riding on horseback; and from smoking.

RELATIONSHIP: *Similar to: Agar., Apis, Ars., Bell., Canth., Croc., Crot-H., Cupr., Ferr., Kali-Br., Kali-P., Lach., Mag-P., Merc., Mygale, Naja, Nat-M., Phos., Plat., Rhus-T., Sec., Stram., Sulph., Verat.* and *Zinc.*

Complementary: Ars.

Antidote: Lach.

Tarantula Cubensis.

COMMON NAME: CUBAN SPIDER; LARGE, DARK-BROWN AND HAIRY SPIDER OF CUBA.

This remedy is indicated in septic conditions, with great prostration (*Ars., Bapt., Kali-P., Lach., Pyrog.*) (Bl.).

The affected parts are of a purplish colour (*Apis, Lach.*) and *there are burning, stinging pains* (*Apis, Ars., Nit-Ac.*) (Bl.).

The agony of a felon compels the patient to walk on the floor for nights (A.).

PRODUCES A PERFECT PICTURE OF SLOUGHING CARBUNCLE, WITH GREAT PROSTRATION AND ATROCIOUS, BURNING PAINS (*Anthrac., Ars., Lach.*) (D.).

Malignant ulcers (*Ars., Carb-Ac., Kreos., Lach., Nit-Ac.*) (A.).

Anthrax (*Apis, Ars., Lach.*) (A.).

Old suppurating, bluish-coloured, offensive buboes (*Carb-An., Lach.*) (N.).

Pruritus, especially about the genitals (*Crot-T., Graph., Merc., Petr., Sulph.*) (Br.).

Bubonic plague, with early and persistent prostration (*Ars., Bell., Ign., Lach., Op., Phos., Rhus-T.*) (Br.).

Retention of urine (*Ars., Caust., Lyc., Nux-V., Op., Puls.*) (Br.).

Cannot hold urine on coughing (*Caust., Nat-M., Puls.*) (Br.).

Sleep prevented by harsh cough (*Lyc., Puls., Sep.*) (Br.)

Loss of appetite, except for breakfast (Br.).

Hiccough after breakfast (*Zinc.*) (K.).

AGGRAVATION: At night; from exertion; from cold drinks.

RELATIONSHIP: *Compare*: *Anthrx., Ars., Lat-M.*

Taraxacum.

COMMON NAME: DANDELION.

The limbs are movable, but it seems to him as if the moving power was obstructed.

Painfulness of all the limbs by touch and a like condition when in an improper position.

Crampy pains in different parts of the body (*Cupr., Mag-P., Sec.*).

Sensation of weakness through the whole body with a desire to lie around.

More symptoms appear while sitting or standing and disappear when walking.

Perspiration in the evening when going to sleep.

Debility and profuse night-sweats, especially when convalescing from bilious or typhoid fever (Chin., Lach., Phos.) (A.).

Sensation of great heat on the top of the head (Ars., Lach., Sulph.).

Gastric headache (*Ant-C., Kali-M., Nux-V., Puls.*) (A.).

Darting pains in the outer parts (G.).

Sterno-cleido mastoid muscle very painful to the touch (Lach.).

Cramp in the left sterno-mastoid muscle.

Tongue covered with a white film with sensation of rawness. This film comes off in patches, leaving dark-red, tender and very sensitive spots (Ran-S.) (A.).

MAPPED TONGUE (*Ars., Kali-B., Lach., Nat-M.*) (D.).

Salivation (Chin., Kali-B., Merc.) (Bl.).

Hawking up of sour mucus.

Sour blood from decayed teeth during toothache.

Collection of water in the mouth (*Colch., Merc., Nit-Ac., Puls., Rhus-T.*).

Loss of appetite (*Chin., Lyc., Puls.*) (A.).

Food tastes sour (Am-C., Ars., Calc., Caps., Chin., Jac-C., Lyc., Nux-V., Podo., Puls., Tab., Tarant.).

Bubbly sensation in the abdomen (*Hell., Lyc., Nat-M., Phos-Ac., Puls., Stann., Sulph-Ac.*).

Sharp, stitching pains in the hepatic region (*Bry., Chel., Kali-C.*) (Bl.).

Liver troubles, with soreness in the region of the liver (*Chin., Merc.,*) (D.).

Difficult evacuation (*Alum., Plb., Sep.*) (Br.).

Bilious diarrhœa (*Bry., Nat-S., Podo.*). (D.).

Tympanites (*Carb-V., Lyc., Puls.*) (Bl.).

JAUNDICE WITH ENLARGEMENT AND INDURATION OF THE LIVER (*Chel., Iod., Lach., Merc., Nat-M., Podo., Sep.*) (A.).

Secretion of urine increased (*Acet-Ac., Gels., Helon., Lyc., Merc., Phos-Ac.*).

Frequent desire to urinate (*Nux-V.*) (C.).

Restlessness of and pain in the thighs and limbs in typhoid and typho-malarial fever (*Rhus-T., Zinc.*) (A.).

Great chilliness after eating, and especially after drinking (*Bell., Caps., Kali-C.*) (A.).

Long-lasting chill (*Chin., Nux-V.*), *when he falls asleep, sweat breaks out, mostly on the head* (A).

Nose, hands and tips of fingers are icy cold (*Sabad., Stann.*) (A.).

Heat in the face, with redness (A.).

Copious sweat at night, with pain in the spleen (*Nat-M.*) (A.).

Neuralgia of the knees (*Bell., Puls.*) (Br.).

Yawning and sleepiness during the day (*Nux-V.*) (C.).

Vivid, unremembered dreams (C.).

Tearing pain in the occiput (C.).

Pustule in the right corner of lips (C.).

AGGRAVATION: When sitting; while standing; from lying down; from fat food; and while resting.

AMELIORATION: When walking; and from moving.

RELATIONSHIP: *Compare*: *Ars., Bry., Chel., Chin., Cupr., Hydr., Kali-M., Lach., Lyc., Merc., Nat-M., Nat-S., Nit-Ac., Nux-V., Podo., Puls., Sep., Sulph., Thuj.* and *Verat.*

Antidote: *Camph.*

Tartarus Emeticus.

COMMON NAME: TARTAR EMETIC; ANTIMONIUM TARTARICUM.

A cardiac depressant; it produces motor and sensory paralysis and loss of reflex action (D.).

On the mucous membranes and skin it produces catarrhal and pustular inflammations (D.).

Often useful in both ends of life—childhood and old age (*Bar-C., Lyc., Sil., Sulph.*) (N.).

Violent pains in the sacro-lumbar region; the slightest effort to move causes retching and cold sweat (N.).

Sneezing with fluent coryza, with loss of taste and smell (*Nat-M., Puls.*) (G.).

FAN-LIKE MOTION OF THE ALAE NASI IN PNEUMONIA (*Am-C., Kreos., Lyc., Phos., Sulph.*) (K.).

Great debility and weakness (*Ars., Kali-P., Lach., Phos., Verat.*).

Internal trembling (*Sulph-Ac.*).

Great sleepiness (*Gels., Nux-M., Op.*) (N.).

Irresistible inclination to sleep with nearly all complaints (*Nux-M., Op.*) (N.).

CONVULSIONS, WHEN SMALL-POX FAILS TO BREAK OUT (*Cupr., Zinc.*) (K.).

Face very pale or cyanotic from unoxidized blood (*Carb-V., Ipec.*) (N.).

General coldness and cold sweat (*Carb-V.*) (N.).

Attacks of fainting and syncope (*Ars., Camph., Kali-P., Laur., Nux-V., Phos., Verat.*).

One-sided complaints (rheumatic pains in the left chest), pulsation in one side of the forehead and one-sided headache.

Convulsive twitches in almost every muscle of the face (*Bell., Cupr., Hyos.*) (N.).

CHILD WANTS TO BE CARRIED (*Acon., Ars., Brom., Carb-V., Cham., Cina, Ign., Lyc.*), AND DOES NOT WISH TO BE TOUCHED (*Ant-C., Arn., Ars., Bell., Bry., Cham., Cina, Kali-C., Lach., Sil.*).

CHILD CLINGS TO THOSE AROUND AND CRIES AND WISHES IF ANY ONE TOUCHES IT; WILL NOT LET YOU FEEL THE PULSE (*Cham., Cina*) (N.).

Cannot keep her eyes open; irresistible drowsiness, and deep, stupefied sleep; when awake, hopelessness and despair, or chill and fever, or vomiting of food (N.).

Diseases originating from exposure in damp basements or cellars (*Aran., Ars., Tereb.*) (A.).

Soreness all over the chest (*Arn., Bry., Ran-B.*).

If children get angry the coughing spell comes on; also after eating (N.).

CONSTANT AND DISTRESSING COUGH, DISPOSED TO BE LOOSE WITH MUCH EXPECTORATION (*Ipec., Kali-S., Puls.*).

Rattling or hollow cough, worse at night, with suffocation; throat full of phlegm; sweat on the forehead; vomiting of food (*Ipec.*) (N.).

A remedy of great utility in cases of pneumonia (*Kali-C., Lyc., Phos.*).

In broncho-pneumonia, second stage, with bronchi loaded with mucus, it is specific (Bt.).

When of service there is rattling of mucus in the chest, catarrhal ophthalmia, and marked gastro-enteric disturbance.

COUGH GROWS LESS FREQUENT; PATIENT SHOWS SIGNS OF CARBONIZED BLOOD (N.).

When the child coughs there appears to be a large collection of mucus in the bronchial tubes; it seems as if much would be expectorated, but nothing comes up (N.).

COARSE RATTLING WITH INABILITY TO EXPECTORATE; IMPENDING PARALYSIS OF THE LUNGS (N.).

PARALYSIS OF THE LUNGS, WITH GREAT DYSPNOEA AND FITS OF SUFFOCATION (*Hyos., Lyc., Op.*) (Bt.).

Coughing and gaping constantly, particularly children (Hn.).

Short, hoarse, weak, nearly suffocating breathing, with whistling noise; thorax expands with great difficulty; head thrown backwards, with great anxiety and prostration;

face livid and cold; forehead and sometimes the whole body covered with cold perspiration; pulse feeble and accelerated (Bt.)

Acute œdema of the lungs (Apis, Ars., Lach., Lyc., Merc-Sulph., Phos.) (Bt.).

CROUP, WITH WHISTLING AND RATTLING EXTENDING INTO THE TRACHEA (D.).

Whooping cough; cough worse when the child is angry, or when eating; it culminates in vomiting of mucus and food (D.).

Asphyxia: Mechanical, as apparent death from drowning; from mucus in the bronchi; from impending paralysis of the lungs; and from foreign bodies in the larynx and trachea (A.).

Asphyxia neonatorum; child at birth pale, breathless, gasping. It relieves the death-rattle (Laur.) (A.).

Sooty or flapping nostrils (*Hyos., Lyc.*) (B.).

Painful urging to urinate; scanty discharge, dark-red, or the last portion bloody; with stitches in the bladder and burning in the urethra (N.).

After checked gonorrhœa, pain in the testes (*Puls.*) (G.).

Severe bearing down in the vagina (*Bell., Murx., Sep.*) (G.).

Leucorrhœa of watery blood, liable to occur in paroxysms, worse while sitting (N.).

Feet "go to sleep" immediately after sitting down (C.).

Insensibility and coldness of the limbs (*Camph., Carb-V.*) (C.).

Dropsy of the legs (*Ars., Ferr., Kali-C.*) (B.).

Rapid, weak and trembling pulse (R.).

Icterus with pneumonia, especially of the right lung (Chel., Merc.) (A.).

Tongue very thinly white with reddened papillæ and red edges particularly with whooping cough (N.).

Tongue red in streaks (Hn.).

The pustular inflammation occurs in the œsophagus, mouth, throat, larynx, stomach and small intestines (Hg.).

Gastro-enteritis characterized by great anxiety, nausea, vomiting of a green, watery, frothy material that contains particles of food (Bl.).

Desire for acids (Ars., Cor-R., Hep.) and fruits (Ars., Calc-S., Phos-Ac., Verat.) (K.).

Extraordinary craving for apples (Aloe; for acids and pickles—Ant-C.) (A.).

Very thirsty day and night (*Ars., Bry., Phos., Sulph.*) (Bt.).

HE COULD LIE ON HIS RIGHT SIDE ONLY; ANY CHANGE FROM THIS POSITION WAS SURE TO PRODUCE VOMITING (Wd.).

Much nausea and vomiting day and night, with drowsiness (*Aeth.*) (G.).

Aversion to milk, and often to all kinds of nourishment (G.).

Violent pains, like cramps in the epigastrium (*Cupr.*) (G.).

Vomiting, until he faints (A.).

NAUSEA WITH FREQUENT VOMITING (*Ant-C., Ars., Ipec., Nux-V.*) OF BITTER, SOUR SUBSTANCES—A MARKED CHARACTERISTIC.

Long-lasting dyspeptic symptoms, with loss of appetite (*Carb-V., Kali-C., Lyc., Nux-V., Puls., Sep., Sulph.*).

Colic, as if the bowels would be cut to pieces; labour-like tearing from above downward, with rumbling and looseness (N.).

Beating and throbbing through the whole body, particularly in the belly or pit of the stomach, with great concern about the future (N.).

INTENSE NAUSEA AND VOMITING, WITH PROSTRATION (*Ipec., Tab., Verat.*) (N.).

Vomiting of large quantities of mucus (Ipec., Phos., Puls.) (Bt.).

Inflamed lids with catarrhal conjunctivitis (*Calc., Euphr., Merc., Puls., Sulph.*).

Purging frequently associated with vomiting (*Ars., Podo., Verat.*) (Bl.).

The stools are profuse and watery, and indications of collapse are present (*Carb-V., Kali-P., Verat.*) (Bl.).

Diarrhœa in association with pneumonia, small-pox, and other eruptive diseases, especially if the eruption has been suppressed (*Sulph.*) (G.).

The stools may be very offensive, watery, bloody, light brownish-yellow, or green as grass (G.).

Intermittent fever with lethargic condition (*Gels.*) (Br.).

Violent vomiting in association with intermittent fever (*Ant-C., Cina, Elat., Ferr., Lyc.*) (K.).

Short chill and long-lasting heat, with somnolency and profuse sweat on the forehead (A.).

Perspiration on the scalp (*Calc., Ipec., Merc., Sil., Tarant.*) *or forehead on coughing* (*Chlor., Ipec., Verat.*) (K.).

Vertigo, with drowsiness (Hn.).

The head trembles, particularly when coughing, with an inward trembling; teeth chattering and drowsiness more in the evening and in the warmth (N.).

Thick eruptions like pocks, often pustular (*Rhus-T.*); *as large as a pea* (*Merc.*) (N.).

Variola, with vomiting of viscid mucus clogging the air-passages; pustules in the larynx, mouth, throat and digestive organs (Bt.).

Great dysphagia; deglutition almost impossible (*Bell., Hep., Lach., Merc., Phos., Sil.*) (G.).

AGGRAVATION: In damp, cold weather; from lying down; at night; from the warmth of the room; from change of weather; in spring; from touch; from anger; and from over-eating.

AMELIORATION: In the open air; from sitting upright; from expectoration; and from lying on the right side.

RELATIONSHIP: In lobar pneumonia and broncho-pneumonia *Tart-Emet.* is very similar to *Lyc.* (In *Lyc.* there are greater and more distressing dyspnœa, many mucous rales, stitching and stabbing pleuritic pain and a tendency to abdominal distension. Over and above in *Lyc.* there is present not only marked weakness, but also there is great struggling on the part of the patient to get his breath, with a flaying of the alæ nasi).

Tart-Emet. is similar to *Verat-Alb.,* in cholera. Both have diarrhœa, colic, vomiting, coldness and craving for acids; but in the latter copious sweating on the forehead is more prominent.

In capillary bronchitis or broncho-pneumonia *Tart-Emet.* corresponds to *Ipec.,* but can be distinguished by its excelling drowsiness or coma from defective respiration. Over and above, you should remember that it supplants *Ipec.,* when the lungs seem to fail, and the cough declines or ceases.

It is called for bad effects of vaccination, when *Thuja* fails and *Silicea* is not indicated.

Children not easily impressed when *Ant-T.* seems indicated in coughs, require *Hep-S.*

Antidotes: *Chin., Ipec., Puls.* and *Sep.*

Terebinthina.

COMMON NAME: TURPENTINE.

Fresh ecchymoses in great numbers occur from day to day (*Sulph-Ac.*) (A.).

Great languor and loss of strength (*Ars., Bapt., Gels., Kali-P.*) (Ho.).

Hæmorrhages from all outlets, especially in connection with urinary or kidney troubles (N.).

Purpurà hæmorrhagica (*Arn., Crot-H., Lach., Phos.*) (N.).

Congestion and inflammation of the urinary organs (*Bell., Ferr-P.*), *with scanty, high-coloured urine* (*Canth., Lyc.*) (Bt.).

Nephritis (*Apis, Canth., Lach., Lyc., Merc.*) (Bl.).

BURNING, DRAWING PAINS IN THE KID-
NEYS (*Zinc.*) (Bt.).

Dull, aching pains in the renal region (*Berb., Lyc.,
Nux-V.*) (D.).

Albuminous urine (*Apis, Canth., Merc-C., Phos., Sep.*)
(N.).

HAEMATURIA (*Canth., Hep., Lach., Merc-C., Sars.*)
(N.).

BLOOD IS THOROUGHLY MIXED WITH THE
URINE, LIKE COFFEE-GROUND SEDIMENT (Bt.).
Urethritis (*Cann-S., Canth., Kali-B.*) (Bl.).

Distressing strangury (*Bell., Canth., Merc-C., Nux-V.,
Puls., Sep.*) (D.).

Burning and smarting on passing urine (*Canth., Caps.*)
(N.).

*Pressure in the bladder, extending up into the kidneys
when sitting, disappearing when walking* (Ha.).

URINE: SCANTY, BLOODY, DARK AND
SMOKY, LOOKING AND SMELLING LIKE
VIOLETS (D.).

Violent burning and cutting in the bladder; tenesmus;
sensitive hypogastrium; cystitis and retention from atony
of the fundus (A.).

Spasmodic retention of urine (*Bell., Canth., Nux-V.*)
(A.).

ALBUMINURIA AFTER DIPHTHERIA, SCAR-
LATINA OR TYPHOID (A.).

Incontinence of urine (*Calc., Sep.*) (R.).

Constant desire to urinate (*Canth., Nux-V.*) (R.).

TONGUE SMOOTH AND GLOSSY, AS IF DE-
PRIVED OF ITS PAPILLAE, IN TYPHOID FEVERS,
(ALSO IN STOMATITIS AND ENTERO-COLITIS)
(Wd.).

TONGUE VERY SORE, RED AND GLOSSY,
BURNING LIKE FIRE (Bt.).

Choking sensation in the throat (*Ign., Lach., Nat-M., Phos.*) (Br.).

Stomatitis (*Bor., Kali-B., Merc.*) (Br.).

Rancid eructation (*Carb-V.*) (R.).

Burning sensation in the stomach (*Ars., Canth., Lyc., Phos., Sulph.*) (R.).

Griping colic (*Bell., Coloc., Mag-P.*) (R.).

Nausea and vomiting (*Colch., Ipec.,*) (Br.).

Burning in the chest along the sternum (*Phos.*).

Complaints from living in basements and damp dwellings (A.).

PERITONITIS (*Apis, Bell., Bry., Lach.*) (R.).

Abdomen extremely sensitive to touch (*Apis, Bell., Lach.*) (A.).

Flatulence (*Aloe, Nat-S., Nux-V., Podo.*) (A.).

IMMENSE TYMPANITES (*Carb-V., Lyc.*) (Bt.).

Stools: Copious, watery, greenish, and very foetid; has motions from ten to twenty from 12 A.M. to 12 P.M.

Entero-colitis, with frequent and exhaustive stools (Ha.).

Griping, pinching colic, with muco-purulent stools (*Merc.*) (Bt.).

Fainting after each stool (*Ars., Calc., Con., Lyc., Nux-M., Phos., Podo., Sulph., Verat.; before stool—Ars., Dig., Glon., Puls., Sars., Sumb.; during stool—Aloe, Coll., Dulc., Dios., Nux-M., Ox-Ac., Puls., Sars., Sulph.*).

BURNING IN THE RIGHT HYPOCHONDRIUM (*Ars., Aur-M., Bry., Chel., Crot-C., Gamb., Kali-C., Lac-C., Lach., Mag-M., Med., Mur-Ac., Nit-Ac., Phos., Sulph.*).

HAEMORRHAGES FROM THE BOWELS IN TYPHOID FEVER (*Kali-P., Lach., Nit-Ac., Phos., Sulph.*) (Bt.).

Burning in the anus and rectum (*Aloe, Ars., Canth., Caps., Graph., Iris, Lach., Nit-Ac., Sulph.*) (A.).

Ascarides, lumbrici or tape-worms (*Calc., Stann., Sulph.*) (A.).

Tickling at the anus (*Aloe, Calc., Merc.*).

Worms, with foul breath, choking (*Cina, Spig.*); dry, hacking, cough (A.).

Irregular chills and flushes of heat (A.).

Coldness and chill in the abdomen (A.).

Heat with great thirst (*Ars., Bry., Sulph.*) (A.).

Copious hæmorrhage, black fluid, from the nose, stomach, kidneys, lungs, bowels, with ulceration of Peyer's patches; great prostration and emaciation (A.).

Low, muttering delirium (*Bry., Hyos., Rhus-T.*) (Bl.).

Cold, clammy sweat over the whole body (A.).

Post-scarlatinal dropsy (or dropsy after scarlatina), with smoky urine (*Apis, Colch., Hell., Lach.*) (N.).

Dryness of the mucous membranes of the air-passages.

Expectoration streaked with blood (*Calc-S., Phos., Sil.*) (R.).

Hæmoptysis (*Acalypha, Ipec., Phos.*) (Br.).

Short, hurried and anxious breathing (*Lach., Lyc., Phos.*) (R.).

Capillary bronchitis (*Ant-T.*) (R.).

Bronchial asthma (*Ant-T., Ipec., Lob.*) (B.).

Hæmoptysis (*Acon., Bell., Ferr-P., Lach., Nit-Ac., Phos., Rhus-T., Sep., Sulph.*) (N.).

Intense burning in the uterine region (*Ars., Lach., Sulph.*) (Br.).

Metritis (*Bell., Lach., Puls., Rhus-T.*) (Br.).

Puerperal peritonitis (*Bry., Lach., Sep.*) (Br.).

Metrorrhagia, with burning in the uterus (*Lach., Phos., Sec.*) (Br.).

Thin, offensive, acrid lochia after miscarriage or childbirth (*Ars., Sec.*) (R.).

Intense pressure and fullness of the head (*Bell., Bry., Nux-V.*) (C.).

AGGRAVATION: From dampness; from cold; at night; from lying down; from pressure; when urinating; and when sitting.

AMELIORATION: From motion; when walking.

RELATIONSHIP: *Compare*: *Alumn.*, *Apis*, *Arn.*, *Ars.*, *Berb.*, *Canth.*, *Dig.*, *Equiset.*, *Ferr-P.*, *Gels.*, *Hell.*, *Ipec.*, *Kali-B.*, *Kali-C.*, *Kali-P.*, *Lach.*, *Lyc.*, *Merc-C.*, *Nit-Ac.*, *Phos.*, *Puls.*, *Rhus-T.*, *Sep.*, *Sulph.*, *Thuj.* and *Verat-V*.

Is recommended as a prophylactic in malarial and African fevers.

Antidote: *Phos.*

Teucrium Marum Verum.

COMMON NAME: CAT THYME.

Useful in worms (*Cina, Merc., Stann.*).

THIS IS A GREAT REMEDY FOR ASCARIDES, WHERE THERE IS GREAT ITCHING OF THE ANUS (Bt.).

Creeping and crawling in the rectum worse during evening and from warmth of bed (Bl.).

Tearing in the limbs, especially in the bones and joints (*Merc.*).

The limbs go to sleep (*Puls., Rhus-T.*).

About noon general sensation of debility.

Nervous, trembling, irritable sensation in the whole body.

Tingling in the nose (All-C.).

Child frequently rubs its nose (*Arg-N., Cina, Sil.*) (N.).

SENSATION AS IF THE NOSTRILS WERE STOPPED; BLOWING NOSE OR SNEEZING DOES NOT REMOVE OBSTRUCTION (*Stict.*) (N.).

POLYPUS NARIUM OR NASAL POLYPUS (*Calc., Lyc., Merc., Phos., Sil.*) (Bt.).

Catarrh, with expectoration of solid chunks from the posterior nares (D.).

Biting sensation in the vicinity of the polypus (Bt.).

Frequent sneezing (*All-C., Ars., Rhus-T.*) (Bl.).

Sensation of crawling in the nose, without coryza (Bl.).

Ingrowing toe-nails (*Graph., Sil.*) (Bt.).

Suppurating grooves in the nails.

Loss of sense of smell (*Nat-M., Puls.*) (Br.).

Desire for open air, which does not fatigue him but improves the condition (*Carb-V., Phos., Puls., Tub.*).

Staggering when walking (*Arg-N., Gels., Nux-V., Stram.*).

POLYPUS IN THE UTERUS OR VAGINA (*Calc., Merc., Petr., Phos-Ac., Puls., Staph., Thuj.*) (K.).

Very indolent; inclined neither to physical nor to mental exertion (*Nux-V., Sil.*) (C.).

Singing involuntarily (*Croc., Lyc., Lyss.*) (K.).

Unusual hunger (*Calc., Cina, Iod., Nat-M., Phos.*); *prevents sleep* (*Abies-N., Chin., Ign., Lyc., Phos., Sanic.*) (C.).

Violent hiccough (*Cic., Lyc., Mag-P., Nat-M., Nux-V., Stram.*) (C.).

Jerking hiccough, after nursing (F.).

Vomiting of large quantities of dark-green masses (Br.).

AGGRAVATION: In the evening; at night; from warmth of bed; when walking; and after nursing.

AMELIORATION: In the open air.

RELATIONSHIP: *Compare*: *Calc., Cic., Cina, Gels., Ign., Kali-B., Lyc., Mag-P., Merc., Nat-M., Nat-P., Phos., Puls., Sep., Sulph.* and *Thuj.*

Complementary: *Calc.* and *Nat-P.*

Theridion Curassavicum.

COMMON NAME: ORANGE SPIDER.

For extreme sensitiveness of puberty; during pregnancy and climacteric years (A.).

Most complaints are accompanied with vertigo (*Kali-P., Phos.*) (Bt.).

Headache: When beginning to move, as of a dull heavy pressure behind the eyes; violent, deep, in the brains, worse from lying down (*Lach.*); very much aggravated from others walking on the floor, or from least motion of the head (A.).

Great aversion to work (*Chin., Lyc., Nux-V., Phos., Sep., Sulph.*) (G.).

ANXIETY ABOUT THE HEART (*Acon., Ars., Aur., Camph., Carb-V., Ign., Kalm., Meny., Naja, Phos., Puls., Spig., Tab.*) (Hr.).

Great inclination to be startled (*Bell., Bor., Gels., Kali-C., Stram.*) (Hr.).

Time seems to pass very rapidly (too slowly—*Arg-N., Cann-I., Nux-M.*) (A.)

Burning in the liver region (*Sulph.*) (Br.).

Nausea and vomiting when closing the eyes (Hr.).

Nausea from least motion (*Bry., Cocc., Kali-C.*); *from fast riding in a carriage* (*Cocc., Petr., Sep.*) (A.).

EVERY SOUND SEEMS TO PENETRATE THROUGH THE WHOLE BODY, CAUSING NAUSEA AND VERTIGO (A.).

Headache behind the eyes (Hr.).

Nausea increased to vomiting during vertigo (*Iris, Kali-B., Tab.*) (Hr.).

VERTIGO ON CLOSING THE EYES (*Lach., Thuja*), FROM ANY, EVEN THE LEAST NOISE (A.).

MENIERE'S DISEASE OR AURAL OR LABRYINTHINE VERTIGO (A.).

Periodical headache; throbbing and shooting, over the left eye: aggravated by the heat of the sun and noise (D.)

Luminous vibrations before the eyes (Br.)

Chronic nasal catarrh (*Calc., Nat-S.*) (A.).

Nasal discharge thick, yellow, greenish and offensive
(*Calc., Kali-S., Merc., Nat-S., Thuj.*) (A.).

SEA-SICKNESS OF NERVOUS WOMEN; THEY CLOSE THEIR EYES TO GET RID OF THE MOTION OF THE VESSEL AND GROW DEATHLY SICK (*Tab.*) (A.).

Scrofulosis, when best remedies fail (*Calc., Iod., Tub.*)
(N.).

Phthisis florida (*in the beginning*) (A.).

Stitch high up (*apex*) *in the left chest to the back* (A.).

Cardiac anxiety and pain (*Ars., Cact., Lach., Naja,
Nat-M., Phos.*) (Bl.).

Inclination to take deep breath (*Bry., Phos.*); to sigh
(*Ign.*) (C.).

*Violent stitches in the upper left chest, below the scapula,
extending to the neck* (*Anis., Myrt., Pix., Sulph.*) (A.).

Pain in the bones all over, as if broken (*Eup-P.*) (A.).

*Great sensitiveness between the vertebræ; sits sideways
in a chair to avoid pressure against the spine* (*Chin-S.*);
aggravated by the least noise and jar of foot on the floor
(A.).

TOOTHACHE: EVERY SHRILL SOUND PENE-TRATES THE TEETH (A.).

Teeth sensitive to cold water (*Ant-C., Calc., Hep., Merc.,
Staph., Sulph.*) (C.).

Salty taste in the mouth (*Puls.*) (C.).

Hysteria during puberty (*Ign., Puls.*) (C.).

Faints after every exertion (*Ars., Cocc., Nux-V., Sep.,
Verat.*) (C.).

AGGRAVATION: From noise; from touch; on clos-
ing the eyes; from least motion; from jar; from riding in a
carriage; from going on board the ship; and from pressure.

AMELIORATION: From rest; and from warmth.

RELATIONSHIP: *Compare*: *Acon.*, *Aran.*, *Bell.*, *Con.*, *Graph.*, *Ign.*, *Lyc.*, *Nat-M.*, *Phos.*, *Spig.*, *Sep.*, *Sil.*, *Tab.*, *Thuj.* and *Zinc.*

Follows well after: *Calc.* and *Lyc.*

Antidotes: *Acon.*, *Graph.* and *Mosch.*

Thlaspi Bursa Pastonis.

COMMON NAME: SHEPHERD'S PURSE.

Albuminuria during gestation (*Apis*) (Br.).

Renal colic (*Berb.*, *Dios.*, *Nux-V.*) (Bl.).

Phosphatic deposit in the urine (*Calc-P.*, *Phos-Ac.*, *Sulph.*) (Bl.).

Spasmodic retention of urine (*Bell.*) (Bl.)

Dysuria (*Canth.*, *Ferr-P.*, *Kali-B.*, *Lyc.*, *Merc.*) (Bl.).

Cystitis (*Apis, Bell.*) (Bl.)

Urine runs away in little jets (Br.).

Brick-dust-like sediment in the urine (*Lyc.*) (Br.).

Profuse hæmorrhage from all parts of the body (*Crot-H.*, *Phos.*, *Sec.*) ; *blood dark and clotted* (*Sab.*, *Sec.*) (A.).

Exhausting hæmorrhage from uterine inertia; scarcely recovers from one period before another begins (*Sec.*) (A.).

Menses: *Too early and too profuse; protracted* (*eight, ten, even fifteen days*) ; *tardy in starting, first day merely a show; second day colic, vomiting, a hæmorrhage with large clots; each alternate period more profuse* (A.).

METRORRHAGIA: WITH VIOLENT CRAMPS AND UTERINE COLIC; AFTER ABORTION, MISCARRIAGE, OR LABOUR; WITH CANCER UTERI (*Phos.*, *Ust.*) (A.).

Hæmorrhage accompanying uterine fibroid (*Calc.*, *Lyc.*, *Nit-Ac.*) (Bl.).

Leucorrhœa before and after menses; bloody, dark, offensive; stains indelibly (Br.).

Vertigo, worse on rising (*Bry., Chin., Phos., Puls., Sep.*) (Br.).

Craves butter-milk (Br.).

Frequent epistaxis (*Carb-V., Lach., Phos.*) (Br.).

Eyes and face puffy (*Apis, Ars., Kali-C., Phos., Sep.*) (Br.).

Spermatic cord sensitive to concussion of walking or riding (Br.)

Mouth and lips cracked (*Graph., Kali-B., Nat-M., Nit-Ac., Sulph.*) (Br.).

AGGRAVATION: On alternate menstrual period; before, during and after menses; during gestation; after abortion, miscarriage, or labour; on rising; on riding; and from walking.

AMELIORATION: From pressure; and from warmth

RELATIONSHIP: Compare: *Chin., Ferr., Kali-P., Lach., Nit-Ac., Phos., Sec., Sinap., Tril., Ust.,* and *Vib.*

Thuja Occidentalis.

COMMON NAME: ARBOR VITAE.

The leading anti-sycotic (the leading anti-psoric—*Sulph.;* the leading anti-syphilitic—*Merc.*) (N.).

Hydrogenoid constitution (*Nat-S.*) (B.).

One-sided complaints (*Caust., Lach., Lyc.*).

Aversion to motion (*Bry.*).

Useful in removing many of the symptoms of gonorrhœa (inferior to *Medorrhinum*)

Especially suited to the treatment of ailments following suppressed gonorrhœa (*Puls., Sep., Staph.*) (N.).

Twitching, especially in the upper part of the body.

Stinging in the limbs and joints (*Apis, Kali-B., Sil.*).

The limbs go to sleep (*Anac., Nux-V., Puls.*).

Painful swelling and redness of the points of the fingers.

BAD EFFECTS FOLLOWING VACCINATION; NEVER WELL SINCE (N.).

White dandruff (*Merc., Sulph.*) (N.).

Hair falling out or grows slowly and splits (N.).

VERTIGO, WHEN CLOSING THE EYES (*Lach., Ther.*) (A.).

Headache is of sycotic origin, with various symptoms (N.).

Intense stabbing pains in the head, driving the patient almost to distraction; must lie down (D.).

Sensation as though a nail were being driven into the vertex or frontal eminences (D.).

Headache, as if a convex button were pressed on the part; worse from sexual excesses, over-heating, or from tea-drinking (A.).

Chronic headache of sycotic or syphilitic origin (A.).

Styes on the eyelids (*Calc., Puls., Sep.*) (N.).

CHALAZAE OR TARSAL TUMOURS (*Staph.*) (N.).

Ophthalmia nenatorum (*Arg-N., Puls.*) (A.).

Large granulations, like warts or blisters on the eyelids (A.).

Eye symptoms are ameliorated by warmth and covering; if uncovered, feels as if a cold stream of air were blowing out through them (A.).

Discharge of pus from the ears (*Calc., Graph., Puls., Sil.*) (N.).

Polypi in the ears (*Calc., Lyc., Puls.*) (N.).

Eyelids agglutinated at night (*Alum., Carb-S., Graph., Lyc., Sep.*) (A.).

Eyelids become dry and scaly on the edges (*Graph., Petr., Sep.*) (A.).

Chronic otitis; discharge purulent, like putrid meat (A.).

RANULA (BLUISH) (*Ambr., Calc., Merc., Nat-M., Nit-Ac., Plb., Staph.*).

Teeth decay at the roots, the crown remaining sound; crumble, turn yellow (N.).

Toothache, worse from tea drinking (*Chin., Coff., Ferr., Ign., Lach., Selen., Sep.*) (K.).

On blowing the nose a pressing pain in the hollow tooth, or at the side of it (Bn.).

Dislike for fresh meat and potatoes (Br.).

Complete loss of appetite (*Chin., Lyc., Puls., Sep.*) (Br.).

Thirst, with a gurgling sound in the œsophagus on drinking (*Ars., Hydro-Ac.*) (D.).

Abdomen enlarged and puffed; protrudes here and there as if from the arm of a fœtus; movements and sensation as if something were alive; no pain (N.).

Fistula in ano (*Berb., Calc-P., Sil.*).

ANUS FISSURED OR SURROUNDED WITH CONDYLOMATA (*Ant-C., Graph., Sil.*) (N.).

Diarrhœa, especially from the effects of vaccination (N.).

LOOSE BOWELS (*Aloe, Calc-P., Nat-S., Podo.*).

Curative in frequent, small and painful bowel movements (*Merc., Nux-V., Sulph.*).

STOOL FORCIBLY EXPELLED (*Calc-P., Gamb.*); COPIOUS, GURGLING LIKE WATER FROM A BUNG-HOLE (*Podo., Sulph.*) (N.).

Oily stool (*Bol., Iod., Pic-Ac.*) (B.).

Constipation: Stools consist of hard, black, balls; stools large; and they recede after being partially expelled (*Sanic., Sil.*) (N.).

Violent pains in the rectum compel cessation of effort (A.).

Piles swollen; pain most severe when sitting (A.).

Face has a greasy or shiny look (*Nat-M.*) (N.).

Diarrhœa, worse in the morning after break-fast, from coffee and onions, with rapid emaciation and exhaustion (D.).

COUGH BY DAY ONLY (*Arg-M., Calc., Euph.*) (B.).

Warts on the outside of the nose (N.).

Catarrh, with thick, green mucous discharge (Kali-B., Nat-S., Puls.) (N.).

Scabs form inside the nose (*Graph., Sep.*) (N.).

Troublesome, slight, long-lasting cough.

Asthma (*Ant-T., Carbo-V., Nat-S.*) (N.).

Short, difficult breathing (*Sulph.*) (B.).

Fixed ideas, as if a strange person were at his side; as if the soul and body were separated; that the body and particularly the limbs were made of glass, and will readily break; as if a living animal were in the adbomen; tells about being under the influence of a superior power (N.).

Insane women will not be touched or approached (N.).

Is always in a hurry (*Arg-N.*), talks hurriedly (*Bell., Hep., Lach.*), moves hurriedly, and is excitable (D.).

Imagines himself double or treble and scattered about (D.).

When walking the limbs feel as if made of wood (A.).

Emotional sensitiveness; music causes weeping and trembling (Br.).

Always chilly from least change of weather (*Hep.*) (A.).

Chill beginning in the thighs (Cedr., Cham., Rhus-T., Ther.) (K.).

Violent shaking chill, for a quarter of an hour, about 3 A.M., followed by thirst; then profuse perspiration all over except on the head (A.).

SHIVERING THROUGH AND THROUGH, FROM THE SLIGHTEST UNCOVERING OF THE BODY IN WARM AIR (A.).

Sweat when he sleeps, stops when he wakes (reverse of Samb.) (A.).

Profuse night-sweat; so that he changes his shirt several times at night (A.).

Sweat on the side not lain on (*Benz., Sanic.*) (A.).

Fetid or sour-smelling sweat at night (A.).

Flesh feels as if beaten, from the bones (*Phyt.;* as if scraped—*Rhus-T.*) (A.).

Dribbling urine (*Bell., Clem., Staph.*) (G.).

FORKED STREAM OF URINE (*Canth., Caust., Merc., Merc-C., Petr., Rhus-T.*) (K.).

Frequent micturition with the pains (*Cann-S., Canth., Merc., Sep.*) (N.).

Severe cutting at close of urination (*Sars.*).

Sensation after urinating, as if urine thickening in the urethra (A.).

URETHRITIS IN SYCOTIC PATIENTS (WHICH *Cann-S.* DOES NOT RELIEVE); STREAM SPLIT; CUTTING AFTER URINATION; DISCHARGE THICK (N.).

Long-lasting gleet after gonorrhœa (but inferior to *Medorrhinum*).

Red, smooth excrescences on the glans penis (Bt.).

Thuja bears the same relation to sycosis (figwarts, condylomata and wart-like excrescences upon the mucous and cutaneous surfaces) that *Sulphur* does to psora, or *Mercury* to syphilis (N.).

Chronic induration of the testicles (*Aur., Clem.*) (Br.).

Gonorrhœa suppressed by injections, and complicated with rheumatism or orchitis (*Clem., Puls., Sil.*) (D.).

Gonorrhœa with thin, greenish discharge (*Merc.*) *and scalding urine* (D.).

Hæmorrhage from the urethra after urination (*Hep., Mezer., Puls., Sars., Sulph., Zinc.*) (K.).

Perspiration, smelling like honey, on the genitals (A.).

Suppressed gonorrhœa causing articular rheumatism, prostatitis, impotence and many other constitutional troubles (A.).

Nocturnal erections (*Canth., Phos.*) (G.).

Retarded menstruation (*Graph., Sep.*) (Hg.).

Vagina is filled with warty excrescences (G.).

Voluptuous formication in the fossa navicularis (C.).

Chancroidal ulcer of the genitals (*Nux-V.,*) (R.).

Ovarian troubles (*Apis, Coloc., Podo., Sep., Sulph.*) (N.).

Distressing, burning pain in the left ovarian region when walking or riding; must sit or lie down (*Croc., Ust.*); worse at each menstrual nisus (A.).

Coition prevented by extreme sensitiveness of the vagina (*Plat.,* prevented by dryness—*Lyc., Lyss., Nat-M.*) (A.).

Abortion at the end of third month (*Sab., Sec.*) (G.).

Profuse, mucous leucorrhœa, which is extremely acrid and excoriates the uterus, vulva and perineum (Bl.).

Nails brittle, distorted, crumbling, misshapen or soft (*Ant-C., Graph.*) (N.).

Bleeding fungous growths (N.).

EPITHELIOMA (*Ars., Lach., Nit-Ac.*) (N.).

Skin looks dirty (*Psor., Sulph.*) (A.).

Brown or brownish-white spots here and there on the skin (A.).

Eruptions only on covered parts; burn after scratching (A.).

SWEAT ONLY ON UNCOVERED PARTS, OR ALL OVER EXCEPT THE HEAD (N.).

PERSPIRATION OF THE UNCOVERED PARTS AND DRYNESS OF THE COVERED PARTS.

Of great usefulness in the cure of warts in any part of the body (*Caust., Nit-Ac., Staph.*).

Wart-shaped excrescences here and there, especially on hands and genitals (*Staph.*) (N.).

Large, seedy, pedunculated warts on the skin (A.).

Pathological vegetations, condylomata, polypi, etc. (N.).

Moistening and suppurating sycotic excrescences (*Sil.*).

AGGRAVATION: In the evening; from the heat of the bed; by extension; in cold, damp air; after vaccination;

from excessive tea drinking; from narcotics; at night; at 3 A.M. and 3 P.M.; from tobacco; and from spirituous liquors.

AMELIORATION: By rest; by drawing up the limbs; from warmth; and in the open air.

RELATIONSHIP: *Compare*: *Cann-S., Canth., Cop., Kali-S., Merc., Nat-S., Puls., Sep., Sil., Staph.* and *Sulph. Follows well after*: *Med., Merc.,* and *Nit-Ac. Cinnab.* is preferable for warts on the prepuce. *Complementary*: *Med., Nat-M., Sab.* and *Sil. Antidotes*: *Camph., Merc.* and *Sil.*

Thyroidinum.

COMMON NAME: DRIED THYROID GLAND OF THE SHEEP.
Rickets (*Calc., Calc-P., Lyc., Nat-M., Sil.*) (Br.).
Rapid emaciation (*Ars., Iod., Nat-M.*) (B.).

CRETINISM (*Aur., Bar-C., Iod.*) (Br.).
Muscular weakness (*Gels., Nat-M., Op., Sil.*) (Br.).
Easy fatigue (*Kali-P., Pic-Ac.*) (Br.).

ARRESTED DEVELOPMENT IN CHILDREN (*Bar-C., Calc-P., Merc., Sil.*) (Br.).
Nose dry, indoors, moist in the open air (*Nux-V.*) (B.).
Palpitation from least exertion (*Ars., Phos.*) (Br.).
Pulse weak and frequent, with inability to lie down (*Lach.*) (Br.).
Cough on entering a warm room from cool air (*Ant-C., Bry., Med., Nat-C., Nux-V.*) (B.).
Dry, painful cough with scanty, difficult expectoration and burning in the pharynx (Br.).
Oily musty sweat (*Merc.*) (B.).

EXOPHTHALMIC GOITRE (*Spong.*) (Br.).

Eyeballs prominent (*Stram.*) (Br.).

Progressive diminution of sight (*Calc., Phos., Sulph.*) (Br.).

Thirst for cold water (*Bry., Calc., Nat-M., Phos., Sulph., Verat.*) (Br.).

DESIRE FOR SWEETS (*Arg-N., Calc., Lyc., Merc., Sulph.*) (Br.).

Polyuria (*Arg-N., Kali-P., Lyc., Merc., Sulph.*) (Br.).

Cold hands and feet (*Calc., Sep., Stram.*) (Br.).

Rolling flatulence with gurgling (*Carb-V., Lyc., Nat-S., Podo.*); then a loose, gassy stool (*Aloe, Calc-P., Nat-S., Podo., Sulph.*) (B.).

Irritable, worse from least opposition (*Aur., Bry., Sulph.*) (Br.).

Goes into a rage over trifles (*Nux-V.*) (Br.).

AGGRAVATION: From least exertion; from cold; on entering a warm room from cool air; and from contradiction.

AMELIORATION: From lying on the abdomen; and from rest.

RELATIONSHIP: *Compare:* *Aur., Bar-C., Calc., Calc-P., Gels., Iod., Kali-P., Lyc., Merc., Nat-M., Nux-V., Op., Phos., Sep., Sil., Verat.,* and *Zinc.*

Trillium Pendulum.

COMMON NAME: WAKE ROBIN.

Active or passive hæmorrhage (*Ferr., Ham., Ipec., Kali-P., Lach.*) (D.).

Hæmorrhage from the nose, lungs, kidneys, and uterus (*Carb-V., Ipec., Lach., Mill., Nit-Ac.*) (A.).

Blood usually bright red (*Acon., Bell., Cact.*) (A.).

Tendency to putrescence of the fluids (*Ars., Bapt., Carb-Ac., Kali-P., Kreos., Lach.*) (A.).

Epistaxis, profuse, passive, or bright red (*Carb-V., Lach., Phos.*) (A.).

Uterine hæmorrhage, after over-exertion or too long a ride (A.).

IS ESPECIALLY USEFUL IN MENSES EVERY TWO WEEKS, LASTING A WEEK AND VERY PROFUSE (*Calc., Nux-V.*) (N.).

FLOODING, WITH FAINTING, FAINT, DIM SIGHT, PALPITATION, OBSTRUCTION AND NOISES IN THE EARS (*Chin.*) (N.).

Menorrhagia from displaced uterus or at the climacteric; blood dark and clotted (A.).

Threatened abortion (*Caul., Sep.*), *with a gush of blood on each movement, with a sensation as if the hips and back were falling apart; relieved by bandaging the hips tightly* (D.).

Post-partum hæmorrhage (*Chin., Ferr-P., Ham., Ipec.; Sec.*) (N.).

Profuse yellow, creamy or bloody leucorrhœa, which renders the patient anæmic (Bl.).

Tendency to uterine prolapsus (*Bell., Nat-M., Sep., Thuj.*) (Bl.).

Hæmorrhages from uterine fibroids (*Calc., Nit-Ac., Thuj.*) (Bl.).

Varices of pregnancy (*Puls., Sep.*) (B.).

Profuse, long-lasting lochial discharges (*Calc., Sec., Sep*). (C.).

Bleeding from the tooth-cavity after extraction of a tooth (*Ham., Kreos.*) (A.).

Painful sinking at the pit of the stomach (*Sep., Sulph., Zinc.*) (A.).

Incipient phthisis, with bloody sputa; in advanced stages with copious, purulent expectoration and troublesome cough (A.).

Diarrhœa: Thin, watery, tinged with blood; often painless (*Podo.*) (C.).

AGGRAVATION: After over-exertion; from too long a ride; from least motion; every two weeks; during the climacteric; after eating; and from sitting erect.

AMELIORATION: From bending forward; from exercise in the open air; and from tight bandage.

RELATIONSHIP: *Compare*: *Arn., Bell., Cact., Calc., Calc-P., Chin., Ferr-P., Ipec., Kali-C., Kali-P., Lach., Mill., Nat-M., Phos., Puls., Sep., Sulph., Thlas.* and *Ust.*

Complementary to: *Calc-P.* (in menstrual and hæmorrhagic affections).

Tuberculinum.

COMMON NAME: PUS FROM A (PULMO-NARY) TUBERCULAR ABSCESS.

Persons with a history of tuberculosis in the family (*Calc., Phos., Sulph.*) (N.).

SYMPTOMS EVER-CHANGING (*Ign., Puls.*), BEGINNING SUDDENLY, CEASING SUDDENLY (*Bell.*) (N.).

LONGS FOR OPEN AIR (*Apis, Phos., Puls.*); WANTS DOORS AND WINDOWS OPEN (*Sulph.*), OR TO RIDE IN STRONG WIND (N.).

Wandering pains in the limbs and joints (*Bell., Ign., Kali-B., Kali-S., Puls.*); *stiff when beginning to move* (*Rhus-T.*); *worse when standing and better from continued motion* (*Rhus-T.*) (N.).

Tubercular arthritis (*Calc., Iod.*) (D.).

Takes fresh cold on least exposure, can't get rid of one before another comes (*Calc., Phos.*) (N.).

Takes cold easily, without knowing when or where (N.).

Constant disposition to catch cold (*Hep., Phos., Sil.*) (D.).

16

Emaciation, even while being well, and so hungry must get up in the night to eat (*Phos., Psor.*) (N.).

Emaciation rapid and pronounced; while he eats well loses flesh rapidly (*Iod., Nat-M.*) (N.).

Tubercular meningitis (*Apis, Calc., Hell., Lyc., Sulph.*) (D.).

Think of this remedy, when with a history of tubercular affections the best-selected remedy fails to relieve or permanently improve (A.).

Ailments first affect one organ, then another—the lungs, brain, kidneys, liver, stomach, nervous system, etc. (A.).

Sensitive, every trifle irritates (*Ign., Staph.*) (B.).

COSMOPOLITAN; NEVER SATISFIED TO REMAIN IN ONE PLACE LONG; WANTS TO TRAVEL (N.).

Active and precocious mentally, but weak physically (*Lyc.*) (A.).

Melancholy, despondent (*Aur., Ign., Puls., Stann.*) (A.).

Morose, irritable, fretful, peevish (*Bry., Cham., Nux-V., Sulph.*) (A.).

Taciturn, sulky (*Bry., Nux-V.*) (A.).

Naturally of a sweet disposition, now on the borderland of insanity (A.).

Everything in the room seemed strange, as though in a strange place (A.).

FEAR OF DOGS (*Bell., Caust., Chin., Hyos., Stram.*) (C.).

Is averse to work (*Nux-V., Phos.*) (C.).

Nocturnal hallucinations; wakes from sleep frightened, screaming (*Stram.*) (A.).

Chronic (tubercular) headache; pain intense, sharp, cutting, from above the right eye to the occiput (A.).

Sensation as of an iron hoop around the head (*Anac., Sulph.*) (A.).

School-girl's headache; aggravated by study, or even slight mental exertion (*Calc-P., Nat-M.*) (A.).

Persistent, offensive otorrhœa (*Calc., Graph., Petr., Tell.*) (C.).

RAVENOUS APPETITE, WITH EMACIATION (*Abrot., Calc., Iod., Nat-M., Petr., Phos., Psor., Sulph.*) (K.).

Aversion to food with hunger (*Cocc., Nat-M., Nux-V., Phos., Sulph.*) (K.).

DESIRE FOR MEAT (*Ferr-M., Kreos., Lil-T., Mag-C., Meny., Nat-M.*), ESPECIALLY SMOKED MEAT (*Calc-P., Caust., Kreos.*) (K.).

Desire for cold milk (*Phel., Phos-Ac., Phos., Rhus-T., Sabad., Staph.*) (K.).

All-gone hungry sensation (*Aloe, Petr., Sulph.*) (C.).

Chilly, yet wants fresh air (*Puls.*) (B.).

Delayed dentition (*Calc., Calc-P., Sil.*) (B.).

Hawks mucus after eating (*Puls.*) (B.).

Menses soon after child-bearing (B.).

Mucus rattles in the chest, without expectoration (*Ant-T., Phos.*) (B.).

Pain through the left upper lung to the back (*Phos.*). *Tubercular deposit begins there* (N.).

Shortness of breath (*Ars., Calc., Kali-C., Phos., Sulph.*) (C.).

Sore spot in the chest (*Puls.*) (B.).

Thick, easy expectoration (*Puls., Stann.*) (C.).

Hard, dry cough during sleep (*Cham., Coff., Mag-S., Nit-Ac., Rhus-T., Sep.*) (C.).

Tabes mesenterica (*Calc., Sulph.*) (C.).

Diarrhœa: Early morning, sudden imperative (*Sulph.*); *stool dark, brown, watery and offensive; discharged with great force* (*Crot-T., Gamb.*); *with great weakness and profuse night-sweats* (A.).

Menses too early, too profuse, and too long-lasting, in patients with a tuberculous history (A.).

Frightful dysmenorrhœa (*Coloc.*) (A.).

Enlarged glands (*Calc., Iod., Merc.*) (B.).

Fiery red skin (*Bell., Sep., Stram.*) (A.).

Escape of immense quantities of white bran-like scales (*Ars.*) (A.).

Intense itching, worse at night, when undressing (*Rumx.*) *and from bathing* (*Rhus-T.*).

Eczema over the entire body (*Graph.*) (A.).

Ringworm (*Rhus-T., Sep., Sulph.*) (A.).

ITCHING, AMELIORATED BY THE HEAT OF THE STOVE (*Rumx.*) (K.).

Oozing behind the ears (*Graph.*), in the hairs (*Viol-T.*) and in the folds of the skin (*Petr.*), with rawness and soreness (A.).

Plica polonica (*Bor., Psor.*) (A.).

Crops of small boils, intensely painful (*Arn., Hep., Lach., Tarant.*), *successively appear in the nose; green fœtid pus* (*Sec.*) (A.).

AGGRAVATION: From beginning to move; from music; before a storm; from cold; in cold, damp weather; from standing; from exertion; in a closed room; at night; in the morning; and during sleep.

AMELIORATION: In the open air; from the heat of the stove; and from continued motion.

RELATIONSHIP: *Complementary*: *Calc., Kali-S., Psor., Puls., Sep.* and *Sulph.*

Bell. for acute attacks, congestive or inflammatory, occurring in tubercular diseases.

Hydra. to fatten patients cured with *Tub.*

Compare: *Abrot., Apis, Bell., Calc., Graph., Hep., Iod., Lyc., Merc., Nat-M., Petr., Phos., Psor., Rhus-T., Sep., Sil., Sulph., Thuj., Ust.* and *Zinc.*

Urtica Urens.

COMMON NAME: DWARF NETTLE.

Nettle-rash, with intolerable itching and burning (G.).

Urticaria alternating with rheumatism (alternating with asthma—*Calad.*) (K.).

Urticaria, worse after bathing (Phos.), after violent exercise (Con., Nat-M., Psor.), and from warmth (Apis, Kali-I., Nat-M., Puls.) (K.).

URTICARIA, DURING RHEUMATISM (*Rhus-T.*) (K.).

VOMITING FROM SUPPRESSION OF URTICARIA (during urticaria—*Apis, Cina*) (K.).

Diarrhœa after suppressed eruptions (Bry., Dulc., Hep., Lyc., Mezer., Psor., Sulph.) (K.).

URTICARIA; THE SKIN BECOMES ELEVATED, WITH A WHITE CENTRAL SPOT AND A RED AREOLA, WITH STINGING AND BURNING, RELIEVED BY RUBBING (N.).

Hives from eating shell-fish (D.).

RED RAISED BLOTCHES, ITCHING AND BURNING, REQUIRE CONSTANT RUBBING (N.).

The upper part of the body enormously swollen, pale and dropsical and covered with confluent, small, transparent vesicles, filled with serum and sudamina (Kg.).

As soon as she lay down again, eruption and itching disappeared entirely, and reappeared immediately after rising again (Ch.).

Absence of milk after confinement, without apparent cause (Calc., Sil.) (D.).

Epistaxis (*Bry., Carbo-V., Ferr-P., Kali-P.*) (Bl.).

Hæmatemesis (*Ipec., Phos., Sep.*) (Bl.).

Sensation of soreness in the bowels while lying down, and on pressure, a sound as if the bowels were filled with water (T.).

STOOLS OF MUCUS AND BLOOD (*Acon., Merc., Nux-V., Rhus-T., Sulph.*).

Burning and itching at the anus (*Calc.*). (C.).

HAEMORRHAGE FROM THE BOWELS, OR LUNGS (*Nit-Ac., Phos.*).

Pruritus of genitals in both sexes (*Petr.*) (C.).

Hæmorrhage from the uterus (*Ipec., Merc., Nit-Ac.*) (Bl.).

Menorrhagia alternating with leucorrhœa (Bl.).

Burns and scalds (*Apis, Ars., Canth., Carb-Ac., Rhus-T., Sulph.*) (Bl.).

Dropsical effusions (*Apis, Dig., Lyc., Nat-M., Sulph.*) (Bl.).

Anasarca following scarlatina (*Apis, Ars., Lach.*) (Bl.).

The kidneys are affected and the urine is suppressed (*Apis, Stram.*) Bl.).

The hands and feet are much swollen (*Ars., Rhus-T.*) (Bl.).

Erysipelatous inflammation of the extremities with burning heat and formication (*Ars., Bell., Rhus-T.*) (Bl.).

Acute gout (*Benz-Ac., Colch., Lyc., Nit-Ac., Rhus-T., Sil.*) (Bl.).

Uric acid diathesis (*Lyc., Sars.*) (B.).

Acrid urine, causing itching (*Nat-M., Nit-Ac., Sulph.*) (B.).

Dull headache, mostly on the right side (*Lyc.*) (C.).

Symptoms return at the same time every year (C.).

AGGRAVATION: After bathing, after suppressed eruptions; from eating shell-fish; after confinement; from rising up; after scarlatina; during rheumatism, and at night.

AMELIORATION: By rubbing; and from lying down.

RELATIONSHIP: *Compare*: *Agn., Apis, Ars., Bell., Benz-Ac., Calc., Canth., Ferr-P., Graph., Hep., Kali-P., Lach., Lyc., Merc., Nat-M., Nit-Ac., Petr., Phos., Puls., Rhus-T., Sep., Sil., Sulph., Thuj.* and *Ust.*

Uva Ursi.

COMMON NAME: BEAR BERRY.

This agent is an astringent, tonic and mild diuretic (Bl.).

The urine contains pus and blood (*Hep., Merc., Sil.*) (Bl.).

With straining discharge of tenacious mucus and large clots of blood (Bl.).

Constant urging to urinate (*Canth.*) (Bl.).

DYSURIA AND STRANGURY (*Apis, Bell.*) (Bl.).

CYSTITIS, WITH BLOODY URINE (*Canth.*) (Bl.).

SLIMY URINE; SLIME PASSES WITH BLOOD (*Equiset., Kali-B., Merc-C.*) (G.).

CATARRH OF THE BLADDER (*Benz-Ac., Coloc., Dulc., Lyc., Nux-V., Puls., Sulph.*) (K.).

Pain in the bladder in the evening (*Ipec., Morph., Pall., Pic-Ac.*) (K.).

Burning pain in the bladder (*Berb., Canth., Caps., Tereb.*) (K.).

Enlargement of the prostate (*Bar-C., Calc., Con., Dig., Puls.*) (K.).

BURNING IN THE URETHRA DURING URINATION (*Arg-N., Bell., Cann-S., Cub., Lil-T., Merc-C., Nit-Ac., Nux-V., Sulph., Tereb., Thuj.*) (K.).

Cloudy urine (*Apis, Berb., Cina*) (K.).

AGGRAVATION: During urination; in the evening; after gonorrhœa.

AMELIORATION: After urination.

RELATIONSHIP: *Compare*: *Apis, Berb., Canth., Dig., Gels., Hep., Kali-B., Lach., Lyc., Merc., Merc-C., Nat-M., Nit-Ac., Nux-V., Puls., Sep., Sulph., Tereb., Thuj.,* and *Verat.*

Vaccininum.

COMMON NAME: VACCINE (COW-POX LYMPH).

This remedy is employed as a prophylactic against, and to modify the course of an attack of small-pox (Bl.).

Vaccine poison is capable of setting up a morbid state of extreme chronicity, named by Dr. Burnett "*Vaccinosis*," the symptoms of which are like those of Hahnemann's "*Sycosis*" (Br.).

Irritable, impatient, ill-humoured, and nervous (*Cham., Cina, Nux-V., Phos., Sulph.*) (Br.).

Frontal headache; forehead and eyes feel as if split (*Bry.*) (Br.).

Inflamed and red lids (*Euphr., Graph., Puls., Sulph.*) (Br.).

Indigestion with great flatulent distension (*Carb-V., Lyc., Nat-S.*) (C.).

Chilliness (*Ars., Gels., Puls., Rhus-T., Sil.*) (Cla.).

Hot and dry skin (*Acon., Bry., Sulph.*) (Br.).

Inveterate skin eruptions (*Graph., Merc., Sulph.*) (Cla.).

Eruption like variola (*Ant-T., Merc., Rhus-T., Sil., Sulph.*) (Br.).

Pimples and blotches on the skin (*Calc., Graph., Sep.*) (Br.).

Neuralgias (*Ars., Bell., Chin.*) (Cla.).

Whooping cough (*Ant-T.. Dros., Indg., Kali-C., Phos., Sil.*) (Br.)

RELATIONSHIP: *Compare*: *Ant-T., Maland., Merc., Sarrac., Sil., Thuj.,* and *Variol.*

For diseases caused by vaccination think of after vaccination *Ant-T.* (for bronchial catarrh), *Mezer.* (itching eruptions after vaccination), *Sil.* (the principal remedy for almost all kinds of diseases, such as diarrhœa, cough, fever, etc.) and *Thuj.* (diarrhœa after vaccination).

Valeriana.

COMMON NAME: VALERIAN.

Acts very beneficially in soothing nervous irritability in the neurotic.

Rheumatic tearing in the limbs, worse during rest after motion, better during motion (*Rhus-T.*).

Violent tearing up and down in the muscles of the extremities.

Nervousness, especially at the climaxis, or at the time of institution of the menstrual epochs.

Twitching, suddenly-appearing pains, relieved by change of position.

Of great value in hysteria (Coff., Scutel., Vib.).

Vertigo, in hysterical females (*Puls.*) (G.).

Red parts become white (*Ferr.*) (A.).

Mental confusion; replies incoherently (*Arn., Bapt., Hyos.*) (A.).

Of great utility in general nervousness, obsessions, night terrors, extreme impressionability and bad effects from impurity of life.

Sleeplessness (Coff., Scutel.).

Suddenly-appearing and disappearing perspiration of the face and forehead.

White lips, body icy cold, with faintness (Camph.) (Bt.).

Afraid of the dark or of being left alone (*Ars., Kali-C., Phos., Stram.*) (C.).

OVER-SENSITIVENESS AND OVER-EXCITABILITY (*Scutel., Vib.*).

FEELS LIGHT, AS IF FLOATING IN THE AIR (*Asar., Lac-C.;* as if the legs were floating—*Sticta*) (A.).

The opposite symptoms of the mind appear alternately (Ign.).

Changeable disposition (Ign., Puls.) (A.).

ILLUSIONS OF SIGHT, HEARING, SMELL, AND TASTE.

Hysterical spasms, fearfulness and tremulousness, with palpitation of the heart (Bt.).

Great nervous excitement and trembling (*Acon., Plat.*) (A.).

Unusually joyous mood (*Coff.*) (C.).

Hysterical dyspnœa (*Ign., Nux-M., Sep.*) and chorea (*Agar., Nat-M., Stram.*) (Bt.).

Neuralgia; the pain is unbearable (*Acon., Cham., Coff.*) (Bt.).

Especially useful for persons in whom the intellectual faculties predominate (*Lyc.*) (A.).

Oversensitiveness of all the senses (*Cham., Nux-V.*) (A.).

Sensation of great coldness in the head (on the vertex— *Sep., Verat.*) (A.).

SCIATICA; THE PAIN IS UNBEARABLE WHILE STANDING, WITH A FEELING AS IF THE THIGHS WOULD BREAK OFF (Ra.).

SCIATIC PAIN WORSE WHEN LETTING THE FOOT REST ON THE FLOOR (*Bell.*), WHEN STRAIGHTENING OUT THE LIMB, AND DURING REST FROM PREVIOUS EXERTION; BETTER WHEN WALKING (A.).

Sensation of light before the eyes in the dark.

SENSATION AS IF SOMETHING WARM RISING IN THE THROAT, ARRESTING BREATHING (G.).

Feels a sensation as if a thread was hanging down in the throat, with tickling deep in her throat (on the tongue— *Nat-M., Sil.*) (A.).

SLIMY TASTE IN THE MOUTH IN THE MORNING, ON WALKING (*Merc-I., Zinc.*) (K.).

Child vomits curdled milk, in large lumps and passes the same with stools (*Aeth.*) ; *it vomits milk as soon as it has nursed, after anger of mother* (A.).

Nausea with hunger (*Cycl., Ign., Lach., Mosch., Phos., Sep., Tab., Verat.*) (Bl.).

Foul eructations (*Arn., Asaf., Graph., Nux-V., Phos., Plb., Puls., Sep., Sulph., Sulph-Ac.*) (Bl.).

Delirium: Hallucinations; sees figures, animals, men; delusions, thinks she is some one else, moves to edge of bed to make room; imagines animals lying near her which she fears she may hurt (A.).

Increase of the urinary secretion, which is limpid like water (*Gels., Helon., Nat-M., Phos-Ac.*).

SPASMODIC ASTHMA (*Ars., Cupr., Hydr-Ac., Ipec., Lob., Mag-P., Mosch., Nux-V., Puls., Spong., Sumb., Tab., Zinc.*) (K.).

Choking on falling asleep (*Bell., Crot-H., Kali-C., Lac-C., Lach., Naja, Nux-V., Sep., Teucr.*) (Bl.).

Suppressed catamenia (*Bry., Ferr., Graph., Nat-M., Puls., Vib.*).

Great nervous irritation, cannot sit still (*Kali-Br., Phos.*) (N.).

Tearing pains and cramps in different places (*Cupr.*) (N.).

Short chill with thirst. Chill begins in the neck and runs down the back (heat begins in the neck and runs down the back—*Paris*), *with fainting during chill* (during heat —*Acon.*) (A.).

Long-lasting, severe heat, with thirst and dull headache; with restlessness and neuralgia of the limbs (A.).

Profuse sweat, worse at night, but not debilitating sweat from exertion. Sweat on the face with heat. Better after sweat (A.).

Urine contains a white, red or turbid sediment (*Lyc.*) (C.).

Sudden stitching in the chest and in the region of the liver, from within outward (C.).

AGGRAVATION: Towards noon; in the first hours of the afternoon; towards evening until midnight; periodically (every two to three months); while standing; when sitting; and on falling asleep.

AMELIORATION: From walking; and after sweat.

RELATIONSHIP: *Compare*: *Aeth., Asaf., Asar., Cham., Croc., Ign., Lac-C., Nat-M., Sil., Spig., Sulph.,* and *Zinc.*

It is useful for the abuse of *Chamomile tea.*

For pain in the heels compare this remedy with *Agar., Caust., Cycl., Led., Mang.,* and *Phyt.*

ANTIDOTES: Camph. and *Coff.*

Variolinum.

COMMON NAME: PUS FROM THE SMALL-POX PUSTULE.

It bears the same relation to small-pox that *Anti-toxin* does to diphtheria (A.).

This remedy is employed as a prophylactic against, and to modify the course of an attack of small-pox (Bl.).

An extended clinical record by competent and reliable observers attests its curative value in vairola—simple, confluent and malignant—as well as in varioloid and varicella (A.).

As a preventive of, or protection against, small-pox, it is far superior to crude vaccination and absolutely safe from the sequelæ, especially septic and tubercular infection (A.).

Delirium with high temperature (*Ars., Bell., Lach., Stram.*) (R.).

Morbid fear of small-pox (C.).

Great restlessness (*Acon., Ars., Phos., Rhus-T.*) (Bl.).

Violent headache (*Acon., Bell., Ferr-P., Glon., Lach., Nat-M., Rhus-T.*) (R.).

Pain in the occiput (*Cocc., Gels., Pic-Ac., Sil.*) (C.).

Herpes zoster (*Canth., Ran-B., Rhus-T.*) (R.).

PUSTULAR ERUPTIONS (*Crot-T., Merc., Rhus-T.*) (B.).

Petechial eruptions (*Arn., Bapt.*) (R.).

Inflamed eyelids (*Ars., Euphr., Merc., Rhus-T., Sulph.*) (C.).

Rheumatic pains in the wrists (C.).

Deafness (*Bar-C., Chin., Kali-P., Lyc., Phos., Puls., Sep.*) (C.).

Chronic catarrh (*Calc., Hydr., Kali-S.*) (C.).

Nausea (*Bry., Kali-M., Nux-V., Puls., Sep.*) (R.).

Oppressed breathing (*Ant-T., Bry., Carb-V.*) (C.).

Cough with thick, viscid, bloody mucus (*Kali-B., Phos., Sulph.*) (C.).

Putrid, coppery taste in the mouth (*Merc.*) (B.).

Pains in the bones of the limbs (*Eup-P.*) (R.).

Sensation as if the throat were closed (*Brom., Kali-B., Lach., Phos.*) (C.).

Sensation as of a lump in the right side of the throat (*Merc-I-F.*) (C.).

EXCRUCIATING BACKACHE (*Bell., Phos., Rhus-T.*) (Bl.).

Aching in the legs (*Bry., Rhus-T.*) (Bl.).

INTENSE FEVER (*Ars., Bell., Stram., Sulph.*) (Bl.).

Profuse, offensive sweat (*Calc., Chin., Merc., Psor., Rhus-T., Sil.*) (Bl.).

Severe chill and coldness (*Acon., Nat-M., Nux-V.*) (R.).

Chilliness, as if cold water were trickling down the back (R.).

AGGRAVATION: On motion; and at night.

AMELIORATION: From rest.

RELATIONSHIP: *Compare*: Apis, Arn., Ars., Bell., Bry., Canth., Ferr-P., Graph., Hep., Iod., Kali-P., Lach., Merc., Nat-M., Phos., Rhus-T., Thuj., Urt. and Verat-V. *Complementary to*: Bell. and Rhus-T.

Veratrum Album.

COMMON NAME: WHITE HELLEBORE.

Difficulty of walking; first the right and then the left hip-joint feels paralytic (Hr.).

SUDDEN SINKING OF STRENGTH (*Ars., Camph., Kali-P., Phos., Sec.*).

Continued great debility and trembling (Ars., Gels., Hyos., Lach.).

Numbness and tingling in the extremities (Acon., Caust., Merc., Rhus-T.).

Stiffness of the limbs, especially in the forenoon and after walking.

Violent tonic spasms—the soles of the feet and palms of the hands are contracted (Cupr., Sec.).

Whole body icy cold (*Carb-V.*) (N.).

Cramps of the limbs, with cold sweat (G.).

Cramps in the calves of legs (*Cupr.*) (N.).

Icy coldness of hands and feet (*Camph., Carb-V.*) (N.).

Attacks of pain, which produce delirium and mania for a short time.

Rheumatism aggravated by the heat of the bed and cold, damp weather—relieved from rising and walking (*Mag-C., Rhus-T.*).

The symptoms of debility are especially aggravated by motion.

Generalized weakness and sudden loss of power (Camph., Hydr-Ac., Phos.).

Dry itch (*Mezr., Sulph.*).

Chill at 6 A.M. (Arn., Bov., Eup-P., Nux-V.) (R.).

Intermittent fever with external coldness and much thirst (Camph., Carb-V.).

Fevers, with great coldness externally, and violent internal heat; pulse thread-like; great craving for cold drinks (Bt.).

Headache causing delirium (G.).

Feels dizzy, staggers about; vision becomes obscure; the pulse is depressed; and complete extinction of nervous power goes on at a fearful rate (Hm.).

SENSATION AS IF A LUMP OF ICE WAS ON THE TOP OF THE HEAD (Ra.).

Sensation as if brain were torn to pieces (A.).

Vertigo in drunkards, opium-eaters, or those who use tobacco, characterized by sudden faintings, collapse of pulse, loss of vision, and cold sweat on the forehead (Bt.).

Nervous headache at each menstrual molimen (Bt.).

Delirium and restlessness (*Ars., Rhus-T.*) (D.).

Anxiety, fear of death, and rage (Ars., Nux-V.)

MANIA, WITH DESIRE TO TEAR OR CUT EVERYTHING (*Bell., Stram.*).

Despair about his position in society; feels very unlucky (Hr.).

Wanders about the house, is very taciturn (Bt.).

Excessive mirthfulness (*Coff.*) (Bt.).

Expression of fright (*Acon.*) (Bt.).

Disposed to talk about fault of others, or silence; but if irritated, scolding and calling names (Hr.).

Lewd in talk (*Hyos., Stram.*) (D.).

Nymphomania, from unsatisfied passion or mental causes (Phos., Plat., Stram.) (Bt.).

LOQUACITY (*Bell., Hyos., Lach., Stram.*) (D.).

Strikes those about him (Bell., Stram.) (D.).

Springs out of the bed (Bell., Hyos., Stram.) (D.).

Religious melancholy (Aur., Puls. Stram.).

Praying and talking about religious things (Stram.) (N.).

DESPAIR OF SALVATION (*Ars., Aur., Calc., Kali-P., Lach., Lil-T., Lyc., Nat-M., Puls., Stram., Sulph., Thuj.*) (D.).

Sullen indifference (*Staph.*) (D.).

Cannot bear to be left alone (*Ars.*), yet persistently refuses to talk (A.).

Thinks she is pregnant, or will soon be delivered (*Ign.; Sabad., Thuj.*) (A.).

Memory weak, or entirely lost (*Calc., Lyc. Sil.*) (G.).

Inconsolable over fancied misfortune, howls and screams; wails and weeps; sits brooding in a corner (R.).

Bad effects of opium-eating, or tobacco-chewing (A.).

Catamenia too early and too profuse, or suppressed (*Graph., Puls., Sep.*).

Puerperal mania and convulsions, with violent cerebral congestion; bluish and bloated face; protruded eyes; wild shrieks, and disposition to tear and bite.

Dysmenorrhœa, with vomiting and purging, or exhausting diarrhœa with cold sweat (Hr.).

Sinking feeling during hæmorrhage (*Chin., Ipec., Sec.;* fainting—*Trill.*) (A.).

COLD FEELING IN THE ABDOMEN (*Colch., Tab.*) (A.).

Icy coldness of face, tip of nose, feet, legs, hands, arms, and many other parts (*Carb-V.*) (A.).

The nose grows more pointed, seems to be longer; face cold and sunken (N.).

Attacks of fainting from least exertion (*Ars., Carb-V. Sulph.*) (A.).

Palpitation, with anxiety and rapid, audible respiration (R.).

Cough with vomiting (*Ipec., Phos., Puls.*).

Cough with much expectoration, blueness of the face, and involuntary micturition (C.).

Stertorous breathing (*Am-C., Arn., Op.*) (Bt.).

Shortness of breath on slightest motion (*Acon., Ars., Dig.*) (C.).

Feeble voice (*Ant-T., Canth., Hep., Stann.*) (Bt.).

ASTHMA, WITH GREAT SUFFOCATION, ANGUISH, AND OPPRESSION ABOUT THE HEART (*Ars., Cupr., Kali-P., Lach.*) (Bt.).

Spasmodic cough with blue face, suffocation and retching (*Cupr., Ipec.*) (Bt.).

Neck too weak to hold the head up, particularly in children with whooping cough (Hr.).

Cold, collapsed face; pinched up, bluish nose; dry and cracked lips; lock-jaw; grating of the teeth (*Ars., Cupr.*) (Bt.).

While in bed, face is red; after getting up it becomes pale (*Acon.*) (Hr.).

Leaden colour of the face, with frequent nausea and vomiting, with great exhaustion (G.).

Sporadic and Asiatic cholera (*Ars., Camph., Cupr., Kali-P., Phos., Podo., Sec.*).

(*In the first stages of the disease Camphor is undoubtedly the remedy of choice, and the same is to be used as Hahnemann first suggested* (*in material doses and frequently repeated*).

Cholera after fright (*Acon.*) (A.).

Cold, bluish skin (*Camph., Carb-V., Cupr., Lach.*).

Rapid, slow, irregular, and at times intermittent pulse (*Nat-M., Phos.*) (R.).

THREAD-LIKE AND SCARCELY PERCEPTIBLE PULSE (*Camph., Carb-V.*).

COLD SWEAT, PRINCIPALLY ON THE FOREHEAD.

Dangerous diarrhœa (*Ars., Kali-P., Sec., Sulph.*).

Chronic diarrhœa (*Aloe, Nat-S., Petr., Podo., Sulph.*).

Some symptoms are accompanied by hunger, thirst, flow of urine, delirium, salivation and oppression of the chest.

Constipation (*Chel., Plb., Sil.*).

17

Large, hard, black stools with faintness; patient strains until covered with cold sweat and then gives it up, and fæces accumulate in large masses in the rectum (D.).

Rectum seems inactive (*Bry., Ign., Op.*) (N.).

Taste in the mouth is like peppermint.

Cold tongue (*Camph., Carb-V., Hydr-Ac.*) (K.).

VERY EXHAUSTING DIARRHOEA; ESPE-CIALLY WEAK AFTER EVERY STOOL (*Ars., Camph., Phos.*); WITH COLD SWEAT ON THE FOREHEAD (G.).

TERRIBLE COLIC (*Bell., Cupr., Mag-P.*), WITH VIOLENT NAUSEA AND VOMITING (*Coloc., Cupr., Nux-V.*) (Bt.).

TERRIBLE COLIC; THE SUFFERING CAUSES A COLD SWEAT TO STAND UPON THE SURFACE, ESPECIALLY ON THE FOREHEAD (G.).

Craves fruits (*Ant-T., Ars., Nat-M.*) (A.).

Aversion to warm things (*Puls.*) (A.).

THIRST, WITH CRAVING FOR THE COLDEST DRINKS (*Acon., Ars., Bry., Cham., Chin., Cina, Eup-P., Merc., Merc-C., Nat-S., Phos., Sec., Sulph.*) (G.).

WANTS ICE (*Elaps, Med., Merc-C., Nat-S.*) (N.).

Unquenchable desire for cold drinks (*Ars., Phos.*) (Bt.).

Craving for acids (*Ars., Puls.*) or refreshing things (*Phos-Ac.*).

Pain in the abdomen preceding stool (*Acon., Coloc., Ipec., Nux-V., Sulph.*) (D.).

Flatulent colic (*Coloc., Lyc., Nux-V., Puls., Sep.*) (G.).

Hunger and appetite between paroxysms of vomiting (A.).

Frequent nausea and vomiting, with laden colour of the face, and cold perspiration especially on the forehead (G.).

VIOLENT RETCHING; WANTS EVERYTHING COLD (*Ars., Cupr., Phos., Sec.*) (Bt.).

Least quantity of liquid excites vomiting (*Ars., Bism., Phos.*) (Bt.).

Motion excites the nausea (*Bry., Cocc., Ipec., Kali-C., Lact-Ac., Op., Sep., Tab.*) (Bt.).

Diseases caused by ice-cream and cold drinks (*Ars., Ipec.*) (Bt.).

Burning and oppression in the epigastrium (*Ars., Carb-V., Phos.*) (Bt.).

Copious, watery diarrhœa, with violent nausea and vomiting (*Crot-T., Podo.*) (Bt.).

WATERY DIARRHOEA, EXPELLED IN A FORCIBLE GUSH, WITH LITTLE OR NO GRIPING (Ra.).

Involuntary, watery stools, without the patient's knowledge (*Aloe*) (Bt.).

Involuntary stools, on coughing and sneezing, or passing flatus (*Bell., Phos-Ac., Sulph.*) (K.).

RETENTION OF URINE, IN CHOLERA (*Camph., Canth., Lach., Op.*) (K.).

Profuse, watery, greenish-like spinach, or bloody stools (*Ipec., Merc.*), with cramps and cutting pains in the abdomen (*Coloc., Cupr.*), with great weakness and fainting (*Ars.*) (D.).

RICE-WATER STOOLS (*Ars., Camph., Carb-Ac., Cupr., Ferr., Iris, Kali-P., Merc-Sulph., Nat-M., Phos-Ac., Phos., Sec.*), ATTENDED WITH PROSTRATION AND COLLAPSE (*Ars., Camph.*) (D.).

Sensation in the abdominal rings as if a hernia would protrude (*Nux-V.*) (D.).

Very dark urine (*Apis, Benz-Ac., Colch.*) (G.).

AGGRAVATION: From least motion; after drinking; before and during menses; during and after stool; when perspiring; after fright; from exertion; and during pain.

AMELIORATION: By pressure on the vertex (headache); from stimulants; and from walking about.

RELATIONSHIP: Often useful after *Arn., Ars., Chin., Cupr., Ipec.* and *Podo.*

May be given after *Camph.*, in cholera and cholera morbus, and after *Am-C., Bov.* and *Carb-V.* in dysmenorrhœa with vomiting and purging.

Complementary: Carb-V.

Veratrum Viride.

COMMON NAME: GREEN HELLEBORE.

Exerts a decided influence upon the brain, especially cerebrellum and cerebral portion of the cord, and also over the muscular system.

It probably acts on the inhibitory nerves of the heart, controlling the heart's action in a remarkable degree.

Congestive stage of inflammation, with great arterial excitement (Acon., Bell., Ferr-P.) (D.).

RAPID, FULL PULSE (*Acon., Bell., Ferr-P., Glon., Phos.*) (D.).

Spasmodic diseases with gastric irritation and much vascular excitement (*Ferr-P.*) (D.).

INTENSE FEVER, WITH TWITCHING AND TENDENCY TO SPASMS (*Acon., Bell., Stram., Sulph.*) (N.).

INTENSE CEREBRAL CONGESTION (*Acon., Bell., Glon., Lach., Meli., Nat-M., Op., Sulph.*) (Bt.).

Feeling as though the head would burst open (*Bell., Cann-I., Glon.*); accompanied with nausea and vomiting (*Bry., Sang.*) (Bt.).

Can hardly hold the head up from paralysis of the muscles of the neck (*Sil.*) (Bt.).

Diplopia, of near objects (*Aur., Bell., Cic., Con., Nit-Ac., Phyt., Stann.;* of distant objects—*Am-C., Bell., Nit-Ac., Plb.*) (*K.*).

Dimness of vision from congestion to the base of the brain (*Gels.*) (Bt.).

Loss of sight, with great faintness (*Phos.*) (Bt.).

Ringing in the ears, from congestion of blood to the head (*Bell., Ferr.*), with nausea and vomiting (Bt.).

Face cold, pale or livid; nose looks pinched, cold and blue (Bt.).

CONGESTION, ESPECIALLY TO THE BASE OF THE BRAIN, CHEST, SPINE AND STOMACH (A.).

SUDDEN SPASMS, FROM INTENSE CONGESTION OF BLOOD TO THE HEAD (*Acon., Bell., Glon., Op.*) (Bt.).

Child trembles, jerks, threatened with convulsions; continual jerking or nodding of the head (*Stram.*) (A.).

BASILAR MENINGITIS; HEAD RETRACTED CHILD ON THE VERGE OF SPASMS (*Tub.*) (A.).

A dry, red streak down the centre of the tongue (D.).

Copious secretion of saliva (*Kali-B., Merc., Tab.*) (Bt.).

Tongue coated yellow (*Chel., Merc-I-F., Nat-S.*) (Bt.).

Vomiting of food, and large quantities of glairy mucus (*Kali-B.*) (Bt.).

VIOLENT AND LONG-CONTINUED VOMITING (*Ars., Ipec., Nux-V., Phos., Verat.*) (Bt.).

Nausea on rising (*Acon., Arn., Bry., Carb-An., Chel., Cocc., Ferr., Nat-S., Phos., Senec., Verat., Zinc.*) (D.).

Frequent and long-continued hiccough (*Ars., Mag-P., Nux-V.*), with a constant sensation as if a ball were rising in the œsophagus (*Arg-N., Asaf., Nux-M.*) (Bt.).

Heavy aching pains in the umbilicus (Bt.).

Acute rheumatism; high fever; full, hard, rapid pulse; severe pains in the joints and muscles (*Bry., Salic-Ac.*); *scanty, red urine* (A.).

CONGESTIVE APOPLEXY; HOT HEAD, BLOOD-SHOT EYES, THICK SPEECH, AND SLOW FULL PULSE, HARD AS IRON (A.).

Involuntary stool and urine (*Kali-P., Phos-Ac., Sulph.*) (A.).

Dropping of the lower jaw (*Hyos., Lyc.*) (A.).

Picking of bed-clothes (*Hyos.*) (A.).

Boring the head into the pillow (*Bell., Hell., Stram.*) (A.).

IS OF SERVICE IN THE CONGESTIVE STAGE OF PNEUMONIA. THE TEMPERATURE IS HIGH, THE PULSE IS HARD, FULL AND RAPID. THE RESPIRATIONS ARE RAPID AND ARE OFTEN ASSOCIATED WITH A GASTRIC IRRITABILITY (Bl.).

Acute bronchitis and asthma associated with severe congestion of the lungs and great difficulty of breathing (Bl.).

Useful in endo-carditis and peri-carditis, when there is great arterial excitement and distress in the præcordial region (Bl.).

HYPER-PYREXIA, OR RAPIDLY OSCILLATING TEMPERATURE (*Ars., Bell., Stram.*) (B.).

Delirious, quarrelsome, striking and kicking with hands and feet (*Bell., Canth., Stram.*) (R.).

Breathing heavy, difficult, slow, short, convulsive, almost to suffocation; constriction of the chest (R.).

Sense of utter prostration (*Ars., Camph., Hydr-Ac.*) (C.).

Violent, (galvanic battery-like) shocks in the limbs (C.).

Menstrual colic, with nausea and vomiting (*Cocc., Ipec., Nux-V., Puls., Sep.*) (Bt.).

Dysmenorrhœa (*Bell., Coloc., Mag-P., Nux-V., Puls., Sep.*) (Bt.).

Puerperal peritonitis or metritis (*Apis, Bell., Bry., Lach., Puls., Rhus-T.*), *with nausea and vomiting* (Bt.).

Puerperal convulsions, with intense congestion of blood to the brain (*Bell., Lach., Stram.*) (Bt.).

Nervous or sick headache; congestion from suppressed menses; intense, almost apopletic, with violent nausea and vomiting (A.).

Heart beats loud and strong, with great arterial excitement (*Acon., Bell.*) (C.).

Tongue feels as if it has been scalded (*Iris, Sang.*) (C.).

AGGRAVATION: From rising up; from motion; from cold; from lying on the back; from suppression of menses; from heat of the sun; from noise; on waking; and in the evening.

AMELIORATION: From rubbing; from lying with head low; and from hot, strong coffee.

RELATIONSHIP: *Compare*: *Acon., Bell., Cupr., Ferr-P., Gels., Glon., Hell., Hyos., Ipec., Kali-P., Lach., Meli., Nat-M., Nux-V., Op., Phos., Rhus-T., Stram., Sulph.* and *Verat.*

Verbascum Thapsus.

COMMON NAME: MULLEIN.

This is an ancient and popular remedy for deafness now used mostly locally in the form of an oil.

Stinging pains in the limbs and neuralgic pain in the left ankle.

The pains are generally accompanied by a benumbing sensation (*Kalm.*).

The symptoms are caused and aggravated by a change of temperature, especially when entering from the open air into the room and vice versa.

Tearing from above downwards.

One-sided shudderings.

Face-ache aggravated by change of temperature and pressure.

Great stiffness in the left ankle-joint and more or less soreness and stiffness in the joints of the lower extremities.

Sensation of heat in the epigastrium, as if from dyspepsia (Carb-V., Lach., Lyc., Sep., Sulph.).

A great deal of belly pain, as if pierced with a lance.

CRAMPS AROUND THE NAVEL; SEEMS AS IF PAIN WAS CAUSED BY THE BOWELS BECOMING TWISTED (*Coloc., Cupr., Plb.*).

Very violent diarrhœa with griping (Aloe, Coloc., Mag-P., Nux-V., Verat.).

Intestinal obstruction from induration of stool (*Alum., Bry., Plb., Sep., Sulph.*) (G.).

Hæmorrhoids (*Aloe, Calc-F., Graph., Hep., Lach., Lyc., Nux-V., Sep., Sil., Sulph.*) (G.).

Cough without waking (*Cham., Lach., Sulph.*) (B.).

Migraine, with a sensation as though the temples were crushed together (Bl.).

Nervous cough ameliorated by deep breathing (*Lach., Puls.*) (B.).

Severe soreness in the pharynx, felt in swallowing and cough during sleep, especially in children.

Catarrhs and colds accompanied by neuralgia and a hoarse, barking cough (D.).

COUGH, DEEP, HOLLOW, HOARSE, WITH SOUND LIKE A TRUMPET (N.).

Bronchial and tracheal irritation (*Ipec., Lob., Seneg.*) (Bl.).

Hoarseness, when reading aloud (Calc-F., Cupr., Med., Naja, Seneg.) (Bl.).

Stitching pain in the chest (*Bry., Chel., Kali-B., Kali-C., Phos., Sil.*) (Bl.).

Want of perspiration (*Sulph.*) (G.).

General lassitude and sleepiness in the morning after rising (*Nux-V.*).

Burning urination with frequency—increase of urine with pressure in the bladder.

Constant dribbling of the urine (*Canth., Caust., Puls., Sep., Thuj.*) (Bl.).

Nocturnal enuresis (*Calc., Kreos., Sep.*) (Bl.).

Sensation as if the ears were obstructed (*Calc., Puls., Sep.*) (C.).

Tearing, drawing pains in the left ear (C.).

Attacks of vertigo, on pressing the left cheek (C.).

Pressing, stupefying headache, principally in the forehead (C.).

Neuralgic pains about the zygoma, ear and temporomaxillary joint upon the left side. These pains are aggravated by a change of temperature, talking, sneezing, or biting the teeth togethr (Bl.).

AGGRAVATION: When sitting; from change of temperature; towards evening; with every cold; when reading aloud; from talking; from sneezing; from biting fhe teeth together; and at the same hour.

AMELIORATION: On rising from a sitting posture; and from deep inspiration.

RELATIONSHIP: *Remedies following*: *Bell., Chin., Lyc., Puls., Rhus-T., Sep.* and *Stram.*

Compare: *Acon., Bry., Calc., Caust., Dros., Gels., Hep., Kali-S., Kali-C., Lach., Lyc., Merc., Mur-Ac., Nat-M., Nit-Ac., Op., Petr., Phos., Rhus-T., Spong., Sulph.* and *Thuj.*

Antidote: *Camph.*

N.B.—The preparation known as *Mullein Oil* comes from this plant, and is used locally for earache and deafness.

Viola Odorata.

COMMON NAME: VIOLET.

Flying, burning pains, now here and then there, as if it was contracting and burning, as from a small flame.

Relaxation of all the muscles (Gels.).

Trembling of the limbs (*Agar., Bel., Gels., Kali-Br., Tarant.*).

Great excitability and nervous debility (*Coff., Nux-V., Tarant.*).

HYSTERICAL AND HYPOCHONDRIACAL COMPLAINTS (*Ign., Nat-C., Nux-M., Nux-V., Sep.*).

Nervous activity, then sudden exhaustion (B.).

FREQUENT SHEDDING OF TEARS (*Nat-M., Puls., Sep.*).

Great weakness of memory (*Agn., Calc., Kali-P., Lac-C., Lyc., Nat-M.*).

Predominance of intellect—judgment over impulses (*Lyc.*).

Congestion of blood to single parts (*Bell., Glon., Sulph.*) (G.).

Eczema capitis; cracks, exudes and wets tne hair (*Calc., Graph., Mezer., Psor., Sulph.*) (N.).

Troubles of, or on the left ear (G.).

Tense scalp (*Apis, Carb-V., Caust.*) (Bl.).

OTORRHOEA (*Graph., Merc., Puls., Sil., Tell.*) (Bl.).

Deafness, with sharp stitching pains in the ear (*Kali-B., Puls.*) (Bl.).

Constipation (*Bry., Caust. Graph., Hydr., Kali-M., Lyc., Merc., Nat-M., Sep., Thuj*).

STRONG URINE, LIKE CAT'S URINE (*Aspar., Caj., Vib.*) (N.).

Milky urine (*Apis Aur., Hep., Lyc., Phos-Ac.*) (B.).

Enuresis (*Calc., Kreos., Sep.*) (B.).

Frontal headache (*Bell., Bry.*) (Bl.).

Burning of the forehead (*Kali-I., Phos.*) (Bl.).

Vertigo (*Calc-P., Con., Ferr., Gels.*) (Bl.).

Oppression of the chest, awaking her at night (*Grind., Lach., Sulph.*).

Sensation of weight on the chest (*Bry Phos.*) (B.).

Pain over brows (*Arg-N., Kali-B., Nat-M., Spig.*) (B.).

Cramp in the eyes (B.).

Craves meat (*Ferr-M., Iod., Kreos., Lil-T., Mag-C., Nat-M., Sanic., Tub.*) (B.).

Itching at the anus (*Calc., Graph., Kali-S., Nat-C., Phos., Sulph., Teucr.*) (B.).

Dry skin, with moist palms (B.).

Cold shoulders (*Arg-N., Caust., Hydr., Kali-B., Kreos., Lyc., Phos., Sep., Strych.*) (B.).

AGGRAVATION: In cloudy weather; in cool air; from music; at night; during sleep; and in the left side.

AMELIORATION: In warm weather.

RELATIONSHIP: *Remedies following*: *Bell., Nux-V.* and *Puls.*

Antidote: *Camph.*

X-Ray.

COMMON NAME: THE VIAL CONTAINING ALCOHOL EXPOSED TO X-RAY.

Repeated exposure to *Roentgen* (*X-Ray*) has produced skin lesions often followed by cancer.

Distressing pain (*Ars., Bell., Kreos.*) (Br.).

Sexual glands are particularly affected; atrophy of the ovaries (*Apis, Bar-M., Carb-S., Con., Helon., Iod., Plb.*) *and testicles* (*Aur., Bar-C., Caps., Carb-An., Gels., Iod., Kali-I., Lyss., Plb., Staph., Zinc.*) (Br.).

Re-establishes suppressed gonorrhœa (*Med., Thuj.*) (Br.).

Sexual desire lost (*Agn., Calad., Graph., Lyc., Nat-M.*) (Br.).

Lewd dreams (*Calc., Kali-P., Phos., Staph.*) (Br.).

Sterility (*Aur., Bor., Nat-C., Nat-M., Sep., Zinc.*) (Br.).

Anæmia and leukæmia (*Apis, Calc-P., Ferr., Graph., Kali-P., Lach., Merc., Nit-Ac., Puls., Sep.*) (Br.).

Throat painful on swallowing (*Bell., Merc., Nit-Ac.*) (Br.).

General tired and sick feeling (*Gels., Kali-P., Lach.*) (Br.).

Palms rough and scaly (*Kali-Ars.*) (Br.).

Rheumatic pains (*Bry., Kali-I., Rhus-T.*) (Br.).

PSORIASIS (*Ars., Kali-Ars., Merc., Sep.*) (Br.).

Warty growths (*Nit-Ac., Thuj.*) (Br.).

Skin dry, wrinkled (*Ars.*) (Br.).

Dry, itching eczema (*Alum., Mezer., Psor., Sep., Tell.*) (Br.).

Painful cracks (*Graph., Nat-M., Petr.*) (Br.).

AGGRAVATION: In the open air; in bed; in the evening; on swallowing; and at night.

AMELIORATION: From warm application.

RELATIONSHIP: *Compare*: *Ars., Aur., Calc., Ferr., Graph., Iod., Kali-Ars., Kali-C., Lach., Lyc., Merc., Nit-Ac., Sep.* and *Thuj.*

Yohimbinum.

COMMON NAME: YOHIMBEHA: YUM-BEHOA.

It is an aphrodisiac (that is, a sexual stimulant) when used in physiological doses (*Bufo, Cann-I., Canth., Phos.*) (Br.).

It greatly increases the sexual desire in men and in animals (Bl.).

Useful for anæmic, thin, nervous and partly impotent men (*Calc-P., Nat-M., Sil.*) (Bl.).

Copious salivation (*Merc., Nit-Ac., Tab.*) (Br.).

Disagreeable, metallic taste in the mouth (*Merc.*) (Br.).

Urethritis (*Apis, Cann-S., Canth., Merc-C., Staph., Thuj.*) (Br.).

STRONG AND LASTING ERECTIONS (*Canth., Fluor-Ac., Phos., Pic-Ac.*) (Br.).

NURASTHENIC IMPOTENCE (*Calc-P., Graph., Kali-P., Phos-Ac., Sulph., Zinc.*) (Br.).

Menorrhagia (*Calc., Ferr-P., Kali-C., Lach., Nit-Ac.*) (Br.).

Hyperæmia of milk glands and stimulation of the function of lactation (Br.).

Bleeding piles (*Aloe, Caps., Graph., Lach., Nit-Ac., Sulph., Thuj.*) (Br.).

Feverish condition (*Gels., Kali-P., Lyc., Sep.*) (Bl.).

Waves of heat and chilliness (Br.).

Sleeplessness (*Coff., Kali-P., Nat-M., Nux-V., Phos., Psor., Sulph.*) (Br.).

Thoughts of events of the whole past life keep him awake (Br.).

AGGRAVATION: At night; from sexual excitement; and during stool.

AMELIORATION: From sleep.

RELATIONSHIP: *Compare*: *Apis, Bell., Cann-I., Canth., Fluor-Ac., Graph., Kali-P., Lach., Lyc., Merc., Nat-M., Nux-V., Op., Phos., Pic-Ac., Sep., Sulph., Thuj.* and *Zinc.*

Zincum Metallicum.

COMMON NAME: ZINC.

Pallor of the body surface, with low fevers (Ferr., Nat-M., Sep.).

Nape of the neck feels weary and tired, from writing or any exertion (N.).

Variableness of the symptoms (Ign., Kali-S., Tub.).

Pain in the back, worse when sitting (*Agar., Arg-M., Rhus-T., Sep., Valer., Zinc.*) (N.).

DEFECTIVE VITALITY, BRAIN OR NERVE POWER TOO WEAK TO DEVELOP—EXANTHE-MATA, OR MENSES; TO EXPECTORATE; TO URINATE; TO COMPREHEND; OR, TO MEMO-RISE (N.).

Twitching of the members (Agar., Bell., Bufo, Cupr., Hell., Ign., Lach., Mosch., Nux-M., Op., Phos., Zinc.).

CANNOT KEEP THE FEET STILL (WHILE SITTING) (*Alum., Bar-C., Puls.*) (N.).

Constant trembling of the limbs with cold extremities (*Stram.*) (N.).

Weakness and trembling of the hands while writing (*Bism., Caps., Chel., Stann.*) (A.).

Spinal irritation (Phos., Pic-Ac., Sil.) (A.).

Cannot bear back touched (Chin-S., Tarant., Ther.) (A.).

Burning along the spine (Phos.) (D.).

Aching about the last dorsal or the first lumbar vertebra, worse when sitting (D.).

Twitching of single muscles all over the body (*Ign.*) (N.).

Violent trembling all over, so as to shake the bed; lost nerve control (N.).

Excessive nervous moving of the feet in bed for hours after retiring, even when asleep (A.).

FIDGETY FEET; MUST MOVE THEM CON-STANTLY (N.).

Feet sweaty and sore about the toes (A.).

Fœtid, suppressed foot-sweat (*Sil.*) (A.).

Chilblains, painful, worse from rubbing (A.).

INCLINATION TO COMA (*Apis, Bell., Hell., Op., Verat-V., Zinc.*).

Mental faculties impaired (*Bar-C., Kali-P., Lyc., Nat-M., Phos-Ac.*) (D.).

Child repeats everything said to it (A.).

Child cries out during sleep; whole body jerks during sleep; wakes frightened, starts and rolls the head from side to side (A.).

Convulsion during dentition, with pale face, no heat, except perhaps in the occiput, no increase in temperature (reverse of *Bell.*); rolling the eyes, gnashing the teeth (*Bell., Cupr., Stram.*) (A.).

Chorea from suppressed eruption or from fright (*Op.*) (A.).

During sweat cannot tolerate any covering (A.).

Cannot take stimulants (*Selen.*) (N.).

Wine greatly aggravates all the symptoms (*Alum., Con., Nux-V.*) (N.).

Symptoms of the chest are ameliorated by expectoration; of bladder, by urinating; of back, by emissions (aggravated by emissions—*Cobalt.*); *and general, by menstrual flow* (N.).

In anæmic subjects, brain exhaustion; not able to develop exanthema (N.).

Cachexia, with prostration, emaciation, etc. (*Calc., Ferr., Nat-M., Sep.*) (D.).

Descending paralysis (*Bar-C., Merc.*; ascending paralysis —*Agar., Ars., Con., Hydr-Ac., Kali-C., Mang.*) (B.).

Somnambulism (*Acon., Anac., Art-V., Bell., Bry., Cic., Hyos., Ign., Kali-P., Lach., Nat-M., Op., Phos., Sü., Stram.*) (K.)

Frequent jerking of the body during sleep (G.).

Varicose veins during pregnancy (*Puls., Sep.*) (Bt.).

COUGH DURING CATAMENIA (*Calc-P., Graph., Lac-C., Nat-M., Phos., Sep., Sulph., Thuj.*) (N.).

Menses flow more at night (*Am-C., Am-M., Bov., Coca, Coc-C., Glon., Mag-C., Mag-M., Nat-M., Sulph.*) (G.).

Menses too early, too profuse (*Calc., Phos., Tub.*); lumps of coagulated blood pass away, mostly when walking (G.).

A constant distressing boring pain in the left ovarian region, only partially relieved by pressure, or during menstruation, but returns again soon after the flow (G.).

During menses, heaviness of the limbs, with violent drawing around the knees, as if they could be twisted off (G.).

Sudden shocks and jerks in the cardiac region (N.).

Vertigo, as if he would fall to the left (*Lach., Nat-M. Sulph.*) (R.).

Chronic sick headache (*Gels., Nat-M., Sil.*) (Bt.).

MENINGITIS, WITH SHARP PAINS THROUGH THE HEAD (*Apis, Bell., Hell., Lach., Lyc., Nat-M., Sep., Sulph.*) (D.).

Child cries out during sleep; rolls the head from side to side; face alternately pale and red (N.).

Impending paralysis of the brain (*Hyos., Lyc.*) (A.).

Symptoms of effusion into the ventricles of the brain (*Apis, Hell., Lyc.*) (A.).

Infantile convulsions (*Bell., Cupr.*) (Bt.).

AUTOMATIC MOTION OF HANDS AND HEAD, OR ONE HAND AND HEAD (*Apoc., Bry., Hell.*) (A.).

Typhoid: Delirium, attempts to get out of bed; complete unconsciousness; sliding down in bed (*Mur-Ac.*); grasping at flocks (*Hyos.*); subsultus; decubitus; involuntary stool and urine (*Kali-P.*) (A.).

Upper eyelids heavy, as if paralyzed (*Caust., Gels.*) (C.).

Agglutination of lids at night (*Merc., Puls.*) (C.).

Inflammation of the conjunctiva, worse in the inner canthi; pains worse during evening and night, as from sand, with frequent lachrymation (N.).

Great weakness of sight (*Calc., Nat-M., Phos., Sep., Sulph.*) (Bt.).

Sticking in the right eye (Bt.).

PTERYGIUM (*Arg-N., Calc., Lach., Sulph.*) (K.).

Itching and stinging in the inner angles of the eyes, with cloudiness of vision (N.).

Sensation of drawing together of the eyes as by a cord (R.).

Dim vision (*Cycl., Kali-P., Phos., Sep.*) (R.).

Photophobia (*Con., Euphr., Nat-M.*) (R.).

Objects appear elongated, sometimes double (R.).

Much burning in the eyes and lids, in the morning and evening (C.).

Cough worse after sweet things (*Med., Spong.*) (Hr.).

Dry, spasmodic cough, morning and evening (*Alumn., Bar-C., Carb-An., Hep., Ign.*) (R.).

DURING THE SPASMS OF COUGH THE CHILD GRASPS THE GENITALS (R.).

Hoarseness (*Alum., Calc., Caust., Phos., Rhus-T.*) (C.).

Tightness and oppression of the chest (*Ars., Carb-V., Kali-C., Lach., Phos., Sulph.*) (C.).

Bloody expectoration (*Hep., Puls., Stann.*) (C.).

Palpitation (*Acon., Kali-P., Lach., Phos., Spig.*) (C.).

Tension and stitches in the præcordial region (C.).

Constriction in the œsophagus during deglutition (*Alum.*) (R.).

Deathly sickness at the stomach, with marked nausea (*Ant-T., Ars., Bry., Ipec., Tab., Verat.*).

Great greediness when eating; cannot eat fast enough (A.).

RAVENOUS HUNGER, ABOUT 11 or 12 A.M. (*Sulph.*) (A.).

Terrible heart-burn after taking sweet things; much nausea and vomiting (G.).

Sweetish rising from the stomach (Bt.).

Flatulent colic; worse towards evening, and from wine (G.).

Great difficulty in expelling stools, which are insufficient (*Anac., Ign., Sep.*) (G.).

Hæmorrhoids, with itching, burning and sticking (*Aesc., Sulph.*) (C.).

Diarrhœa with great debility (Chin., Phos.) (C.).

Constant urging to pass water; only when sitting and bending backward can he discharge the same (can only urinate lying—*Kreos.,*); *much sand in the sediment* (N.).

Pressive, cutting about the kidneys (B.).

Retention of urine (*Caust., Op., Verat.*) (R.).

Partial paralysis of the bladder (*Arn., Caust., Op.*) (R.).

INVOLUNTARY URINATION WHILE WALKING, COUGHING AND SNEEZING (*Caust., Nat-M., Phos., Puls., Sep.*) (C.).

Acute drawing in the forepart of the urethra and in penis (C.).

Urine turbid or loam-coloured in the morning (C.).

Sexual desire several times in the night (*Canth., Phos.*) (G.).

Irresistible desire for onanism (*Nux-V., Phos-Ac., Staph.*) (G.).

Drawing up of the testicles with pain and swelling (R.).

EMISSIONS AT NIGHT WITH LASCIVIOUS DREAMS (*Canth., Nux-V., Phos. Sulph.*) (R.).

Long-lasting and violent erections (*Canth.*, *Phos.*, *Pic-Ac.*) (C.).

Easily excited (*Nux-V.*, *Phos.*) (C.).

The emission during an embrace is too rapid (*Nux-V.*, *Sulph.*), or difficult and almost impossible (*Graph.*) (C.).

ALL HER OTHER COMPLAINTS DURING MENSES FEEL QUITE WELL WHILE THE FLOW IS ON (N.).

AGGRAVATION: After dinner; towards evening; from urine; while sitting; after being heated; from suppressions; from noise; from touch; and from exhaustion.

AMELIORATION: During the menses; by restoration or development of eruptions; from expectoration; from seminal emission; from restoration of discharges; from walking about (backache); from motion; from hard pressure; and in the open air.

RELATIONSHIP: *Compare*: *Apis*, *Bell.*, *Cic.*, *Cupr.*, *Gels.*, *Hell.*, *Lach.*, *Lyc.*, *Op.*, *Phos.*, *Rhus-T.*, *Sil.*, *Sulph.* and *Tub.*, in incipient brain diseases from suppressed eruptions.

Inimical to : *Cham.* and *Nux-V.* (should not be used before or after).

Is followed well by Ign. (but not by *Nux-V.*, which disagrees).

Complementary: *Puls.*

Antidotes: *Camph.*, *Hep.* and *Ign.*